May 12, 1986

Male Contraception:
Advances and Future Prospects

PARFR Series
on Fertility Regulation

Proceedings of an International Workshop
on Male Contraception:
Advances and Future Prospects,
May 28–31, 1985, Geneva, Switzerland

Sponsored by the Program for Applied Research
on Fertility Regulation,
Northwestern University, Chicago, Illinois

Male Contraception: Advances and Future Prospects

edited by

Gerald I. Zatuchni, M.D., M.Sc.

Professor, Department of Obstetrics and Gynecology,
Northwestern University Medical School;
Director of Technical Assistance, Program for Applied Research on Fertility Regulation,
Northwestern University, Chicago, Illinois

Alfredo Goldsmith, M.D., M.P.H.

Associate Professor, Department of Obstetrics and Gynecology,
Northwestern University Medical School;
Head, Research Project Development, Program for Applied Research on Fertility Regulation,
Northwestern University, Chicago, Illinois

Jeffrey M. Spieler, M.Sc.

Biologist, Research Division,
Office of Population,
Agency for International Development,
Washington, D.C.

John J. Sciarra, M.D., Ph.D.

Professor and Chairman, Department of Obstetrics and Gynecology,
Northwestern University Medical School;
Program Director, Program for Applied Research on Fertility Regulation,
Northwestern University, Chicago, Illinois

**Prepared with the technical assistance of
Carolyn K. Osborn**

With 93 contributors

HARPER & ROW, PUBLISHERS
PHILADELPHIA

Cambridge   London
New York   Mexico City
Hagerstown   São Paulo
San Francisco   Sydney

1817

Acquisitions Editor: Lisa A. Biello
Sponsoring Editor: Sanford J. Robinson
Manuscript Editor: Mary K. Smith
Indexer: Julia Schwager
Design Director: Tracy Baldwin/Anne O'Donnell
Production Supervisor: Kathleen P. Dunn
Production Assistant: Susan Hess
Compositor: Tapsco, Inc.
Printer/Binder: Haddon Craftsmen

6 5 4 3 2 1

Library of Congress Cataloging-in-Publication Data

International Workshop on Male Contraception: Advances and Future Prospects (1985: Geneva, Switzerland)
  Male contraception, advances and future prospects.

  (PARFR series on fertility regulation)
  Bibliography: p.
  Includes index.
    1. Infertility, Male—Congresses.   2. Oral
contraceptives, Male—Congresses.   3. Generative
organs, Male—Effect of drugs on—Congresses.
4. Vasectomy—Congresses.   I. Zatuchni, Gerald I.,
1933–   II. Northwestern University (Evanston,
Ill.). Program for Applied Research on Fertility
Regulation.   III. Title.   IV. Series.
RC889.I6 1985   616.9′4   86-2845
ISBN 0-06-142907-4

The authors and publisher have exerted every effort to
ensure that drug selection and dosage set forth in this
text are in accord with current recommendations and
practice at the time of publication. However, in view of
ongoing research, changes in government regulations,
and the constant flow of information relating to drug
therapy and drug reactions, the reader is urged to check
the package insert for each drug for any change in indications and dosage and for added warnings and precau-
tions. This is particularly important when the recommended agent is a new or infrequently employed drug.

FOREWORD

It has been only 25 years since women assumed the major responsibility for fertility control. Prior to the introduction of the pill and IUD, most couples managed to control their fertility by sexual abstinence, coitus interruptus, condom use, and illegal abortion; except for the latter, the man assumed the responsibility. It is unfortunate that improved male methods of fertility control have not been developed, for it is clear that in most societies, the man does bear the major responsibility for fertility control. Reasons for the lack of new methods include incomplete understanding of male reproductive physiology, fewer biologic target areas (as compared to the female) for contraceptive action, the proximity of hormone-producing cells to the gametes, the complicated cycling of spermatogenesis, lack of financial support from foundations and public sector agencies, reluctance of the pharmaceutical industry, and male chauvinistic factors.

The proceedings of this PARFR Workshop on Male Contraception indicate that for the short-term of the next 5 to 10 years, condom use and vasectomy will remain the major methods of male fertility control. As is evidenced, however, from the research described in this volume, new methods for male use or at least methods directed against sperm are in advanced stages of development. Simpler technical procedures for vas deferens obstruction, good prospects for pharmacologic post-testicular sperm inhibition, devices for vas obstruction with potentially easy reversibility, and vaccines directed against specific sperm components are described and discussed by leading international scientists. These scientists conclude that it is likely that with continuing and additional funding support, several of the research efforts will culminate in approved products for the control of male fertility, thereby adding significantly to the meager contraceptive choices now available.

PREFACE

Today, male contraception is limited to the use of condoms, coitus interruptus, or vasectomy. Although these methods find modest acceptance, their disadvantages have prevented their wholehearted acceptance by couples for the control of male fertility. The search for improved methods that act on the male reproductive system began about 1950, but as yet no method has been found that is fully effective, fully safe, fully reversible, and fully acceptable.

Research efforts to find an appropriate male method have been constrained by several factors. Foremost among these are the incomplete understanding of the biology and physiology of the male reproductive system and the relative lack of suitable targets for fertility interference in the male as opposed to the female. Additional constraints are imposed by the relative disinterest of the pharmaceutical industry in developing a male method, owing to the tremendous costs and time involved, inadequate patent life, and liability issues.

Despite these real constraints, international research continues in this important field, as documented by the collection of papers in the PARFR workshop series. Several research approaches to male fertility control offer promises of new and improved methods that could be available within the next 5 to 10 years. Other research leads could take longer, but as an outgrowth of dramatic new technologies, especially in the fields of molecular and cellular biology and genetics, a fuller knowledge of the male reproductive system will create opportunities for more rapid development of better methods of male contraception.

Gerald I. Zatuchni, M.D., M.SC.
Alfredo Goldsmith, M.D., M.P.H.
Jeffrey M. Spieler, M.SC.
John J. Sciarra, M.D., PH.D.

ACKNOWLEDGMENTS

The editors express deep appreciation to Diane Krier-Morrow, M.B.A., Director of Administration of the Program for Applied Research on Fertility Regulation, for her excellent management of the diverse elements of this international conference so that the scientific aims of the meeting could be achieved.

Carolyn K. Osborn is especially grateful to Ruvenia Thomas for her tireless and highly skilled assistance in typing the manuscript.

PARFR extends sincere thanks to the following organizations for their assistance in supporting this International Workshop:

Northwestern University Medical School
Organon International BV
Ortho Pharmaceutical Corporation
Stolle Research and Development Corporation
Syntex USA, Inc.
United States Agency for International Development

The Program for Applied Research on Fertility Regulation is staffed by the following persons:

John J. Sciarra, M.D., Ph.D., Director
Gerald I. Zatuchni, M.D., M.Sc., Director of Technical Assistance
Alfredo Goldsmith, M.D., M.P.H., Head, Research Project Development
Diane Krier-Morrow, M.B.A., Director of Administration

The discussion summaries were written by Carolyn K. Osborn.

CONTENTS

IMMUNOLOGIC APPROACHES

Overview

1

Male Contraception in Family Planning Programs

D. MALCOLM POTTS

Men are the forgotten 50% of family planning. The male role in family planning is often misunderstood, and clinical services focus almost exclusively on women. There have been no improvements in male methods of family planning since the 19th century.

The anatomically male methods of coitus interruptus and condoms were the first methods of birth control to be practiced in Europe. In many parts of the world, they remain commonly used techniques. The demographic transition, as Wrigley has pointed out

> . . . was achieved largely by preindustrial methods, by coitus interruptus and by the procuring of abortion . . . The tremendous growth in the use of contraception to limit family size in the late nineteenth century onwards was due to a much wider employment of means long known to European society rather than to the opportunity offered to them by the development of new techniques.[27]

Ideally, contemporary family planning programs need both new male methods of contraception and services that are more accessible to men. The latter may prove more achievable than the former.

DECISION MAKING

Contraceptives can be categorized according to the sex of the user or the sex of the person most directly involved in the decision to use the method. Categorization by the second criterion is more difficult but perhaps more useful in the design of family planning programs. It prompts the question, what is a male method of contraception? For example, in Japan, 20% of total condom sales are made by women to women. Armies of saleswomen descend on Japanese homes every day. One firm, Mainichi Shoji, employs 2,000 such women. In this instance, the woman plays an equal or more dominant role in method selection. At the same time, the majority of condoms in Japan continue to be sold by men to men.[5] Conversely, in Bangladesh nearly all oral contraceptives are sold by men to men. In a society where purdah is widespread, men play a significant role in both the decision making and acquisition of contraceptive methods.[15]

In Iran in 1972, Siassi found that when Iranian women were given oral contraceptives, the continuation rate at 6 months was only 12%. When the same method was given to the husbands of the same group to be passed on to their wives, the continuation rate at 6 months was more than 90%.[24] Distributing the method to women apparently challenged the social structure, whereas involving men seems to have enhanced family decision making.

Many aspects of the use, or nonuse, of contraception are the outcome of both implicit and explicit negotiation between the two partners;[16] nevertheless, in this negotiation, one partner often takes the dominant role. Sociologists divide married couples into role-sharers and role-dividers. Role-sharers are emancipated men and women who discuss major family decisions about money or family size. The man is expected to satisfy his wife as well as himself sexually. Role-dividers in the West are usually unemancipated, blue-collar class workers jealous of their specific marital roles. The wife may not know her husband's income. Friends of the marital partner do not know one another, and sexual encounters generally occur with the lights off. The man can both initiate contraceptive use and veto his wife's use of a method.[3] In an otherwise developing world, most couples continue to be deeply divided in sexual roles within marriage.

Vasectomy, condoms, and coitus interruptus seem common in European marriages in which sex roles are divided. To test this hypothesis, Deys offered vasectomy in a coal mining community in the English midlands. Coal miners observe strict marital role division.[6] Vasectomy proved highly acceptable; 82.7% of the coal mining community chose condoms and only 4.1% female diaphragms.[14]

Many health planners share these attitudes about marital roles. As a consequence, they may misjudge the potential acceptability of contraceptive methods. If men are excluded from family planning services because the experts "know" they will not use them, then the beliefs of family planning providers become a self-fulfilling prophecy. In contraception, as elsewhere, men and women generally conform to the roles that society creates for them. Organizers of family planning services often assume that men will refuse any role in fertility control.[7]

Many men in the third world, especially those without the privilege of education, are ambivalent about male contraception.[25] The best response to such ambivalence is provision of well-designed services. A satisfied minority of users will offer reassurance for the ambivalent majority.

METHODS

Condoms were first described in 1564 and vasectomy was begun in the 19th century. Coitus interruptus (male withdrawal) is mentioned in the Bible, the Talmud, and the Koran. In developed countries, male methods of contraception account for 20% to 80% of contraceptive devices among couples of reproductive age, making it all the more remarkable that male methods receive so little emphasis in structural family planning programs in either developed or developing countries.[26]

Coitus interruptus is the oldest method of contraception known,[21] but is sometimes overlooked in KAP (knowledge, attitude, and practice) surveys. It remained the most common single method in Europe until after World War II and is still the leading contraceptive used in Italy.[22] The United States is unusual among industrialized societies in having a low rate of coitus interruptus.[8]

Failure rates of coitus interruptus probably overlap those of condoms, spermicide, and periodic abstinence. The 1949 British Royal Commission on Population reported no difference in average family size among users of appliances and users of nonappliance methods, predominantly coitus interruptus.[21] Although sperm have been found in the preejaculatory fluid, there is no evidence that they are viable or in concentrations sufficient for fertilization.

Coitus interruptus is like a buffalo cart or a bicycle: There may be better ways of getting around the world as there may be better methods of contraception, but for many people these methods represent a practical solution to an everyday problem.

Condoms are an effective, easy-to-distribute method of contraception. Consistently used, they have a low failure rate. They also provide some protection against sexually transmitted diseases. The addition of color and of a spermicide as a lubricant enhances acceptability. The social marketing program in Bangladesh now sells 5 million condoms a month to the men of one of the poorest, yet most religiously conservative, nations of the world. Americans buy half a billion condoms a year, and the method appears to appeal to adolescents, probably because anonymous access to condoms is possible.

In a study of inner-city black adolescents aged 12 to 16, 80% were sexually experienced and 60% used a method of contraception at last intercourse. Of this number, 40% used condoms, 15% withdrawal, and 23% pills.[4] Among married couples in Japan, the condom remains the single most important method of contraception (5).

A male analogue to the female pill is needed. According to Keith and associates, 70% of American men would accept such an invention if it were perfected.[13] Unfortunately, over the past 20 years, the possibility of a male pill has diminished. In 1969, the London *Times* reviewed progress towards a male pill and concluded such a method was unlikely "within 5 years or so."[2] Today, it appears unlikely within 10 to 15 years, unless there is a marked increase in investment in reproductive research and/or changes of policies relating to drug regulation and manufacturers' liability. If progress is to be made, it may well derive from efforts to interrupt sperm maturation or interfere with the accessory glands,[11] rather than through suppression of spermiogenesis. Federal investment in all aspects of male fertility research has varied between 12% and 22% of total outlays.[9]

Vasectomy is already such a simple operation that few improvements are possible. Six million vasectomies were performed in the United States in the 1970s,[26] and the method has been more widely used than any other in India. Work on percutaneous methods of male sterilization is promising.[1]

SERVICES

Men often have a more positive attitude to family planning than many health professionals believe.[2,12,19,23] In many countries, family planning clinics have evolved into stylized medical services, often staffed by women and usually focused on helping women. The clinic staff often feel threatened by male clients. In 1981, a male medical student in Britain approached 12 family planning clinics and asked for a supply of condoms. He writes:

> On entering the clinics I was always the only male in the room and I felt self-conscious. If I was met with surprise, or worse, giggling, I became very embarrassed and uncomfortable. If I was met with suspicion, and even accused of trying to obtain condoms for resale, my self-consciousness turned to guilt.[12]

In the United States in 1979, the Department of Health and Human Services spent $242 million on family planning, of which only $0.75 million went to specifically male clinics. Today even that support has been discontinued. Advertising directed toward men often is opposed in developed countries. In Britain, the commercial television act of 1954 permits the promotion of anything from candy to tampons, except "contraceptives, matrimonial agencies, fortune tellers and undertakers."[20] In the Sudan, a survey of 250 men interviewed in the marketplace, in mosques, and in governmental offices, found that three fifths of those sampled wished to use family planning services but only one fifth were using an effective method, and only 2.8% were currently using clinic services.[18]

Nowhere is the attitude of services more important than in the provision of vasectomy. For many years it was assumed, although never tested, that Latin American men would not accept vasectomy. But Dr. Marcus de Castro in Sao Paulo, Brazil, demonstrated that when vasectomy was promoted properly, it was acceptable. Of nearly 500 men seeking vasectomy in Colombia and Costa Rica, the operation was most popular among blue-collar workers.[10]

CONCLUSIONS

Condoms should be made available and aggressively promoted in all family planning programs. Vasectomy is a simpler and safer operation to perform than female sterilization. Coitus interruptus is a widely used traditional method of contraception that can serve as an essential first step in contraceptive usefulness.

In male-dominant societies, anatomically female methods such as the pill should be made available to men to pass on to their wives. Male methods such as condoms also can be promoted to women. In short, heterosexual channels of contraceptive distribution always need exploring. The greater the number of contraceptive choices available to society, the higher the prevalence of contraception; therefore, the addition of a male systemic method of contraception would be a welcome step forward in family planning. In all cultures men can make a trusting, open contribution to a sexual partnership.

REFERENCES

1. BLACK T: Personal communication, 1984
2. Birth Control Trust: Men, Sex and Contraception. London, Birth Control Trust/Family Planning Association, 1984
3. BORIA-BERNA MC: Husband's role in birth control acceptance. Med Aspects Hum Sexuality 129:48, 1972

4. CLARK SD, ZABIN LS, HARDY JB: Sex, contraception and parenthood: Experience and attitudes among urban black young men. Fam Plann Perspect 16:77–82, 1984
5. COLEMAN S: Family Planning in Japanese Society. Princeton, NJ, Princeton University Press, 1983
6. DENNIS N, HENRIQUES F, SLAUGHTER C: Coal Is Our Life: An Analysis of a Yorkshire Mining Community, 2nd ed. London, Tavistock Publications, 1969
7. DELVIN D: Man and contraception. Br J Fam Plann 10:101, 1985
8. DEYS CM, POTTS M: Condoms and things. Adv Biosci 10:286–297, 1973
9. DRILLER L, HEMBREE W: Male contraception and family planning: A social and historical review. Fertil Steril 28:1271–1279, 1977
10. GOLDSMITH A, GOLDBERG R, ECHEVERRIA G: An in-depth study of vasectomized men in Latin America: A preliminary report. J Reprod Med 10:150, 1973
11. HOMONNAI ZT, SHILON M, PAZ GF: Phenoxybenzamine: An effective male contraceptive pill. Contraception 29:479–489, 1984
12. HOWARD G, WHITTAKER I: Difficulties in obtaining condoms in the NHS. Br J Fam Plann 7:12–15, 1981
13. KEITH L, KEITH D, BUSSEL R, WELLS J: Attitudes of men toward contraception. Arch Gynaecol 22:89, 1975
14. KOYA Y, KUBO H, OGINO H, YUASA S: Five-year experiment on family planning among coal miners in Japan. Population Studies 13(2):157–163, 1959
15. LOUIS T, CISZEWSKI R: Social marketing. In Potts DM, Bhiwandiwala P (eds): Birth Control. Lancaster, England, MTP Press, 1979
16. LUKER K: Taking Chances: Abortion and the Decision Not to Contracept. Berkeley, CA, University of California Press, 1975
17. MADRIGAL V, EDELMAN DA, GOLDSMITH A: Male sterilization in El Salvador. J Reprod Med 14:167, 1975
18. MUSTAFA MAB, MUMFORD SD: Male attitudes toward family planning in Khartoum, Sudan. J Biosoc Sci 16:437–449, 1984
19. NOBBE CE, OKRAKU IO: Male–female differences in family size preferences among college students. Social Biol 21:279–289, 1974
20. POTTS DM: Coitus Interruptus. In CORSON SL, DERMAN RJ, TYRER LB (eds): Fertility Control, pp 299–305. Boston, Little Brown & Co, 1985
21. POTTS DM, DIGGORY P: Textbook of Contraceptive Practice, 2nd ed. Cambridge, England, Cambridge University Press, 1983
22. RIPHAGEN FE, VAN DER VURST J, LEHERT P: Contraception in Italy. Geneva, International Health Foundation, 1985
23. RYSER P, SPILLANE WH: The effect of education and significant others upon contraceptive behaviour of married men. J Bios Sci 6:305–314, 1974
24. SIASSI I: The psychiatrist's role in family planning. Am J Psychiatry 128(1):48–53, 1972
25. Social Marketing Update: Focus groups reveal consumer ambivalence. Social Marketing Update 3(4):4–6, 1982
26. STOKES B: Men and Family Planning. Worldwatch Paper 41, Washington, DC, 1980
27. WRIGLEY EA: Population and History. London, Weidenfeld & Nicolson, 1969

2

The International Experience with Vasectomy

DOUGLAS H. HUBER

SAWON HONG

JOHN A. ROSS

Voluntary sterilization is one of the world's leading methods of family planning; however, there have been considerable differences in the balance between male and female sterilization from country to country and within countries over time. In general, female sterilization has been more popular than male sterilization. Because vasectomy and tubectomy may be direct substitutes for one another, it is useful to examine the incidence and prevalence of vasectomy in the context of both male and female procèdures.

We will review the most current experience with male and female sterilization as well as selected recent trends, considering the safety, effectiveness, and reversibility of vasectomy as criteria for standards against which new methods can be measured. We will also review a recently reported experience with chemical occlusion of the vas in the People's Republic of China.

INCIDENCE AND PREVALENCE OF VASECTOMY AND TUBECTOMY

The information contained in Tables 2-1 and 2-2 on Acceptance and Prevalence of Sterilization is summarized from *Voluntary Sterilization: An International Factbook.*[5] We will focus primarily on the most recent data; trends over time are documented in the *Factbook.* For some countries, data were only available for male and female sterilization combined. (When this occurs for either incidence or prevalence rate, inferences about the role of vasectomy can still be drawn if the alternate measure includes sex specific rates.)

The incidence of vasectomy equals or exceeds tubectomy in two countries, the Netherlands and Hong Kong. Vasectomy incidence is half or more the incidence of tubectomy in another eight countries (by rank order): China, New Zealand, United States, Sri Lanka, Denmark, Australia, Nepal, and Norway. There are also several countries reporting vasectomy acceptors as zero or less than 1% of tubectomies: Dominican Republic, El Salvador, Honduras, Jamaica, and Tunisia. Some other Latin American countries have recently expanded vasectomy services: Brazil, Colombia, and Mexico.[1]

(Text continues on p. 13)

TABLE 2-1. Number of Sterilization Acceptors, by Sex:
Selected Countries and Years[1]

COUNTRY AND YEARS	TOTAL (in 000s)	MALE (in 000s)	FEMALE (in 000s)
Australia[3]			
1979–1980	58.7	23.0	35.7
Bangladesh			
1982–1983	363.2	88.5	274.6
Botswana			
1976	0.2		
China, People's Republic of			
1977	5,392	2,616	2,776
Colombia[2]			
1983	51.3[2]	0.7	50.6
Costa Rica			
1969	2.1		
Denmark[4]			
1981	11.8	4.7	7.1
Dominican Republic			
1983[5]	12.9	0	12.9
Ecuador			
1982	4.4		4.4
El Salvador			
1983[6]	14.6	0.1	14.6
England and Wales			
1978	97.7	22.4	75.2[7]
Fiji			
1980	1.1		
Finland			
1982	4.7	0.2	4.5
Guatemala			
1982	9.8	1.3	8.5
Honduras			
1982	5.0[2]	0.0	4.9
Hong Kong			
1980	1.2	0.6	0.6
India			
1982–1983	3,981	590	3,391
Indonesia			
1983–1984	110.0	16.6	93.4
Iran			
1977	1.6	0.4	1.2
Jamaica			
1975	3.2	0	3.2
Japan			
1982	8.0	0.1	7.9
Korea, Republic of			
1981	196.1	31.3	164.8
Malaysia			
1980	5.1	0.2	4.9
Mexico			
1979	136		

TABLE 2-1. *(continued)*

COUNTRY AND YEARS	TOTAL (in 000s)	MALE (in 000s)	FEMALE (in 000s)
Nepal			
1982–1983	45.0	16.5	28.5
Netherlands			
1981	75.0	42.0	33.0
New Zealand			
1982	8.4	3.6	4.7
Norway			
1977	6.3	2.3	4.0
Pakistan			
1979	24.9	0.7	24.2
Panama			
1975	0.8		
Philippines			
1981	63.5	1.8	61.7
Puerto Rico			
1975	9.0		
Scotland			
1978	14.1	3.0	11.1
Singapore			
1980	5.7	0.4	5.3
Sri Lanka			
1983	103.8	44.8	59.0
Taiwan			
1983	53.1	3.0	50.1
Thailand			
1982	167.0	23.4	143.6
Tunisia			
1982	9.6	0	9.6
United States			
1983	1,077	455	622
Venezuela			
1973	0.1		
Zimbabwe			
1975	0.1		

[1] Males and females may not add exactly to total because of rounding.

[2] These estimates are for IPPF affiliates only. They do not reflect total number of sterilization acceptors in the country.

[3] Figures come from the medical benefits (rebates) provided by the Commonwealth Department of Health. They exclude services rendered in hospitals to standard ward patients free of charge; thus, they are considered underestimates.

[4] All men treated as outpatients since 1977 are not included. For example, 3,000 male outpatients in 1979 were excluded.

[5] October to December estimated.

[6] Estimates based on statistical data January to June 1983.

[7] This is an estimate of sterilizations performed in National Health System hospitals. If we account for those carried out privately, the female total is probably around 100,000 a year or even more.

TABLE 2-2. Prevalence of Sterilization and Number of Users, by Sex: Selected Countries and Years[1]

COUNTRY AND YEAR	PREVALENCE (%)		
	TOTAL	MALE	FEMALE
Argentina			
1964 (Buenos Aires)[2,3]	0.3		
Australia			
1979 (Canberra)[3,6]	22.2	6.4	15.8
Bangladesh			
1983	7.4	1.2	6.2
Barbados			
1980–1981[5]	14.7	0.3	14.4
Belgium			
1975–1976[8]	5.1	0.0	5.1
Botswana			
1976			0.2
Brazil			
1980 (Bahia)	9.6		
1980 (Paraiba)	15.7		
1980 (Pernambuco)	18.9		
1980 (Rio Grande do Norte)	17.4		
1981 (Parana)	19.7		
1981 (S. Region)	14.6		
1981 (Rio Grande do Sul)	11.3		
1981 (Santa Catarina)	10.9		
1982 (Amazonas, urban)	33.1		
1982 (Piaui)	19.5		
Bulgaria			
1976	1.5	0.8	0.8
Canada[10,11]			
1982 (Quebec)	41.2	9.7	31.5
China, People's Republic of			
1982[12]	24.5	6.9	17.6
Colombia			
1980[5]	10.8	0.3	10.5
Costa Rica			
1981	18.0	1.0	17.0
Cuba			
1980 (Arroyo Naranjo)[5]	15.8		15.8
Czechoslovakia			
1977[10]	2.9	0.0	2.9
Denmark			
1975[10,13]	12.8		
Dominican Republic			
1980	21.0	0.0	21.0
Ecuador			
1982	12.4	0.0	12.4
Egypt			
1982[5]	1.2	0.0	1.2
El Salvador			
1978[5]	18.0	0.2	17.8

TABLE 2-2. *(continued)*

COUNTRY AND YEAR	PREVALENCE (%)		
	TOTAL	*MALE*	*FEMALE*
England and Wales			
1976[8]	16.2	8.5	7.7
Fiji			
1978	17		
Finland			
1977[10,14]	4.8	0.8	4.0
France			
1978[3,7,15]	7.3		
Ghana			
1979[5]	0.5	0.0	0.5
Guadeloupe			
1976[3,5]	7.8		7.8
Guatemala			
1983[9]	11.2		
Guyana			
1975[5]	8.5	0.0	8.5
Haiti			
1977[15]	0.3	0.1	0.2
Honduras			
1981	8.2	0.2	8.0
Hong Kong			
1981	17.7	1.2	16.5
Hungary			
1978[13,16]	2.8		
India[2,4]			
1981–1982	20.6		
Indonesia			
1981	1.0		
Iran			
1978	0		
Iraq			
1974[5]	0.6		0.6
Italy			
1979[10]	0.7	0.0	0.7
Jamaica			
1979	9.8	0.0	9.8
Japan			
1979[5]	4.0	1.1	2.9
Jordan			
1983[11]	3.8	0.1	3.7
Kenya			
1977–1978[15]	0.9	0.0	0.9
Korea, Republic of			
1982	28.4	5.2	23.2
Lebanon			
1971[5]	1.1	0.0	1.1
Lesotho			
1977[5]	0.7	0.0	0.7

(continued)

TABLE 2-2. (*continued*)

COUNTRY AND YEAR	PREVALENCE (%)		
	TOTAL	*MALE*	*FEMALE*
Malaysia			
1981[5]	5.0		
Martinique			
1976[3]	9.0		9.0
Mexico			
1982	13.7		
Morocco			
1981	1.0		1.0
Nepal			
1981	5.3	2.9	2.4
Netherlands			
1982	20	10	10
New Zealand			
Late 1970s	30.0		
Norway			
1977[3,10]	5.0	1.7	3.3
Pakistan			
1980	0.6		
Panama			
1979–1980	29.7	0.4	29.3
Paraguay			
1979[5]	2.8	0.1	2.7
Peru			
1981[5]	4.5	0.0	4.5
Philippines			
1982	11.8	0.7	11.1
Poland			
1977[4,8]	4.9		
Portugal			
1979–1980[5]	1.0	0.1	0.9
Puerto Rico			
1982[9]	45.6		
Singapore			
1977	22.0	1.0	21.0
South Africa			
1975–1976	5.2	0.0	5.2
Spain			
1977[5,11]	0.3		
Sri Lanka			
1982[5]	20.7	3.6	17.1
Sudan (North)			
1979[15]	0.3	0.0	0.3
Syria			
1978[5]	0.4	0.1	0.3
Taiwan			
1981	19.6	1.6	18.0
Tanzania			
1976	0		

TABLE 2-2. *(continued)*

COUNTRY AND YEAR	PREVALENCE (%)		
	TOTAL	*MALE*	*FEMALE*
Thailand			
1981	22.9	4.2	18.7
Trinidad and Tobago			
1977[5]	4.5	0.2	4.3
Tunisia			
1982[5]			4.5
Turkey			
1978	0.7	0.2	0.6
United States			
1982	27.9	10.4	17.4
1982[7]	38.9		
Venezuela			
1977	7.7	0.1	7.6
Yemen Arab Republic			
1979[2,6]	0.2	0.1	0.1
Yugoslavia			
1976[7,14]	10.0		10.0

[1] Unless otherwise specified, prevalence is based on currently married women 15–44 years old
[2] 20–50 years old
[3] All women
[4] Less than 45 years old
[5] 15–49 years old
[6] 18 years old and over
[7] Noncontraceptive sterilizations are included.
[8] 16–44 years old
[9] Preliminary and unweighted data for currently married women 15–49 years old. Noncontraceptive sterilizations add about 6% to the total figure.
[10] 18–44 years old
[11] Ever-married women
[12] Currently married women aged 15–49
[13] Confined to women who were still in the first marriage
[14] 20–44 years old
[15] 15–50 years old
[16] 15–39 years old
[17] Currently married men 17–51 years old

Figure 2-1 shows the trends in incidence from 1979 to 1983 for 17 countries. Countries were included that had information on the incidence of vasectomy and tubectomy for at least 3 years between 1979 and 1983. There are seven countries in which tubectomy has increased and six in which vasectomy has increased. This picture is somewhat different from a similar assessment for twelve of these developing countries (all developing countries in Fig. 2-1

Male Sterilization	Down	Female Sterilization Same or irregular	Up
Down	Netherlands	Thailand	
Same or irregular	USA	Denmark El Salvador Guatemala Sri Lanka Taiwan	Colombia Finland Philippines
Up	Korea	Hong Kong	Bangladesh India Indonesia Nepal

FIG. 2-1. Trends in male and female sterilization acceptance by country (1979–1983).

except Nepal) by Ross and Huber.[6] For this previous assessment, based on 1977 to 1980 data, 10 of the 12 countries had increases in tubectomy incidence, whereas only 2 had increases in vasectomy incidence. Therefore, since our assessment 2 years earlier, 9 countries have shifted towards a category of higher vasectomy incidence and only 2 have moved toward a category of higher female sterilization. This shift is in part a result of several having upward trends in female sterilization for the earlier period, and therefore any change would be downward in this framework. It is also a reflection that the downward trends in vasectomy for several countries have now been reversed. This is consistent with a previous conclusion that the acceptance of vasectomy is highly dependent on provider variables, particularly the availability of services and the emphasis on vasectomy as an option.[6]

Fluctuations in vasectomy acceptance over time have been striking in several countries. For example, in India, vasectomy led tubectomy from 1960 through 1972 and 1973, and then tubectomy took the lead for 2 years. This was reversed by a vasectomy increase in the period from 1975 to 1976 and the emergency period of 1976 to 1977. This was followed by a dramatic decline in vasectomy with a gradual increasing trend from 188,000 in 1977 to 1978 to 590,000 in 1982 to 1983. During these 6 years tubectomy increased from 761,000 to 3,391,000.

In the United States, vasectomy led tubectomy in the late 1960s and early 1970s; however, tubectomy began increasing in 1973 and 1974 and clearly surpassed vasectomy from 1975 through 1983. A decline in U.S. vasectomy incidence in 1981 and 1982, followed by an apparent rebound in 1983, may be a result of publicity, first about concerns related to the long-term safety of vasectomy published in 1979 through 1981, and followed by the reports published in 1982 through 1984 of several large-scale epidemiologic studies reconfirming the safety of vasectomy. The experience in China is notable because of the much wider acceptance of vasectomy in Sichuan Province than in the remainder of China. The ratio of vasectomy to tubectomy was 4:1 in

Sichuan Province over a 13-year period from 1971 to 1983. Vasectomy was widely used and had an important demographic effect in Sichuan Province.[7]

The prevalence of sterilization is a reflection of the incidence of vasectomy and tubectomy over several years. Voluntary sterilization provides a long period of effectiveness (usually 10–20 yr) for most couples before the woman reaches menopause. The age distribution of acceptors, as well as the incidence, will influence prevalence rates 10 to 20 years later. Prevalence is therefore the reflection of long-term acceptance patterns. The country with the highest vasectomy prevalence rate in Table 2-2 is the United States at 10.4% (prevalence is given as the percentage of currently married women 15 to 44 years old protected by the method, unless otherwise stated). Although we do not have recent male and female prevalence data for India, it is plausible that vasectomy is half of the 20.6% prevalence for male and female combined.[4] Therefore, India is a leading country in prevalence of vasectomy use, although the higher acceptance rates for tubectomy since 1977 mean that tubectomy prevalence will be increasing relative to vasectomy. Closely following the United States in order of rank are: the Netherlands, Canada, England and Wales, China, Australia, Korea, Thailand, Sri Lanka, and Nepal. The countries with the highest current level of vasectomy use are therefore consistently in North America, Europe and Asia.

Countries in which the prevalence of vasectomy is greater than or equal to tubectomy include Nepal, England and Wales, the Netherlands, Yemen Arab Republic, Bulgaria, and probably India. In Yemen Arab Republic and Bulgaria, however, the prevalence of both male and female sterilization is low. Other countries in which vasectomy prevalence equals 50% or more of the tubectomy prevalence include the United States, Norway, and Haiti. Male sterilization prevalence in China is slightly less than half of the female rate.

In conclusion, vasectomy plays an important role in the contraceptive practice for several countries. The prevalence rate is 5% or more of fertile couples in several of the large population countries, including China, India, and the United States.

SAFETY, EFFECTIVENESS, AND REVERSIBILITY OF VASECTOMY

Vasectomy is one of the safest of all surgical procedures. During the first 12 years, the Association for Voluntary Sterilization (AVS) supported international projects (1971–1983) in a large number of developing countries. Only two fatalities have been attributed to vasectomy in over 160,000 procedures.[5] In the Bangladesh national program, when excess mortality was reported with vasectomy (7 deaths among 22,526 men), the institution of meticulous aseptic technique was followed by a prompt decline in mortality. In the United States, vasectomy usually is performed on an outpatient basis or as an office procedure. No vasectomy fatalities have been reported in over 6 million procedures, although there is no systematic effort to identify vasectomy fatalities in the United States.[2,5]

The most common complaints following vasectomy surgery are pain, bruising, and swelling of the scrotum. Some bleeding under the skin is common and most often of little consequence. Complications of more importance, such as hematoma or infection, generally occur in fewer than 3% of men.[5] Hematoma usually is reported in fewer than 1% of men, and this rate apparently can be reduced to a considerably lower level when careful attention is placed on hemostasis.[5] Likewise, without careful attention to bleeding and careful postoperative instructions, the reported incidence also may be higher.

Infection rates usually are reported to be fewer than 2%. Skin infections at the site of the incision and around the sutures are most common. Infection of a hematoma may lead to a more serious complication. Therefore, aseptic technique and careful attention to surgical detail, including hemostasis, are both important in preventing serious infections.[2,5]

Epididymitis usually is reported in fewer than 1% of vasectomized men. In a recent large study in the United States, epididymitis or orchitis was reported more frequently by vasectomized men than by their carefully matched controls but only by an excess of 1.5% among vasectomized men.[3] Symptomatic granulomas have been reported by 0% to 3% of vasectomized men. During reversal procedures, however, granulomas at the vasectomy site have been reported in 15% to 40% of men.[6] In most instances the symptomatic granulomas can be treated successfully with mild analgesics. If this treatment is ineffective, the granuloma can be removed surgically.

The long-term safety of vasectomy has been reaffirmed by several large-scale epidemiologic studies, which have failed to show an association with atherosclerotic heart disease in men. These studies have strengthened the conclusion that vasectomy poses no identifiable long-term risks to physical or mental health.[8]

Failure rates for vasectomy based on sperm in the semen range from 0% to 2.2% in various studies, and most report fewer than 1%.[2] Vasectomy effectiveness is usually computed as a crude rate of failures per 100 procedures rather than life table rates, however. It is therefore difficult to compare effectiveness of vasectomy with female sterilization techniques. Pregnancy rates among wives of vasectomized men are usually similar to the rate for female sterilization and lower than currently available reversible methods however.

Reversibility of vasectomy, as measured by pregnancy rates, is usually reported in the range of 30% to 60%, with some even higher.[2] Several factors may affect the success of attempted reversals, including the fecundity of the woman, the method of occlusion, length of vas removed, the skill and technique of the surgeon performing the reversal, and the length of time since the vasectomy. The occurrence of normal sperm counts may be more frequent when the reversal is performed within 10 years of vasectomy.[9] The availability of services for vasectomy reversal is limited in many countries. The surgery is considerably more complicated and much more expensive than the initial vasectomy. Current estimates are that 1 to 3 per 1000 vasectomized men will request a reversal later.[2,5]

In summary, vasectomy has become a widely accepted method of male fertility control with high effectiveness and low complication rates in several countries. These characteristics make it a practical standard against which to measure new methods of male fertility regulation. There seems little likelihood that reversibility of vasectomy will be improved dramatically. Therefore, vasectomy will continue to be offered as a permanent method, and men should consider it permanent in their decision-making process.

NEW METHODS OF VAS OCCLUSION

Experimental devices have been utilized to make vas occlusion more reversible. Intravasal devices that could be removed or opened to allow sperm passage were studied in the United States, India, and South Korea in the 1970s.[2] Problems occurred with intravasal devices, and at the same time microsurgical methods improved, resulting in less interest in these devices. The surgical technique for implanting valves and intravasal devices was sometimes more difficult than anticipated. Only a few projects remained active in 1980.[2] Percutaneous techniques for vas occlusion have held great interest because these presumably would be more widely accepted than would vasectomy. Pain, complications, and fear of surgery are important barriers for vasectomy acceptance in many countries. Percutaneous occlusion techniques have employed chemical agents, electrocoagulation, or thermocoagulation.

A promising percutaneous method is a chemical occlusion technique extensively used in China.[2,7] Since 1972, approximately 500,000 men have received this percutaneous chemical occlusion technique, making use of phenol and cyanoacrylate as the sclerosing agent.[8] Under local anesthesia, the vas deferens is fixed with a specially designed clamp. A sharp needle is used to pierce the skin and vas sheath. A blunt needle then is advanced through the puncture site into the vas lumen, where 0.02 ml of the chemical agent is delivered. In more recent applications, the chemical is restricted to a 1-cm segment by digital compression of the vas below the puncture site. The chemical mixture solidifies within 20 seconds and the needle is then withdrawn.

Prior to chemical injection, two tests may be used to ensure that the needle is within the vas lumen. First, Congo red dye is injected into the vas on one side. On the opposite side, methylene blue is instilled. After the procedure the man voids. Successful placement of the needle on both sides results in a mixture of the two dyes, turning the urine brown. If the color remains unchanged, both sides were unsuccessful, if the urine is "orange red", or "apple green" there has been failure to enter the lumen on one side only. This side is then reinjected or ligated by conventional vasectomy.[8]

A second test for entry into the lumen is an "air pressure test," in which the vas is compressed digitally at two points and a syringe with 4 ml of air is attached to the needle, compressed to 2 ml for 2 seconds, and then released. If the needle tip is in the lumen, the plunger will return to its original position. If it does not return, the vas was not compressed effectively or the puncture failed, in which case subcutaneous emphysema appears around the needle site.[8]

In one Chinese follow-up study 8 years postprocedure, including semen analysis for 404 men, azoospermia occurred in 389 (96.3%). Including other men who did not have semen analysis, a total of 577 couples were followed up, among whom 14 had a pregnancy. For nine of these couples, the husband was azoospermic, however. The other five were considered method failures.

(Three of the five had sperm in the semen and two were not examined.) By these criteria, the pregnancy rate attributable to method failure was 0.9%. These results are an improvement over earlier techniques, which did not restrict the chemical agent to a 1- to $1\frac{1}{2}$-cm segment of the vas. Confining the chemical to a short segment also may improve the chances of a successful reversal procedure.[8]

One complication, a painful nodule, was reported with this technique, among 829 cases studied over 10 years. No long-term complications were reported among another group of 577 men followed up at 8 years. The developers of this technique feel that for practitioners skilled in vasectomy, the injection technique can be mastered by performing 30 cases in a training program.

CONCLUSION

Vasectomy has become a popular and demographically important method of fertility control in several countries. It has proven safe and highly effective as performed in a large number of countries with widely differing health care systems. The wide variation in vasectomy use within the same region suggests that provider variables strongly influence the level of use. The international experience implies that vasectomy could play a greater role in the programs of many countries than it now does. For safety and effectiveness it is a useful standard against which to assess other male methods. Because it must be considered a permanent method and because it involves surgery, however, vasectomy is unacceptable to some men. Nonsurgical, percutaneous vas occlusion techniques using chemicals or electrocoagulation could have a potentially important role in many programs. A chemical vas occlusion technique has been widely used in Sichuan Province in the People's Republic of China. If such a technique proved to be safe and effective in other countries, we expect it would be rapidly adopted.

REFERENCES

1. LISKIN L, PILE JM, QUILLAN WF: Vasectomy: Safe and simple. Population Reports, Series D, No. 4, 1983
2. MASSEY FJ, BERNSTEIN GS, SCHUMAN LM, O'FALLON WM: Results from the Collaborative Vasectomy Study. Paper read at the 111th Annual Meeting of the American Public Health Association, Dallas, November 13–17, 1983
3. Population Crisis Committee: Briefing Paper on Contraceptive Technology (in press).
4. ROSS JA, HONG S, HUBER DH: Voluntary sterilization: An international factbook. Association for Voluntary Sterilization (in press)
5. ROSS JA, HUBER DH: Acceptance and prevalence of vasectomy in developing countries. Stud Fam Plann 14(3):67–73, 1983
6. SHUN-QIANG L: Experience in the training of vasal sterilization. Presented at the International Training Workshop of the World Federation for Voluntary Surgical Contraception, Rio de Janeiro, Brazil, September 26–29, 1984
7. SHUN-QIANG L, JIN-BO Z: Nonoperative sterility research with intravasal injecting drug (clinical report). Presented at the International Training Workshop of the World Federation for Voluntary Surgical Contraception, Rio de Janeiro, Brazil, September 26–29, 1984
8. SILBER SJ: Vasectomy and vasectomy reversal. In WALLACH EE, KEMPERS RD (eds): Modern Trends in Infertility and Conception Control. Baltimore, Williams & Wilkins, 1979

3

Discussion Summary: Overview

MODERATOR: JOHN J. SCIARRA

WHAT DETERMINES ACCEPTANCE OF VASECTOMY IN VARIOUS CULTURES?

The first vasectomies in a country where the method is virtually nonexistent are the most difficult, in terms of acceptability, because understanding of the procedure is poor. After the method becomes known, however, especially by word of mouth—an important factor in vasectomy programs—acceptance levels may accelerate. In countries where the traditional wisdom has been that vasectomy would be totally unacceptable to men in that culture but program implementers are enthusiastic and willing to offer a high-quality vasectomy service that is well attuned to the concerns of men, vasectomy has become well accepted. Where program implementers have been half-hearted or have used inadequate anesthesia or huge incisions, or have been unfamiliar with the more refined techniques, vasectomy has been poorly accepted.

WILL ENLISTING THE WOMAN'S SUPPORT OF VASECTOMY INCREASE ITS ACCEPTANCE?

A comprehensive answer is difficult. The figures suggest that as women progress in society, vasectomy becomes more acceptable to couples, but provider attitudes and other factors may be more important. It has been observed that vasectomy is not always a liberating procedure for women. In some traditional societies, vasectomy is sometimes sought by men who would not accept sterilization of their wives out of the concern that the women subsequently would be less faithful. In such a society, a man may have the vasectomy and tell his wife about it afterward. At the other end of the spectrum, in some Western societies, a man may have a vasectomy as a loving gesture to his wife or because he has been asked by his wife to have the operation. Deciding which

Panelists: D. Malcolm Potts, Douglas Huber; *Discussants:* Nancy J. Alexander, Alfredo Goldsmith, Walter L. Herrmann, Lila Mehra, Sherman J. Silber, Jeffrey M. Spieler, Emil Steinberger, Michel Thiery, P. A. Van Keep

partner uses a contraceptive method, particularly a permanent one, is a complex issue, one about which we do not have adequate information at this time.

WHAT INFLUENCE DOES COST HAVE ON ACCEPTABILITY OF VASECTOMY VERSUS FEMALE STERILIZATION?

For government programs, the fact that vasectomy usually costs considerably less than female sterilization is an important factor in determining selection of fertility control methods.

Information is scanty about the importance of cost factors to people making a decision about vasectomy. In the United States, vasectomy costs anywhere from one fourth to one half what a female sterilization costs; outpatient laparoscopy, the most commonly used interval procedure, costs $1200 on an average. In England, desire for vasectomy is so great that many men are willing to pay the equivalent of $75 (U.S. currency) for a vasectomy so that they can avoid the long wait to have the procedure performed free of charge at the National Health Service.

IS THE TIME RIGHT FOR PROMOTION OF CONDOMS, NOT ONLY FOR CONTRACEPTION BUT ALSO AS A DETERRANT TO SEXUALLY TRANSMITTED DISEASES (STD)?

In the late 1960s and early 1970s, condoms were provided in some family planning programs with the idea that they could be effective both for contraception and for prevention of STD. Then, during the late 1970s, the idea of linking the prevention or control of STD with a family planning method like condoms went out of vogue because administrators of many programs felt that relating a negative aspect of sex to family planning was undesirable. Now, in newly emerging countries in Africa and elsewhere, where sexually transmitted disease is rampant, possibly promoting the double action of condoms may again be useful. In the Middle East, however, where societies are more traditionally chaste, promoting the double benefit of condoms is not appropriate, and the major need is to promote condoms to married couples as a reasonable method of contraception.

WHAT IS THE NO-TOUCH TECHNIQUE OF VASECTOMY?

With this technique, described by the International Planned Parenthood Federation and widely used in England, only instruments touch an aseptically prepared scrotum. As the program evolved in Bangladesh, however, instructions, perhaps poorly translated, did not emphasize the importance of asepsis, and so neither was the scrotum prepared with an aseptic solution nor was there any attention paid to using only sterile instruments; unwashed hands and fingers frequently were used in the vasectomy incision for manipulating tissues, with disastrous results.

HOW CAN ONE EXPLAIN THE INABILITY OF SOME WESTERN INVESTIGATORS TO REPEAT THE CHINESE RESULTS WITH METHYL CYANOACRYLATE?

A study to repeat the Chinese work with methyl cyanoacrylate was conducted in the United States with the assistance of investigators from China, using the dog model. The results with the U.S.-manufactured cyanoacrylate were unsuccessful. One possibility is that the Chinese add something to the cyanoacrylate, such as formaldehyde or phenyl cyanoacrylate.

One would expect that among some of the 500,000 procedures performed in China over an 11-year period, there has been variation in the sclerosing agent and the carrier, but these have not been carefully documented in the literature, either in China or elsewhere. The influence of variations in purity and technique requires more careful documentation and understanding.

Vasectomy and Reversal: Clinical Issues

4

Epidemiologic Studies of Vasectomy

DIANA B. PETITTI

Concern about the possibility of long-term effects of vasectomy on health in men stems from observations that vasectomy increases levels of circulating antisperm antibodies,[4,19,22,33] and from reports that vasectomy is associated with more extensive and severe atherosclerosis in some species of monkeys.[1,6] In 1978, when reports of more severe atherosclerosis in vasectomized monkeys were first published, few epidemiologic studies of the effects of vasectomy on disease risk in man had yet been published. In 1985, the situation is different, and recent growth in our knowledge about the effects of vasectomy on health in men has been great. In this chapter, the results of epidemiologic studies of vasectomy are reviewed, with special attention to their limitations and to remaining important questions about the long-term safety of vasectomy.

CARDIOVASCULAR DISEASE

Because of reports of accelerated atherosclerosis in vasectomized monkeys,[1,6] most epidemiologic studies of vasectomy have centered on the possibility of its affecting the risk of cardiovascular disease. Studies of cross-sectional, case-control, and cohort design have all addressed this subject. Their designs and results are summarized in Table 4-1.

The earliest epidemiologic study that assessed the association of vasectomy with cardiovascular disease in man was published by Goldacre and colleagues in 1978.[8] This study was a retrospective cohort study based on computer record linkage. It compared the incidence of hospitalization for acute myocardial infarction, stroke, hypertension, and all cardiovascular disease, considered as a group, in 1764 men who had had vasectomies in hospitals participating in the Scottish Hospital In-Patient Statistics System with the incidence of hospitalization for the same diseases in men who had had other minor surgery in the same hospitals. Disease risk was not elevated in vasectomized men for any of the cardiovascular disease groupings examined. A serious limitation of this early study was the short duration of vasectomy in the men studied, however; the mean was only 2.5 years. In a later analysis from the same retrospective cohort based on somewhat longer durations of follow-up,[10] there also was no association of vasectomy with increased risk of cardiovascular disease. In later studies of similar design based on much larger numbers of vasectomized men, longer durations of vasectomy, and more cases of cardiovascular disease at follow-up, Massey and co-workers,[13] Petitti and colleagues,[17] Walker and others,[26-28] and preliminary analysis of the World Health Organization Collaborative Study,[32] also found no increase in the risk of cardiovascular disease in vasectomized men.

Table 4-2 shows separately the estimated risk of cardiovascular disease in men with vasectomies of long duration based on the studies of Petitti and colleagues,[17] and Walker and associates.[28] The table shows that even in men, the risk of cardiovascular disease is not elevated. The confidence intervals for the relative risk estimates are narrow, and the studies exclude increases in the risk of cardiovascular disease of 1.6 or greater in men vasectomized for 10 years.

Case-control studies of the possible association of vasectomy with cardiovascular disease also have been done. Goldacre, Holford, and Vessey found that 2.4% of 1512 men under 55 years who had died or been hospitalized with acute myocardial infarction, stroke, or hypertension had had a vasectomy prior to death or hospitalization, whereas 2.7% of men the same age and residence admitted to the same hospital with diseases other than cardiovascular disease had had vasectomies.[9] They estimated on the basis of their study that the risk of acute myocardial infarction, stroke, and hypertension considered together was 0.9, a risk that was not significantly different from 1.0. The risk of acute myocardial infarction estimated separately was 1.1, of stroke 0.8, and of hypertension 0.4. In a case-control study that included 55 men with documented coronary heart disease and a control group of 55 age-matched, first-degree relatives of these men, Wallace and colleagues similarly estimated that the relative risk of acute myocardial infarction in vasectomized men less than 50 years of age was 1.0.[29]

Two cross-sectional studies of cardiovascular disease prevalence or symptoms are consistent with the findings of the cohort and case-control studies. Rimm determined the vasectomy status of 7429 men who had been referred for coronary angiography because of cardiovascular symptoms and found no association of vasectomy with a greater degree of angiographically determined coronary occlusive disease.[20] The mean angiographically determined coronary occlusion score of men with vasectomies for less than 10 years was 114, compared with 140 for age-matched controls. The mean score of men with vasectomies for 10 or more years was 121, compared with 150 for their age-matched controls. In a multivariate analysis in which investigators controlled statistically for differences between the vasectomized and nonvasectomized men in use of alcohol, cigarette smoking, history of diabetes, education, a measure of obesity, triglyceride and cholesterol concentrations, and age, there was no significant association of duration of vasectomy with a higher coronary occlusion score. Petitti and co-workers studied the frequency of self-reported symptoms of coronary heart disease in 4385 vasectomized and 11,155 age- and race-matched nonvasectomized men, all of whom were having comprehensive multiphasic health check-ups as members of a prepaid medical care program.[18] The percentages of vasectomized and age- and race-matched nonvasectomized men who reported having chest pain brought on by activity and relieved by rest were 6.5 and 6.9, respectively. The percentages of vasectomized and age- and race-matched nonvasectomized men who reported a history of coronary heart disease, hypertension, or stroke prior to the examination also were virtually identical.

TABLE 4-1. Summary of Designs and Findings of Epidemiologic Studies of the Association of Vasectomy with Cardiovascular Disease

STUDY	DESIGN	SIZE OF STUDY POPULATION	OUTCOME OR OUTCOMES STUDIED	RESULTS
Fahrenbach et al (7)	Cross-sectional	41 vasectomized 112 nonvasectomized	Hypertensive and athero-sclerotic retinal vascular changes	Significant association of vasec-tomy with mild degree of changes in retinal vessels only in men 40 years or younger
Goldacre et al (9)	Case-control	1,512 cases 3,024 controls	Death from hospitalization for myocardial infarction, stroke, hypertension	No association of vasectomy with increased risk of these outcomes; significant trend of increasing risk with longer time since vasectomy
Goldacre et al (6, 8, 9)	Cohort	1,764 vasectomized 16,641 controls not known to have vasectomy	Hospitalization for myocardial infarction, stroke, hyper-tension; all cardiovascular disease as a group	No association of vasectomy with increased risk of these outcomes
Linnet et al (12)	Cross-sectional	46 vasectomized	Atherosclerotic retinopathy	No significant association of va-sectomy with distribution of atherosclerotic retinopathy grading
Massey et al (13)	Cohort	10,590 vasectomized 10,590 nonvasectomized	Physician documented myo-cardial infarction; all car-diovascular disease as a group	No association of vasectomy with increased risk of these outcomes

Study	Design	Population	Outcome	Result
Petitti et al (17)	Cohort	4,385 vasectomized 13,155 age- and race-matched nonvasectomized	Hospitalization for myocardial infarction; all atherosclerotic disease, all cardiovascular disease as a group	No association of vasectomy with increased risk of these outcomes
Petitti et al (18)	Cross-sectional	4,385 vasectomized 13,155 age- and race-matched nonvasectomized	History of myocardial infarction; symptoms of coronary heart disease	No significant difference between vasectomized and nonvasectomized men in reporting of history of coronary heart disease or symptoms of coronary artery disease
Rimm et al (20)	Cross-sectional	370 vasectomized 7,050 nonvasectomized	Severity of angiographically proven coronary artery disease	No significant association of vasectomy with higher score measuring extent of coronary occlusion
Walker et al (26–28)	Cohort	4,800 vasectomized 24,000 controls not known to have vasectomy	Hospitalization for myocardial infarction; all cardiovascular disease as a group	No significant association of vasectomy with increased risk of these outcomes
Wallace et al (29)	Case-control	55 cases 55 close relative controls	Symptomatic coronary heart disease	No significant association of vasectomy with increased risk of coronary heart disease
W.H.O. Collaborative Group (32)	Cohort	5,000 vasectomized 5,000 nonvasectomized	Positive exercise test, ECG abnormalities, atherosclerotic retinal vascular changes	Consistent pattern of better health status in vasectomized men (preliminary data)

(From Petitti DB: Long-Term Health Risks of Vasectomy. In Sciarra JJ (ed): Gynecology and Obstetrics. Philadelphia, JB Lippincott, 1985)

TABLE 4-2. Incidence and Risk of Two Cardiovascular Outcomes in Men With Long Duration
of Vasectomy and Their Nonvasectomized Controls

STUDY	DURATION OF VASECTOMY (yr)	OUTCOME	INCIDENCE*		RELATIVE RISK (95% CONFIDENCE LIMITS)
			VASEC-TOMIZED	NONVASEC-TOMIZED	
Walker et al (32)	9–19	Myocardial infarction	2.3	2.6	0.9 (0.5, 1.7)
Petitti et al (17)	≥10	Myocardial infarction	1.3	1.8	0.7 (0.3, 1.8)
		Other ischemic heart disease	4.5	5.3	0.8 (0.4, 1.6)

* Rate per 1000 man-years

Three groups of investigators approached the question of vasectomy and cardiovascular disease by studying retinal vasculature in vasectomized men and a control group. Fahrenbach and associates used ophthalmologic examinations to evaluate the extent of hypertensive and atherosclerotic retinal vascular changes in 41 vasectomized and 112 nonvasectomized men 60 years or younger.[7] Overall, the vasectomized group did not differ significantly from the nonvasectomized group in the extent of atherosclerotic retinal damage; however, the percentage of vasectomized men 40 years of age or younger who had a Keith–Wagener score of one or two was 53.3, whereas only 20.0% of nonvasectomized men under age 40 had a score of one or two. In contrast, the percentage of vasectomized and nonvasectomized men over age 40 who had Keith–Wagener scores of one or two was almost identical. Linnet and colleagues studied the distribution of ophthalmoscopically determined gradings of atherosclerotic retinopathy in 46 men aged 33 to 53 who had been vasectomized for 5 years, and in 46 men of the same age without vasectomies.[12] In this study, the percentage of men with atherosclerotic retinopathy gradings of one, two, or three was 46 in the vasectomized subjects and 52 in the nonvasectomized controls. In men younger than age 40, the percentage with high retinopathy gradings was 35 in both the vasectomized and nonvasectomized subjects. Results of the World Health Organization Collaborative Study, in which retinal photographs were compared in 2000 vasectomized and 2000 nonvasectomized Chinese men, are still pending.[32]

AUTOIMMUNE DISEASE

The observation that vasectomy causes increases in detectable levels of circulating antisperm antibodies has generated concern about the possibility that vasectomy might increase the risk of autoimmune diseases.[4,19,22,33] This concern is largely theoretical because several studies have failed to detect an important change in the presence of antibodies to a large number of antigens other than sperm antigens in men with vasectomies.[5,11,14,21] Conversely, there have been recent reports of changes in cell-mediated immune response,[30] decreased levels of circulating immunoglobulins,[15] and increases in circulating immune complexes,[31] in vasectomized men. These observations have heightened concern about the possibility of an association of vasectomy with diseases that are linked with the immune response. The rarity of autoimmune disease in men limits the ability of epidemiologic studies to address the question of autoimmune disease in vasectomized men. Similarly, the lack of a complete understanding of how disease risk might be affected by alterations in cell-mediated immunity hampers efforts to study the possibility of an effect of vasectomy on conditions related to such alterations. The possibility of immune-related and autoimmune disease in vasectomized men continue to be topics of research.

To date, the most comprehensive evaluation of the possibility of an association of vasectomy with immune diseases was done by Massey and co-workers.[13] This study, the results of which on cardiovascular disease were summarized in Table 4-1, was a retrospective cohort study of 10,590 vasectomized men and 10,590 nonvasectomized men who were individually matched by age and residence with the vasectomized men. Diagnoses of illness were ascertained by self-report and then validated by contacting the subjects' physicians. A special attempt was made to ascertain the occurrence of diseases possibly related to immune dysfunction. The study's comparisons of immune disease in vasectomized and nonvasectomized men are summarized in Table 4-3. Vasectomy was not associated significantly with an increase in the risk of any of the specific immune diseases examined or with any of the groupings of diseases classified by pathophysiologic mechanism. On the other hand, the number of cases of myasthenia gravis, periarteritis, polymyalgia rheumatica, polymyo-

TABLE 4-3. Summary of Results of Comparison of Immune-Related Diseases in Retrospective Cohort Study of Massey and Colleagues

GROUPING	NUMBER OF CASES	PAIRS IN WHICH VASECTOMIZED MAN HAD DISEASE (%)*	Z†
Ig-E mediated diseases	182	50	0.00
Diseases associated with immune complexes	96	44	−1.22
Serum sickness-like syndromes	397	52	0.85
Diseases caused by cross-reactions with tissue antigens	17	53	0.24
Autoimmune endocrine disorders	108	49	−0.19
Autoimmune nonendocrine disorders	143	48	−0.42
Multiple sclerosis	13	54	0.28
Asthma	117	53	0.65

* Or had the disease first

† Standardized Z score; if /Z/ > 1.96 then p < 0.05.

(From Massey FJ, Bernstein GS, O'Fallon WM, Schuman LM, Coulson AH, Crozier R, Mandel JS, Benjamin RB, Berendes HW, Chang PC, Detels R, Emslander RF, Korelitz J, Kurland LT, Lepow IH, McGregor DD, Nakamura RN, Quiroga J, Schmidt S, Spivey GH, Sullivan T: Vasectomy and health: Results from a large cohort study. JAMA 252:1023, 1984)

sitis, polyarteritis nodosa, scleroderma, Sjögren's syndrome, temporal arteritis, Hashimoto's disease, regional enteritis, sarcoidosis, and systemic lupus erythematosus was not large enough to consider the possibility of an association of vasectomy with each disease specifically.

CANCER

Anderson and associates reported in 1983 that 63% of 24 mice vasectomized at 3 months and necropsied at 30 months had grossly detectable hepatomas, hepatoblastomas, hemangiomalike lesions, or alveologenic carcinomas, whereas only 14% of 14 sham-vasectomized mice had such tumors.[2] In a second study of 171 vasectomized and 97 sham-vasectomized mice, these investigators found a statistically significant association of vasectomy with the prevalence of hepatic tumors but no association with lung tumors.[2] In one study, leukocytes from vasectomized men were found to react more frequently to three or more tumor-associated antigens than were leukocytes from nonvasectomized men. This observation provides a plausible biologic explanation for an increase in the risk of neoplasm in association with vasectomy.[3] Table 4-4 shows the risk of malignant and nonmalignant neoplasms in vasectomized and nonvasectomized men in three of the large retrospective cohort studies.[10,17,26] In none of them was vasectomy associated with an increased risk of malignant or nonmalignant neoplasms; however, the number of cases of hepatoma was undoubtedly small, and none of the studies examined the possibility of an association of vasectomy separately with hepatoma. Thus, at this time, an association of vasectomy with tumor types found in excess in vasectomized mice cannot be evaluated. Future analyses of data from large cohort studies should address the question of vasectomy and hepatoma to the extent that the number of cases of this rare tumor permits such analysis. Data on hepatoma in men in the World Health Organization Collaborative Study would be of particular interest because hepatoma is of much higher incidence in China than in the United States or the United Kingdom.

PROSTATIC DISEASE

A number of investigators have found that vasectomy alters the composition of seminal fluid.[16,24] Specifically, vasectomy decreases prostatic secretory function. This observation has lead to speculation that vasectomy might alter the risk of prostatic hypertrophy or prostatic carcinoma. In an as yet unpublished study, Sidney found no association of vasectomy with benign prostatic hypertrophy or with prostatic cancer.[23] The number of cases of prostatic cancer was only 17, however. The risk of prostatic cancer in vasectomized men is another important topic for future research.

IMPOTENCE

In a widely publicized but unpublished study, Korenman and colleagues reported an association of vasectomy with impotence.[33] Massey and others found that the incidence of impotence was 1.9 per 1000 man-years of obser-

TABLE 4-4. Summary of Results of Three Retrospective Cohort Studies of Disease in Vasectomized Men and Comparison Subjects

ICDA-8 CODE	ICDA-8 DESCRIPTION	STUDY*	RISK RATIO IN VASECTOMIZED MEN (95% CONFIDENCE LIMIT†)	NUMBER OF CASES IN VASECTOMIZED MEN
140–209	Malignant neoplasm	Oxford	0.6‡	9
		Puget Sound	1.0 (0.6, 1.6)	31
		Kaiser	0.8 (0.5, 1.3)	21
210–228	Benign neoplasm	Oxford	0.6‡	4
		Puget Sound	1.5 (0.9, 2.5)	34
		Kaiser	0.9 (0.3, 2.1)	6
240–279	Endocrine, nutritional,	Oxford	1.0‡	12
	and metabolic	Puget Sound	0.5 (0.3, 0.8)	32
	diseases	Kaiser	0.8 (0.6, 1.0)	5
290–318	Mental disorders	Oxford	0.3‡	5
		Puget Sound	0.3 (0.1, 0.5)	14
		Kaiser	0.6 (0.3, 1.4)	8
390–548	Diseases of the	Oxford	1.0‡	76
	circulatory system	Puget Sound	0.8 (0.6, 1.0)	111
		Kaiser	1.1 (0.8, 1.4)	77
460–519	Diseases of the	Oxford	0.8‡	46
	respiratory system	Puget Sound	0.8 (0.6, 1.1)	77
		Kaiser	1.0 (0.6, 1.7)	21
520–577	Diseases of the	Oxford	0.8‡	90
	digestive system	Puget Sound	1.0 (0.9, 1.3)	194
		Kaiser	0.8 (0.6, 1.0)	79
580–611	Diseases of the	Oxford	0.6‡	21
	genitourinary	Puget Sound	1.6 (1.2, 2.0)	116
	system	Kaiser	1.2 (0.8, 1.9)	28
710–739	Diseases of the	Oxford	0.7‡	47
	musculoskeletal	Puget Sound	1.3 (1.0, 1.6)	121
	system and	Kaiser	1.1 (0.7, 1.7)	26
	connective tissue			

* References 10 (Oxford), 17 (Kaiser), and 26 (Puget Sound)

† Where it was calculated

‡ Ratio of standardized first-event rate in vasectomized men to average of standardized first-event rates in the three comparison groups

vation in men with vasectomy and 1.7 per 1000 man-years in nonvasectomized men, a difference that was not statistically significant.[13]

OTHER DISEASES

Three of the five retrospective cohort studies examined the association of vasectomy with many diseases other than cardiovascular disease and presented their comparisons of disease risk in vasectomized and nonvasectomized men in identical groupings, according to the International Classification of Diseases.[10,17,25,26] This allows the results of the three studies to be compared directly for several disease categories (Table 4-4). The table shows that vasectomy is not associated consistently with increased risk of any of the categories of disease. It is of note that the risk of hospitalization for mental disorders is substantially lower in vasectomized men in each of the studies. This suggests that mentally more stable men may elect vasectomies because it is unlikely that vasectomy prevents mental disorders.

CONCLUSIONS

Several epidemiologic studies of vasectomy have been published in recent years. These studies have been methodologically diverse, have been conducted by several groups of investigators in the United States, in the United Kingdom, and in China. The studies are consistent in finding no increase in the risk of cardiovascular or other disease in vasectomized men. Continued follow-up of vasectomized men to evaluate further the possibility of adverse effects of vasectomy is probably wise, however. At this time, epidemiologic studies of vasectomy in man are strongly reassuring.

REFERENCES

1. ALEXANDER NJ, CLARKSON TB: Vasectomy increases the severity of diet-induced atherosclerosis in Macaca fascicularis. Science 201:538, 1978
2. ANDERSON DJ, ALEXANDER NJ, FULGHAM DL, PALOTAY JL: Spontaneous tumors in long-term vasectomized mice: Increased incidence and association with antisperm immunity. Am J Pathol 111:129, 1983
3. ANDERSON DJ, ALEXANDER NJ, FULGHAM DL, VANDENBARK AA, BURGER DR: Immunity to tumor-associated antigens in vasectomized men. JNCI 69:551, 1982
4. ANSBACHER R: Sperm-agglutinating and sperm-immobilizing antibodies in vasectomized men. Fertil Steril 22:629, 1971
5. BULLOCK JY, GILMORE LL, WILSON JD: Autoantibodies following vasectomy. J Urol 118:604, 1977
6. CLARKSON TB, ALEXANDER NJ: Long-term vasectomy: Effects on the occurrence and extent of atherosclerosis in rhesus monkeys. J Clin Invest 65:15, 1980
7. FAHRENBACH HB, ALEXANDER NJ, SENNER JW, FULGHAM DL, COON LJ: Effect of vasectomy on the retinal vasculature of men. J Androl 1:299, 1980
8. GOLDACRE M, CLARKE JA, HEASMAN MA, VESSEY MP: Follow-up of vasectomy using medical record linkage. Am J Epidemiol 108:176, 1978
9. GOLDACRE MJ, HOLFORD TR, VESSEY MP: Cardiovascular disease and vasectomy: Findings from two epidemiologic studies. N Engl J Med 308:805, 1983
10. GOLDACRE M, VESSEY M, CLARKE J, HEASMAN J: Record linkage study of morbidity following vasectomy. In LEPOW IH, CROZIER R (eds): Vasectomy: Immunologic and Pathophysiologic Effects in Animals and Man, p 567. New York, Academic Press, 1979
11. HESS EV, HERMAN JH, HANK JL, MARCUS ZH: Studies on the immune system in human vasectomy. In LEPOW IH, CROZIER R (eds): Vasectomy: Immunologic and Pathophysiologic Effects in Animals and Man, p 509. New York, Academic Press, 1979
12. LINNET L, MOLLER NPH, BERNTH-PETERSEN P, EHLERS N, BRANDSLUND I, SVEHAG S: No increase in arteriosclerotic retinopathy or activity in tests for circulating immune complexes 5 years after vasectomy. Fertil Steril 37:438, 1982
13. MASSEY FJ, BERNSTEIN GS, O'FALLON WM, SCHUMAN LM, COULSON AH, CROZIER R, MANDEL JS, BENJAMIN RB, BERENDES HW, CHANG PC, DETELS R, EMSLANDER RF, KORELITZ J, KURLAND LT, LEPOW IH, MCGREGOR DD, NAKAMURA RN, QUIROGA J, SCHMIDT S, SPIVEY GH, SULLIVAN T: Vasectomy and health: Results from a large cohort study. JAMA 252:1023, 1984
14. MATTHEWS JD, SKEGG DC, VESSEY MP, KONICE M, HOLBOROW EJ, GUILLEBAND J: Weak autoantibody reactions to antigens other than sperm after vasectomy. Br Med J 2:1359, 1976

15. MUMFORD DM, MCCAULEY MJ, BLACK D, SUNG JS, MCCORMICK N, GORDON HL, ANSBACHER R: Serum immunoglobulin levels in vasectomized men: Preliminary report. Fertil Steril 23:749, 1977
16. NAIK VK, JOSHI UM, SHETH AR: Long-term effects of vasectomy on prostatic function in men. J Reprod Fertil 58:289, 1980
17. PETITTI DB, KLEIN R, KIPP H, FRIEDMAN GD: Vasectomy and the incidence of hospitalized illness. J Urol 129:760, 1983
18. PETITTI DB, KLEIN R, KIPP H, KAHN W, SIEGELAUB AB, FRIEDMAN GD: A survey of personal habits, symptoms of illness, and histories of disease in men with and without vasectomies. Am J Public Health 72:476, 1982
19. PHADKE AM, PADUKONE K: Presence and significance of autoantibodies against spermatozoa in the blood of men with obstructed vas deferens. J Reprod Fertil 7:163, 1964
20. RIMM AA, HOFFMAN RG, ANDERSON AJ, GRUCHOW HW, BARBORIAK JJ: The relationship between vasectomy and angiographically determined atherosclerosis in men. Prev Med 12:262, 1983
21. ROSE NR, LUCAS PL: Immunological consequences of vasectomy: Two-year summary of a prospective study. In LEPOW IH, CROZIER R (eds): Vasectomy: Immunologic and Pathophysiologic Effects in Animals and Man, p 553. New York, Academic Press, 1979
22. SHULMAN S, ZAPPI E, AHMED U, DAVIS JE: Immunologic consequences of vasectomy. Contraception 5:269, 1972
23. SIDNEY S: Personal communication, January, 1985
24. THAKUR AN, SHETH AR, RAO SS, THACKER PV: Effect of vasectomy on the prostatic function as indicated by seminal maltase activity. Contraception 11:155, 1975
25. Vasectomy and impotence linked. Med World News 24:39, 1983
26. WALKER AM, JICK H, HUNTER JR, DANFORD A, ROTHMAN K: Hospitalization rates in vasectomized men. JAMA 245:2315, 1981
27. WALKER AM, JICK H, HUNTER JR, DANFORD A, WATKINS RN, ALHADEFF L, ROTHMAN KJ: Vasectomy and nonfatal myocardial infarction. Lancet i:13, 1981
28. WALKER AM, JICK H, HUNTER JR, MCEVOY J: Vasectomy and nonfatal myocardial infarction: Continued observation indicates no elevation of risk. J Urol 130:936, 1983
29. WALLACE RB, LEE J, GERBER WL, CLARKE WR, LAVER RM: Vasectomy and coronary disease in men less than 50 years old: Absence of an association. J Urol 128:182, 1981
30. WHITE AG, WATSON GS, DARG C, EDMOND P: Lymphocytotoxins in vasectomized men. J Urol 114:240, 1975
31. WITKIN SS, ZELIKOVSKY G, BONGIOVANNI AM, GELLER N, GOOD RA, DAY NK: Sperm-related antigens, antibodies, and circulating immune complexes in sera of recently vasectomized men. J Clin Invest 70:33, 1982
32. World Health Organization Collaborative Study: Personal communication, January, 1985
33. ZAPPI E, AHMED U, DAVIS J, SHULMAN S: Immunologic consequences of vasectomy. Fed Proc 29:374, 1970

5
Psychosocial Consequences of Vasectomy in Developed and Developing Countries

ROCHELLE N. SHAIN

Other chapters in this volume have discussed vasectomy's surge in popularity during the past 15 years (see Potts, Chap. 1 and Huber et al, Chap. 2). Male sterilization is safe and effective, with minimal surgical complications or physical sequelae (see Petitti, Chap. 4). What then prevents it from being more universally accepted? This is a complex question, and only one component will be addressed herein: the possible development of sexual and psychosocial sequelae.

What are the likely sexual and psychosocial consequences of vasectomy, and how do these vary cross-culturally? Answering these questions is hampered by the absence of comparability across studies and by basic methodologic shortcomings in most existing work. Comprehensive reviews of male and/or female sterilization have discussed these flaws in detail.[45,54,57,76,87] Consequently, only three will be mentioned now: retrospective design, absence of suitable controls, and failure to use multivariate statistical analyses.

1. Without collecting baseline data prospectively, determining which conditions predated the procedure is impossible. Retrospective design leads to problems because individuals may reevaluate prior experience in the light of a more recent event. For example, a man who regrets having undergone vasectomy may overestimate his previous sexual pleasure.
2. Without employing suitable controls or comparison groups, it is impossible to determine if given changes resulted from the procedure or were due to chance, to specific life events, or to the aging process itself. For many people, surgery is paired with other medical and psychological occurrences. Because vasectomy is a major life event, there may be a tendency for persons to attribute any subsequent changes to it. Consequently, the effects of vasectomy cannot be evaluated unequivocally without comparison to a suitable control group.[76]
3. Without the use of multivariate statistical analyses, it is impossible to determine which factors are both significantly and independently associated with the dependent variables, in this case psychosocial sequelae of vasectomy.

Because most studies in this area suffer from all three major flaws, forming definitive conclusions from the literature is impossible. Nonetheless, several overall patterns concerning the development of psychosocial sequelae of vasectomy are discerned and discussed. These will be discussed first, relative to studies conducted in developed countries; however, the primary focus is on work from the developing world.

DEVELOPED COUNTRIES

The vast majority of studies in the United States,[8,15-17,23,31,36,37,42,44,48,51,56,70,78,83,98] Canada,[24-26] England,[2,35,94] Australia,[40,86] France,[5] Denmark,[52] and Germany[53] indicate a high level of satisfaction with vasectomy: regret is rarely reported by more than 5% of respondents and deterioration in some aspects of sexuality or the marital relationship is rarely reported by more than 3% to 5% of men without preexisting problems. Most men and/or their wives report improvements or no change in these areas; improvements are largely attributed to reduced anxiety, once the fear of pregnancy is removed. (See Philliber and Philliber[54] for the most recent comprehensive review in this area.)

Even childless men appear to undergo minimal detrimental effects. Brown and Magarick conducted a study of 44 childless, vasectomized males and 51 vasectomized parents, matched in age, education, and time of vasectomy.[6] Sample members had undergone surgery up to 2 years before their interview. Ninety percent of both groups reported that vasectomy was a "very good" means of birth control and no subject said the method was less than "good." Eighty percent of both groups said they would definitely repeat the procedure, and another 15% said that they probably would do so. Only one person in each group reported a decrease in sexual sensitivity or pleasure. There were no group differences in measures of psychologic adjustment or marital satisfaction. Interestingly, the only differences that did exist were unrelated to vasectomy: the childless group indicated a greater capacity for independent thought and action, more geographic mobility, and less religious affiliation. They also showed a greater tendency to experiment and were less tied to tradition. The authors conclude that vasectomy is an appropriate procedure for relatively young, married men who are firmly committed to childlessness and whose wives agree to the procedure.

Problems that arise postvasectomy usually are associated with prior marital, sexual, or psychologic instability.[8,15,28-30,32,38,51,84,94] For example, Howard studied 145 couples in England before and from 1 year to 18 months after vasectomy. Cases were selected randomly, and all couples underwent a follow-up interview, regardless of whether they actually had obtained the procedure. Results indicate that the majority of marriages improved postvasectomy. Exceptions occurred in the case of couples with severe preexisting problems. Whereas couples experienced improvement of minor sexual problems related to extreme fears of pregnancy or to disruption of spontaneity due to condom use, long-standing sexual difficulties appeared to be exacerbated. This was especially true when the husband had believed that vasectomy would improve his impotence or his wife's frigidity. The greatest anger and resentment was found among men who felt that they had "given everything" and it had been a "dead loss." Apparently, their wives had used fear of pregnancy as a defense against sexuality; however, after vasectomy, these basic sexual problems could no longer be denied.[28,30] Rodgers and Ziegler have also described this latter finding.[63]

Another factor that may contribute to negative sequelae is disagreement with one's spouse over the appropriateness of the procedure. Ferber, Tietze, and Lewit interviewed 73 men who had undergone vasectomy in the preceding 5 years.[15] According to their clinical impressions, spousal disagreement was the strongest contraindication for vasectomy. Only four men in their sample had disagreed with their wives, and two of these subjects exhibited the most negative sexual sequelae. Only two of the nine couples studied by Poffenberger and Poffenberger provided any negative responses to vasectomy.[55] In one case there was evidence that the wife had been coerced, and in the other, the husband. Rodgers and Ziegler also mention spousal disagreement as a contraindication.[63] Our own prospective study of female sterilization, using a control group of wives married to vasectomized males, indicates that the factor most strongly correlated with women's preoperative (both vasectomy and tubal sterilization) ambivalence,[46,73] and poststerilization dissatisfaction[75] is spousal control over the decision-making process. A related contraindication, choice of vasectomy to satisfy needs of others as opposed to oneself, also is noted by researchers.[11,39,63,93] Unresolved anxiety about the operation itself, either because of inadequate information or its equation with castration, also contributes to negative outcomes.[63,84]

The most basic challenge to the "clean bill of health" given to vasectomy in the literature derives from the controlled, prospective work of Rodgers, Ziegler, and associates in California during the period from 1961 to 1968.[60–66,96,97] Their first study, prospective in design but using no controls, involved interviewing and administering psychological tests (primarily the Minnesota Multiphasic Personality Inventory [MMPI]) to 35 men preoperatively and 1 year postoperatively. Although 34 respondents reported satisfaction with the vasectomy, 7 noted decreased sexual functioning. Moreover, psychological test results indicated increased psychological disturbance in 15 men. The authors therefore suggested that vasectomy may produce negative emotional sequelae that earlier retrospective surveys were unable to detect.

In a second study, 42 couples were followed prospectively for 4 years and compared to a control group that was using oral contraception. Because of attrition, reported sample size varies by year of publication. By the fourth follow-up year, reports are based on two matched groups, each consisting of 22 couples.

At the 2-year follow-up interval, almost all vasectomy couples were satisfied with their decision but displayed greater marital tension and dissatisfaction than did the controls. The authors attribute this to a heightened concern about masculinity and an increase in "masculine" behavior on the part of some vasectomized males; the authors hypothesize that respondents were trying to prove that the operation had not been demasculinizing and, in so doing, placed greater pressure on their wives. Although coital frequency increased somewhat in both groups, it rose more in the study group.

The strong emphasis on masculine behavior may have put increased strain on marriages during the first 2 postoperative years but largely disappeared by the 4-year follow-up interview. Even then some vestiges of earlier concerns appear to have remained, however: although the vasectomized sample did not report a higher incidence of impotence than did the controls, impotence was greatest among the vasectomized couples who reported the highest coital frequency, whereas the reverse was true for the control group. The authors theorize that several vasectomized men tried to prove their masculinity through unusually high rates of intercourse, which they could not physiologically maintain over long intervals and thus developed partial impotence. They suggest that the need to prove masculinity may result from a confusion of vasectomy with castration or the risk of castration.

In an attempt to explain overt satisfaction with vasectomy by the same men who show indications of increased psychological disturbance, Rodgers and Ziegler refer to the process of *dissonance reduction:* some respondents may reduce their inner conflict, resulting from having made an unalterable but incorrect decision, by exaggerating their satisfaction with the procedure.

In a very comprehensive review, Wiest and Janke[87] challenged the Rodgers and Ziegler findings. They note that nine changes were observed at the 2-year follow-up on four of the MMPI and five of the California Personality Inventory (CPI) scales. Because changes were measured for husbands, wives, and husbands and wives combined, the number of possible comparisons would be 93. Wiest and Janke suggest that the "probability of finding nine statistically significant differences with two-tailed tests is not impressively different from what is expected under the null hypothesis" (p. 445).[87] Consequently, they argue that the vasectomized males may not have actually changed. They also argue that differences between study and control group scores were small and could have resulted from having marked only one or two more items in the direction scored and thus may not be clinically significant. They further stress failure to use a blind review process and the disappearance of differences at the 4-year follow-up. Whereas they acknowledge that Rodgers and Ziegler's "psychological threat hypothesis" may be based on clinical impressions, they feel that it is neither confirmed nor contradicted by existing research data.

Janke and Wiest conducted their own study of 33 vasectomized men and a matched group of 33 nonvasectomized males at the Kaiser Foundation Hospital in Portland, Oregon.[31] All were part of a 5% random sample of subscribers. The study was based on previously collected data, unrelated to vasectomy and sexual functioning. The advantage of such an approach is that it does not sensitize respondents to vasectomy; however, its major disadvantage is failure to obtain critical items of information. Study results did not support the Rodgers and Ziegler hypothesis that vasectomized men exaggerate their masculinity as a defensive maneuver; men obtaining a vasectomy showed as many masculine traits prior to the procedure as after it. Vasectomized males experienced no greater marital, job, or general living stress than did the controls. In fact, their psychosocial adjustment appeared superior; the authors believe this is due to reduced anxiety concerning unwanted pregnancy.

Mixed support for the Rodgers and Ziegler hypothesis is found in other work.[3,92] Results of a prospective study of 224 subjects—vasectomized males, their spouses, sterilized women and their spouses—indicate that at 6 months' follow-up, sterilized males are no more likely than nonsterilized males to report an increase in sexual desire. Consequently, little support is provided therein for the compensatory hypothesis, that is, that vasectomized men feel that their masculinity is threatened and attempt to compensate by overemphasizing masculine behaviors (*e.g.*, sexual activity).[3] Exploring these data further, however, Williams and colleagues found that among vasectomized males, the more highly masculine subjects were more likely to report increases in sexual desire postprocedure than were less masculine males.[92] The authors of this study note that this result is consistent with the idea that the more stereotypically masculine males may feel more psychologically threatened by sterilization and thus respond through compensatory processes such as increasing coital desire.

Indirect support for the psychological threat hypothesis derives from our own research, which indicates that a perceived threat to sexual integrity is a major reason for rejecting male sterilization. Close to 39% of married women in the tubal sterilization sample chose the female procedure because their husbands had refused or were apprehensive about vasectomy. Moreover, 41% of tubal sterilization patients reported that their husbands had been unwilling to undergo vasectomy, compared with 21% of vasectomy wives who were unwilling to be sterilized themselves. When asked to explain why their husbands refused vasectomy, one third of the women reported fear of sexual side-effects.[74]

Data from other researchers indicate that vasectomy involves a complex decision-making process,[50] and that social support is a more important factor for men than for women in their sterilization decision.[9,10] Results from our study support the latter finding: choice of vasectomy, unlike female sterilization, is significantly related to having many friends or relatives who had undergone the procedure already, that is, wives or their husbands either had sought out men who had a vasectomy or already knew such men and thus felt comfortable with the decision. Moreover, wives of men about to undergo vasectomy discussed sterilization with their husbands more often and discussed it with more people than did women scheduled for sterilization. This additional deliberation suggests that the decision to undergo vasectomy involves a more extensive social process and may be the more difficult one of the two to make.[74]

Social attitudes affect and are affected by individual perceptions of vasectomy and its relationship to masculinity. There are strong indications in the literature that vasectomy was negatively regarded in the 1960s. Rodgers, Ziegler, and Levy[65] assessed the attitudes of churchgoers and undergraduate psychology students toward a brief description of a hypothetical couple. Approximately half the subjects were told the couple was using vasectomy and the remaining half, oral contraceptives. Although subjects did not produce stereotypical characterizations of either couple, significantly more favorable attitudes were expressed towards the pill-users than the vasectomy-users. Eisner and associates conducted a survey among Cornell students and faculty in 1969.[14] Only 6% mentioned vasectomy as a preferred method of birth control, and the majority said that they would never be sterilized for contraceptive purposes. Nearly half the respondents either misunderstood or did not know the consequences of male sterilization.

In view of these survey results, it is not surprising that satisfied vasectomy acceptors have sometimes been reluctant to disclose their sterilization. Ferber and associates report that 71 of their 73 subjects stated they would recommend the operation to others; nonetheless, only 35 had actually done so.[15] Further investigation indicated widespread reluctance to disclose their vasectomy. This subject area was an especially "charged" one: subjects, even those who said they were indifferent, were observed to flinch and show tension during questioning. The authors feel that most men assumed a loss of status following sterilization and "were reluctant to face the disapproval of others" (p. 362).[15] Respondents told investigators that significant others in their lives felt vasectomy was a form of castration, affecting potency. Poffenberger and Poffenberger also reported some disclosure hesitation among several subjects.[55] Kohli and Sobrero reported that 98% of their patients were pleased with vasectomy and were willing to recommend it to others. Only 86%, however, had actually discussed the operation with friends, and of this group, one third had received negative feedback.[36]

There seems little doubt that derogatory societal attitudes affect the self-concept of men undergoing vasectomy.[84] There is also little doubt, as noted by Pohlman,[57] that attitudes change with time. Consequently, in order to resolve the issue of psychosocial consequences of vasectomy, not only do we need large-scale, prospective, controlled studies, collecting comparable information, we need them repeated every 5 or 10 years.[57]

DEVELOPING COUNTRIES

Studies from developing countries are reported here in greater detail than those from the developed world. The former are in greater need of fertility regulation and, to develop contraceptive methods and educational programs appropriate to non-Western people's needs, it is first necessary to understand individual reactions to methods currently in use.[43,58,72]

LATIN AMERICA

Vasectomy is significantly less popular than tubal sterilization in Latin America.[47,67–69] This is consistent with cultural beliefs that women undertake contraceptive responsibility, the apparently still-persistent need on the part of some males not to tamper with any aspects of their masculinity, and a greater institutional commitment to female procedures.[20–22,68]

Research undertaken in Latin America on the psychosocial consequences of vasectomy, albeit limited, indicates that those men who select sterilization appear pleased with the results. Findings from studies conducted in Colombia, Costa Rica, Guatemala, and Mexico are summarized below.

Goldsmith and colleagues interviewed 172 Colombian and 77 Costa Rican men who had undergone vasectomy at least 3 months earlier.[22] An adaptation of the questionnaire developed by Ferber and associates was used.[15] Results indicated overall satisfaction: 98% would repeat the decision, and as shown in Table 5-1, most men felt that their physical and emotional health as well as their sexual and marital satisfaction either improved or did not change. Change in coital frequency was attributed almost always to the vasectomy. Some husbands also reported an increase in wives' initiation of sexual activity. Positive consequences of vasectomy are attributed to generally feeling more

TABLE 5-1. Psychosocial Sequelae of Vasectomy (Costa Rican/Colombian Study)

	IMPROVED (%)	NO CHANGE (%)	WORSENED (%)
General happiness	80.7	18.1	1.2
Physical health	16.9	81.5	1.6
Emotional health	22.9	71.9	5.2
Sexual satisfaction	61.4	32.9	5.7
Quality of sexual relations	43.8	49.0	6.8
Coital frequency	39.8	51.0	8.8
Marital relationship	46.1	51.8	2.1

(Data from Goldsmith A, Goldberg R, Echeverria G: An in-depth study of vasectomized men in Latin America: A preliminary report. J Reprod Med 10:150–155, 1973)

personally and/or sexually relaxed and, specifically, to removal of the fear of an unwanted pregnancy.

The importance of appropriate counseling and provision of full information is stressed. Before counseling, over 35% of men feared that vasectomy would lead to impotence, castration, and loss of virility or sexual satisfaction; an additional 6% believed there would be other negative sequelae. By the time of the research interview, only 3% of respondents still expected some type of sexual, mental, or physical change.[22]

The authors conclude that despite the influence of the Catholic church (approximately 80% of subjects and wives were Catholic), and still-prevalent ideal of machismo, vasectomy is highly acceptable to some Latin American men. In a related publication, Goldsmith and Goldberg note, "Most men who really fear the operation simply do not choose to have it; therefore, the process of self-selection will exclude many men who should not have a vasectomy" (p. 288).[21] Returning to the study sample, we note that it is an especially motivated group: over 90% of men and their wives feared another pregnancy, 57% had experienced a contraceptive failure, and 92% had used contraceptives before the operation. The latter characteristic alone distinguishes these subjects from the norm in their respective countries. Given prevailing cultural beliefs in Latin America, however, it is possible that even highly motivated men would report negative results. The Goldsmith study demonstrates that this is not the case.

The Guatemala City study involved interviewing 500 (out of a possible 872) men 12 to 36 months postvasectomy.[69] Results indicate a high level of satisfaction: over 97% of the men reported they had never regretted their decision; 93% would recommend the procedure to others, and only 8% would be bothered if their friends knew about the vasectomy. Regrets, expressed by 2.6% of the sample, were based on desire for another child, dissatisfaction with sexual performance, procedure failure, and divorce. As shown in Table 5-2, other aspects of life tended to remain unchanged or improve. Additionally, 30% of men noticed some increased sexual responsiveness on the part of their wives.

The authors tried to determine which factors were correlated with regret. Given little intragroup variability—only 2.6% expressed regret—it is not

TABLE 5-2. Psychosocial Sequelae of Vasectomy (Guatemala City Study)

	IMPROVED (%)	NO CHANGE (%)	WORSENED (%)
General health	12.8	85.4	1.8
Work capacity	5.0	92.2	2.8
Sexual relationship (marital)	38.0	60.0	2.0
Sexual desire	26.4	68.4	5.2
Sexual satisfaction	40.2	57.6	2.2
Quality of orgasms	16.6	79.2	4.2

(Data from Santiso R, Pineda MA, Marroquin M, Bertrand JT: Vasectomy in Guatemala: A follow-up study of five hundred acceptors. Soc Biol 28:253–264, 1981)

surprising that no sociodemographic factor or preoperative event had predictive power. Regret was, rather, related to procedure failure and to perceived negative effects on health and sexuality.

Conclusions drawn from this study are similar to those from Colombia and Costa Rica.[22] The importance of counseling and education are stressed; over 97% of the sample felt they knew exactly what vasectomy entailed before having it performed. Because close to 80% of subjects were Roman Catholic, results also point to the diminished influence of the Catholic church in contraceptive matters. Finally, the educational level attained by this sample was higher than the norm, and, most important, respondents were highly motivated to limit family size: 79% reported contraceptive use before vasectomy.[69]

Results from Mexico also indicate a favorable outcome among a highly motivated sample.[19] Most subjects had been using contraceptive methods before vasectomy, and of 500 couples, only 1% complained of reduced libido and less than 1%, of decreased potency. On the basis of the Colombian and Costa Rican, Guatemalan, and Mexican studies, it can be argued that vasectomy has predominantly positive psychosocial sequelae among self-selected Latin American couples, highly motivated to limit their fertility.

ASIA

Results from follow-up investigations in Asia are generally more negative, but vary by country and study. A 1973 study conducted in Thailand[7,49] used an adaptation of the Ferber and associates questionnaire.[15] One hundred and eighty-five males (out of a possible 292), who had been vasectomized between January 1970 and March 1973, were interviewed between May and July 1973. Sample members were better educated than the average Bangkok resident but had relatively low mean incomes.

Results indicate overall satisfaction. Most respondents (97%) reported that their health was the same or improved since the vasectomy; however, 10% noted they were more easily fatigued and could not work as hard. Weakness was most often mentioned by men over 40. All subjects reported that since the operation they were either as happy as or happier than they had been previously. Marital relations remained unchanged and the few sexual changes tended to be improvements: 70% of respondents noted no change in their sexual response, whereas 22% reported an improvement, and 8%, a deterioration. Eighty-six percent reported that their wives' sexual response had not changed, 12% noted an improvement and only 1%, a deterioration. Responses to questions about erection, duration of intercourse, ability to control orgasm, and response to orgasm indicated minimal change as well: between 4% and 10% of respondents indicated a deterioration, and between 14% and 23%, an improvement. When coital frequency rates were age standardized, there was a small (not significant) increase in average number of coital episodes per month (from 11.2 to 11.7). The authors constructed an index of overall change in sexual satisfaction: 2.7% of the men showed a great deal of deterioration, 14%, slight deterioration, and the remainder varied between no change and a great deal of improvement.

The relative absence of negative psychosocial sequelae may be attributed to various factors; however, in the absence of multivariate statistical analyses, it is impossible to determine independent association. The authors note that the educational level of their sample was above average for the country, but that income levels were relatively low. Consequently, this "status inconsistency" may have led to a strong desire to terminate childbearing. In fact, 90% of respondents indicated that their primary motivation was economic. Moreover, subjects had reached or surpassed their stated ideal family size, and there was considerable worry over additional pregnancies. Sixty-eight percent of the sample used a contraceptive method before vasectomy; although only eight percent reported a method failure, all respondents expressed some dissatisfaction with their particular method. Additionally, the majority of men were self-motivated, and only 3% indicated that their spouses had coerced them into the procedure. Ninety-three percent had discussed vasectomy with their wives preoperatively, and in only one case was there any disagreement. Consequently, as in the case of both the Guatemalan and Colombian and Costa Rican samples, these men represent a highly motivated group and, as such, experienced generally satisfactory outcomes.

Follow-up studies in other parts of Asia, particularly India and Bangladesh, generally produced less favorable results. One hundred seventy-six patients from Chandigarh, India who had undergone vasectomy 6 to 8 months earlier were interviewed and administered psychological tests.[90] Most subjects were poor and semiliterate. Over 31% complained of some symptom that they attributed to their vasectomy. Age, education, occupation, income, religion, type of family, number of children alive, and age of youngest child did not differ from the symptomatic to the asymptomatic group. Prevalence of symptoms was slightly higher among the lower social classes. The factors that accounted for group differences, in order of importance, are self motivation versus persuasion by others to undergo surgery (p = 0.01) and immediate complications (p = 0.01).

Complaints were divided into physical, sexual, and psychological symptoms. Some of the physical symptoms seemed to be closely related to the procedure: pain or swelling at the operative site and a dragging sensation while walking. Others were more difficult to explain: weakness; pain in the back, abdomen, or legs; weight loss; and insomnia. Approximately 14% of the sample reported negative sexual symptoms, including decreased coital frequency and sexual desire, poor erection, and decreased coital duration. These changes were very distressing to the majority of patients. Included among psychological symptoms were excessive worrying, insomnia, nervousness, poor concentration, and feelings of depression. Of the 55 men who reported symptoms, 31% regretted their decision.

In a second study undertaken by Wig and colleagues, a prospective design was used and a total of 130 sample members were recruited from rural and urban populations.[89] Follow-up interviews were scheduled 3 to 6 months after the vasectomy and 90% of patients completed both preoperative and postoperative interviews. Most subjects were poor and semiliterate.

At the postoperative interview, 22% of the sample complained of some symptom. Physical symptoms included pain at the operative site; general weakness; loss of weight; and pain in back, legs, and abdomen. Sexual symptoms included weakness and decreased desire; psychological symptoms included nervousness, depression, insomnia, bad health, and loss of ability to work. Most symptoms were physical in nature, as opposed to psychological or sexual, probably because of the short interval between surgery and the postoperative interview.[89]

The authors again separated the symptomatic and nonsymptomatic groups and tried to determine factors correlated with complaints. Age, education, profession, income, religion, type of family, and number of children alive did not significantly discriminate between the two groups. Self-motivation versus persuasion and/or coercion by others strongly (p = 0.01) differentiated between the groups, however. Approximately 31% of the sample had been persuaded or coerced by others to undergo vasectomy. The development of immediate postsurgical complications also was correlated (p = 0.01) to later problems. It is impossible, however, to determine the extent to which the development of immediate problems also was correlated with persuasion and coercion. Interestingly, preoperative psychological test results could not predict the development of postoperative complaints. Because the sample population was largely illiterate in Hindi, however, the researchers were confined to those tests that could be understood and translated readily into local languages. Additionally, the widespread influence of coercion may have masked other effects.

Investigation of 107 men with postvasectomy psychiatric symptoms was conducted in Jhansi, India.[77] The most common psychiatric diagnoses were sexual inadequacy and neuroses. Approximately 5% of men had more severe problems, either psychotic depression or schizophrenia. The investigators learned that only 21% of the men had been "properly persuaded" and had undergone vasectomy voluntarily. Pressure had been used in 79% of cases. Most significantly, severity of illness was related directly to degree of coercion. Consequently, the authors stress appropriate selection of candidates without coercive tactics.

Gandotra and colleagues interviewed 200 men from southern Delhi and administered various psychologic tests 6 months to 3 years postvasectomy.[18] Sample members were more highly literate and occupied higher-status jobs than did the rest of the population. Results indicate that 71% of men perceived no change in their general health, 11% noticed an improvement and 18% a deterioration. Close to 13% complained of general weakness. Of the men claiming a deterioration in health, in the case of half, further examination revealed a probable cause other than vasectomy. Approximately 70% of the sample perceived no change in mental health, close to 15% noted improvement, and 15%, deterioration. Symptoms such as irritability, sadness, and anxiety were noticed. Five percent of complainers attributed these perceived changes to factors other than vasectomy. Six percent of men in the sample reported an increase in coital frequency and 12%, an increase in sexual desire; 26% reported a decrease in coital frequency, and 11%, a decrease in desire. Only 4% described a change in ejaculation; however, 23% noted a decrease, and only 1.5% noted an increase in their ability to have erections. In general, 46% of the sample complained of some deterioration in sexual activity. Approximately half of these men reported that these changes did not affect their actual sexual enjoyment, however. In only 3% of cases was the wife perceived to be disturbed with her husband's sexual performance. Of the men perceiving any type of sexual deterioration, half attributed it to the vasectomy. Despite the various problems that the men in the sample associated with vasectomy, over 86% were satisfied with the procedure.

The authors determined that the following factors were associated with the development of problems: low literacy, occupational levels and income; immediate postoperative complications; poor preoperative knowledge; and negative reactions from significant others. Physical and mental problems were more common in the younger age groups, whereas sexual problems were more prevalent among older men. Parity, wife's age or level of literacy, interval since operation, and previous use of contraceptives were not related to postoperative problems. No details were provided on prevalence of contraceptive use, however. If that figure is very low, there may not be sufficient variability to distinguish between groups. Sample members who stated that the vasectomy decision was voluntary had the fewest problems, as did men whose wives fully shared in the decision. Cases in which the wife either had not been informed or had voiced opposition were associated with maximal physical, mental, and sexual problems.

Because multivariate statistical analyses were not used, it is impossible to determine which factors are independently associated with the development of problems. Lower socioeconomic status, nonvoluntary acceptance of vasectomy, and inadequate preoperative information were associated with the greatest level of problems. It is impossible, however, to discern the extent to which these factors are intercorrelated. The role of financial incentives was not examined.

Sinha and colleagues, conducting a study in Lucknow, noted the prevailing cultural beliefs surrounding vasectomy:

> . . . there are widespread fears and apprehensions about the operation. People are naturally suspicious and afraid about surgical operations in general and in particular about surgery on sexual organs. It is widely believed that such an operation leads to sexual aberration, instability, mental derangement, physical debility, change in sexual relations and even to impotence. It is not infrequently confused with castration (p. 134).[79]

Of a possible 337 men, 242 were interviewed 3 months postoperatively. Over 82% perceived no change in general health, 8% noted an improvement, and 10%, a deterioration. Improvement was marked by the disappearance of body pain following coitus and deterioration, primarily by general weakness, early tiredness, and body pains. Changes in sexual activity were assessed in detail. Overall, 71% of men perceived no change, 12% indicated an increase, and 17%, a decrease. Seventy-nine percent of the sample perceived no change in sexual desire; 9% perceived an increase, and 12% a decrease. Over 83% of the sample noted no change in either duration of or satisfaction from coitus; 7% noted an increase and 10% a decrease. Only 5% of the sample reported a decrease in the amount of seminal discharge; the remainder perceived no change. Decrease in sexual activity was correlated with low educational level, preoperative fears or apprehensions, and immediate postoperative complications. Tests of significance were not, however, performed.

Slightly over 80% of the sample were satisfied with their vasectomy, whereas 14% regretted their decision. Reasons for dissatisfaction included postoperative complications, sexual weakness, and loss of wages. Over 16% of respondents had not disclosed their procedure to friends because they feared loss of status. Of the men who had done so, 15% met with disapproval. Unfavorable reactions took the form of "making fun, criticism of interfering in natural phenomenon, and of being fed up with children" (p. 138).[79] One sample member had to stave off a physical attack by his wife's relatives when they learned of his vasectomy. Close to 79% of men agreed to recommend vasectomy to others; however, some indicated they would do so without disclosing their own procedure.

Although motivation and nonvoluntary acceptance of vasectomy are not discussed, the authors note the tendency of professional motivators to coerce others into accepting the procedure solely for monetary gain to both parties. The danger inherent in this practice is underscored.

A study in Malaysia, primarily of Indian subjects working on rubber estates, was conducted by Wolfers and colleagues.[95] Two hundred and forty-six men were interviewed between 1 and 4 years postvasectomy. Ninety-one percent of the sample had no regrets, 89% had no fears, 88% did not feel a loss of libido, and 96% had no marital problems as a result of the vasectomy. Parity (specifically, having more than 5 children) was negatively correlated with the dependent variable, regret. Absence of daughters (all respondents had at least one son) was associated with negative effects, but only when the two dependent variables, regret and fears, were combined. Joint decision-making was negatively correlated with both regrets and fears, either considered individually or jointly, and its absence was the strongest predictor of overall anxiety. Results are compared to those of Ferber and colleagues, who found that the strongest contraindication for vasectomy was a man's disagreement with his wife over its advisability.[15]

As in most other studies of Indian subjects, general body weakness was reported by a considerable number of men (17%). The in-depth interviews provided some ethnographic information to help explain this belief. Some men felt that, after vasectomy, sperm may be absorbed by the body, resulting in weakness, fatness, and flabbiness. There was also a belief expressed by some respondents that vasectomy caused an increase in libido; the resulting increased frequency of sexual intercourse then depleted the body of strength.[95]

Apte and Gandhi interviewed 168 men 1 to 4 years postvasectomy about their feelings at the first postoperative year.[1] These subjects were representative of the 337 men who had been sterilized in the greater Bombay area between 1964 and 1967. Results were generally positive. Over 70% of respondents perceived no change in their general health, 12% noted an improvement, and 18%, a deterioration. The most commonly perceived negative health change was weakness (10% of the sample). The authors note that there is a widespread belief that, after vasectomy, a man becomes withdrawn, irritable, and depressed. However, 74% of the sample reported no temperamental change; 21% noted an improvement, in that they had become more relaxed and sociable, and 5% reported a negative change, in that they had become primarily more nervous and irritable.

Most males perceived either no change or an increase in sexual desire; only 6.5% noted a decrease. Close to 69% of the sample perceived no change in coital frequency, 14% experienced an increase, and 17%, a decrease. Although fear of losing masculine vitality postvasectomy was prevalent in Bombay, 95% of respondents reported no change in perceived virility; 2% noted an increase, and 3%, a decrease.

In general, subjects reported fewer negative sequelae than in other studies of Indian subjects. Because very few sociodemographic variables were examined, it is difficult to determine exactly why this is the case. The following factors, however, form the basis for an explanation. Over 85% of subjects used contraception preceding their operation; thus, sample members were highly motivated to control their fertility. Moreover, 58% of contraceptive users were dissatisfied with either the reliability or acceptability of their prior method. This may have made them especially motivated to undergo vasectomy. The authors also note that subjects faced relatively little opposition from significant others. Of the 114 men who informed friends, relatives or parents preoperatively, 11% received negative feedback. Over 39% of the sample were self-motivated, 33% were motivated by friends and relatives, and 23% by doctors or social workers. No information on financial incentives is provided. Most significantly, the authors note that vasectomy was primarily "a decision between husband and wife" (p. 13).[1] This indicates that coercion was likely to have been minimal.

Devi compared the relative popularity of male and female sterilization in two rural areas of Tamil Nadu, India.[13] The following five comparison groups, each consisting of 71 respondents, were used: 1) vasectomy acceptors, 2) their wives, 3) tubal sterilization adopters, 4) their husbands, and 5) currently married women within similar age and parity categories who had not chosen sterilization. Thus, three subsamples consisted of women, and two of men. No information was provided as to why the fifth category consisted only of females. Nor is information provided as to the interval between the interview and sterilization. Twenty-one physicians were interviewed independently as a separate substudy.

Results indicate that tubal sterilization was more often approved than vasectomy (92% vs 73%). The majority (74%) of respondents considered tubal sterilization the superior method; only 17% felt vasectomy was preferable. Whereas 100% of the women who underwent tubal sterilization felt that it was best, only 63% of the vasectomized males felt that their procedure was preferable. Men who underwent vasectomy despite their preference that their wives be sterilized did so primarily because of the cash incentive or the desire to keep sterilization secret.

Generally, vasectomy was believed to be associated with more negative consequences than female sterilization. Coupled with this belief was the assumption that men, as breadwinners, should take fewer risks with their health and that women could always rely on their husbands in case of illness. Those who favored vasectomy mentioned among other reasons its relative lack of complications, its simplicity, and the fact that it can be readily hidden from friends and relatives. Moreover, nearly 10% of the vasectomy acceptors were motivated solely by the financial incentive. Eighty-three percent of women married to vasectomy acceptors would have preferred tubal sterilization; most reported that their husbands underwent the procedure without their knowledge.

The 21 physicians confirmed that tubal sterilization was the more popular of the two procedures. Whereas all agreed that vasectomy was simpler and associated with fewer complications, they stressed nonmedical criteria for acceptability. Fourteen physicians feared that vasectomy would reduce potency and physical vigor. Stress also was placed on the male's economic role, and consequently the need to give his health and welfare priority. Many physicians saw no need to counter popular beliefs and offered female sterilization simply because it inspired greater confidence among patients. Consistent with these results, Philliber and Philliber found, in their comprehensive literature review, that regret rates in Asia are clearly higher for male (average of 15%) than female (average of 4%) sterilization.[54]

A 1-year follow-up study of 304 vasectomy acceptors in two Bangladesh cities (Shibtur and Shalna) was based on a random selection of clients, a high participation rate (88%–92%), and a case-control design (controls were matched in all vital aspects except that they were more often landholders).[34] Thus, it is one of the more comprehensive investigations in this area.

Results indicate a high rate of dissatisfaction (between 45% in Shibtur and 49% in Shalna). Reasons mentioned most frequently include decreased ability to work (20%) and nonpayment of promised incentives (11%). Interestingly, whereas vasectomized men frequently complained about decreased ability to work and sexual "weakness," so did the controls: 58% and 55% of the latter group reported, respectively, that they were less able to work and had become sexually weaker in the last year. Thus, vasectomized subjects appear to be attributing to vasectomy culturally conditioned patterns of behavior that are independent of the procedure. Why, then, was there so much dissatisfaction?

Examination of certain subject characteristics and motivation for vasectomy helps clarify the issue. The majority of subjects had no formal education (the average educational level was 1.0 and 1.6 years) and were agricultural or unskilled laborers. Although most vasectomy clients reported that they wanted no additional children, only between 3% and 7% had used contraceptives preoperatively. Although fewer than 10% of respondents reported that they were coerced into surgery, 40% and 60% noted that their primary motivation was receipt of a financial incentive. Moreover, only 18% considered themselves the most influential factor in the vasectomy decision; in fact, 75% of Shibtur's subjects were recruited by motivators, police, or councilmen.

Some recruiters misinformed potential clients regarding the amount of incentive payments. Thus, although direct coercion was relatively infrequent, indirect pressure through financial incentives was prevalent. Frequency of dissatisfaction was greatest among "agent"-recruited subjects: 89% of these men reported dissatisfaction, compared to between 30% and 50% of their counterparts motivated by family planning workers, neighbors, relatives, or councilmen. The authors of this study also note that financial incentives were particularly attractive to the most destitute members of society—the people most likely to have preexisting problems with their health, sexual performance, and marital relationships. As noted earlier, the study group differed from the controls in that the latter were more frequently landholders.

Finally, vasectomy was not accepted socially among the subjects' peers. Between 75% and 84% of clients discussed their procedure with other men; the majority met with disapproval. This is not because there is a cultural proscription against sterilization in general. A study of tubal sterilization by a similar research team in Bangladesh indicated that only 5% of women regretted their procedure.[81] Almost all women who expressed regrets did so because they had lost a child since their sterilization. Although 7% to 9% of male respondents experienced a child death postvasectomy, this was not cited as a reason for regret.[34] Consequently, dissatisfaction with vasectomy in this study appears to result not from permanent termination of childbearing per se but from direct and indirect forms of coercion, culturally conditioned attitudes against male sterilization, and attraction of the most destitute elements of the population. These patients are most prone to experience problems that are independent of vasectomy and to attribute them to the procedure, out of ignorance or misinformation.

The psychosocial consequence described most frequently in the literature, and thus having the greatest cross-cultural comparability, is change in coital frequency. Table 5-3 categorizes this information according to country and amount and direction of change. These data indicate that, in general, the least favorable results are found in India. Studies discussed thus far indicate that, in addition to cultural attitudes against vasectomy, negative sequelae result from insufficient motivation, inadequate preoperative information, absence of spousal communication and/or joint-decision-making, and, most importantly, from coercion prior to surgery (also see references 16, 23, 54).

N. N. Wig, a pioneering Indian psychiatrist in psychosocial research, wrote in 1979:

> We began with the "clinic approach" hoping that people will themselves come for family planning advice. When that did not happen, we began the "field era" by extending family planning services down to every primary health center, establishing an extensive network of paraprofessionals. When enough people refused to be persuaded by our slogans and incentives, we brought in political pressure and coercion. The result was not the breaking of people's resistance but the breaking up of the political system. At present we are all sitting numb—not knowing which way to go (p. 16).[88]

In an even more critical indictment of coercive tactics in India, Vicziany describes the pervasiveness and influence of the financial incentive system.[85] She notes that, on the average, incentives were equal to half of 1-month's

TABLE 5-3. Relationship Between Vasectomy and Frequency of Intercourse (Sexual Desire)*

AUTHORS	FREQUENCY OF INTERCOURSE			NATION
	MORE	*SAME*	*LESS*	
				Asia
Apte and Gandhi, 1970	14	69	17	India
Bhatnagar, 1964	19	70	12	India
Dandekar, 1963	12	35	54	India
Gandotra et al, 1978	6	68	26	India
Kakar, 1972	18	41	41	India
Poffenberger and Sheth, 1963	15	59	10	India
Rathore, 1970	4	76	20	India
Saxena et al, 1965	7	73	20	India
Sinha et al, 1969	12	71	17	India
Wig and Singh, 1972	NR	NR	5	India
Wig et al, 1970	NR	NR	10	India
Lee, 1970	Average frequency: 1.92/wk before 1.70/wk after			Korea
Burnight et al, 1975 (age-standardized)	Average frequency: 11.21/mo before 11.71/mo after			Thailand
Hassan, 1975	6	64	30	Pakistan
				Latin America
Goldberg et al, 1974	38	51	11	Colombia
Goldsmith et al, 1973	40	51	9	Colombia and Costa Rica
Santiso et al, 1981 (desire)	26	68	5	Guatemala
				North America
Ferber, Tietze, and Lewit, 1967	Average frequency: 8.4/mo before 9.8/mo after			United States
Freund and Davis, 1973	68	32	0	United States
Kohli and Sobrero, 1973	36	61	3	United States
Landis and Poffenberger, 1965 (desire)	38	60	2	United States
Nash and Rich, 1972 (desire)	21	75	4	United States
Sobrero and Kohli, 1975	34	60	5	United States
Truesdale, 1965 (desire)	24	73	3	United States
Uehling and Wear, 1972 (desire)	32	65	3	United States
Zufall, 1980 (desire)	8	88	4	United States

* If coital frequency data are not reported and sexual desire data are available, the latter are substituted.

(Adapted from Philliber WW, Philliber SG: Social and psychological perspectives on voluntary sterilization: A review. Stud Fam Plann 16:1–29, 1985 and Sinha SN et al., A sociomedical study of urban sterilized males in Lucknow, J Indian Med Assoc 53:134–141, 1969)

earnings and in some cases were over double an average monthly wage. Moreover, she documents that sterilization campaigns tended to coincide with job shortages in agriculture and attracted the poorest, most illiterate classes, who often did not know what was happening to them and were unaware of their civil rights. The motivator–canvasser was paid for each vasectomy acceptor; he often brought pressure on the potential adopter and frequently used fraudulent methods. She concludes that members of lower socioeconomic groups were sterilized not out of conviction but because they had no real choice.

Given the pervasiveness of coercion in India, it is surprising that results are as positive as they are; however, until studies are conducted on populations accepting vasectomy voluntarily, it will be impossible to determine the true psychosocial sequelae of this procedure in many countries, or to make valid cross-cultural comparisons. Where coercion is absent and vasectomy is chosen freely by highly motivated couples who agree about the procedure's advisability—whether in the United States, Colombia, or Thailand—psychosocial outcomes tend to be neutral or positive.

REFERENCES

1. APTE JS, GANDHI VN: A follow-up study of vasectomy cases. J Fam Welfare 17:3–17, 1970
2. BARNES MN, BLANDY JP, ENGLAND HR, GUNN SIR G, HOWARD G, LAW B, MASON B, MEDAWAR J, REYNOLDS C, SHEARER RJ, SINGH M, STANLEY-ROOSE DG: One thousand vasectomies. Br Med J 4:216–221, 1973
3. BEAN FD, CLARK MP, SOUTH S, SWICEGOOD G, WILLIAMS D: Changes in sexual desire after voluntary sterilization. Soc Biol 27:186–193, 1980
4. BHATNAGAR NK: Vasectomy: A study of effect and reaction. J Fam Welfare 11:1–3, 1964
5. BOURGET F, LE DANOIS A, CONNEHAYE P: Analysis of a series of 272 vasectomies: Medical and psychological sequelae. Concours Medical 104:5907–5921, 1982
6. BROWN RA, MAGARICK RH: Psychological effects of vasectomy in voluntary childless men. Urology 14:55–58, 1979
7. BURNIGHT RG, MUANGMUN V, COOK MJ: Male sterilization in Thailand: A follow-up study. J Biosoc Sci 7:377–391, 1975
8. CASS AS: Unsatisfactory psychosocial results of vasectomy resulting in modification of preoperative counseling. Urology 14:588–591, 1979
9. CLARK MP, BEAN FD, SWICEGOOD G, ANSBACHER R: The decision for male versus female sterilization. Fam Coord 28:250–254, 1979
10. CLARK MP, SWICEGOOD G: Husband or wife: A multivariate analysis of decision making for voluntary sterilization. J Fam Issues 3:341–360, 1982
11. COETZEE T: The nonreproductive consequences of vasectomy. S Afr Med J 61:472–475, 1982
12. DANDEKAR K: Aftereffects of vasectomy. Artha Vijnana 5:212–224, 1963
13. DEVI SDR: Comparative popularity of vasectomy and tubectomy. J Fam Welfare 26:79–91, 1980
14. EISNER T, VAN TIENHOVEN A, ROSENBLATT F: Population control, sterilization and ignorance. Science 167:337, 1970
15. FERBER AS, TIETZE C, LEWIT S: Men with vasectomies: A study of medical, sexual, and psychosocial changes. Psychosom Med 29:354–366, 1967
16. FRANCES M, KOVACS GT: A comprehensive review of the sequelae of male sterilization. Contraception 28:455–473, 1983
17. FREUND M, DAVIS JE: A follow-up study of the effects of vasectomy on sexual behavior. J Sex Res 9:241–268, 1973
18. GANDOTRA VK, JOSEPH G, MOHAN JD, RAMACHANDRAN K: A follow-up study of 200 cases of vasectomy. Indian J Med Res 68:620–630, 1978
19. GINER J, ZAMORA G, ORTIZ S, PEDRON N: Vasectomia: Estudio clinico de 500 parejas. Ginecol Obstet Mex 39:405–411, 1976

20. GOLDBERG R, GOLDSMITH A, ECHEVERRIA G: Vasectomy as a contraceptive choice in Latin America. Paper presented at the Eleventh Annual Scientific Meeting, American Association of Planned Parenthood Physicians, Houston, Texas, April, 1973
21. GOLDSMITH A, GOLDBERG RJ: Psychosocial aspects of vasectomy in Latin America. J Sex Res 10:278–292, 1974
22. GOLDSMITH A, GOLDBERG R, ECHEVERRIA G: An in-depth study of vasectomized men in Latin America: A preliminary report. J Reprod Med 10:150–155, 1973
23. GONZALES B: Psychosexual aftermath of voluntary sterilization. Adv Plann Parenthood 14:137–143, 1979
24. GRINDSTAFF CF, EBANKS GE: Male sterilization in Canada. In GALLAGHER JE, LAMBERT RD (eds): Social Process and Institution: The Canadian Case, pp 396–414. Toronto, Holt, Rinehart & Winston, 1971
25. GRINDSTAFF CF, EBANKS GE: Vasectomy: Canada's newest family planning method. Can Ment Health 21:3–5, 1972
26. GRINDSTAFF CF, EBANKS E: Male sterilization as a contraceptive method in Canada—An empirical study. Popul Stud 27:443–455, 1973
27. HASSAN R: A follow-up study of vasectomized clients in three towns of the Punjab. Pakistan, The Family Planning Association of Pakistan, 1975
28. HOWARD G: Attitudes to Vasectomy. International Planned Parenthood Federation Medical Bulletin 15:1–3, 1981
29. HOWARD G: Motivation for vasectomy. Lancet i:545–548, 1978
30. HOWARD G: The quality of marriage before and after vasectomy. Br J Sex Med 6:13–14, 1979
31. JANKE LD, WIEST WM: Psychosocial and medical effects of vasectomy in a sample of health plan subscribers. Int J Psychiatr Med 7:17–34, 1976–1977
32. JOHNSON M: Social and psychological effects of vasectomy. Am J Psychiatry 121:482–486, 1964
33. KAKAR DN: After-effects of vasectomy on sex behavior: An exploratory investigation. J Fam Welfare 19:37–46, 1972
34. KHAN AR, SWENSON IE, RAHMAN A: A follow-up of vasectomy clients in rural Bangladesh. Int J Gynaecol Obstet 17:11–14, 1979
35. KING M, PULLEN D: Vasectomy in a national health service clinic. Br J Fam Plann 5:8–10, 1979
36. KOHLI KL, SOBRERO AJ: Vasectomy: A study of psychosexual and general reactions. Soc Biol 20:298–302, 1973
37. LANDIS JT, POFFENBERGER T: The marital and sexual adjustment of 330 couples who chose vasectomy as a form of birth control. J Marriage Fam 27:57–58, 1965
38. LEAR H: Psychosocial characteristics of patients requesting vasectomy. J Urol 108:767–769, 1972
39. LEAVESLEY JH: Vasectomy: Psychological effects and preoperative counseling. Aust Fam Physician 5:142–150, 1976
40. LEAVESLEY JH: Study of vasectomized men and their wives. Aust Fam Physician 9:8–10, 1980
41. LEE HY: Effects of vasectomy on medical and psychosocial aspects. J Popul Stud 11:145–182, 1970
42. LISKIN L: Vasectomy—Safe and simple. Popul Rep, Series D, (4): 1983
43. MARSHALL JF: Acceptability of fertility regulating methods: Designing technology to fit people. Prevent Med 6:65, 1977
44. MASCHHOFF TA, FANSHIER WE, HANSEN DJ: Vasectomy: Its effect upon marital stability. J Sex Res 12:295–314, 1976
45. MILLER WB: Psychosocial aspects of contraceptive sterilization in women. In NEWMAN SH, KLEIN ZE (eds): Behavioral–Social Aspects of Contraceptive Sterilization, pp 119–136. Lexington, MA, Lexington Books, 1978
46. MILLER WB, SHAIN RN: Married women and contraceptive sterilization: Factors that contribute to presurgical ambivalence. J Biosoc Sci 17:471–479, 1985
47. MORRIS L, LEWIS G, POWELL D, ANDERSEN A, WAY A, CUSHING J, LAWLESS G: Contraceptive prevalence surveys: A new source of family planning data. Popul Rep, Series M, (5): 1981
48. MOSS WB: Attitudes of patients one year after vasectomy. Urology 6:319–322, 1975
49. MUANGMUM V, MUANGMAN D, GOJSENI P, VISETHSINDH V, LEOPRAPHAI B, BURNIGHT RG: Follow-up study of vasectomized Thai males. J Med Assoc Thailand 57:500–507, 1974

50. MUMFORD SD: The vasectomy decision-making process. Stud Fam Plann 14:83–88, 1983
51. NASH JL, RICH JD: The sexual aftereffects of vasectomy. Fertil Steril 23:715–718, 1972
52. NIELSEN CM, GENSTER HG: Male sterilization with vasectomy: The effect of the intervention on sexual function. Ugeskr Laeger 142:641–643, 1980
53. PETERSEN P: Surgical contraception versus sterilization: Psychohygenic aspects of counseling for vasectomy and tubal ligation. Pro Familia Information 1:11–16, 1976
54. PHILLIBER WW, PHILLIBER SG: Social and psychological perspectives on voluntary sterilization: A review. Stud Fam Plann 16:1–29, 1985
55. POFFENBERGER T, POFFENBERGER SB: Vasectomy as a preferred method of birth control: A preliminary investigation. Marriage Fam Liv 25:326–330, 1963
56. POFFENBERGER SB, SHETH DL: Reactions of urban employees to vasectomy operations. J Fam Welfare 10:1–17, 1963
57. POHLMAN E: Psychosocial effects of vasectomy: A research progress report and critical review of past and proposed research. Paper presented to the workshop on research on the Behavioral Aspects of Surgical Contraception, Center for Population Research, Bethesda, Maryland, June 1973
58. POLGAR S, MARSHALL JF: The search for culturally acceptable fertility regulating methods. In MARSHALL JG, POLGAR S (eds): Culture, Natality and Family Planning, Monograph 21, p. 204. Chapel Hill, NC, Carolina Population Center, University of North Carolina, 1976
59. RATHORE SHS: After-effects of vasectomy and its social acceptance. J Fam Welfare 17:20–25, 1970
60. RODGERS DA, ZIEGLER FJ: Changes in sexual behavior consequent to use of noncoital procedures of contraception, Psychosom Med 30:495–505, 1968
61. RODGERS DA, ZIEGLER FJ: Psychological reactions to surgical contraception, pp 306–326. In FAWCETT JT (ed): Psychological Perspectives on Population. New York, Basic Books, 1973
62. RODGERS DA, ZIEGLER FJ: Effects of surgical contraception on sexual behavior, pp 161–166. In SCHIMA ME, LUBELL I, DAVIS JE, CONNELL E, COTTON DWK (eds): New York, American Elsevier Publishing Company, 1974
63. RODGERS DA, ZIEGLER FJ: Psychological aspects of surgical contraception. In HAFEZ ESE (ed): Human Semen and Fertility Regulation in Men, pp 525–529. St. Louis, CV Mosby, 1976
64. RODGERS DA, ZIEGLER FJ, ALTROCCHE J, LEVY N: A longitudinal study of the psychosocial effects of vasectomy. J Marriage Fam 29:59–64, 1965
65. RODGERS DA, ZIEGLER FA, LEVY N: Prevailing cultural attitudes about vasectomy: A possible explanation of postoperative psychological response. Psychosom Med 24:367–375, 1967
66. RODGERS DA, ZIEGLER FJ, ROHR P, PRENTISS RJ: Sociopsychological characteristics of patients obtaining vasectomies from urologists. Marriage Fam Liv 25:331–335, 1963
67. ROSS JA, HUBER DH: Acceptance and prevalence of vasectomy in developing countries. Stud Fam Plann 14:67–73, 1983
68. SANTISO R, BERTRAND JT, PINEDA MA: Voluntary sterilization in Guatemala: A comparison of men and women. Stud Fam Plann 14:73–82, 1983
69. SANTISO R, PINEDA MA, MARROQUIN M, BERTRAND JT: Vasectomy in Guatemala: A follow-up study of five hundred acceptors. Soc Biol 28:253–264, 1981
70. SAVAGE PM: Vasectomy and psychosexual damage. Health Serv Reports 87:803–804, 1972
71. SAXENA SR, CHITRE KT, LOBO JA: Follow-up of vasectomy. J Fam Welfare 11:1–12, 1965
72. SHAIN RN: Acceptability of contraceptive methods and services: A cross-cultural perspective. In PAUERSTEIN CJ, SHAIN RN (eds): Fertility Control: Biologic and Behavioral Aspects, pp 299–312. Hagerstown, Harper & Row, 1980
73. SHAIN RN, MILLER WB, HOLDEN AEC: The decision to terminate childbearing: Differences in preoperative ambivalence between tubal ligation women and vasectomy wives. Soc Biol 31:40–58, 1984
74. SHAIN RN, MILLER WB, HOLDEN AEC: Factors associated with married women's selection of tubal sterilization and vasectomy. Fertil Steril 43:234–244, 1985
75. SHAIN RN, MILLER WB, HOLDEN AEC: Married women's dissatisfaction with tubal sterilization and vasectomy at first-year follow-up: Effects of perceived spousal dominance. (submitted for publication)

76. SHAIN RN, MILLER WB, SHEPARD MK, DALTERIO SL, ASCH RH: Cultural dimensions in obstetrics, gynecology and neonatology. In SHIMKIN DB, GOLDE P (eds): Clinical Anthropology. A New Approach to American Health Problems?, pp 47–74. Lanham, MD, University Press of America, 1983
77. SHUKLA GD, NIGAM P, VERMA DL: Psychiatric complications of vasectomy. Health and Population Perspectives and Issues 1:243–249, 1978
78. SIMON POPULATION TRUST: Vasectomy: Follow-up of a thousand cases. In LADER L (ed): Foolproof Birth Control, pp 131–141. Boston, Beacon Press, 1972
79. SINHA SN, JAIN PC, PRASAD BG: A sociomedical study of urban sterilized males in Lucknow, Part II. J Indian Med Assoc 53:134–141, 1969
80. SOBRERO AJ, KOHLI KL: Two years' experience of an outpatient vasectomy service. Am J Public Health 65:1091–1094, 1975
81. SWENSON IE, KHAN AR, JAHAN FA: A follow-up of tubectomy clients in Kaliakair, Dacca and Kustia, Bangladesh, No. 11. Dacca, Bangladesh, The Johns Hopkins Fertil Res Proj, June 1977
82. TRUESDALE CW: Assessment of vasectomy as a means of voluntary sterilization. J-Lancet 85:155–156, 1965
83. UEHLING DT, WEAR JB: Patient attitudes towards vasectomy. Fertil Steril 23:838–840, 1972
84. VAUGHN RL: Behavioral response to vasectomy. Arch Gen Psychiatry 36:815–821, 1979
85. VICZIANY M: Coercion in a soft state: The family planning program of India. Part 2: The sources of coercion. Pacific Affairs 55:577–592, 1983
86. WHITBY RM, BROWN IG, SEENEY NC: Vasectomy: Follow-up of 831 cases. Med J Aust 1:164–167, 1975
87. WIEST WM, JANKE D: A methodological critique of research on psychological effects of vasectomy. Psychosom Med 36:438–449, 1974
88. WIG NN: Mental health and population growth. Indian J Psychiatry 21:12–33, 1979
89. WIG NN, PERSHAD D, ISAAC RP: A prospective study of symptom and nonsymptom groups following vasectomy. Indian J Med Res 61:621–626, 1973
90. WIG NN, SINGH S: Psychosomatic symptoms following male sterilization. Indian J Med Res 60:1386–1392, 1972
91. WIG NN, SINGH S, SAHASI G, ISAAC RP: Psychiatric symptoms following vasectomy. Indian J Psychiatry 12:169–176, 1970
92. WILLIAMS D, SWICEGOOD G, CLARK MP, BEAN FD: Masculinity–femininity and the desire for sexual intercourse after vasectomy: A longitudinal study. Soc Psychol Quart 43:347–352, 1980
93. WOLFERS D, WOLFERS H: Psychology of the vasectomy candidate. In WOLFERS D, WOLFERS H (eds): Vasectomy and Vasectomania, pp 208–225. London, Mayflower, 1974
94. WOLFERS H: Psychological aspects of vasectomy. Br Med J 4:297–300, 1970
95. WOLFERS H, SUBBIAH N, BIN MAZURKA A: Psychological aspects of vasectomy in Malaysia. Soc Biol 20:315–322, 1973
96. ZIEGLER FJ, RODGERS DA, KRIEGSMAN SA: Effect of vasectomy on psychological functioning. Psychosom Med 28:50–63, 1966
97. ZIEGLER FJ, RODGERS DA, PRENTISS RJ: Psychosocial response to vasectomy. Arch Gen Psychiatry 21:46–54, 1969
98. ZUFALL R: Vasectomy: Five- to ten-year follow-up of 200 cases. Urology 15:278–279, 1980

6

Microsurgery for Vasectomy Reversal and Vasoepididymostomy

SHERMAN J. SILBER

Because of its simplicity and effectiveness, vasectomy is the most popular method of birth control in the world today. Irreversibility has traditionally been its major drawback. A small fraction of men, no matter how well counseled and permanent their original resolve, eventually have cause to regret their vasectomy. Making vasectomy more readily reversible would thus give it greater appeal to many segments of the world community.

There are now very encouraging data in over 2200 patients undergoing microsurgical reversal of vasectomy. The first requirement for success is an anatomically accurate microsurgical reanastomosis. The second is to recognize pressure-induced epididymal ruptures and blockage, and bypass them when present with a very delicate microsurgical vasoepididymostomy. The third requirement is that in the future all vasectomies should be performed in an "open-ended" fashion to prevent this pressure-induced epididymal damage. This would allow 98% of vasectomies to be reversed more easily by a simple vas reanastomosis and also would obviate the 10% risk of pressure-induced congestive epididymitis.

Our accurate microsurgical techniques have allowed a dramatic improvement in success rate for vasectomy reversal, and a better understanding of the pathophysiology of obstruction.

CONVENTIONAL APPROACH TO VASECTOMY REVERSAL

Conventional techniques for reanastomosis of the vas have led to sperm leakage and granuloma, with poor alignment of the vas mucosa, causing total or partial obstruction.[11,13,15,29,32,34,36–38,61] These conventional techniques have yielded a 30% to 70% incidence of sperm in the ejaculate, with only 5% to 20% of wives achieving pregnancy.[13] Many of the patients in these series were incorrectly referred to as having "patent tubes," (because of the presence of "sperm in the ejaculate") despite very poor sperm counts with poor or no motility. The documentation of data in most conventional series was very weak; a few dead sperm per high-power field were mistakenly considered a sign of patency and technical success. It is no surprise that the pregnancy rate was low.

An accurate microscopic technique for reconnecting the vas not only increases the fertility rate dramatically but also clarifies what other factors may

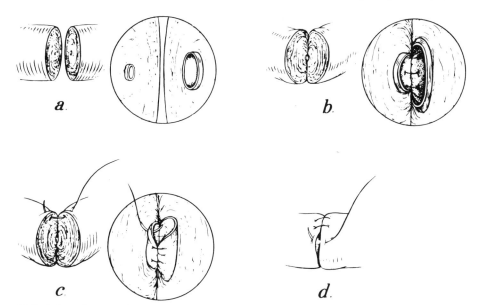

FIG. 6-1. Microscopic two-layer vasovasostomy. Steps in microscopic technique of vasovasostomy. a) The lumen is inspected for patency. b) and c) Mucosal anastomosis. d) Separate anastomosis of muscalaris.

be operating. Anyone who examines the anastomotic site after conventional vasovasostomy under the microscope ceases to wonder why success rates in the past were so low. Vasograms of failed vasovasostomy (as well as histologic sections) demonstrate strictures and blockage even though there may be some sperm present in the ejaculate. After reoperation with microsurgery, the sperm counts and motility in these patients improve dramatically in 90% of cases.

MICROSURGICAL APPROACH

We have performed the microscopic technique in over 2,000 patients.[43,45–47,49,52–54,56–59] It is advisable to practice in the animal before doing such surgery on patients. Accurate mucosal alignment is the key to success. For the best mucosal approximation (particularly when lumens are of different diameter because of chronic obstruction and increased pressure), a non-splinted, *two-layer* approach is advisable (Fig. 6-1). With a one-layer anastomosis there is clearly a much poorer mucosal approximation when lumen diameters differ, which is why such techniques frequently scar down. A splint of any kind should never be used because it is only an excuse for not being certain that one has obtained a good anastomosis. It results in sperm leakage, inflammation, and scarring.

It is unnecessary to determine preoperatively what type of vasectomy had been performed on the patient. We have learned to expect almost any kind of vasectomy. Often a very large segment has been removed, and in the majority of our cases the vasectomy has extended well into the convoluted portion. Such cases would have been considered impossible to approach with conventional techniques. With the techniques to be described, it merely means a little more dissection but essentially no change from a standard routine.

The preparation of the two ends of the vas deferens for the microscopic anastomosis is best performed with $2\frac{1}{2}$ times loupe magnification. The healthy ends of the vas deferens above and below the fibrosis are "freed up" several centimeters (more than that if a large gap has to be bridged). The more one frees up the healthy vas deferens from surrounding attachments, the more easily the two ends will bridge any gap between them. It is critical to have a tension-free anastomosis. No effort at anastomosis should be made until the two ends above and below the obstruction have been freed adequately. One generally need not fear devascularizing the vas deferens. The blood supply around the outer muscularis of the vas is quite extensive and, contrary to conventional thinking, we have found that freeing the vas a good distance will do nothing to injure the blood supply.

The beginner will immediately wonder why performing the anastomosis with the loupes is not easy, as it avoids the encumbrance of a microscope. Actually, use of a microscope makes the operation easier and more accurate, not more difficult. Loupes can at best provide $2\frac{1}{2}$ to 4 times magnification. To visualize the inner lumen of the vas deferens adequately for easy and accurate placement of stitches requires 16× magnification. The advantage of the microscope, in addition to providing higher power magnification, is that the depth of focus is much deeper, light is constantly supplied directly to the subject, and the microscope is resting on a stand and is therefore immobile. One can thus move one's head or neck without in any way disturbing the steadiness of the view on the subject.

The fibrotic portion of the vas deferens is excised under the microscope until healthy lumen is reached. The testicular side lumen is dilated because of the chronic high pressure caused by obstruction. The abdominal side lumen will be tiny by comparison. A microcatheter is placed in the dilated end of the lumen on the testicular side of the vasectomy site, allowing sperm fluid to enter by capillary action. This fluid then is examined under a laboratory microscope for the presence or absence and characterization of sperm. Microscopic characterization of the sperm in the vas fluid is extremely accurate in predicting success or failure, and in alerting one to the likelihood of secondary epididymal blockage. Therefore it is important to obtain enough fluid from the vas for it to be a representative sample of the sperm content of the entire length of the proximal vas. It is possible for a hasty smear to show no sperm even though a larger sample of fluid coming from a more proximal area in the vas may show many sperm.

Semen analysis is obtained every month for the first 4 months, then at 8 months, 1 year, $1\frac{1}{2}$ years, and 2 years postoperatively. The sperm count and sperm quality gradually improve with time. If the anastomosis is poor, the sperm count may increase at first but then eventually scar down to oligospermia or aspermia. If the patient is azoospermic at 3 months or more following the vasovasostomy, then either the vas anastomosis or the epididymis is obstructed.

For patients who remain azoospermic after vasovasostomy, the interpretation of where the problem lies depends strictly on the quality of sperm found in the vas fluid at the time of surgery. The sperm findings in the vas fluid tell whether there is continuity in the epididymis (with fresh sperm continuing to come through and reach the vasectomy site), or whether there is a blockage in the epididymis which prevents sperm from reaching the vas. As will be discussed in more detail, if there are numerous long-tailed sperm in the vas fluid, the epididymal tubule is intact and the vasovasostomy should be successful.

We will now present the results (and the conclusions that we can draw from these results) of our studies on the effect of vasectomy on the testis and epididymis, and the practical consequences of this information, which may help those patients who remain infertile after what should have been a successful vas anastomosis.

RESULTS WITH TWO-LAYER MICROSCOPIC TECHNIQUE

Between 1975 and 1978, the first 400 patients subjected to the two-layer technique for vasovasostomy were carefully studied both preoperatively and postoperatively in an effort to determine which factors affect recovery of fertility.[46] The overall pregnancy rate after $1\frac{1}{2}$ years of follow-up on the first 42 unselected patients was 71%. The 5-year follow-up yielded an 82% pregnancy rate. The causes for the failures will become apparent in the rest of this section. We now have performed over 2000 such cases, with similar results throughout. Not many patients become pregnant before 3 months, and most of the pregnancies occur between 6 months and 2 years. Thus an accurate assessment of pregnancy rate is usually not possible before a series has been followed for 2 to 3 years. Although some patients achieve good sperm counts within the first few months and impregnate their wives quickly, this is certainly the exception.

Most of the confusion in the literature on vasovasostomy stems from the lack of documentation of preoperative sperm quality in the vas fluid, inadequate postoperative semen analyses, sparse observations of the epididymal ductal system, and poor testis biopsy studies in vasectomized patients. The group that we operated upon were very carefully studied. Seminal fluid was sampled from the testicular side of the obstructed vas for each patient at the time of reanastomosis. The degree of dilatation of the vas lumen on the testicular side of the vasectomy site was measured in all patients. Appearance and quantity of vas fluid, as well as sperm morphology (electron micrograph and light microscopy), quantity, and motility also were recorded and correlated with postoperative results. The age of the patient, the time since the vasectomy, the type of vasectomy performed, as well as the area in which it was performed, were correlated to subsequent sperm count and pregnancy of the spouse. Sperm counts were measured at monthly intervals after surgery for the first 4 months and then at intervals 4 months apart during the entire follow-up period. No patient was accepted for surgery who did not agree in advance to provide this careful follow-up.

Over 300 of the patients were subjected to a quantitatively meticulous testicle biopsy at the time of vasovasostomy, and the findings correlated with successful and unsuccessful postoperative results.[60] This was particularly important when there was no sperm in the vas fluid and the patient remained azoospermic postoperatively, despite a successful vas anastomosis.

Sperm counts were arbitrarily considered normal when there was a concentration of more than 10 million sperm per ml, 50% motility with good progression, and greater than 70% normal forms, according to the criteria of MacLeod and Gold.[27] It is recognized that lower sperm counts sometimes can be found in fertile men and higher counts in infertile men. The semen of most of the patients with "normal" counts actually had in excess of 30 million sperm per ml. All semen samples with good motility had >70% normal forms. The follow-up on these patients in most cases was superb.

With this kind of careful investigation, in patients subjected to as meticulous a microsurgical anastomosis as possible, physiological data of greater reliability were obtainable. These data revealed that spermatogenesis is not harmed significantly by obstruction, and that failure to achieve fertility after an accurate vasovasostomy is caused by dilation and subsequent perforation of the epididymal duct with subsequent secondary epididymal obstruction. We also noted that there appeared to be an improved quality of sperm in the vas fluid in patients who had minimal dilation of the testicular side lumen and in patients who had a sperm granuloma at the site of the vasectomy.

In 32% of the early patients, an obvious sperm granuloma could be seen at the vasectomy site. That is a much higher incidence than in more recent patients, a change probably due to the increasing use of cautery for sealing the vas more effectively at the time of vasectomy. There were no particular symptoms of discomfort related to the sperm granuloma. The sperm granuloma represented a continual leakage of sperm fluid at the vasectomy site.

In the group with sperm granuloma, all had abundant morphologically normal sperm in the vas fluid. Even when the vasectomy had been performed over 10 years earlier, none of the patients with sperm granuloma had poor quality sperm in the vas fluid. No matter how long ago the vasectomy had been performed, the presence of a sperm granuloma ensured a high quality of sperm in the vas fluid at the time of vasovasostomy.

The internal diameter of the testicular side lumen of the vas deferens was almost always $\frac{3}{4}$ mm or less in vasa with sperm granuloma. In patients without sperm granuloma, the internal diameter of the testicular side lumen was usually 1 mm or more. Thus, the presence of sperm granuloma was associated with less dilation of the vas deferens on the testicular side of the obstruction.

In patients who had unilateral sperm granulomas, the sperm quality was always satisfactory on the side with the sperm granuloma but usually of poorer quality on the opposite side. Thus, a dramatic benefit was conferred on the side with sperm granuloma that was not conferred to the side without granuloma. These data favored the postulate that a failure to recover fertility after an accurate anatomic reconnection of the vas deferens is due to the local effects of high pressure created by the vasectomy. The presence of a sperm granuloma at the vasectomy site represents persistent and continual leakage of sperm, which alleviates the deleterious high intravasal and epididymal pressure that otherwise always occurs after vasectomy.

EFFECTS OF VASECTOMY ON THE TESTIS AND EPIDIDYMIS

Despite the fact that vasectomy is one of the most popular operations performed in the United States, there has been a great deal of controversy in the scientific literature about its effects, both in humans and in animals. Many of the differences in experimental results in the early literature are related to the use of different animal models and different techniques of vasectomy. However, much of the controversy is simply a result of sloppy methodology. A 1978 review of the data available at the time, organized according to species, to elucidate the effect of pressure increase after vasectomy on the testis and epididymis,[54] revealed many contradictions. The last 6 years have brought a clearer understanding.

There is no question about the marked dilation of the vas deferens and epididymal tubule that occurs consequent to vasectomy in all species. Observation of the epididymis in humans undergoing reversal reveals marked tubular dilation, with blow-outs and leakages in weak points of the epididymal tubule consequent to the pressure buildup, resulting in secondary epididymal obstruction. There is no longer any controversy about the presence of these epididymal changes in virtually all species.[16,19,24,25,28]

Bedford studied in great detail the effects of vasectomy in four different species of animals.[8] He noted rupture of the epididymal duct with leukocytic infiltration in all four species. He believed that sperm were continually produced after vasectomy, but no reabsorption occurred until there was an epithelial rupture somewhere within the ductal system. By 8 months postvasectomy, the corpus epididymis began to show signs of dilation, and a series of ruptures and scars could be seen in the epididymis. Only after epithelial rupture had occurred did leukocytic infiltration and invasion appear, with reabsorption of sperm.

Although there is substantial pressure damage to the epididymis, there is no discernible effect on spermatogenesis or testicular architecture. The testicle biopsy showed normal spermatogenesis in all patients who had no sperm in the vas fluid, and therefore we felt that the problem had to be epididymal blockage. We reasoned that if the problem was secondary epididymal obstruction caused by rupture and sperm extravasation in the epididymis, much more sophisticated microsurgery, bypassing epididymal blockage, might restore fertility even in these least favorable cases.

To resolve this question, we explored patients who had azoospermia for at least 2 years after a patent vasovasostomy.[44] These patients, of course, had no sperm (or only sperm heads) in the vas fluid at the time of vasovasostomy; however, normal sperm were found in the epididymal fluid despite absence of sperm in the vas fluid. Epididymal histology distal to this site revealed extensive interstitial sperm granulomas, resulting from rupture of the epididymal duct, similar to what Bedford observed in four animal species.[8]

Once the epididymal rupture and subsequent blockage occurs, the fluid that had accumulated previously in the vas deferens is trapped and isolated. The sperm in that vas fluid die of "old age" and then eventually degenerate, the tails fall off, and the heads finally deteriorate into amorphous debris. Thus, the absence of sperm in the vas fluid just proximal to the vasectomy site indicates that there is secondary epididymal blockage from epididymal rupture and blockage. The presence of morphologically intact sperm in the vas fluid indicates an intact ductal system with relatively fresh sperm continuing to reach the vas. That is why the most accurate vasovasostomy cannot result in a success if there is no sperm in the vas fluid. To treat such failures successfully, one would have to bypass the secondary blockage in the epididymis.

We now have experience in over 2000 cases and can state that in every case in which there is no sperm in the vas fluid and the patient is azoospermic after an accurate vasovasostomy, sperm can be found somewhere in the epididymal tract proximal to a point of secondary blockage; occasionally, this may be as high as the vasa efferentia. Fortunately, most of the blockages are limited to the region of the junction of the corpus and tail of the epididymis. Therefore, most bypass vasoepididymostomy procedures can be performed either at the distal or the midcorpus region of the epididymis, where epididymal length is long enough for good maturation of sperm.[31–35]

The duration of time since vasectomy correlates with the likelihood of pressure-induced rupture of the epididymis in these patients, just as it did in the laboratory animal studies of Bedford. In humans, however, the time range is expanded considerably. For example, in humans, whenever reversal was performed within 1 year of vasectomy, high-quality sperm were always found in the vas fluid, and normal semen analyses were obtained after surgery.

There was no sudden period of time after which an epididymal blow-out would occur predictably. Rather, the risk of epididymal blow-out on each side gradually increases as the years progress. The chances of finding no sperm in the vas fluid on one side at 10 years was 75%. The chances of finding no sperm on *both* sides at 10 years was about 50%, however. At 5 years postvasectomy, the chances of finding no sperm on one side was 25%, but the chances of finding no sperm on both sides was only 6%. In every case in which no sperm were found in the vas fluid, the testicle biopsy was normal. The absence of sperm was not caused by a disruption of spermatogenesis but rather by epididymal ruptures and secondary blockage.

Examination of the epididymal histology shows dilated epididymal ducts, sperm extravasation into the interstitium, sperm granuloma formation, and many macrophages, sperm heads, and inspissated protein within the tubular lumen. Distal to this transition point, the epididymal tubules are empty and devoid of sperm. There may be some macrophages noted in the fluid, and possibly some cellular debris, but no sperm.

The sperm count and the quality of motility gradually rise during the first 12 months after successful vasovasostomy while the epididymis recovers from the partial disruptions in the epithelium and the chronic dilatation. Most patients with high sperm counts after vasovasostomy eventually develop normal motility as the epididymis recovers. Patients who persist in having oligospermia and poor motility more than 1 year after vasovasostomy have continued blockage (partial) either at the vasovasostomy site or in the epididymis.

VASAL AND EPIDIDYMAL FLUID: INTERPRETATION

What should be done when the fluid from the vas at the time of vasovasostomy has no sperm in it? What about when there are sperm heads only but no normal sperm? Is motility important? What about macrophages or debris? Knowledge of the appearance of the sperm, if any, in the vas fluid is critical for intelligent management.

To make a proper interpretation of the vas fluid, an adequate collection must be obtained. Some very serious mistakes in clinical judgment are made because of an improper collection of fluid from the cut end of the vas deferens. We recommend that a No. 22 Medicut catheter (or smaller) be inserted into the proximal cut end of the vas deferens, and the fluid allowed to rise up by capillary action. Occasionally this can be assisted by gentle fingertip massage of the vas. The fluid will be drawn into the tube, providing a copious specimen for examination and interpretation. It cannot be emphasized enough how important it is to obtain the specimen in this fashion. Not only will it give a clear answer whether the fluid is transparent, but it will provide enough fluid for the pathologist to view under phase contrast, dilute if necessary, or stain for greater detail, and will provide a more representative sample of all the fluid that has built up in the vas.

There have been scattered reports of successful results from vasovasostomy in patients who supposedly have "no sperm" in nontransparent vas fluid. On talking directly to the physicians who had this experience, we found that the specimen was only smeared on a slide, not diluted when necessary, not stained, and often observed under a very poor quality microscope on a table in the operating room. When these physicians began to obtain more complete collections of fluid from the vas and to submit these better specimens to a pathologist to characterize the sperm more accurately, they verified what we have observed in over 2000 well-documented cases: When there is no sperm in the vas fluid, and the fluid is not transparent, the patient does not have a successful vasovasostomy. The only exception to this finding is when the fluid is clear and voluminous. In these cases in which there is no sperm in the vas fluid, if one is unprepared to perform a vasoepididymostomy, the patient should be advised of the poor prognosis after his vasovasostomy and referred to a specialist who can perform vasoepididymostomy.

It is senseless to open the tunica vaginalis and explore the epididymis to try to see if there are epididymal blow-outs. One cannot tell whether there is epididymal ductal continuity just by observing the outside of the epididymal duct. The epididymis is always dilated and filled with inspissated material at various levels, owing to the pressure buildup created by the vasectomy, but this observation gives no clue to whether the epididymis is blocked. The decision about whether there is epididymal blockage can be made reliably only on the basis of interpretation of the vas fluid. To open the tunica vaginalis and explore the epididymis without actually being able to perform the vasoepididymostomy at the same time allows the formation of extensive adhesions that will make a subsequent vasoepididymostomy more difficult. A vasoepididymostomy should not be performed until the surgeon is extremely experienced with very advanced microsurgical techniques.

We have found that if the vas fluid has many sperm with long tails, the prognosis for normal sperm count after vasovasostomy is over 90%, depending on the skill and accuracy of the surgeon's microsurgical technique. Whether the sperm are motile has had no influence on the prognosis. If there are no sperm in the vas fluid (with the exception of transparent fluid), none of the patients has a good postoperative result. The only exception is that if the vas fluid is transparent and voluminous, the presence or absence of sperm is irrelevant. These patients usually can be expected to have a good prognosis if an accurate vasovasostomy is performed. The reason for this exception is not altogether clear.

With new understanding of the morphologic changes of senescent sperm, it becomes easier to interpret findings in the vas fluid in cases that are not so clear-cut as simply "many long-tailed sperm" or "no sperm." The in-between findings include varying proportions of sperm with short tails, sperm heads only, sperm heads with macrophages and debris, or sperm heads with debris but no macrophages. We have found that if there are no sperm with long tails, but only short-tailed sperm and sperm heads, the prognosis is very guarded; it is hard to say whether the patient will have good results after vasovasostomy. If there are greater than 20% sperm with normal long tails, then the presence of sperm heads and sperm with short tails will not hurt the prognosis. If there are no long-tailed sperm but only sperm heads, the prognosis is also very guarded. Furthermore, when we have found only sperm heads in the vas fluid and the fluid is curdy, the patient will be sure to have an unsuccessful result after vasovasostomy. Only in cases in which the fluid was still translucent or liquid in appearance did the patient with sperm heads only have chances of good results after vasovasostomy. In a similar vein, the presence of a large number of macrophages or debris is worrisome and portends a bad prognosis in the presence of only sperm heads or short-tailed sperm. If there are many long-tailed sperm, however, we expect successful results even if the fluid is loaded with macrophages and debris.

SPERM ANTIBODIES

There has been considerable speculation about the role of autoantibodies to sperm in preventing subsequent restoration of fertility after an accurate vaso-vasostomy. Most studies report about a 60% incidence of agglutinating antibodies and a 40% incidence of immobilizing antibodies in the serum of vasectomized men.[1-5,7,14,21,35,42] Despite the fact that many studies have demonstrated the formation of antisperm antibodies, most have been unable to show a strong association between the formation of antibodies and subsequent infertility.[1-5,7,14,21,35,42]

Bedford, on the basis of experiments in unilaterally vasoligated animals, has stated that he does not believe that sperm antibodies have any important role in subsequent fertility.[8,10] In his classic paper on the effects of vasectomy in four different species,[8] Bedford showed in rats and rabbits that unilaterally vasectomized animals suffered no loss of fertility. He concluded that "vasectomy has no general immunologically mediated suppressive effect on the potential fertility of these species." In humans, also, we know that unilateral blockage (as in inguinal hernia cases, in which one vas is ligated; vasectomy cases, in which only one side is patent; and vasectomy cases, in which only one side recanalizes) does not interfere with fertility (Fig. 6-2).

Clearly the pressure effects of obstruction on the epididymal system in humans are such that purely physical factors are probably the major ones

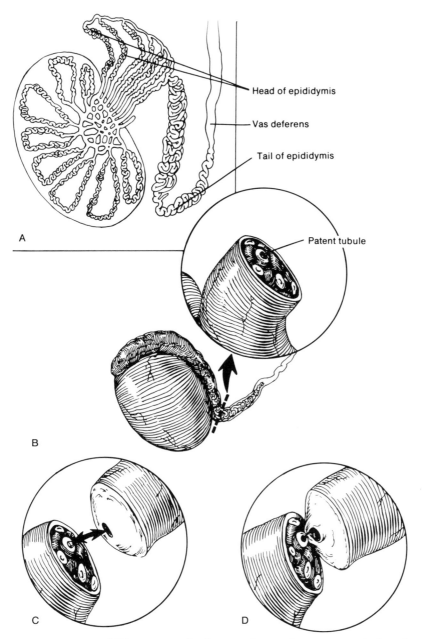

FIG. 6-2. Vasoepididymostomy for bypass of secondary pressure-induced epididymal blockage.

(rather than autoimmunity) affecting the recovery of normal semen analysis and fertility. Thomas has found *no* correlation between pregnancy or lack of pregnancy and serum agglutinating or immobilizing antibody titers.[62] Sperm antibodies were present in the semen in only 3.9% of cases, but even in those couples there were pregnancies but possibly some decrease in fertility.[26] Although more work needs to be done on this interesting problem of sperm antibodies, it is clear that the major obstacle to recovering fertility is persistent obstruction, whether partial or complete, either at the vasovasostomy site or in the epididymis.

MICROSURGICAL VASOEPIDIDYMOSTOMY

The epididymis is a 20-foot long coiled tubule with myriad intricate convolutions. It is squeezed into a 2-inch length with pleats similar to those of an accordion. Because the epididymal tubule is so tiny, even by microsurgical standards, the results with conventional surgery for this type of obstruction have been very poor. Schoysman has reported the best pregnancy rate with conventional vasoepididymostomy, (25%).[39,40] In other series, 36% achieved some sperm in the ejaculate after vasoepididymostomy, and only 18% had good semen quality.[6] There were very few pregnancies. Hanley reported only one pregnancy after 83 vasoepididymostomies.[22] The procedure used by Hanley and that described by Hotchkiss formed the basis for the usual conventional vasoepididymostomy still performed by most urologists today.[23] Although this conventional procedure was the best that could be performed in the 1950s, modern microsurgical facilities have rendered it obsolete, and these patients now can be given a much better prognosis with extremely exacting microsurgical procedures.

I first developed and described the microsurgical "specific tubule" technique for vasoepididymostomy in 1978.[48,50,51,55] This idea had never been considered previously because anastomosing a specific epididymal tubule to the vas deferens required microsurgical expertise not yet developed. Over the past 5 years I have refined the microsurgical technique and now have experience with over 1000 such cases.

After the scrotal sac is entered, the vas is freed up, the tunica vaginalis is opened, and the testis and epididymis are exposed. The dilated epididymal tubule is usually about 0.1 ml to 0.2 ml in diameter. The epididymal duct is extraordinarily delicate, with a wall thickness of about 30 μ. If one were to employ the usual conventional approach and make a deep longitudinal incision into the outer epididymal tunic, one would see what appeared to be many tiny cut tubules. Without the benefit of microscopic observation, there is an illusion that sperm fluid is welling up from all of these tubules, but in truth the fluid is coming from only one of them. The other tubules are just blind loops disconnected from continuity with the testis by this incision. The ideal approach for reestablishing continuity of the ductal system is to anastomose directly the inner lumen of the vas deferens, specifically to the one epididymal tubule that is leaking sperm.

Rather than a conventional longitudinal incision, a *transverse* section of the epididymis is made at the most distal point (*i.e.*, at the junction of the cauda and corpus epididymis). With this approach one can slice off portions of the epididymis more and more proximally until sperm are recovered at the most distal possible level but proximal to the area of obstruction. Under the operating microscope, three to ten cut tubules are usually visible on the transected surface of the epididymis, and all are examined carefully for efflux of sperm fluid. Material from this cut surface of the epididymis is smeared on a slide and observed under a standard laboratory microscope or phase-contrast microscope for the presence and quality of sperm (described in the previous section). Sometimes no fluid at all is observed, and in those cases one must transect more proximally. The presence of fluid does not necessarily mean the presence of sperm, however. One must wait for the report on the fluid before deciding whether to do the anastomosis at that point or to transect more proximally. The anastomosis is performed at the distal-most level, where normal sperm are found in the epididymal fluid, which allows for the maximal possible length of epididymis.

For the first stitch, the epididymis is held between the thumb and the forefinger, facing the microscope. A slight milking action sometimes may be necessary to promote a continual efflux of fluid for one to continue to see which is the correct tubule to anastomose. We use a 9-0 or 10-0 monofilament nylon on a GS-16, a BV-9 needle, or the new Silber V-100 (Ethicon). Ethicon designed the Silber V-100 needle especially for this procedure. The first suture is placed from the outside to the inside of the specific epididymal tubule that is leaking the sperm fluid. After the first suture has been placed in this fashion, the epididymis is put into one jaw of the Silber vasovasostomy clamp and the vas is inserted into the other jaw. A piece of blue plastic then is placed underneath the epididymis and vas, which are held in the two jaws of the vasovasostomy clamp. From this point, the specific anastomosis of the vas lumen to the epididymal tubule can be performed in a fashion somewhat similar to vasovasostomy; however, instead of six sutures as in vasovasostomy, four sutures are adequate.

The first stitch was placed *before* the epididymis was put in the jaws of the vasovasostomy clamp because it is extremely difficult to locate the specific tubule leaking the fluid in any other way. The gentle milking action that the thumb and forefinger can provide is helpful in making sure that the fluid is continuing to flow from the tubule to which suturing is to be done. After placement of the first suture, the tubule is now easily identified at all times. Three more perfect mucosa-to-mucosa sutures are then placed to achieve an accurate anastomosis of the vas lumen to the epididymal tubule.

FERTILITY AFTER VASOEPIDIDYMOSTOMY

What can be expected of sperm that have not progressed completely through the epididymis? It is certainly well known that sperm from the cauda epididymis are mature and capable of fertilizing the ovum. A large percentage of sperm from the corpus epididymis are also capable of impregnating and have good, active, progressive motility. In the head of the epididymis in animal models, however, sperm have not yet obtained maturity, and motility consists only of weak vibratory motions.

In the human, as long as the sperm have had an opportunity to pass through some small portion of the corpus epididymis, there is a good proportion of fertile sperm. Thus, when the anastomosis is anywhere along the corpus epididymis, prognosis is good; however, prognosis is not as good in a patient whose anastomosis was performed in the head of the epididymis. Schoysman, with long-term follow-up, has had pregnancies in only 11% of patients with a patent anastomosis at the head of the epididymis.[41] That is still greater than what would have been predicted from the animal studies, however.

All of the animal data on sperm maturity in the epididymis come from sperm that were sampled from an intact epididymis. Whether remaining segments of the epididymal tubule and vas deferens would be able to promote sperm maturation in the physiologic context of vasoepididymostomy could not be answered by any of the animal experiments that form the basis of our understanding of epididymal function.

For example, in the rabbit, Gaddum sampled spermatozoa from the seminiferous tubules, the ductuli efferentes, and various levels of the epididymis, to determine intrinsic motility and fertilizing capability.[17] Spermatozoa from the seminiferous tubules and ductuli efferentes showed only weak vibratory movements with no forward progress. Spermatozoa from the proximal head of the epididymis showed very irregular, erratic motility with no forward progression. Traversing the corpus epididymis, however, increasing numbers of spermatozoa began to show forward movement with proper longitudinal rotation as they progressed distally toward the cauda epididymis. Similar studies have been performed by Bedford in the rabbit and by Orgebin-Crist in the rabbit.[9,30]

In an effort to see whether the increase in spermatozoal maturity was merely a function of the time required for passage of spermatozoa through the epididymis, or whether it was dependent on specific areas of the epididymis, various authors ligated different portions of the epididymis in rabbits and examined samples of the spermatozoa from each portion at intervals after the ligation.[18,20,33] After interruption of sperm flow, epididymal spermatozoa, which had poor motility in the caput region of the epididymis, now showed good motility.

Because of the pathologic nature of the chronic obstruction created by such an experimental model, however, all of these sperm once again lost their motility by 3 weeks. These researchers believed that it was possible for spermatozoa to mature at any level of the epididymal duct, but their experimental approach created such an abnormal environment that this hypothesis could not be tested adequately. Obstruction to the flow of spermatozoa within the epididymis clearly has been shown to result in stagnation of epididymal spermatozoa. Thus, the increased time allowed for maturation in that experiment was counterbalanced by the abnormally obstructed environment.

Orgebin-Crist first suggested to us that in cases of human vasoepididymostomy it was theoretically possible that sperm might be mature and fertile after vasoepididymostomy, even to proximal portions of the epididymis. The remaining epididymal tubule might undergo compensatory changes, or spermatozoa might have more time to mature after coming out of proximal regions of the epididymis than they would in the previously alluded to experimental models.[31] Our results in humans with vasoepididymostomy for proximal epididymal obstruction indicate that this is true and that after a prolonged period of time, the remaining segment of a shortened epididymis allows motility and fertility to spermatozoa in a region where under normal circumstances there would be none. In most patients undergoing vasoepididymostomy, the proximal-most obstruction will be somewhere in the corpus region, usually in the distal corpus. We see no significant difference in pregnancy rates thus far at any particular point along the corpus epididymis.

Ninety percent of patients undergoing vasoepididymostomy with this technique have a sperm count of greater than 10 million per ml and directional motility of greater than 50%. It appears to take longer in many cases for motility to reach high levels in vasoepididymostomy patients than in vasovasostomy patients, and the sperm count may not come up to normal levels until a year and a half postoperatively. This indicates that a considerable period of time is required in some of these patients for sperm transport mechanisms to recover completely. Nonetheless, by $1\frac{1}{2}$ years 90% of the patients have an adequate semen analysis.

About 60% of these patients impregnate their wives within 2 to 3 years. It is too early to know what the eventual pregnancy rate will be because it does seem that fertilizing capacity per monthly cycle of sexual exposure is less in these patients than the normal population. Furthermore it seems that with time the fertility of these patients gradually increases, making difficult a life table type analysis. Thus, it will take more followup before we can state with assurance how high the pregnancy rate will be. Thus far it appears that there will be no serious discrepancy between good semen analysis and eventual pregnancy.

OPEN-ENDED VASECTOMY

With this new understanding of the pathophysiology of obstruction due to vasectomy, we have recommended and will continue to recommend an "open-ended" vasectomy. I coined the term 5 years ago, and subsequent experience of Moss in California, Shapiro in Ottawa, and Errey in Australia, confirm that it is safe and effective. It reduces the otherwise 10% incidence of congestive epididymitis after vasectomy and makes subsequent reversal of vasectomy easier because it lessens the otherwise inevitable likelihood of secondary, pressure-induced epididymal blockage.

There has been a reluctance on the part of some urologists to leave the testicular side lumen of the vas "open" after vasectomy as I have suggested, but this reluctance is unnecessary. So long as the abdominal side is sealed with a cautery needle of 2 cm rather than 1 cm, the risk of recanalization is no different than with a closed-ended cautery procedure.

The open-ended vasectomy that I have developed offers much greater ease of reversibility to less experienced reversal surgeons. If advocated in the developing world of Africa and Asia, where infant mortality rate is so high, it could make vasectomy much more popular and thus have a greater impact on controlling runaway overpopulation.

REFERENCES

1. ALEXANDER NJ: Immunologic and morphologic effects of vasectomy in the rhesus monkey. Fed Proc 34:1692, 1975
2. ALEXANDER NJ: Morphological consequences of vasectomy. Primate News 12:2, 1974

3. ALEXANDER NJ: Vasectomy and vasovasostomy in rhesus monkeys: The effect of circulating antisperm antibodies on fertility. Fertil Steril 28:526, 1977
4. ALEXANDER NJ, SCHMIDT SS: Incidence of antisperm antibody levels and granulomas in men. Fertil Steril 28:655, 1977
5. ALEXANDER NJ, WILSON BJ, PATTERSON GD: Vasectomy: Immunologic effects in rhesus monkeys and men. Fertil Steril 25:149, 1974
6. AMELAR RD, DUBIN L: Commentary on epididymal vasostomy, vasovasostomy and testicular biopsy, pp 1181–1185. In Current Operative Urology. New York, Harper & Row, 1975
7. ANSBACHER R: Sperm agglutinating and sperm immobilizing antibodies in vasectomized men. Fertil Steril 22:629, 1971
8. BEDFORD JM: Adaptation of the male reproductive tract and the rate of spermatozoa following vasectomy in the rabbit, rhesus monkey, hamster and rat. Biol Reprod 14:118, 1976
9. BEDFORD JM: Development of the fertilizing ability of spermatozoa in the epididymis of the rabbit. J Experimental Zool 163:312, 1966
10. BEDFORD JM: PARFR Conference on Sterilization Reversal. San Francisco, December 5, 1977
11. CAMERON CS: Anastomosis of the vas deferens. JAMA 127:119, 1945
12. CHARNY CW: Testicular biopsy: Its value in male sterility. JAMA 115:1429, 1940
13. DERRICK FC Jr, YARBROUGH W, D'AGOSTINO J: Vasovasostomy: Results of questionnaire of members of the American Urological Association. J Urol 110:556, 1973
14. DOMINIQUE GJ, HARRISON RM, HEIDGER PM, ROBERTS JA, SCHLEGEL JU: Vasectomy in rhesus monkeys. II. Failure to demonstrate humoral and cellular immune response specific for sperm. Urology, 9:645, 1977
15. DORSEY JW: Anastomosis of the vas deferens to correct post vasectomy sterility. J Urol 70:515, 1953
16. FRIEND DS, GALLE J, SILBER SJ: Fine structure of human sperm, vas deferens epithelium and testicular biopsy specimens at the time of vasectomy reversal. Anat Rec 14:584, 1976
17. GADDUM P: Sperm maturation in the male reproductive tract: Development of motility. Anatomic Record 161:471, 1969
18. GADDUM P, GLOVER TD: Some reactions of rabbit spermatozoa to ligation of the epididymis. J Reprod Fertil 9:119, 1965
19. GALLE J, FRIEND DS: Fine structure and cytochemistry of the guinea pig epididymis and vas deferens after vasectomy. Am J Pathol (in press)
20. GLOVER TD: Some aspects of function in the epididymis. Experimental occlusion of the epididymis in the rabbit. Internat J Fertil 14:215, 1969
21. HALIM A, ANTONIOU D: Autoantibodies to spermatozoa in relation to male infertility and vasectomy. Br J Urol 45:559, 1973
22. HANLEY HG: The surgery of male sub-fertility. Ann R Coll Surg 17:159, 1955
23. HOTCHKISS RS: Surgical treatment of infertility in the male. In CAMPBELL MF, HARRISON HH (eds): Urology, 3rd Edition, p 671. Philadelphia, WB Saunders, 1970
24. HOWARDS SS, JESSEE S, JOHNSON A: Micropuncture and microanalytic studies of the effect of vasectomy on the rat testis and epididymis. Fertil Steril 26:20, 1975
25. JOHNSON AL, HOWARDS SS: Intratubular hydrostatic pressure in testis and epididymis before and after vasectomy. Am J Physiol 228:556, 1975
26. LINNET L, HJORT T: Sperm agglutinins in seminal plasma and serum after vasectomy: correlation between immunological and clinical findings. Clin Exp Immunol 30:413, 1977
27. MACLEOD J, GOLD RZ: The male factor in fertility and infertility. IV. Sperm morphology in fertile and infertile marriage. Fertil Steril 2:394, 1951
28. MACMILLAN EW: Observations on the isolated vasoepididymal loop and on the effects of experimental subcapital epididymal obstructions. In Studies on Fertility, Vol 6, pp 57–64, Oxford, Blackwell, 1954
29. O'CONNOR VJ: Anastomosis of the vas deferens after purposeful division for sterility. JAMA 136:162, 1948
30. ORGEBIN-CRIST MC: Sperm maturation in rabbit epididymis. Nature 216:816, 1967
31. ORGEBIN-CRIST MC: Studies of the function of the epididymis. Biol Reprod 1:155, 1969
32. PARDANANI DS, KOTHARI ML, PRADHAN SA, MAHENDIAKAR MN: Surgical restoration of vas continuity after vasectomy: Further clinical evaluation of a new operation technique. Fertil Steril 25:319, 1974

33. PAUFLER SK, FOOTE RH: Morphology, motility and fertility in spermatozoa recovered from different areas of ligated rabbit epididymis. J Reprod Fertil 17:125, 1968
34. PHADKE GM, PHADKE AG: Experiences in the reanastomosis of the vas deferens. J Urol 97:888, 1967
35. RUMKE TH: Sperm agglutinating autoantibodies in relation to male infertility. Proc R Soc Med 61:275, 1968
36. SCHMIDT SS: Anastomosis of the vas deferens: An experimental study. II. Successes and failures in experimental anastomosis. J Urol 81:203, 1959
37. SCHMIDT SS: Anastomosis of the vas deferens: An experimental study. IV. The use of fine polyethylene tubing as a splint. J Urol 85:838, 1961
38. SCHMIDT SS: Vas anastomosis: A return to simplicity. Br J Urol 47:309, 1975
39. SCHOYSMAN R: Presentation to American Fertility Society Meeting. Miami Beach, Florida, April, 1977
40. SCHOYSMAN R, DROUART JM: Progrès récents dans la chirurgie de la stérilité masculine et feminine. Acta Clin Belg 71:261, 1972
41. SCHOYSMAN R, STEWART BH: Epididymal causes of male infertility. Monogr Urol, 1:April/May:1, 1980
42. SHULMAN S, ZAPPI E, AHMED U, DAVIS JE: Immunologic consequences of vasectomy. Contraception 5:269, 1972
43. SILBER SJ: Compensatory and obligatory renal growth in babies and adults. Austral NZ J Surg, 44:421, 1974
44. SILBER SJ: Epididymal extravasation following vasectomy as a cause for failure of vasectomy reversal. Fertil Steril 31:309, 1979
45. SILBER SJ: Growth of baby kidneys transplanted into adults. Arch Surg 111:75, 1976
46. SILBER SJ: Microscopic technique for reversal of vasectomy. Surg Gynecol Obstet 143:630, 1976
47. SILBER SJ: Microscopic vasectomy reversal. Fertil Steril 28:1191, 1977
48. SILBER SJ: Microscopic vasoepididymostomy: Specific microanastomosis to the epididymal tubule. Fertil Steril 30:565, 1978
49. SILBER SJ: Perfect anatomical reconstruction of vas deferens with a new microscopic surgical technique. Fertil Steril 28:72, 1977
50. SILBER SJ: Reversal of vasectomy in the treatment of male infertility. J Androl 1:261, 1980
51. SILBER SJ: Reversal of vasectomy in the treatment of male infertility: role of microsurgery, vasoepididymostomy, and pressure induced changes of vasectomy. Urol Clin North Am 8:53, 1981
52. SILBER SJ: Successful autotransplantation of an intra-abdominal testicle to the scrotum using microvascular anastomsis. J Urol 115:452, 1976
53. SILBER SJ: Transplantation of rat kidneys with acute tubular necrosis into salt loaded and normal recipients. Surgery 77:487, 1975
54. SILBER SJ: Vasectomy and vasectomy reversal. Fertil Steril 29:125, 1978
55. SILBER SJ: Vasoepididymostomy to the head of the epididymis: recovery of normal spermatozoa motility. Fertil Steril 34:149, 1980
56. SILBER SJ, CRUDOP J: A three kidney rat model. Invest Urol 11:466, 1974
57. SILBER SJ, CRUDOP J: Kidney transplantation in inbred rats. Am J Surg 125:551, 1973
58. SILBER SJ, MALVIN RL: Compensatory and obligatory renal growth in rats. Am J Physiol 226:114, 1974
59. SILBER SJ, GALLE J, FRIEND D: Microscopic vasovasostomy and spermatogenesis. J Urol 117:299, 1977
60. SILBER SJ, RODRIGUEZ-RIGAU LJ: Quantitative analysis of testicle biopsy: Determination of partial obstruction and prediction of sperm count after surgery for obstruction. Fertil Steril 36:480, 1981
61. SOONAWALA FP: Recanalization of the vas deferens. Bombay, India, Family Planning Association of India, 1977
62. THOMAS AJ, PONTES JE, ROSE NR, SEGAL S, PIERCE JM: Microsurgical vasovasostomy: Immunologic consequences and subsequent fertility. Fertil Steril 35:447, 1981

7
Discussion: Vasectomy and Reversal: Clinical Issues

MODERATOR: ALFREDO GOLDSMITH

AMONG MEN WITH VASECTOMY, DO SMOKERS HAVE A HIGH RELATIVE RISK OF MYOCARDIAL INFARCTION OR LUNG CANCER IF THEY SMOKE FOR A MEAN OF 6 YEARS ONLY?

The risk of myocardial infarction in cigarette smokers is not a function of duration of smoking but is an acute effect of smoking. The risk of lung cancer in smokers of 6.6 years is dependent on the age at which smoking begins; for someone who smokes for 6 years starting at age 18 and then quits, the risk is probably close to 1. If the person were to begin smoking at about age 55 and smoke for 6 years, however, the risk probably would be approximately 2.5.

A consistent finding in the epidemiologic studies in men is of lower rates of cancer in vasectomized men in spite of higher rates of cigarette smoking, and more intense cigarette smoking in vasectomized men in most populations in which it has been studied. A continued look at cancer rates in vasectomized men, with a view perhaps towards finding something that is in keeping with the leukocyte studies reported by Anderson, probably would be useful.

IS THERE ANY EVIDENCE, FROM EPIDEMIOLOGIC STUDIES, THAT BENIGN NODULAR HYPERPLASIA OF THE PROSTATE IS REDUCED IN MEN WHO HAVE HAD VASECTOMY?

In a recently completed study of benign prostatic hypertrophy and prostatic cancer in relation to prior vasectomy, no association, either positive or negative, was found with either condition.

HOW CAN ONE EXPLAIN THE GREAT VARIATION IN RESULTS AMONG COUNTRIES WITH REGARD TO PSYCHOSOCIAL SEQUELAE OF VASECTOMY?

This variation may be caused not by vasectomy itself but perhaps by inappropriate candidate selection or program approach to providing vasectomy. For example, quite unfortunate results were reported from Bangladesh in 1976,

---

Panelists: Diana B. Petitti, Rochelle N. Shain, Sherman J. Silber; *Discussants:* Nancy J. Alexander, Deborah J. Anderson, B. Norman Barwin, Timothy Farley, Douglas Huber, B. Leibendgut, C. Alvin Paulsen, Kenneth S. K. Tung, P. A. Van Keep, John P. Wiebe, Gerald I. Zatuchni

where perhaps 45% of men were dissatisfied with their vasectomy. Markedly improved results were achieved just a few years later when a follow-up study was undertaken of a national vasectomy campaign in which similar compensation was offered to men, but correct information, appropriate candidate selection, and no social pressure were the essential features. The dissatisfaction rate this time was 10% or less.

IN THE OPEN-ENDED VASECTOMY TECHNIQUE IS THE VAS FULGURATED?

Yes, the vas is fulgurated on the abdominal side. In the past, when the vas was fulgurated for only half a centimeter with a little vasector probe, the failure rate was 4%. When it is fulgurated as Schmidt originally suggested, with a longer needle electrode or with a longer vasector, these failures do not occur.

IS AGE A SIGNIFICANT FACTOR IN THE DESIRE FOR STERILIZATION REVERSAL?

Women under age 30 are more likely to request a reversal of sterilization than are women over 30; with men, age seems to be not so important a factor in requesting reversal. One investigator has noted that men are much more likely to request a reversal of sterilization than women, no matter the age; men in their late sixties have requested reversal of sterilization because they have a younger wife, whereas a woman who is 42 and remarried is not likely to want to have a child. One estimate is that 1% of vasectomized men request sterilization reversal, but reliable data are not easily available.

WHAT IS THE INCIDENCE OF ANTIBODY GENERATION IN THE OPEN-ENDED VASECTOMY?

One study of patients with and without sperm granuloma showed a small increase of sperm granuloma in men with open-ended vasectomy, but the open-ended technique is not likely to create any significantly greater immune consequences. In addition, the presence of sperm granuloma does not necessarily indicate that antibodies will develop.

IS THERE ANY LIMIT TO THE PERIOD FOLLOWING VASECTOMY DURING WHICH REVERSAL CAN BE PERFORMED?

Reversal has been performed in men as late as 30 years or more following vasectomy. If vasectomy is not open ended, with each passing year there is a greater chance of epididymal blocking, but there is no restriction on when one may seek reversal, as long as a vasoepididymostomy is possible. Even in the hands of a skilled surgeon, however, when the vasectomy is greater than 10 years old, there is a 60% chance of failure, despite excellent vasovasostomy technique.

IS ANYTHING KNOWN ABOUT THE INCIDENCE OF HYSTERECTOMY IN THE WIFE AFTER THE HUSBAND HAS BEEN STERILIZED?

Investigators are now in the fourth year of data collection on a 5-year follow-up study of the consequences of tubal sterilization, in which they are looking at women preoperatively and following them postoperatively with two control groups. One of the findings from the initial data is that women who undergo tubal ligation are much less fearful of surgery in general, and of reproductive surgery in particular, than are wives of men who are scheduled for vasectomy.

Fear of surgery probably is one of the key predictors of whether couples choose vasectomy or tubal sterilization. When the woman fears surgery more, chances are that the couple will choose vasectomy as opposed to a tubal sterilization.

Male Reproductive Physiology and Contraception

8

Sites for Disruption of Male Fertility

NANCY J. ALEXANDER

Male reproduction can be affected through the hypothalamus-pituitary axis, testes, epididymides, and vasa deferentia. Figure 8-1 depicts possible sites of disruption of male fertility. Except for blockage of the vasa deferentia (vasectomy), there are few safe and effective methods of controlling male fertility. The male reproductive system seems less amenable to interference than does that of the female. Several phenomena work to maintain a reproductively intact and fertile state. First, because the spermatogenic cycle is 74 days, months pass before a drug is effective. Second, because reproductive hormones are generally in a steady state in men, interruption of cyclicity is not an effective contraceptive approach. Third, because the testes are protected by a blood–testis barrier, many agents cannot reach the site of spermatogenesis.

STEROIDS

The possibility of the equivalent of "the Pill" for men has long been considered enticing. Such a pill could affect pituitary function, spermatogenesis, or sperm maturation. Development of a pill for men has followed the lines of efforts used to develop a pill for women. Various steroid combinations have been considered. Excellent reviews already have been published on aspects of male contraception. Therefore, this review will be short and simple. For more details about pharmacologic agents, see the review by Lobl et al.[11]

Estrogens stop spermatogenesis and are indeed used to treat men with prostate cancer. For a healthy man, however, estrogens are unacceptable because they have feminizing effects. Long-acting gestagens such as medroxyprogesterone acetate have been considered.[17] Because gestagens diminish libido and potency, however, they must be administered with either testosterone implants,[22,23] or testosterone enanthate.[2,21] Long-term use of androgens may result in liver damage[8,25] and hepatic tumors.[7,15] Another disadvantage of this approach is that the onset of azoospermia or oligozoospermia takes several months, and recovery takes from 3 months to several years. There always has been the concern that men with oligozoospermia

The work described in this chapter, Publication No. 1390 of the Oregon Regional Primate Research Center, was supported by National Institutes of Health Grant RR-00163.

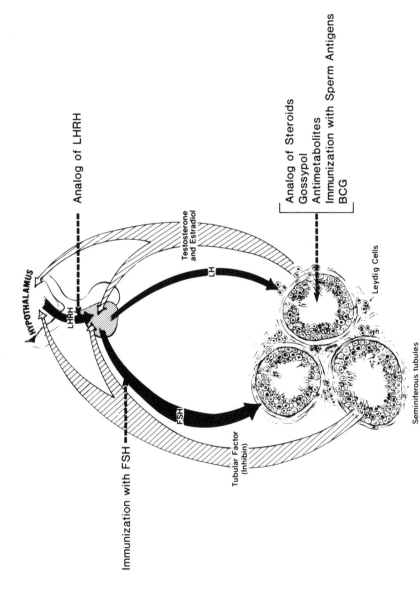

FIG. 8-1. A diagram of hormonal feedback interactions between the testis and brain. Sites of attack by various contraceptive approaches are indicated by dotted lines and arrows. (Alexander NJ, Naz RK: Targets for a male contraceptive. In Sciarra JJ (ed): Gynecology and Obstetrics, Vol 6, Chap. 13. Philadelphia, Harper & Row, 1985)

might not be sterile because theoretically it only takes one spermatozoon to cause fertilization.[3]

Recently, the anabolic steroid nandrolone has been tested on 20 volunteers as an alternative means of steroidal contraception.[20] The World Health Organization is now sponsoring a clinical trial with nandrolone.[30]

GONADOTROPIN SECRETION

Spermatogenesis is regulated by gonadotropins, that is, luteinizing hormone (LH) and follicle-stimulating hormone (FSH), which are secreted by the anterior pituitary. Recent experiments with highly purified material have demonstrated that both FSH and LH are necessary to maintain testicular growth after hypophysectomy in immature rats and rams; LH is thought to act through Sertoli cells, whereas FSH affects the germinal epithelium. Because LH stimulates Leydig cells to produce testosterone, this hormone indirectly affects spermatogenesis.

It is known that FSH is necessary for the initiation of spermatogenesis in rats,[14] as well as for the initiation and maintenance of spermatogenesis in rhesus macaques.[26,27] The precise involvement of FSH in human spermatogenesis still is not completely defined, however. Passive immunization with antibodies specific to FSH and active immunization of male monkeys with purified FSH both reduce FSH levels but do not change testosterone levels. Although sperm counts and motility are reduced, azoospermia is observed only occasionally.[12]

Inhibin feedback hormone appears to be the ideal candidate for suppression of spermatogenesis because it specifically inhibits FSH secretion and does not affect androgen production. Isolation and characterization of inhibin have proved difficult, however. An inhibinlike substance has been isolated from reproductive tissues as well as from ovarian follicular fluids of various animal species; however, these inhibin peptide preparations have been reported to inhibit not only FSH secretion but also LH secretion.[4] Whether FSH is needed to maintain spermatogenesis in adults, especially men, is controversial.

Secretion of LH and FSH is regulated by secretion of gonadotropin-releasing hormone (GnRH) from the basal hypothalamus. On the basis of various studies, scientists have considered using GnRH to prevent conception. Two types of GnRH analogues—agonists and antagonists—have been studied. Antagonists to LH-releasing hormone (LHRH) have seemed the most reasonable because they block the effects of LHRH. Agonists may desensitize the pituitary and inhibit GnRH secretion, desensitize gonadal receptors, or directly inhibit steroidogenesis. Treatment does result in reduced sperm counts but is accompanied by impotence and a loss of libido.[10,18] Because testicular function is reduced when either LHRH agonists or antagonists are used, androgen support therapy is necessary. With androgen support, however, some sperm are produced. The paradox of GnRH administration is that if androgens are given to alleviate side-effects, they may undo the desired effect. Although reversibility is theoretically possible, Pelletier and associates have found that testicular recovery in the rat is not always complete after cessation of LHRH treatment.[16]

DRUGS AFFECTING SPERMATOGENESIS

GOSSYPOL

The polyphenolic dinaphthyl dicarboxaldehyde *gossypol* became the focus of interest after an announcement in 1978 that infertility without ill effects developed in 4,000 Chinese men given gossypol. A dosage of 60 mg to 70 mg daily for 35 to 42 days results in a progressive increase in immotile sperm, followed by oligozoospermia and azoospermia. The substance, which is found in cotton seeds, also causes fatigue and gastrointestinal upset. Hypokalemia has been severe enough to cause paralysis, muscle weakness, and electrocardiogram changes in 170 of more than 8,000 men tested. Efforts are under way to determine whether potassium supplementation can eliminate these dangers. The contraceptive effects of gossypol are not always reversible; about 25% of men do not regain sperm counts in the normal range. This finding may preclude widespread use of gossypol in developed countries. Studies on animals indicate that there are great species differences in the response to gossypol. This finding has made study of the drug more difficult. Suitable analogues are being screened to determine whether an effective but less toxic compound can be developed.[9] The probable mode of gossypol action involves inhibition of lactate dehydrogenase isoenzyme C.[13] Gossypol has a direct spermicidal effect.[24] Its use as a vaginal contraceptive has been studied in monkeys[5] and women.[19] A more complete article on gossypol can be found in *Research Frontiers in Fertility Regulation.*[29]

α-CHLOROHYDRIN

Various glucose analogues have been used to prevent fertility. Among the chlorol sugars, α-Chlorohydrin has been shown to decrease fertility in all tested animals, including nonhuman primates. Treated animals continue to mate as frequently as controls but become infertile after less than a week. Fertility returns about 2 weeks after the cessation of treatment. α-Chlorohydrin and its metabolites are toxic, however. Greater concentrations are found in cerebrospinal fluid. The metabolites may inhibit glucose transfer mechanisms and thus cause the toxicity. (6-chloro-6-D-oxysugars and chlorohydrin act through the same mechanism.) Until drugs of lesser toxicity can be developed, the use of glucose analogues is precluded in humans.

STERILIZATION

Cutting and tying or fulgurating the vas are important approaches to sterilization throughout the world. A simple outpatient surgical procedure can be performed on men under local anesthesia. Although previously there was concern that vasectomy might have systemic effects, epidemiologic studies have not supported this concern, and vasectomy must be considered the best method of permanent contraception for men. Acceptance of this procedure has not reached the level hoped for by some. The reasons include fear of castration or of surgical intervention in the scrotal area, and cultural or political belief that women should play the major role in contraception. New vas occlusive plugs and prostheses have been attempted. The Shug[28] and various other flexible valves are under investigation. One of the stumbling blocks has been the fact that surgical implantation of reversible devices may require manipulation of the vas sheath and nerve supply, that is, much greater surgical skill than that required for vasectomy.[28] Percutaneous injection of ethanol and formaldehyde, another possible approach, has several advantages: 1) reduced risk of postsurgical hemorrhage, 2) reduced risk of postoperative infection, and 3) low cost. Changes in procedures must be considered to reduce the failure rate, however.[6]

IMMUNOLOGIC APPROACHES

Some infertile men have naturally occurring antibodies to their own sperm that can impede cervical mucus penetration or sperm–egg interactions.[1] Researchers currently are trying to assess which antigens are important in fertilization and can be affected by antibodies (see Chapter 40 by Anderson and Chapter 41 by Alexander on the contraceptive potential of antisperm antibodies).

CONCLUSION

The epididymis would seem to be an ideal site of action for a contraceptive if disruption of normal sperm motility can be accomplished there. Spermatozoa remain in the efferent duct system for a long enough time for various agents to act. Except for vasectomy and the condom, there are no methods currently available on a worldwide basis for men. It is to be hoped that this situation will soon change.

REFERENCES

1. ALEXANDER NJ: Antibodies to human spermatozoa impede sperm penetration of cervical mucus or hamster eggs. Fertil Steril 41:433–439, 1984
2. BAGHERI SA, BOYER JL: Peliosis hepatitis associated with androgenic anabolic steroid therapy: A severe form of hepatic injury. Ann Intern Med 81:610–618, 1974
3. BARFIELD A, MELO J, COUTINHO E, ALVAREZ-SANCHEZ F, FAUNDES A, BRACHE V, LEON P, FRICK J, BARTSCH G, WEISKE W-H, BRENNER P, MISHELL D Jr, BERNSTEIN G, ORTIZ A: Pregnancies associated with sperm concentrations below 10 million/ml in clinical studies of a potential male contraceptive method, monthly depot medroxyprogesterone acetate and testosterone esters. Contraception 20:121–127, 1979
4. BRAUNSTEIN GD, SWERDLOFF RS: Effect of aqueous extracts of bull and rat testicles on serum FSH and LH in the acutely castrate male rat. In TROEN P, NANKIN HR (eds): The Testis in Normal and Infertile Men, pp 281–291. New York, Raven Press, 1977

5. CAMERON SM, WALLER DP, ZANEVELD LJD: Vaginal spermicidal activity of gossypol in the *Macaca arctoides*. Fertil Steril 37:273–274, 1982

6. DAVIS JE: New methods of vas occlusion. In ZATUCHNI GI, LABBOK MH, SCIARRA JJ (eds): Research Frontiers in Fertility Regulation, pp 252–261. Hagerstown, Harper & Row, 1980

7. FALK H, THOMAS LB, POPPER H, ISHAK KG: Hepatic angiosarcoma associated with androgenic-anabolic steroids. Lancet ii:1120–1123, 1979

8. FARRELL GC, JOSHUA DE, UREN R, BAIRD PJ, PERKINS KW, KRONENBERG H: Androgen-induced hepatoma. Lancet i:430–432, 1975

9. KIM IC, WALLER DP, MARCELLE GB, CORDELL GA, FONG HHS, PIRKLE WH, PILLA L, MATLIN SA: Comparative in vitro spermicidal effects of (±)-gossypol, (+)-gossypol, (−)-gossypol and gossypolone. Contraception 30:253–259, 1984

10. LINDE R, DOELLE GC, ALEXANDER N, KIRCHNER F, VALE W, RIVIER J, RABIN D: Reversible inhibition of testicular steroidogenesis and spermatogenesis by a potent gonadotropin-releasing hormone agonist in normal men: An approach toward the development of a male contraceptive. N Engl J Med 305:663–667, 1981

11. LOBL TJ, BARDIN CW, CHANG CC: Pharmacologic agents producing infertility by direct action on the male reproductive tract. In ZATUCHNI GI, LABBOK MH, SCIARRA JJ (eds): Research Frontiers in Fertility Regulation, pp 146–168. Hagerstown, Harper & Row, 1980

12. MADHWA RAJ HG, SAIRAM MR, NIESCHLAG E: Immunologic approach to regulation of fertility in the male. In CUNNINGHAM GR, SCHILL WB, HAFEZ ESE (eds): Regulation of Male Fertility, p 209. The Hague, Martinus–Nijhoff, 1980

13. MAUGH TH: Male "pill" blocks sperm enzyme. Science 212:314, 1981

14. MURTY GSRC, SHEELA RANI CS, MOUDGAL NR, PRASAD MRN: Effect of passive immunization with specific antiserum to FSH on the spermatogenic process and fertility of adult male bonnet monkeys (*Macaca radiata*). J Reprod Fertil (Suppl) 26:147–163, 1979

15. PAULSEN CA, BREMNER WJ, LEONARD JM: Male contraception: Clinical trials. In MISHELL DR Jr (ed): Advances in Fertility Research, Vol 1, pp 157–170. New York, Raven Press, 1982

16. PELLETIER G, CUSAN GL, BÉLANGER A, SÉGUIN C, KELLY PA, LABRIE F: Further studies on the inhibitory effect of (D-Ala^6, des-Gly-NH$_2$^{10})LHRH ethylamide on spermatogenesis and steroidogenesis in the rat: Reversibility and effect of androgen administration. J Androl 1:171–181, 1980

17. PRASAD MRN, SINGH SP, RAJALAKSHMI M: Fertility control in male rats by continuous release of microquantities of cyproterone acetate from subcutaneous Silastic capsules. Contraception 2:165–178, 1970

18. RABIN D, LINDE R, DOELLE G, ALEXANDER N: Experience with a potent gonadotropin releasing hormone agonist in normal men: An approach to the development of a male contraceptive. In ZATUCHNI GI, SHELTON JD, SCIARRA JJ (eds): LHRH Peptides as Female and Male Contraceptives, pp 296–306. Philadelphia, Harper & Row, 1981

19. RATSULA K, HAUKKAMAA M, WICHMANN K, LUUKKAINEN T: Vaginal contraception with gossypol: A clinical study. Contraception 27:571–576, 1983

20. SCHÜRMEYER T, KNUTH UA, BELKIEN L, NIESCHLAG E: Reversible azoospermia induced by the anabolic steroid 19-nortestosterone. Lancet i:417–420, 1984

21. SKAKKEBAEK NE, BANCROFT J, DAVIDSON DW, WARNER P: Androgen replacement with oral testosterone undecanoate in hypogonadal men: A double-blind controlled study. Clin Endocrinol 14:49–61, 1981

22. STEINBERGER E, SMITH KD: Effect of chronic administration of testosterone enanthate on sperm production and plasma testosterone, follicle-stimulating hormone, and luteinizing hormone levels: A preliminary evaluation of a possible male contraceptive. Fertil Steril 28:1320–1328, 1977

23. SWERDLOFF RS, PALACIOS A, MCCLURE RD, CAMPFIELD LA, BROSMAN SA: Male contraception: Clinical assessment of chronic administration of testosterone enanthate. Int J Androl (Suppl) 2:731–747, 1978

24. WALLER DP, ZANEVELD LJD, FONG HHS: In vitro spermicidal activity of gossypol. Contraception 22:183–187, 1980

25. WESTABY D, OGLE SJ, PARADINAS FJ, RANDELL JB, MURRAY-LYON IM: Liver damage from long-term methyltestosterone. Lancet ii:261–263, 1977

26. WICKINGS EJ, SRINATH BR, NIESCHLAG E: An immunological approach to male fertility control using antibodies to FSH. In JEFFCOATE SL, SANDLER M (eds): Progress Towards a Male Contraceptive, pp 79–91. Chichester, John Wiley & Sons, 1982

27. WICKINGS EJ, USADEL KH, DATHE G, NIESCHLAG E: The role of follicle-stimulating hormone in testicular function of the mature rhesus monkey. Acta Endocrinol 95:117–128, 1980

28. ZANEVELD LJD, BEYLER SA, PRINS G, TAFT FS, GOODPASTURE JC, REDDY JM, ANDERSON RA Jr, ANDERSON CH: Reversible vas deferens occlusion: A new device. In SCIARRA JJ, ZATUCHNI GI, SPEIDEL JJ (eds): Reversal of Sterilization, pp 81–90. Hagerstown, Harper & Row, 1978

29. ZATUCHNI GI, OSBORN CK: Gossypol: A possible male antifertility agent. Report of a workshop. In ZATUCHNI GI (ed): Research Frontiers in Fertility Regulation, Vol. 1, No. 4, pp 1–14. Chicago, Northwestern University Medical School, 1981

30. ZIPORYN T: Search for male contraceptive complicated by adverse effects. JAMA 252:1101–1103, 1984

9

Endocrine Control of Human Spermatogenesis: Possible Mechanisms for Contraception

WILLIAM J. BREMNER

ALVIN M. MATSUMOTO

Human spermatogenesis requires the stimulatory actions of the pituitary gonadotropins, luteinizing hormone (LH) and follicle-stimulating hormone (FSH).[2] FSH has been thought to be primarily responsible for sperm production whereas LH controls testosterone production. Much effort has been devoted to developing methods for the selective suppression of FSH secretion, leaving LH unchanged, in hopes of inhibiting sperm production without affecting testosterone levels.

We have performed a series of studies on normal men, designed to assess the role of FSH in the control of human spermatogenesis.[1,3-5] Three of these studies were designed to determine whether normal blood levels of FSH are necessary for human spermatogenesis.[1,3,5] We hoped to provide evidence as to the likelihood that selective FSH suppression would be an effective male contraceptive.

METHODS

STUDY 1

Five normal men were studied.[1] The first 3 months of the study constituted a control period during which observations and measurements (see below) were performed in each subject, but no hormones were administered. After the control period, testosterone enanthate (Delatestryl) administration was begun (200 mg IM wkly). The injections of testosterone enanthate (T) alone were continued until three successive seminal fluid analyses (obtained every 2 wk) revealed sperm counts <5 million/ml. At this point, while the injections of T were continued, administration of hCG (Profasi) (5000 IU IM 3× wkly) was added. The combined hCG and T injections were continued in all five men until three successive sperm counts were within the person's control range, or a minimum of 17 weeks.

At this time, to demonstrate that the increases in sperm counts found were due to hCG and not to a decline in the suppressive effect of testosterone, hCG injections were stopped in two subjects and T alone was continued until sperm counts were again suppressed to very low levels. Then T was discontinued and the two subjects entered a post-treatment control period lasting until three successive sperm counts were within the subject's control range.

During each month of the study, each subject submitted two seminal fluid specimens obtained by masturbation after 2 days of abstention from ejaculation. In addition, monthly venous blood samples were obtained for measurement of LH, FSH, and testosterone levels.

STUDY 2

This investigation in four normal men was similar in design to study 1 except that human LH was used instead of hCG.[5] The same 3-month control period was followed by testosterone injections (200 mg IM wkly) until three successive sperm counts were below 5 million/ml. Then, while the T injections were continued, hLH (1100 IU daily SC for 4–6 mo) was added. The hLH used was LER 1549 (batch A-3, provided by the National Pituitary Agency) and contained less than 0.2% FSH activity in the rat ovarian augmentation bioassay for FSH.

To demonstrate that any increases in sperm concentrations during the administration of LH plus T were due to an effect of hLH administration and not the result of a decline in the suppressive effects of exogenous T, seven men served as control subjects. After the T suppression period, these subjects continued to receive T alone at the same dosage for an additional 6 months (*i.e.*, total of 9 months altogether and subjects received no LH).

Monthly blood samples for measurement of LH, FSH, and T levels, as well as twice monthly seminal fluid samples, were obtained throughout the study.

STUDY 3

This study was designed to determine whether prolonged gonadotropin suppression would allow demonstration of a requirement for FSH to restimulate spermatogenesis. This work, undertaken in four normal men, was similar in design to study 1 except that the T-induced suppression of spermatogenesis was maintained for 9 months prior to adding hCG (5000 IU IM 3× wkly).[3] All four men demonstrated sperm counts <3 million/ml by the end of the first 3 months of T suppression and were azoospermic by 9 months.

Measurement Techniques

LH, FSH, and T were measured by previously described radioimmunoassays.[1] LH was measured in some samples by the *in vitro* Leydig cell bioassay.[1] Seminal fluid analysis was performed as described previously.[1]

RESULTS

STUDY 1

Following the 3-month control period, administration of testosterone led to severe inhibition of sperm production (Fig. 9-1). Three subjects became azoospermic, whereas two consistently exhibited sperm counts of less than 3

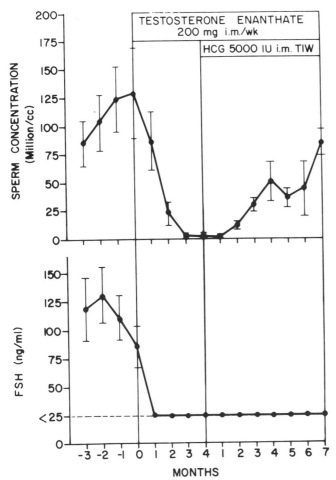

FIG. 9-1. Monthly sperm concentrations and serum FSH data in five normal men during the control, testosterone administration alone, and hCG plus testosterone phases of the study (mean ± SE). Note the increase in sperm concentration induced by hCG in spite of very low serum levels of FSH. Taken from Bremner WJ et al: J Clin Invest 68:1044–1052, 1981. Used by permission of Rockefeller University Press, New York.

million/ml. While the testosterone injections were continued, hCG was added (5000 IU IM, 3× wkly). Sperm counts (Fig. 9-1) increased markedly during hCG administration (p < 0.001 compared with testosterone injections alone). In two subjects, sperm counts during hCG plus T injections returned into the normal control range for each man. In the other three men, although sperm counts increased markedly on hCG plus T, reaching mean levels of 12, 13, and 94 million/ml, they did not consistently reach the men's control ranges. Medication records revealed that the two men with the lowest counts did not receive all their scheduled hCG injections. Serum FSH values (Fig. 9-1) were normal (111 ± 10 ng/ml) in the control period and were suppressed to undetectable levels (<25 ng/ml) in the T alone and in the hCG plus T phases of the study.

Following the hCG plus T phase of the study, in which all men participated, two men received only T injections for 2.5 and 4.0 months. Sperm counts during the T injections alone returned to azoospermic or severely oligospermic levels.

STUDY 2

Seminal Fluid Parameters

After the 3-month control period, exogenous T enanthate administration (200 mg, IM wkly) resulted in a marked suppression of sperm production to under 5 million/ml after 3 to 4 months in all subjects. In the four experimental subjects, sperm concentrations were reduced to 0.7 ± 0.7 million/ml (mean $\pm$ SEM) after the initial 12 weeks of T administration, compared with 98 ± 7 million/ml during the control period. Three of the four experimental subjects (subjects 1–3) became azoospermic, while the remaining man (subject 4) had sperm concentrations consistently below 4 million/ml. While continuing exogenous T at the same dosage, the experimental subjects simultaneously received hLH (1100 IU, SC, daily) for 4 to 6 months (for 4 mo in subject 3, for 5 mo in subject 2, and for 6 mo in subjects 1 and 4). Sperm concentrations increased significantly in all subjects with the addition of hLH to T (Fig. 9-2), reaching a mean of 19 ± 4 million/ml after 3 months of hLH plus T administration (p < 0.001 compared to T alone). Although sperm concentrations increased during hLH plus T therapy, they did not consistently reach the person's control range in any subject. The means of the last three sperm concentrations during the hLH plus T period for subjects 1 to 4 were 36, 34, 8, and 15 million/ml, compared to ranges of sperm concentrations during the control period of 55 to 173, 25 to 126, 40 to 143, and 25 to 180 million/ml, respectively. The maximum sperm concentrations achieved during the hLH plus T period were 64, 80, 19, and 29 million/ml, for subjects 1 through 4, respectively. Three men (subjects 1, 2, and 4) achieved at least one sperm concentration within their control range during hLH plus T administration. Sperm motility and morphology at the end of the hLH plus T period were normal in all four experimental subjects.

Similar to the experimental subjects, exogenous T administration resulted in marked suppression of sperm concentrations in all seven control subjects (data not shown). In these men, sperm concentrations after the initial 12 weeks of T administration were reduced to 2 ± 1 million/ml, compared to 65 ± 9 million/ml during the control period. Four of the seven control subjects became azoospermic, whereas the remaining men had sperm concentrations consistently below 3 million/ml after 3 to 4 months of T treatment. In contrast with that of the men who received hLH and T, sperm concentrations remained suppressed in all control subjects to fewer than 3 million/ml $(0.9 \pm 0.5$ million/ml) throughout the entire experimental period. By the end of this period of prolonged T treatment, all seven control subjects were azoospermic.

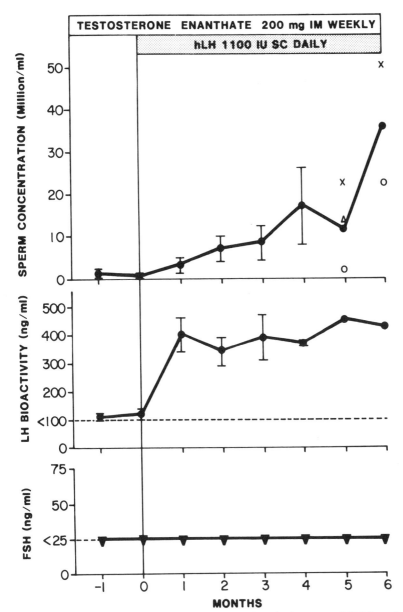

FIG. 9-2. Mean monthly sperm concentration (*top*), serum LH bioactivity (*middle*), and serum FSH level (*bottom*) in subjects 1 to 4 during the last 2 months of the T suppression period and the first 4 months of the hLH plus T period (mean ± SEM). In the last 2 months of the hLH plus T period, mean monthly sperm concentrations are presented for each subject remaining in the study. X, Δ, and O represent mean monthly sperm concentrations for subjects 1, 2, and 4. Addition of hLH to T treatment increased LH bioactivity into the physiologic range and stimulated sperm production, despite continued undetectable FSH levels. Broken line (---) represents the limits of detectability of the LH and FSH assays. Taken from Matsumoto AM et al: J Clin Endocrinol Metab 59:882–887, 1984. Used by permission of the Endocrine Society.

Hormone Levels

Serum LH and FSH levels (Fig. 9-2) were suppressed into the nondetectable or prepubertal range by testosterone administration. With the addition of hLH replacement, LH levels returned to the normal physiologic range, while FSH remained nondetectable. Similarly, urinary FSH determinations revealed that the men both while receiving T alone and while receiving T plus hLH demonstrated FSH excretion rates consistently in the range found in prepubertal children.

STUDY 3

Following the control period, exogenous T enanthate administration (200 mg IM wkly) resulted in severe suppression of sperm production to under 3 million/ml by 3 months. Sperm concentrations remained suppressed below this level for 6 months in all subjects (Fig. 9-3). Sperm concentrations were reduced to 0.8 ± 0.5 million/ml after the initial 12 weeks of T administration ($p < 0.001$ compared to control values). Seminal fluid volume was unchanged (2.6 ± 0.4 ml) and total sperm count was reduced to 2 ± 1 million/ml during this period. All four subjects became azoospermic by the end of the prolonged T suppression period.

While continuing the same dosage of T, subjects then simultaneously received hCG (5000 IU IM 3× wkly). Sperm concentrations increased significantly in all subjects with addition of hCG to T (Fig. 9-3), reaching a mean of 25 ± 4 million/ml after 12 weeks of hCG administration ($p < 0.01$ compared to T alone). Seminal fluid volume was unchanged (2.6 ± 0.2 ml) and total sperm count increased to 65 ± 9 million per ejaculate during this period. Although sperm concentrations increased markedly in all four subjects during hCG plus T administration, no subject achieved sperm concentrations consistently in his control range. Individual sperm concentrations for Subjects 1 to 4 during hCG plus T averaged 35, 16, 30, and 20 million/ml, respectively and the maximum sperm concentrations achieved during this period were 75, 31, 47, and 31 million/ml, respectively. Sperm motility and morphology were consistently normal in all men during hCG plus T.

Hormone Levels

Again, serum LH and FSH levels and urinary FSH excretion were severely suppressed by T administration. FSH remained at these very low levels during hCG administration.

DISCUSSION

Taken together, the results of these three studies demonstrate unequivocally that spermatogenesis in men can be stimulated to a degree almost certainly allowing fertility despite prepubertal levels of FSH. This was true whether the stimulatory agent was hCG or hLH and was found even following prolonged (9-month) gonadotropin suppression. Importantly, spermatogenesis was stim-

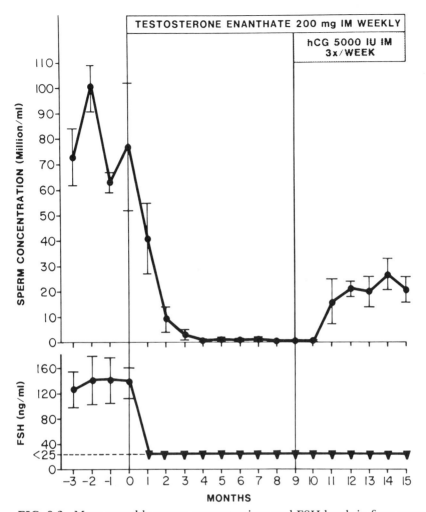

FIG. 9-3. Mean monthly sperm concentrations and FSH levels in four normal men during the control, prolonged T suppression, and hCG plus T periods of the study (mean ± SEM). Prolonged exogenous T administration markedly suppressed sperm concentrations to severely oligospermic levels for 6 months and reduced serum FSH to undetectable levels (▼) for 9 months. Note the increase in sperm concentration with the addition of hCG to T, despite continued undetectable serum FSH levels. Broken line (---) represents the limit of detectability of FSH RIA. (From Matsumoto AM, Bremner WJ: J Androl 6:137–143, 1985)

ulated even when hLH was used in a dosage that produced normal, physiologic levels of LH bioactivity (study 2).

The levels of FSH in blood during T and gonadotropin administration were undetectable in a sensitive radioimmunoassay, which can detect levels in all normal subjects. Urinary excretion of FSH, which is much more sensitive in assessing low levels, demonstrated that FSH was in the range found in prepubertal children and less than that usually found in hypopituitary subjects. While FSH production was presumably not totally eliminated (at least as measured by radioimmunoassay), it was as low as is likely to be achieved by agents potentially useful as male contraceptives, particularly those designed to suppress FSH selectively.

Our results do not lend support to the concept that selective suppression of FSH secretion, while LH levels remain normal, is likely to lead to an effective male contraceptive. Sperm counts in men with this hormonal milieu were in the range almost certainly consistent with fertility. The question arises whether these were normal sperm or whether the FSH deficiency could alter them somehow, rendering them incapable of inducing fertility. As assessed by motility and morphology, these sperm were normal. Furthermore, in the few samples tested, the hamster ovum penetration assay result was normal using these sperm. Although we do not have data concerning true fertility rates in normal men with selective FSH suppression, it seems very likely that they would be fertile.

It remains an open question, deserving of much more study, whether suppression of both LH and FSH levels by agents acceptable for use in normal men can reliably reduce sperm production sufficiently to cause infertility. Although clinical trials of steroid administration have not been able to achieve consistent azoospermia, it is possible that LHRH analogues, particularly antagonists, may be capable of attaining this elusive goal. It is also of great interest whether an agent must produce complete azoospermia to be an acceptable male contraceptive. There are essentially no data available on the fertility rates of men made azoospermic or severely oligospermic by contraceptive agents. This important area remains open for investigation.

REFERENCES

1. BREMNER WJ, MATSUMOTO AM, SUSSMAN AM, PAULSEN CA: Follicle-stimulating hormone and human spermatogenesis. J Clin Invest 68:1044–1052, 1981
2. DIZEREGA GS, SHERINS RJ: Endocrine control of adult testicular function. In BURGER H, DEKRETSER D (eds): The Testis, pp 127–140. New York, Raven Press, 1980
3. MATSUMOTO AM, BREMNER WJ: Stimulation of sperm production by human chorionic gonadotropin after prolonged gonadotropin suppression in normal men. J Androl 6:137–143, 1985
4. MATSUMOTO AM, KARPAS AE, PAULSEN CA, BREMNER WJ: Reinitiation of sperm production in gonadotropin-suppressed normal men by administration of follicle-stimulating hormone. J Clin Invest 72:1005–1015, 1983
5. MATSUMOTO AM, PAULSEN CA, BREMNER WJ: Stimulation of sperm production by human luteinizing hormone in gonadotropin-suppressed normal men. J Clin Endocrinol Metab 59:882–887, 1984

10

Sperm Maturation and the Potential for Contraceptive Interference

WILLIAM CHRISTOPHER LIBERTY FORD

GEOFFREY M. H. WAITES

A male contraceptive to be used by humans must be both effective and safe. Thus it must completely incapacitate spermatozoa or prevent their production and at the same time must have no significant effect on other cells in the body. The extreme specialization of spermatozoa, together with their isolation in a special environment, offers opportunities for the development of drugs with sufficiently selective methods of action.

THE SPECIALIZATION OF SPERMATOZOA

FUNCTION

Spermatozoa carry the genetic contribution of the male to the egg. They must be motile and able to recognize the egg, bind to its surface, and penetrate its investments after undergoing a complex series of changes known as *capacitation*.[1] To fulfil these roles, the sperm cell exhibits marked structural and biochemical specializations.

STRUCTURE

The mammalian spermatozoon is regionally specialized, with a head containing the highly condensed haploid nucleus, a midpiece that contains the mitochondria, and a long flagellum, or tail.[45] The acrosome contains hydrolytic enzymes and is applied to the anterior end of the head. The acrosomal "cap" consists of a sac bounded by the inner and the outer acrosomal membrane, the latter lying immediately beneath the plasma membrane covering the head. The central structure of the tail is a classical 9×2 doublet system similar to that found in the cilia of other cells but with the addition of a system of nine outer dense fibers, one associated with each of the nine microtubule doublets. The mitochondria are arranged in a spiral around the elements of the flagellum in the midpiece. The cytoplasm of the cell is sparse.[3]

The authors' research has been supported by grants from the U.K. Medical Research Council, the World Health Organization, and the U.K. Agricultural Research Council.

BIOCHEMISTRY

The extremely condensed state of the chromatin in the sperm nucleus depends on the replacement of somatic histones by arginine-rich basic proteins with a high cysteine content.[46] The hydrolytic enzymes present in the acrosome include the trypsinlike protease, acrosin, found only in spermatozoa[45] and sperm-specific isoenzymes of hyaluronidase.[70] Sperm also contain unique isoenzymes of lactate dehydrogenase and phosphoglycerate kinase,[3] phosphodiesterase,[66] and enolase,[16] and also possess an adenyl cyclase that lacks the coupling component.[66] Unique antigens are present in specific regions of the sperm surface, and their presence and distribution may change as the spermatozoa mature or capacitate.[2,7,41]

Some of the sperm lactate dehydrogenase (LDH-X or LDH-C$_4$) is located in the mitochondrion, and this provides pathways for the transport of reducing equivalents into the organelle via a lactate–pyruvate shuttle,[9] and for the anaerobic oxidation of pyruvate to succinate.[72] Spermatozoa contain high concentrations of carnitine, and acetyl carnitine is a major end product of the metabolism of glucose or pyruvate.[6,11] Futile substrate cycling in the glycolytic pathway proceeds at a high rate in spermatozoa especially when the energy demand of the cell is low.[34]

DIFFERENTIATION OF SPERMATOZOA

MORPHOLOGY

During spermiogenesis, the principal changes in the postmeiotic cells are the condensation of the nucleus, formation of the acrosome, development of the flagellum, the arrangement of the mitochondria into the characteristic helix in the midpiece, and the elimination of most of the cytoplasm with a large part of the plasma membrane. These changes occur in a strict temporal sequence and are aligned with other events in the spermatogenic cycle (Fig. 10-1).[3,60,63]

BIOCHEMICAL ASPECTS

Sperm differentiation begins at the pachytene spermatocyte stage because soluble proteins characteristic of spermatozoa, including LDH-X, are first detected at this time, as are certain sperm specific antigens (Fig. 10-1). Other proteins appear only after meiosis; these include cysteine-rich basic nuclear protein, phosphoglycerate kinase, and the acrosomal enzymes hyaluronidase and β-galactosidase (Fig. 10-1). Postmeiotic protein synthesis may depend on the delayed translation of stored memory RNA (mRNA) or on the transcription of haploid DNA.[3] The existence of the latter mechanism was confirmed recently by the use of a cloned DNA (cDNA) probe to mouse testis α-tubulin.[15]

Thus, during spermiogenesis, genetic material is handled differently than in the development of somatic cells. Because proteins characteristic of spermatozoa first appear in the primary spermatocytes, the postmeiotic cells should

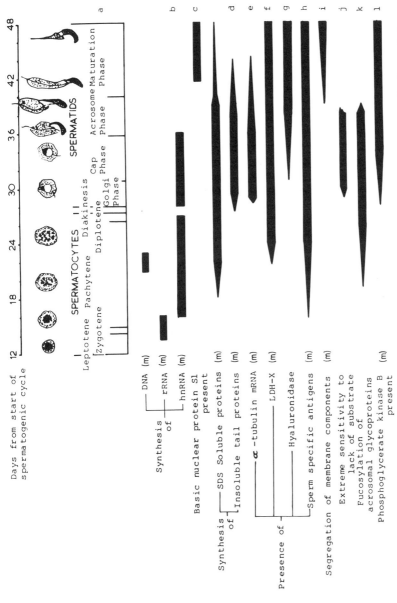

FIG. 10-1. The timing of some biochemical events during spermatogenesis. The time scale shown is for the rat but some data (shown by *m*) have been taken from experiments with mice and the timing adjusted to coincide with the appropriate cell types. For this reason and because the precision of the experimental techniques used varies widely, the positions of the bars should be regarded as only a general guide to the sequence of events: a, 60; b, 43; c, 46; d, 53; e, 15; f, 47; g, 70; h, 48; i, 49; j, 28; k, 30; l, 71

be susceptible to selective drug action as previously proposed for spermatozoa.[20,25,75]

THE ROLE OF THE SERTOLI CELL

The germ cells are in an intimate relationship with the Sertoli cells and depend on them for the maintenance of the specialized environment required for spermatogenesis.[18,61,74] The Sertoli cells are responsible for maintaining the blood–testis barrier and for mediating endocrine effects on spermatogenesis. The latter function includes control of the supply of androgens[14] and of substrates[29,52] to the germ cells. Spermatids are extremely sensitive to lack of substrate, and inhibition of energy metabolism or of the synthesis of lactate and pyruvate by the Sertoli cells could form the basis for a postmeiotic contraceptive.[28]

THE BLOOD–TESTIS AND THE BLOOD–EPIDIDYMIS BARRIER

The composition of the fluid environment of the seminiferous tubules and of the epididymis is regulated by permeability barriers constituted by specialized junctions between the Sertoli cells[18] or the epithelial cells.[18,36] One vital function of these barriers is to isolate the postmitotic germ cells and spermatozoa from the immune system of the body. The barriers also enable the luminal fluid to maintain a composition very different from blood plasma; thus, seminiferous tubule fluid, rete testis fluid, and epididymal fluid all have a higher K^+/Na^+ ratio and contain organic constituents in very different concentrations than in blood plasma.[45,76] Epididymal fluid is discussed below.

Compounds can be divided into three classes with respect to their ability to cross the blood–testis barrier: 1) those whose concentration in tubular fluid rapidly equilibrates with those in plasma (*e.g.*, tritiated water, urea); 2) those that fail to penetrate the lumen of the tubule to any appreciable extent (*e.g.*, inulin, sucrose, [^{51}Cr]EDTA, para-aminohippurate, albumen); and 3) those that enter the tubule slowly (*e.g.*, K^+, Na^+, amino acids, glucose, various drugs). Hydrophilic substances of the last class are probably transported by carrier-facilitated diffusion; the entry of lipophilic substances depends on their relative solubility in organic solvents and water.[55,64,76]

SPERM MATURATION IN THE EPIDIDYMIS

THE EPIDIDYMIS

The epididymis is a long, tightly coiled duct that transports spermatozoa from the testis to the vas deferens. The proximal regions of the duct produce a milieu for fluid absorption and later sperm maturation, whereas the distal region acts as a reservoir for sperm storage.[5,45] It may be considered to have three regions, termed the *caput, corpus,* and *cauda* (Fig. 10-2). These correlate to some extent with function. The duct is surrounded by layers of smooth muscle, only a few in the caput region but relatively many in the cauda, and is lined with a regular, columnar epithelium, about 60 μm high in the caput and

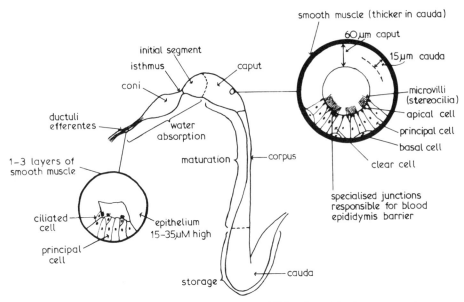

FIG. 10-2. The principal regions of the rat epididymis, with diagrammatic cross-sections of an efferent duct and a tubule from the caput epididymidis. (From Hamilton DW: Structure and function of the epithelium lining the ductuli efferentes, ductus epididymidis and ductus deferens in the rat. In Hamilton DW, Greep RO (eds): Handbook of Physiology, Section 7, Vol 5, Male Reproductive System, pp 259–301. Washington, American Physiology Society, 1975.)

about 15 μm high in the cauda region (rat). The apical surface of the epithelial cells bears many microvilli (or stereocilia), but no true cilia are present (see Fig. 10-2).[31] The epithelial cells are joined by junctional complexes close to their luminal end to form *zona occludentes*, which constitute the blood–epididymis barrier.[36] The structure and function of the epididymis are dependent on androgens; a component of the supply to the initial segment may come from testicular fluid.[5]

SPERM MATURATION

Testicular spermatozoa lack progressive motility, whereas spermatozoa taken from the cauda epididymidis are highly motile.[5,13,38] By contrast, testicular spermatozoa that have been demembranated with Triton X-100 beat vigorously in the presence of ATP and cAMP, but a lower percentage than of cauda spermatozoa were activated, and the nature of the movement was different.[50,68,79] In demembranated spermatozoa, the activation of motility by cAMP is associated with the phosphorylation of specific proteins.[66] In the bull, caput spermatozoa could be induced to show flagellar activity by elevating their cAMP content with theophylline, but they did not become progressively motile unless a "forward motility" protein that is present in bovine seminal plasma also was added.[38]

The fertility of caput spermatozoa is virtually zero, whereas insemination with spermatozoa from the cauda epididymidis results in pregnancy in more than 80% of trials; spermatozoa from the corpus have an intermediate degree of fertility.[13,51] Lack of fertility does not stem solely from a lack of motility but depends on changes in sperm membranes that allow binding to the egg.[13,62] These changes include:

1. The redistribution of membrane components evidenced by changes in the distribution of particles[37]
2. Changes in the terminal sugars of the glycan component of surface glycoproteins and glycolipids, notably an increase in the amount of sialic acid in this position[3,37]
3. Incorporation of proteins secreted by the epididymal epithelium[3]
4. The loss of phospholipid and cholesterol from the membranes and an increase in the unsaturation of the esterified fatty acids[3,45]

In the course of maturation, the cytoplasmic droplet moves from the proximal to the distal end of the midpiece, and the nucleus becomes stabilized by further $-S-S-$ bonds.[3,33] Boar or ram spermatozoa develop an enhanced metabolic rate when they become motile, although this could reflect simply an increased energy demand for motility.[13,40] In the guinea pig and the bull, sperm maturation is associated with a large increase in the amounts of glucose converted to lactate.[26,73] The activity of glyceraldehyde 3-phosphate dehydrogenase in spermatozoa, measured in conditions that should exclude allosteric effects, changed during maturation,[22] and changes in the activity of other glycolytic enzymes,[32] lipase and alkaline phosphatase,[67] Na^+/K^+ ATPase[12] and acetylcholinesterase,[17] as well as an increased affinity of the glucose transport for glucose,[35] have been reported. Decreases in enzyme activity might be explained by selective proteolysis. Increases are unlikely to be due to de novo enzyme synthesis and must be caused by posttranslational modifications. A sperm-specific form of glucose phosphate isomerase probably arises by this mechanism.[8] Spermatozoa contain cAMP-dependent and independent protein kinases and protein phosphatases, some of which may be regulated by Ca^{2+},[66] protein carboxymethylase,[4] and protein methylesterase,[27] which could catalyze such events, and the activities of which themselves change during maturation.[27,57]

THE FLUID ENVIRONMENT IN THE EPIDIDYMIS

The fluid present in the cauda epididymidis is remarkable for a high K^+/Na^+ ratio and a low ionic strength, the osmolarity of the medium being made up with a wide range of organic substances.[5,45] This fluid is derived by the absorption of both water and other materials from the rete testis fluid, which occurs principally in the efferent ducts and caput epididymidis, and by the secretion of substances into the lumen.[31] Leaving aside proteins, some of which have been mentioned above, some of the more interesting substances to be secreted are carnitine, glycerylphosphorylcholine, phosphorylcholine, and inositol. Carnitine attains 60 mM in the cauda epididymal plasma of the rat, a concentration of 2000X greater than in blood plasma.[5] The epididymis is unable to synthesize carnitine, and it is taken up by a stereospecific active transport system.[80] The greatest increase in carnitine concentration occurs in the distal caput and corpus epididymidis.[5] Glycerylphosphorylcholine also begins to accumulate in the distal caput epididymidis and reaches a maximum concentration of about 40 mM. It is synthesized in the epithelium from precursors in blood lipoproteins.[5] Phosphorylcholine arises by the hydrolysis of glycerylphosphorylcholine. The greatest increment in inositol concentration occurs in the proximal cauda epididymidis, where it may be synthesized by the epithelium.[5] The epididymis also will concentrate the drug para-aminohippuric acid, which may reflect similarities between the epididymis and the renal tubules associated with their common embryonic origin.[78]

DIRECTING MALE CONTRACEPTIVE ACTION TOWARD DEVELOPING SPERMATOZOA

OPPORTUNITIES FOR SELECTIVE ACTION

Spermatozoa have features that are unique when compared with those of other cells. These include enzymes and other proteins, which may provide potential drug receptors not found elsewhere in the body and so allow a totally selective action on spermatozoa. Some of the unusual metabolic features of spermatozoa could assist in this. Some special proteins appear at a stage as early as the pachytene spermatocytes, and so it is possible to consider a selective attack on spermatids as well as on spermatozoa. Both spermatids and spermatozoa exist in isolated body compartments, and the composition of the fluid in these compartments is regulated carefully by the cells surrounding them. A drug could be concentrated into the ducts or cleared more slowly from these compartments than from the body as a whole, so that the spermatozoa would be exposed to it to a greater extent than would other cells. Spermatozoa are also unable to turn over their proteins to a significant extent, so that damaged enzyme molecules would not be replaced.

ADVANTAGES OF AN ACTION ON SPERMATIDS OR ON SPERMATOZOA

A chemical attack on mature spermatozoa and late-stage germ cells should minimize the risk of damage to the genetic material because cell divisions are complete and the DNA is in a highly condensed state. Spermatozoa damaged in the epididymis will be expelled from the body by the muscular contractions of the walls of the duct.[45] The Sertoli cell should be able to dispose of damaged spermatids by phagocytosis.

An attack during spermiogenesis or later ensures a more rapid action than an attack at an earlier stage and would require only short periods of treatment before unprotected intercourse became safe.

Interruption of the normal function of the Sertoli cells or the principal cells could be a route to a contraceptive action. In our view, however, a complete and reversible action can be achieved best by direct action on spermatozoa or spermatids because they could be irreversibly disabled without affecting the prospects of reversing the antifertility effect. If the "supporting" cells were

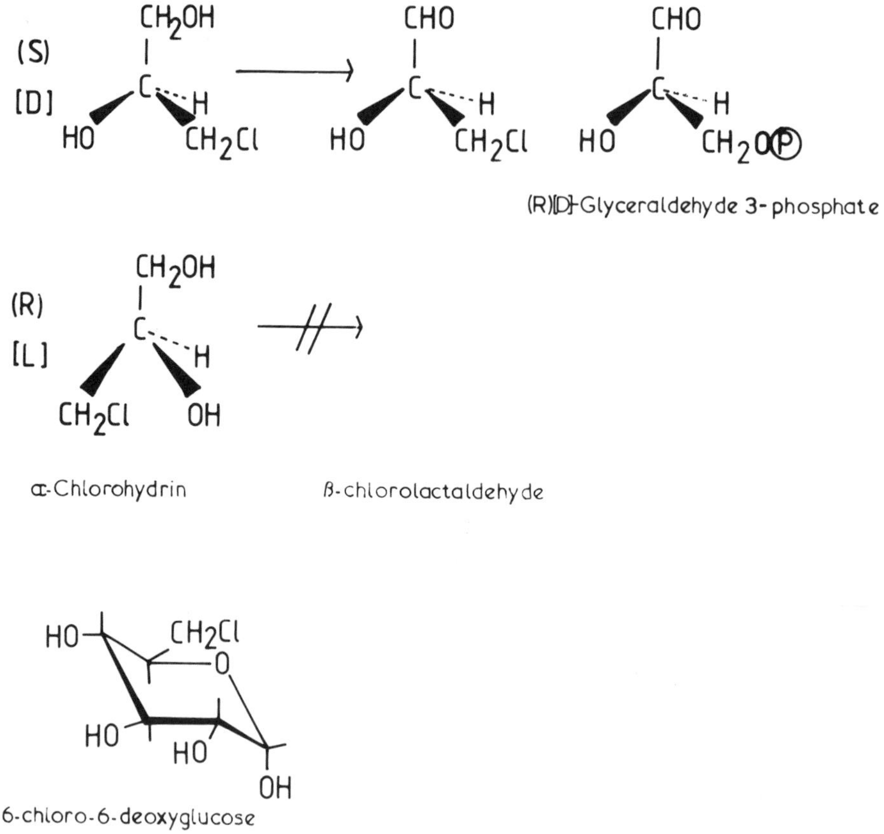

(R)[D]-Glyceraldehyde 3-phosphate

α-Chlorohydrin   β-chlorolactaldehyde

6-chloro-6-deoxyglucose

FIG. 10-3. The structures of α-chlorohydrin and 6-chloro-6-deoxyglucose and the analogy between the structures of S-β-chlorolactaldehyde and R-glyceraldehyde 3-phosphate.

affected, it would be necessary to compromise between a complete effect, which might then be irreversible, and a reversible effect, which might not be complete.

The mode of action of several male contraceptive compounds that are believed to act on spermatids or on epididymal spermatozoa will be discussed to illustrate the concepts described above.

α-CHLOROHYDRIN AND THE 6-CHLORO-6-DEOXYSUGARS

BIOLOGICAL ACTIVITY

Male animals treated daily with a suitable oral dose of one of these compounds (Fig. 10-3) become infertile within 1 week and recover their fertility about 2 weeks after treatment is withdrawn. Subcontraceptive doses may decrease the size of the litters sired by the treated males (Table 10-1).[20,42] α-Chlorohydrin

TABLE 10-1. The Effect of 6,6'-Dichloro-6,6'-Dideoxysucrose on the Fertility of Male Rats*

TREATMENT	WEEKS SINCE FIRST (FINAL) DOSE	IMPLANTATIONS PER FEMALE (INCLUDING RESORBING EMBRYOS)	AVERAGE CONCEPTION RATE (%)†
Control	1	17.3	86
(water 1 ml/kg/day)	2	15.32	89
	3	10.9	69
	7 (3)	13.8	91
	10 (6)	15.0	97
6,6'-Dichloro-6-6'-dideoxysucrose	1	5.2	27
(120 µmol/kg/day)	2	5.4	32
	3	8.3	
	7 (3)	9.5	56
	10 (6)	14.0	93
6,6'-Dichloro-6-6'-dideoxysucrose	1	0.3	0.3
(240 µmol/kg/day)	2	0	0
	3	0.9	4.7
	7 (3)	12.3	70
	10 (6)	13.8	95

* Treated daily for 28 days and paired with a fresh virgin female for 7 days at the end of the weeks indicated.

† Implantations/corpora lutea ×100

is effective in rats, hamsters, guinea pigs, gerbils, dogs, rams, boars, and rhesus monkeys, and the 6-chloro-6-deoxysugars were effective in rats and marmoset monkeys. Neither class of compounds was effective in mice or rabbits. Commercial α-chlorohydrin is a racemic mixture and the S-enantiomer is responsible for the antifertility effect. Many of its side-effects, notably its effect on the rat kidney, may depend on the R-enantiomer.[42] All experiments with the 6-chloro-6-deoxysugars have been done with pure D sugars. Unfortunately, high doses of S-α-chlorohydrin or of 6-chloro-6-deoxysugars are neurotoxic in mice or marmoset monkeys, precluding their development for use by humans.[20] High doses also induce spermatocoele formation in the efferent ducts of the rat, leading to permanent sterility,[20] but these compounds remain the best example of how a selective post-testicular effect on spermatozoa may be achieved.

BIOCHEMICAL EFFECT ON SPERMATOZOA

Spermatozoa taken from rats or rams treated with α-chlorohydrin or with 6-chloro-6-deoxysugars are unable to metabolize glucose or other sugars through the glycolytic pathway.[20,42] Low concentrations (≤1 mM) of α-chlorohydrin but not of 6-chloro-6-deoxysugars will inhibit glycolysis in spermatozoa in vitro. The ability of the spermatozoa to oxidize other substrates is not impaired. The decreased rate of glycolysis depends on the inhibition of glyceraldehyde 3-phosphate dehydrogenase; triose phosphate dehydrogenase also is inhibited, but this is probably less significant. Glyceraldehyde 3-phosphate dehydrogenase in other tissues is unaffected.[20]

Spermatozoa inhibited by α-chlorohydrin may be infertile because they are unable to obtain energy from sugar metabolism. Thus, in incubations with 2 mM-glucose, the ATP concentration in and the motility of spermatozoa from rats treated with α-chlorohydrin were the same as in control spermatozoa when they were measured immediately after the spermatozoa were removed from the epididymis, but declined more rapidly during subsequent incubations.[25] Spermatozoa from rats treated with 6-chloro-6-deoxyglucose rapidly became immotile, with a low energy charge, when they were incubated with glucose but survived quite well and maintained their energy charge when pyruvate plus lactate was given as the substrate.[21] Ram spermatozoa incubated with 1 mM-α-chlorohydrin remained motile, with a high energy charge, unless glucose was present when there was a rapid decline in motility with a concomitant conversion of ATP to AMP (Fig. 10-4).[24] Thus, as well as blocking the normal pathway of glucose utilization, α-chlorohydrin causes the sperm to dissipate ATP in the presence of glucose.

The decrease in ATP concentration is paralleled by the accumulation of large concentrations of glycolytic intermediates (Fig. 10-5).[23] Although it is possible that the lost ATP is consumed in the production of sugar phosphates or that the high concentrations of these intermediates are cytotoxic, it is more likely that they increase the rate of futile substrate cycling in the glycolytic pathway.[24] Alternatively, the intracellular pool of inorganic phosphate could be depleted to a critically low level by the formation of glycolytic intermediates.

FORMATION OF AN ACTIVE METABOLITE

Although α-chlorohydrin will inhibit glycolysis in spermatozoa incubated with it in vitro, it will not inhibit glyceraldehyde 3-phosphate dehydrogenase extracted from spermatozoa,[42] and it is probable that α-chlorohydrin is converted to an active metabolite by the spermatozoa. Rat and boar spermatozoa metabolize S-α-chlorohydrin to S-β-chlorolactaldehyde and β-chlorolactate. S-β-chlorolactaldehyde has the same configuration as does R-glyceraldehyde 3-phosphate, the substrate for glyceraldehyde 3-phosphate dehydrogenase (see Fig. 10-3).[42] Rabbit spermatozoa are unaffected by α-chlorohydrin and did not metabolize it to β-chlorolactaldehyde, but β-chlorolactaldehyde did inhibit glyceraldehyde 3-phosphate dehydrogenase in rabbit spermatozoa. Glycerol can protect spermatozoa against inhibition by α-chlorohydrin and

$\longrightarrow$

FIG. 10-4. The concentrations of ATP (■), ADP (▨) and AMP (▩), the energy charge (ATP + $\frac{1}{2}$ADP)/(ATP + ADP + AMP) (□), and the motility (▲) of ram cauda epididymal spermatozoa incubated for 10 minutes at 34°C with 1 mM-α-chlorohydrin or without it (controls) before the addition of various substrates and incubation for a further 4 hours at 34°C.

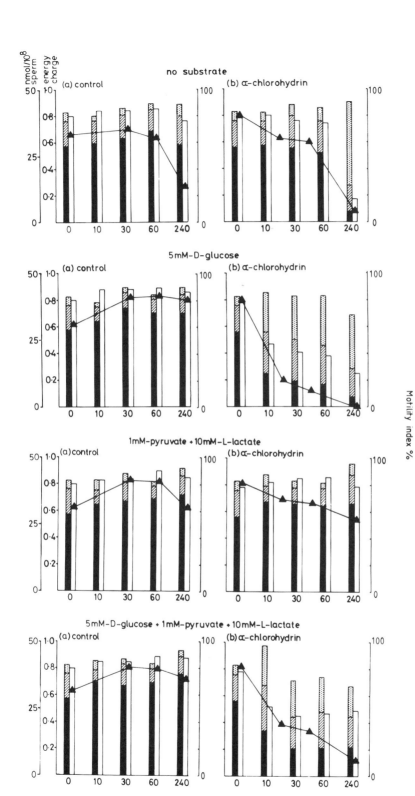

no substrate

(a) control (b) α-chlorohydrin

5mM-D-glucose

(a) control (b) α-chlorohydrin

1mM-pyruvate + 10mM-L-lactate

(a) control (b) α-chlorohydrin

5mM-D-glucose + 1mM-pyruvate + 10mM-L-lactate

(a) control (b) α-chlorohydrin

Time (min)

Motility index %

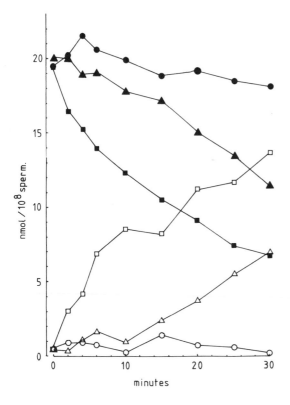

FIG. 10-5. The concentration of ATP (●▲■) and of fructose 1,6-bisphosphate plus glyceraldehyde 3-phosphate plus dihydroxyacetone phosphate (○△□) in boar spermatozoa incubated at 34° C with 0 (○●), 0.05 (△▲), or 1.0 (□■) mM-α-chlorohydrin for 10 minutes before the addition of 0.1 mM-D glucose (0 minutes on abscissa) and further incubation for 30 minutes.

(y-axis label: nmol / 10^8 sperm.; x-axis label: minutes)

also prevent its oxidation to β-chlorolactaldehyde. It was proposed that the oxidation is catalyzed by a NADP-linked glycerol dehydrogenase.[42]

The 6-chloro-6-deoxysugars also could be metabolized to β-chlorolactaldehyde by known pathways, but some of the steps involved must take place elsewhere in the body because these compounds do not affect spermatozoa in vitro.[20]

ACCUMULATION OF THE ANTIFERTILITY AGENT IN THE EPIDIDYMIS

When α-chlorohydrin labeled with ^{14}C was given to rats, radioactivity accumulated in the epididymis but radioactivity from [^{36}Cl] α-chlorohydrin did not. No ^{14}C radioactivity accumulated in the mouse epididymis.[20] In rats, hamsters, and guinea pigs treated with α-chlorohydrin or with 6-chloro-6-deoxyglucose, glyceraldehyde 3-phosphate dehydrogenase was inhibited to a greater extent in spermatozoa from the cauda than in those from the caput or corpus epididymidis. If the antifertility agent entered the duct by simple diffusion, then it would be expected to reach a higher concentration in the caput than in the cauda region because the former has a higher blood flow and is also supplied by means of the rete testis fluid. Thus, it is probable that the agent is actively accumulated in the cauda epididymidis.[22]

The specificity of α-chlorohydrin for spermatozoa depends on a number of factors that might be exploitable with other drugs: 1) the presence of a susceptible form of glyceraldehyde-3-phosphate dehydrogenase; 2) the potential for

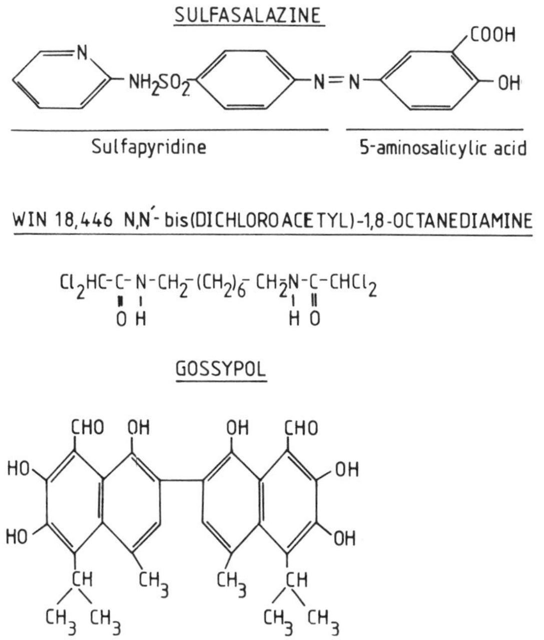

SULFASALAZINE

Sulfapyridine   5-aminosalicylic acid

WIN 18,446 N,N´-bis(DICHLOROACETYL)-1,8-OCTANEDIAMINE

GOSSYPOL

FIG. 10-6. The structures of the male contraceptives: Sulfasalazine, WIN18,446, and gossypol.

futile substrate cycling; 3) the ability to convert α-chlorohydrin and an unknown product derived from the 6-chloro-6-deoxysugars to an active metabolite (probably β-chlorolactaldehyde); 4) the accumulation of the antifertility agent or a close precursor by the cauda epididymidis.

SULFASALAZINE

Sulfasalazine (Fig. 10-6) has been used for decades to control ulcerative colitis, but in the last 5 years investigators have recognized that it can induce infertility in men, producing a diminished sperm count, impaired sperm motility, and an increased proportion of abnormal sperm in ejaculates. The contraceptive effect is reversible.[44] The antifertility action is produced by the sulfapyridine portion of the sulfasalazine molecule because 1) sulfapyridine but not 5-aminosalicylic acid could decrease the fertility of male rats;[44] 2) men treated with 5-aminosalicylic acid did not become infertile.[10]

The mode of action of sulfasalazine as a male contraceptive is unknown. It produced infertility in male rats about 3 weeks from the start of treatment and the rats recovered their fertility 2 to 3 weeks after the drug was withdrawn.[44] It therefore must affect epididymal spermatozoa or late-stage spermatids. In the rat, sulfasalazine does not affect the number of spermatozoa present in the cauda epididymidis, their motility, the ATP concentration in the cells, or the ability to metabolize [U¹⁴C] glucose,* and most sulfonamides are nontoxic to sperm.[45] In humans, mice, and hamsters, spermatozoa from treated subjects

---

* O'Morain C, Ford WCL, Harrison A: Unpublished data, 1985.

performed badly in the denuded hamster egg penetration test, and in the laboratory animals the acrosome reaction was blocked.[54] Semen from men taking sulfasalazine contained a higher than normal proportion of spermatozoa with large heads.[39] Both of these observations might be explained if sulphasalazine produced a lesion in the maturation of the sperm head at a late stage of spermiogenesis.

Sulfasalazine exhibits the rapid onset of and recovery from infertility that is expected of a drug attacking spermatids or spermatozoa, and is of considerable interest because of its long history of clinical use and the possibility that other sulfonamides may have contraceptive properties.

BIS-(DICHLOROACETYL) DIAMINES

These compounds were introduced as amebicides, but they soon were discovered to have a male antifertility effect. The most active was N,N'-*bis* (dichloroacetyl)-1,8-octanediamine (WIN 18,446, Fig. 10-6). In men, azoospermia was achieved 8 to 11 weeks after starting treatment and was fully reversible, but trials were abandoned when a strong Antabuse-like effect with alcohol was revealed. Treatment of rats with WIN 18,446 led to a progressive loss of germ cells and decline in testicular weight but spermatids were the earliest cells to be affected.[45,56,63] In the guinea pig, spermatids were the first cells to be affected, and the drug interfered with the development of the acrosome and the condensation of the nucleus. Two to 3 weeks later, spermatocytes became damaged and vacuoles appeared in Sertoli cells.[19] A decade has elapsed since the diamines were actively investigated and the biochemical basis of their effect on spermatids was never elucidated convincingly. Now that methods are available for the separation and culture of many testicular cell types, these compounds should be reexamined in the hope that an understanding of their mode of action will reveal ways in which a selective contraceptive action on spermatids could be attained.

GOSSYPOL

Gossypol (see Fig. 10-6) has a number of effects on the energy metabolism of spermatozoa (*e.g.,* inhibition of glycolysis and motility[65,77] and uncoupling of oxidative phosphorylation[69]). Most authors believe its primary action is on spermatids and pachytene spermatocytes,[58] and this may result from the great sensitivity of these cells to the interruption of their energy supply.[28]

CONCLUSIONS

The examples described demonstrate that it is possible to achieve a reversible male contraceptive action by an effect on spermatids or on epididymal spermatozoa. α-Chlorohydrin, the 6-chloro-6-deoxysugars, and sulfasalazine exemplify the rapid onset of and recovery from infertility that should be a feature of this site of action. On the other hand, the recovery is not so fast that missed doses would result in unwanted pregnancies.

All of these compounds have undesirable side-effects that will prevent them from being freely used by men worldwide. The specificity of male contraceptive compounds for their target cells must be increased. The improvement of our knowledge of the unique biologic features of spermatozoa and of the differentiation and development of these cells will help to achieve this. The perturbation of normal function by existing contraceptive agents could be a valuable tool to illuminate these processes and also will help to develop our concepts of how a specific antifertility effect can be achieved.

REFERENCES

1. BEDFORD JM: Fertilization. In AUSTIN CR, SHORT RV (eds): Germ Cells and Fertilization, pp 128–163. Cambridge, Cambridge University Press, 1982
2. BELLVE AR, MOSS SB: Monoclonal antibodies as probes of reproductive mechanisms. Biol Reprod 28:1, 1983
3. BELLVE AR, O'BRIEN DA: The mammalian spermatozoon: Structure and temporal assembly. In HARTMAN JF (ed): Mechanism and Control of Animal Fertilization, pp 55–137. New York, Academic Press, 1983
4. BOUCHARD P, GAGNON C, BARDIN CW: Protein carboxymethylase in rat testes and spermatozoa. In STEINBERGER A, STEINBERGER E (eds): Testicular Development, Structure and Function, pp 441–446. New York, Raven Press, 1980
5. BROOKS DE: Epididymal functions and their hormonal regulation. Aust J Biol Sci 36:205, 1983
6. BROOKS DE, HAMILTON DW, MALLEK AM: Carnitine and glycerylphosphorylcholine in the reproductive tract of the male rat. J Reprod Fertil 36:141, 1974
7. BROOKS DE, TIVER K: Analysis of surface proteins of rat spermatozoa during epididymal transit and identification of antigens common to spermatozoa, rete testis fluid and cauda epididymal plasma. J Reprod Fertil 71:249, 1984
8. BUEHR M, MCLAREN A: An electrophoretically detectable modification of glucose phosphate isomerase in mouse spermatozoa. J Reprod Fertil 63:169, 1981
9. CALVIN J, TUBBS PK: Mitochondrial transport processes and oxidation of NADH by hypotonically treated boar spermatozoa. Eur J Biochem 89:315, 1978
10. CANN PA, HOLDSWORTH CD: Reversal of male infertility on changing treatment from sulphasalazine to 5-aminosalicylic acid (letter). Lancet i:1119, 1984
11. CASILLAS ER, ERICKSON BJ: The role of carnitine in spermatozoon metabolism: Substrate-induced elevations in the acetylation state of carnitine and coenzyme A in bovine and monkey spermatozoa. Biol Reprod 12:275, 1975
12. CHULAVATNATOL M, YINDEPIT S: Changes in surface ATPase of rat spermatozoa in transit from the caput to the cauda epididymidis. J Reprod Fertil 48:91, 1976
13. DACHEUX JL, PAQUIGNON M: Relations between the fertilizing ability, motility and metabolism of epididymal spermatozoa. Reprod Nutr Devel 20:1085, 1980
14. DE KRETSER DM: Sertoli cell–Leydig cell interaction in the regulation of testicular function. Int J Androl (Suppl) 5:11, 1981
15. DISTEL RJ, KLEENE KC, HECHT NB: Haploid expression of a mouse testis α-tubulin gene, Science 224:68, 1984
16. EDWARDS YH, GROOTEGOED JA: A sperm-specific enolase. J Reprod Fertil 68:305, 1983
17. EGBUNIKE GN: Changes in the acetylcholinesterase activity of mammalian spermatozoa during maturation. Int J Androl 3:459, 1980
18. FAWCETT DW: Ultrastructure and function of the Sertoli cell. In HAMILTON DW, GREEP RO (eds): Handbook of Physiology, Section 7, Vol 5, The Male Reproductive System, pp 21–55. Washington, American Physiology Society, 1975
19. FLORES MN, FAWCETT DW: Ultrastructural effects of the antispermatogenic compound WIN-18446 (*bis*-dichloroacetyl diamine) (abstr). Anat Rec 172:310, 1972
20. FORD WCL: The mode of action of 6-chloro-6-deoxysugars as antifertility agents in the male. Curr Topics Reprod Endocrinol 2:159, 1982
21. FORD WCL, HARRISON A: The effect of 6-chloro-6-deoxysugars on adenine nucleotide concentrations in and the motility of rat spermatozoa. J Reprod Fertil 63:75, 1981

22. FORD WCL, HARRISON A: The activity of glyceraldehyde 3-phosphate dehydrogenase in spermatozoa from different regions of the epididymis in laboratory rodents treated with α-chlorohydrin or 6-chloro-6-deoxyglucose. J Reprod Fertil 69:147, 1983

23. FORD WCL, HARRISON A: Low concentrations of glucose precipitate a rapid dephosphorylation of ATP in ram spermatozoa exposed to α-chlorohydrin. Biochem Soc Trans 12:691, 1984

24. FORD WCL, HARRISON A: The presence of glucose enhances the lethal effect of α-chlorohydrin on ram and boar spermatozoa *in vitro*. J Reprod Fertil 73:197, 1985

25. FORD WCL, WAITES GMH: Chlorinated sugars: A biochemical approach to the control of male fertility. Int J Androl (Suppl) 2:541, 1978

26. FRENKEL G, PETERSON RN, FREUND M: Changes in the metabolism of guinea pig sperm from different segments of the epididymis. Proc Soc Exp Biol Med 143:1231, 1973

27. GAGNON C, HARBOUR D, DECHAMIRANDE E, BARDIN CW, DACHEUX JL: Sensitive assay detects protein methylesterase in spermatozoa: Decrease in enzyme activity during epididymal maturation. Biol Reprod 30:953, 1984

28. GROOTEGOED JA, JANSEN R, VAN DER MOLEN HJ: The role of glucose pyruvate and lactate in ATP production by rat spermatocytes and spermatids. Biochim Biophys Acta 767:248, 1984

29. GROOTEGOED JA, JUTTE NHPM, JANSEN R, HEUSDENS FA, ROMMERTS FFG, VAN DER MOLEN HJ: Biochemistry of spermatogenesis: The supporting role of Sertoli cells. In VAN DER MOLEN HJ et al (eds): Hormonal Factors in Fertility, Infertility and Contraception, pp 169–183. Amsterdam, Excerpta Medica, 1981

30. GROOTEGOED AJ, KRUGER-SEWNARIAN BC, JUTTE NHPM, ROMMERTS FFG, VAN DER MOLEN HJ: Fucosylation of glycoproteins in rat spermatocytes and spermatids. Gamete Res 5:303, 1982

31. HAMILTON DW: Structure and function of the epithelium lining the ductuli efferentes, ductus epididymidis and ductus deferens in the rat. In HAMILTON DW, GREEP RO (eds): Handbook of Physiology, Section 7, Vol 5, Male Reproductive System, pp 259–301. Washington, American Physiology Society, 1975

32. HAMMERSTEDT RH: Tritium release from [2-³H] D-glucose as a monitor of glucose consumption by bovine sperm. Biol Reprod 12:545, 1975

33. HAMMERSTEDT RH, HAY SR, AMANN RP: Modification of ram sperm membranes during epididymal transit. Biol Reprod 27:745, 1982

34. HAMMERSTEDT RH, LARDY HA: The effect of substrate cycling on the ATP yield of sperm glycolysis. J Biol Chem 258:8759, 1983

35. HIIPAKKA RA, HAMMERSTEDT RH: Changes in 2-deoxyglucose transport during epididymal maturation of ram sperm. Biol Reprod 19:1030, 1978

36. HOFFER AP, HINTON BT: Morphological evidence for a blood epididymis barrier and the effects of gossypol on its integrity. Biol Reprod 30:991, 1984

37. HOLT WV: Membrane heterogeneity in the mammalian spermatozoon. Int Rev Cytol 87:159, 1984

38. HOSKINS DD, BRANT H, ACOTT TS: Initiation of sperm motility in the mammalian epididymis. Fed Proc 37:2534, 1978

39. HUDSON E, DORE C, SOWTER C, TOOVEY S, LEVI AJ: Sperm size in patients with inflammatory bowel disease on sulphasalazine therapy. Fertil Steril 38:77, 1982

40. INSKEEP PB, HAMMERSTEDT RH: Changes in metabolism of ram sperm associated with epididymal transit or induced by exogenous carnitine. Biol Reprod 27:735, 1982

41. ISAHAKIA M, ALEXANDER NJ: Interspecies cross-reactivity of monoclonal antibodies directed against human sperm antigens. Biol Reprod 30:1015, 1984

42. JONES R: Antifertility actions of α-chlorohydrin in the male. Aust J Biol Sci 36:333, 1983

43. KIERSZENBAUM AL, TRES LL: RNA transcription and chromatin structure during meiotic and postmeiotic stages of spermatogenesis. Fed Proc 37:2512, 1977

44. LEVI AJ, TOOVEY S, SMETHURST P, ANDREWS B: Sulphasalazine and male infertility. Curr Top Reprod Endocrinol 2:209, 1982

45. MANN T, LUTWAK-MANN C: Male Reproductive Function and Semen. Berlin, Springer–Verlag, 1981

46. MEISTRICH ML, BROCK WA, GRIMES SR, PLATZ RD, HNILICA LS: Nuclear protein transitions during spermatogenesis. Fed Proc 37:2522, 1977

47. MEISTRICH ML, TROSTLE PK, FRAPART M, ERICKSON RP: Biosynthesis and localisation of lactate dehydrogenase-X in pachytene spermatocytes and spermatids of mouse testes. Dev Biol 60:428, 1977

48. MILLETTE CF, BELLVE AR: Temporal expression of membrane antigens during mouse spermatogenesis. J Cell Biol 74:86, 1977

49. MILLETTE CF, BELLVE AR: Selective partitioning of plasma membrane antigens during mouse spermatogenesis. Dev Biol 79:309, 1980

50. MOHRI H, YANAGAMACHI R: Characteristics of motor apparatus in testicular, epididymal and ejaculated spermatozoa. Exp Cell Res 127:191, 1980

51. MOORE HDM, HARTMAN TD, PRYOR JP: Development of the oocyte-penetrating capacity of spermatozoa in the human epididymis. Int J Androl 6:310, 1983

52. NAKAMURA M, HINO A, KATO J: Stimulation of protein synthesis in round spermatids from rat testis by lactate. 2. Role of ATP. J Biochem 90:933, 1981

53. O'BRIEN DA, BELLVE AR: Protein constituents of the mouse spermatozoon. II. Temporal synthesis during spermatogenesis. Dev Biol 75:405, 1980

54. O'MORAIN CA, SMETHURST P, HUDSON E, LEVI AJ: Further studies on sulphasalazine induced male infertility (abstr). Gastroenterology 82:1140, 1982

55. OKUMURA K, LEE IP, DIXON RL: Permeability of selected drugs and chemicals across the blood testis barrier of the rat. J Pharmacol Exp Ther 194:89, 1975

56. PATANELLI DJ: Suppression of fertility in the male. In HAMILTON DW, GREEP RO (eds): Handbook of Physiology, Section 7, Vol 5. Male Reproductive System, pp 245–258. Washington, American Physiology Society, 1975

57. PURVIS K, CUSAN L, ATTRAMADAL H, EGE A, HANSSON V: Rat sperm enzymes during epididymal transit. J Reprod Fertil 65:381, 1982

58. QIAN SZ, WANG ZG: Gossypol: A potential antifertility agent for males. Ann Rev Pharmacol Toxicol 24:329, 1984

59. ROBINSON R, FRITZ IB: Metabolism of glucose by Sertoli cells in culture. Biol Reprod 24:1032, 1981

60. ROOSEN-RUNGE EC: The process of spermatogenesis in mammals. Biol Rev 37:343, 1962

61. RUSSELL LD: Sertoli-germ cell interactions: A review. Gamete Res 3:179, 1980

62. SALING PM: Development of the ability to bind to zona pellucidae during epididymal maturation: Reversible immobilization of mouse spermatozoa by lanthanum. Biol Reprod 26:429, 1982

63. SETCHELL BP: The Mammalian Testis. London, Paul Elek, 1978

64. SETCHELL BP, WAITES GMH: The blood–testis barrier. In HAMILTON DW, GREEP RO (eds): Handbook of Physiology, Section 7, Vol 5. The Male Reproductive System, pp 143–172. Washington, American Physiology Society, 1975

65. STEPHENS DT, CRITCHLOW LM, HOSKINS DD: Mechanism of inhibition by gossypol of glycolysis and motility of monkey spermatozoa *in vitro*. J Reprod Fertil 69:447, 1983

66. TASH JS, MEANS AR: Cyclic adenosine 3'5' monophosphate: Calcium and protein phosphorylation in flagellar motility. Biol Reprod 28:75, 1983

67. TERNER C, MACLAUGHLIN J, SMITH BR: Changes in lipase and phosphatase activities of rat spermatozoa in transit from the caput to the cauda epididymidis. J Reprod Fertil 45:1, 1975

68. TREETIPSATIT N, CHULAVATNATOL M: Effect of ATP, cAMP, and pH on the initiation of flagellar movement in demembranated models of rat epididymal spermatozoa. Exp Cell Res 142:495, 1982

69. TSO WW, LEE CS: Effect of gossypol on boar spermatozoa *in vitro*. Arch Androl 7:85, 1981

70. TURKINGTON RW, MAJUMDER GG: Gene action during spermatogenesis. J Cell Physiol 85:495, 1975

71. VAN DER BERG JL, COOPER DW, CLOSE PJ: Testis specific phosphoglycerate kinase B in mouse. J Exp Zool 198:231, 1976

72. VAN-DOP C, HUTSON SM, LARDY HA: Pyruvate metabolism in bovine epididymal spermatozoa. J Biol Chem 252:1303, 1977

73. VOGLMAYR JK: Metabolic changes in sperm during epididymal transit. In HAMILTON DW, GREEP RO (eds): Handbook of Physiology, Section 7, Vol 5. Endocrinology, pp 437–451. Washington, American Physiology Society, 1975

74. WAITES GMH: Functional relationships of the mammalian testis and epididymis. Aust J Biol Sci 33:355, 1980

75. WAITES GMH: Sperm maturation and the epididymis: new targets. In ANAND-KUMAR TC, WAITES GMH (eds): Methods for the Regulation of Male Fertility, pp 107–118. Bombay, Indian Council of Medical Research, 1985

76. WAITES GMH, GLADWELL RT: Physiological significance of fluid secretion in the testis and blood testis barrier. Physiol Rev 62:624–671, 1982

77. WICHMANN K, KAPAYO K, SINERVIRTA R, JANNE J: Effect of gossypol on the motility and metabolism of human spermatozoa. J Reprod Fertil 69:259, 1983

78. WONG PYD: Active accumulation of para-aminohippuric acid by the rat epididymis. J Reprod Fertil 73:306, 1985

79. YEUNG CH: Effects of cAMP on the motility of mature and immature hamster epididymal spermatozoa studied by reactivation of the demembranated cells. Gamete Res 9:99, 1984

80. YEUNG CH, COOPER TG, WAITES GMH: Carnitine transport into the perfused epididymis of the rat: Regional differences, stereospecificity, stimulation by choline and the effect of other luminal factors. Biol Reprod 23:294, 1980

11

Discussion: Male Reproductive Physiology and Contraception

MODERATOR: R. JOHN AITKEN

WHEN SPERMATOGENESIS WAS SUPPRESSED WITH hCG ALONE, WAS THERE ANY DOWN REGULATION OF TESTOSTERONE LEVELS IN THE MEN STUDIED?

The testosterone levels increased from mean values of approximately 6 to means of approximately 10, and the estradiol levels increased significantly. It is open to question whether the testosterone levels would have been even higher if the estradiol levels had not risen, but down regulation, expressed as low testosterone levels, was not seen.

DID FSH STIMULATE TESTOSTERONE PRODUCTION?

Testosterone blood levels were measured carefully during the time follicle-stimulating hormone (FSH) was given. FSH had no effect on them or on luteinizing hormone (LH), as measured by bioactivity in the same specimens.

WERE SIDE-EFFECTS SEEN IN THE MEN WHO EXPERIENCED ELEVATED ESTRADIOL LEVELS WHILE THEIR SPERMATOGENESIS WAS SUPPRESSED WITH hCG?

Occasionally, in some of the earlier studies, a mild but palpable gynecomastia, similar to the symptoms reported by a fairly high percentage of normal men who are given hCG, occurred, but this was not seen in the present study. None of the men who were given testosterone at the same time they were given estradiol developed gynecomastia; possibly the testosterone had some antagonistic effect. No other side-effects were seen.

Panelists: Nancy J. Alexander, William J. Bremner, William C. L. Ford; *Discussants:* Shalender Bhasin, Larry M. Ewing, Erwin Goldberg, Douglas Huber, Ulrich A. Knuth, Eberhard Nieschlag, C. Alvin Paulsen, Sherman J. Silber, Jeffrey M. Spieler, Anna Steinberger, Emil Steinberger, Gerald I. Zatuchni

CAN TESTOSTERONE ENANTHATE BE GIVEN IN SUCH A WAY THAT IT WILL CONSISTENTLY CAUSE AZOOSPERMIA?

If testosterone enanthate could cause azoospermia successfully in a large number of men, it could provide a very simple form of contraception. Among normal men, however, only 30% to 50% have become azoospermic in most series under the conditions in which testosterone has been administered. Continuing research is aimed at increasing the percentage of men who become azoospermic with this approach.

In the present study, the investigators, once they had identified the 30% to 50% of men who became azoospermic with the testosterone enanthate, studied those men further to assess the effects of replacement.

No investigator has as yet looked at the effect of chronic low-dose administration of testosterone enanthate rather than the usual administration of testosterone enanthate or another ester, intramuscularly, every 2, 3, or 4 weeks.

PARFR investigators have developed a testosterone microcapsule that will produce low levels of testosterone in a zero-order release for at least 90 days following one injection. Whether that approach will increase the achievement of azoospermia remains to be seen.

WHAT IS THE MECHANISM BY WHICH LH REINITIATES SPERMATOGENESIS?

This is an important question. Testosterone is known to stimulate spermatogenesis. There are data that suggest that LH administration, as it was done in the present studies, leads to marked increases in intratesticular testosterone. This seems perplexing, unless one considers that peripheral testosterone administration, by "turning off" LH and FSH, leads to very low levels of intratesticular testosterone, so that despite the fact that testosterone is being administered, intratesticular testosterone is markedly suppressed when compared to normal. When hCG or LH is given again, it leads to increases in intratesticular testosterone. That may be the most important factor, but there may be other factors as well.

WHAT WOULD HAPPEN IF, DURING THE RECOVERY PERIOD, INSTEAD OF ADMINISTRATION OF hCG, FSH, OR LH, SUPPRESSION OF THE TESTOSTERONE ENANTHATE WERE SIMPLY DISCONTINUED?

The length of time until sperm counts begin to rise once again appears to be similar in either case, but a close comparison of sperm count recovery has not been done. The levels attained are different, of course. After suppression is stopped, sperm levels return to the control range, whereas when hCG or LH is given sperm levels reach the 30 or 40 million range, as described; so that the rapidity with which recovery occurs is probably similar, but the total quantitated amount is less.

Merely giving testosterone does not mean that the same levels and the same suppression are achieved in each subject. What probably happens is that by administering testosterone enanthate, we are unable to maintain a steady, suppressive effect, and when the levels drop, a small amount of LH, sufficient to increase the intratesticular testosterone, may enter the bloodstream. Possibly with the new developments of the slow-release testosterone, more will be learned about this question.

ARE THERE PROBLEMS OF REVERSIBILITY FOLLOWING SUPPRESSION OF SPERMATOGENESIS?

When suppressive treatment was withdrawn, the sperm count was found to be somewhat lower in those men in whom spermatogenesis had been suppressed for 9 months than it was in those men who had been treated for shorter periods. This finding is probably not of great significance, however, because there were only four or five men in each study and the counts were not dramatically different (*e.g.*, 20 versus 35 million per ml). All of the men in these studies, even those with low initial sperm counts, experienced a return to sperm counts generally comparable to what they had been prior to treatment when they were taken off all suppressive therapies.

Since 1949, infertile men have been treated with testosterone suppression and these men have apparently not had problems with return at least to pretreatment sperm levels, unless there was surgical intervention (*e.g.*, testicular biopsy with complications).

SHOULD WE CONCENTRATE RESEARCH EFFORTS ON PRODUCING EFFECTS ON SPERMATOZOA AT THE CELL–CELL LEVEL?

Although the sites of attack are reasonable and the idea of specificity is important, we may not have yet gained the understanding needed for these approaches to be effective. For example, the specificity of some of the sperm enzymes or isoenzymes is becoming well documented; however, the specificity is still not great enough. Gossypol was mentioned as an example of a compound that possibly affects the $LDH-C_4$ system. Part of its mechanism of suppressing spermatogenesis may be due to $LDH-C_4$; more likely, gossypol affects all NAD-dependent d-hydrogenases. Another example is α-chlorohydrin, which probably has a general metabolic poisoning effect; our specificity is not precise enough.

If we want to affect spermatogenesis, the spermatid stage would be an ideal place for interfering at a molecular level. We are beginning to learn, but we need to know more about what kind of specificity occurs after the first meiotic division, and about the interaction and the transport of materials between Sertoli cells and spermatids. Such questions are difficult to answer. Perhaps we should be gearing our attack at these levels, looking at the specificity of hormonal receptors and seeing if we could manipulate hormonal therapy on the basis of up- or down-regulation of receptors.

IS THERE A POSSIBLE ADVANTAGE TO AN IRREVERSIBLE CHEMICAL MALE CONTRACEPTIVE?

Yes. Although a reversible chemical contraceptive is desirable in those cultures in which vasectomy is unacceptable because of widespread fear of surgery, an irreversible chemical male contraceptive might provide an acceptable alternative to vasectomy.

WHAT WILL BE THE FIRST NEW METHOD OF MALE CONTRACEPTION?

It is well established that a great deal more money has been spent to study female reproduction than male reproduction. The first scientific society devoted to research on male fertility, the American Society for Andrology, was not started until 1975. The number of research articles being published every year on male reproduction is now rapidly increasing in relation to those on females, and we are acquiring more information and gaining a better understanding of basic male physiology.

The most likely developments probably will be some kind of barrier method, a new type of vasectomy approach, such as vas occlusion by a percutaneous approach, or some kind of vas valve (*e.g.,* the SHUG). Some type of steroid combination might be acceptable before we could do all the steps necessary for a contraceptive vaccine, simply because of the numerous safety studies that will have to be conducted prior to the initiation of the vaccine approach. This does not mean that a vaccine approach should not be attempted; it has tremendous possibilities for developing countries. Nonetheless, it will take a great deal of time before immunocontraception can be initiated, developed, and tested. Excluding surgical and nonsurgical sterilization, the next generation of male contraception is likely to be some kind of combination steroid.

IS THERE ROOM FOR A MALE CONTRACEPTIVE THAT IS PERHAPS LESS EFFECTIVE THAN VASECTOMY AND PERHAPS ALSO NOT FULLY REVERSIBLE?

Most surveys, at least from developing countries, show that of all couples accepting a contraceptive method at present, the majority do so to terminate childbearing. Therefore, although reversibility is important, it perhaps should not be an absolute factor barring other contraceptive developments.

There seems to be a tremendous gap between effectiveness of vasectomy and condoms, which are really the only available alternatives. Other methods that might be intermediate in terms of effectiveness, difficulty of delivery, and perhaps toxicity and side-effects, might be reasonable options for some men who for one reason or another cannot or will not accept vasectomy, so that in the spirit of making options and free choice available for people based on needs, values, and culture, there would be room perhaps for less effective methods than vasectomy that also were not fully reversible.

In thinking of developing a contraceptive vaccine, most investigators would probably think first of developing one that was safe, and even if it were not reversible, it would be very useful and it would produce less morbidity and mortality because surgical intervention was not required. Only subsequently would the investigators be concerned about reversibility.

ARE ANIMAL MODELS ADEQUATE FOR INVESTIGATING MALE CONTRACEPTION?

Animal models are not perfect, but they are the best substitute at present. If one were to look in any physiology textbook and circle everything that happens to human beings that does not happen to rats, there would be very few circles. In many ways, physiological and biochemical activities in animals are very similar to human beings, but there are always exceptions (*e.g.*, the best model for gossypol is man).

Assessment of
Sperm Function

12

Semen Analysis as a Tool in the Search for a Male Contraceptive

RUNE ELIASSON

In a research program on human male contraceptives that do not induce azoospermia or total immotility of the spermatozoa, there is a need for 1) analytic methods that can assess functional properties of the spermatozoa, and 2) knowledge about the relation between these properties and the potential fertility of the semen donor. In "routine" semen analysis for evaluation of men with a barren union, few of the tests can be classified as "functional," and correlation between predicted fertility and results of semen analysis is poor, particularly when only a few samples have been examined, the observation period has been short, and men with extremely poor semen (*e.g.*, azoospermia, total lack of acrosomes, immotile cilia syndrome, and severe tail defects in most spermatozoa) have been excluded.[1,2,10,11,17,21,31,32]

There are many reasons why it is difficult to predict fertility from the results of semen analysis. There is a poor correlation between the number of spermatozoa per milliliter of semen (or per ejaculate) and male fertility, because there are so many different reasons for a "low" count. Too few functional analyses have been developed and used under a variety of conditions, making establishing normal values for different groups of men difficult. Several research techniques cannot be used on humans without prior testing on animals, and too little is known about the relationship between specific semen qualities from different species to know what animal model to use as a relevant reference for problems related to human males. In addition, it is almost impossible to test the fertility of a human male objectively in a monogamous society (at least if such a testing involved more than a few men).

These special problems warrant serious attention if we are to design investigations that in the future will give us test models for effective research on potential male contraceptive drugs. Drug-induced changes in functions of the male reproductive organs are not only of interest from a contraceptive point of view but also in relation to andrologic pharmacology in general, however. It would be most unfortunate for the scientific development of andrology if all drug-induced effects on the male reproductive organs were discussed only in terms of fertility or infertility.[13,14,26,28,37]

In this chapter, methods and problems will be discussed in the light of this philosophy.

PRINCIPLES AND DEFINITIONS

From a sociologic point of view a man can be classified either as "father" or "fertility not known." A medical examination can result in a definite diagnosis of "sterile," for example, hypergonadotropic hypogonadism with azoospermia. The main problems come when we want to classify men as "fertile" or "infertile." In this presentation, a man who for more than 1 year lives in an involuntary barren union is classified as "infertile." For rational rather than scientific reasons, a man whose wife has recently (<4 mo) become pregnant is classified as "fertile" unless there are special reasons not to do so. It is important that a man is never classified in any of these groups on the basis of semen qualities. We cannot study the relation between semen qualities and male fertility if we at the same time use semen qualities to classify the men as fertile or infertile.

Classification of semen sample follows the same philosophy. The semen will not be referred to in terms of fertility, but only as being "within" or "outside of" the normal range for a relevant population of samples. The usual way of defining "normal range" is to give the 90% or 95% confidence limits.[27]

The man and his semen thus will be treated as separate entities. When we know normal ranges for specified semen variables in relation to different male populations, then, but not before, we may be able to assess on a statistical basis the fertility potential of a semen or its donor.

STANDARDIZATION

A scientific approach to such a difficult problem as the relation between human semen qualities and fertility will be unsuccessful if not *all* methods used for assessing the functions of the male genital organs fulfill modern requirements with regard to standardization, precision, accuracy, and reproducibility.

In clinical laboratory work related to chemistry or cytology of blood, urine, and most other body fluids, generally it is accepted that the procedures for collection and analysis must be strictly standardized if the results are to be used for an evaluation of cell or organ function(s). There is no reason to adopt other principles for semen analysis. If the time between ejaculations can influence the results, this variable must be standardized.

Research on potential reversible contraceptives for men will most likely be carried out over a long period on each man. Infections, vaccinations, allergic reactions, and many other factors can cause changes in the semen samples from a given person over such an observation period. To assess the results in relation to given treatment, controlled studies are necessary.[4,15,25,36]

COLLECTION OF SEMEN

The time between ejaculations influences the volume and number of spermatozoa. The capacity of the testes to produce spermatozoa (all men participating in an experimental study are assumed to have patent ducts) is reflected by the sperm output (here meaning total number of spermatozoa in the ejaculate). The secretory capacity of the various accessory genital glands is similarly reflected by the total content or activity of organ or cell-specific markers in the ejaculate. The time interval between ejaculations therefore must be known. For studies on potential contraceptive drugs, an abstinence period of 2 to 4 days seems suitable, provided reference values are obtained under similar conditions.

Masturbation is the only acceptable method of collection. The withdrawal technique (coitus interruptus) is unreliable because a part of the ejaculate can easily be lost and the spermidical acid fluid from the vagina may contaminate the semen sample. (Collection usually is not a major problem because men who cannot accept masturbation are unlikely to be volunteers in a research program for male chemical contraceptives.)

Laboratory personnel should make sure that plastic materials, which can come in contact with the semen, do not interfere with any of the variables under study.

EXAMINATION OF THE EJACULATE

MACROSCOPIC EXAMINATIONS

Liquefaction should be finished within 30 minutes. The functional significance of the coagulation–liquefaction process is not understood, but a reduced liquefaction can impede sperm motility and trap the spermatozoa. A slow or absent liquefaction usually indicates a prostatic dysfunction, but the occurrence of abnormal proteins from the seminal vesicles can give a similar effect. After liquefaction has taken place, the seminal plasma may still have a high viscosity, but this is a rare condition. Accurate measurement of viscosity of the seminal plasma is difficult; for clinical work it is described as decreased, normal, increased, and highly increased, respectively.

The *volume* should be measured in a graded centrifuge tube or by weighing the bottle used for collection. If the semen is transferred to a graded tube, liquefaction should be completed first.

The color of the semen should be recorded. An abnormal color can be because of chemicals excreted into the semen, or to pyospermia or hemospermia.

MICROSCOPIC EXAMINATION

Number

The sperm count depends on the time of abstinence and the size of the testes. In longitudinal studies on individual subjects, only the days of abstinence need to be controlled, but in studies including comparison of different groups of men, both factors should be known. The sperm count should therefore be expressed in terms of

$$\text{Millions} \times (\text{ml testicular volume})^{-1} \times (\text{days of abstinence})^{-1}$$

This unit is much more informative than is the number of spermatozoa per ejaculate.* Studies on 100 Swedish men whose wives were in early pregnancy showed that the normal range (95% confidence limits) for sperm output was $0.5 - 7$ millions $\times$ ml^{-1} $\times$ day^{-1}. In this study, the testicular size was assessed with orchidometers† according to Pader.[35] There is no reason to believe that the normal testicular size will be the same in different ethnic groups.[15,38]

Motility

Routine analysis of sperm motility is important. Motility should be assessed with regard to both the percentage of motile spermatozoa and the quality of the progressive motility. The latter is frequently expressed as a progressive motility score (*e.g.,* none, poor, medium, and good). Many laboratories express the motility with *one* score, for example, number of progressively motile spermatozoa in millions per ejaculate per ml semen. This method does not give information on the quality of motility. Another method is to multiply the percent motile spermatozoa with a motility score (*e.g.,* 60% $\times$ score 3 /3 = good/ = 180). This method is not scientifically correct because one cannot multiply a number representing a measurement (%) with a nominal number, which represents an ordering or ranking significance (poor, good). In addition, the index gives no real information because there are several combinations that can give the same value. Unfortunately, these two methods have won an acceptance that does not correspond to their value.

There are now objective methods for assessment of sperm motility, and they should be used whenever possible in research programs on male contraceptives.[34]

Viability

There are several supravital staining methods to differentiate between dead and live spermatozoa. Some of these methods are not useful for human cells, however (*e.g.,* 5% eosin + 10% nigrosin). The supravital staining technique should be used whenever it is important to establish if immotile spermatozoa are dead or alive.[4,10]

---

* From a functional point of view, the number of spermatozoa per milliliter of semen does not give any information of value. The semen volume (normal range 2 ml–5 ml) depends mainly on the secretory activity of two independent glands (prostate and seminal vesicles). The secretory functions of these two glands are not correlated to the spermatogenic activity in the testis. To give the ratio between two (or more) independent variables (ml per million spermatozoa or million spermatozoa per ml) does not give meaningful information as far as function is concerned.

† Remcat Trade AB, POB 5011, S-16205 Stockholm, Sweden.

Morphology

A spermatozoon has a head, a midpiece, and a tail. All three parts must be functionally normal for the spermatozoon to reach and fertilize the ovum in vivo. The common practice to present only the head forms should not be accepted in a research program on potential male contraceptives. A report on sperm morphology should specify the real percentage of defects in heads, midpieces, and tails, respectively. To do this, one can first divide the spermatozoa into two groups: normal and abnormal. The percent normal + the percent abnormal is 100. Each abnormal spermatozoon then should be specified with regard to all its defects (*e.g.*, amorphous head, too large a protoplasma droplet, too short a tail). The number of subgroups is limited only to what is possible to handle from a practical point. With the counters* available on the market today there is a limit of 10 to 15 subgroups, depending on the counter, but with computerized techniques the number of subgroups can be larger.[4,10]

There are reports on sperm morphology in which an abnormal spermatozoon has been classified by only one defect; that is, a spermatozoon with an abnormal tail is counted as such only if the head and midpiece are normal. With this classification the sum of percent normal + percent abnormal heads + percent abnormal midpieces + percent abnormal tails will be 100. For obvious reasons such figures cannot be used for any statistical evaluations, and the method must be rejected.

Another common way to present information on morphology is to give only the percent normal spermatozoa (sometimes only the percent oval heads of normal size). With such a presentation one neglects the fact that different types of abnormalities have different causes and can have different effects on the fertility potential. From the experience by veterinarians, bull or boar semen with more than 25% defective sperm tails is subfertile; if there are more than 50% defective sperm tails, the animal is regarded as sterile. In addition, for the human semen more than 25% defective sperm tails indicates subfertility.[5,10,39] A man with 50% normal spermatozoa and 40% tail defects therefore has a poor fertility prognosis, whereas a man with 50% normal spermatozoa and less than 10% defects in the midpiece and tail, respectively, has a better prognosis when such an assessment is done only in relation to sperm morphology. For these reasons, evaluation of sperm morphology should include the total picture and not only the normal spermatozoa.

With a "normal" spermatozoon the whole cell has a morphologic form that fulfills some defined criteria. We refer not to function but to shape.

Drugs, heat, and other stress factors can induce not only a decrease in sperm production but also an increase in the percent abnormal forms. In contrast to sperm count, sperm morphology is a stable variable for a healthy man, and an increase in the proportion of abnormal spermatozoa over a period is a clear warning that something has induced a dysfunction in the germinal epithelium. In the follow-up of men exposed to xenobiotic factors, sperm morphology can be a sensitive "dosimeter" if properly analyzed.[6,8,20,25,28,37]

---

* Analys Instrument AB S-11347 Stockholm, Sweden, for example.

Other Cellular Elements

The identification of the different cellular elements that can be present in semen frequently is difficult, and there is a need for more specific methods, for example, specific staining methods or monoclonal antibodies against components specific for only one type of cell.[4,29]

The occurrence of spermatocytes and/or spermatids in the semen is another sign of "stress" or germinal cell dysfunction. The quantitative assessment of these cells is therefore a semifunctional analysis, particularly if the number of "immature" forms are presented in relation to the number of spermatozoa.

The presence of leukocytes in the semen indicates an inflammatory reaction in the genital system, usually in the prostate or seminal vesicles. Leukocytes also are seen when the time of sexual abstinence is long (usually more than 10 days) and in response to allergic reactions, however. The absence of leukocytes does not exclude that the man has adnexitis.

The number of immature forms and leukocytes should be reported as total per ejaculate to allow a statistical evaluation and comparisons between laboratories. This has not been the case in the past, and for that reason no well-founded limits can be given for normal values.[4]

BIOCHEMICAL ANALYSES

SPERMATOZOA

The ejaculated spermatozoa are biochemically very complex cells, but in one way or another their chemical properties reflect the functional competence of the cells contributing to the semen. It is therefore a major challenge to identify properties reflecting the function of specific parts in the male reproductive system. Knowledge in this field is very limited.

Nuclear Chromatin Decondensation

When testicular spermatozoa are exposed to the detergent sodium dodecyl sulphate (SDS), the heads rapidly undergo nuclear chromatin decondensation (NCD). Ejaculated spermatozoa from all examined subhuman mammalian species are resistant under similar conditions. Ejaculated human spermatozoa respond in a most heterogeneous way, but on the average NCD is less pronounced in semen from "fertile" than from "infertile" men. The resistance to SDS develops in transit through the epididymis, and if a chemical compound induces a reduced resistance to SDS this would indicate an epididymal dysfunction.[22–24]

NCD in the presence of SDS is a very interesting test but cannot for the moment be regarded as unique for epididymal function. For example, NCD of human ejaculated spermatozoa is also related to the ratio of zinc to fructose in the seminal plasma. One possible explanation could be a relation between prostatitis (causing a low secretion of zinc) and epididymitis (causing a disturbed maturation of the spermatozoa), both of which could be subclinical or totally asymptomatic.[30] Other factors to consider are degenerative processes in the germinal epithelium[41] and incorporation of chemicals (*e.g.*, heavy metals) into the chromatin during spermatogenesis; these chemicals later could interact with the formation of S—S bridges. Factors secreted into the seminal plasma at the time of ejaculation likewise could interact with the spermatozoa and affect the stability (or instability) of the chromatin.

DNA Content or Compaction

During spermiogenesis there is a condensation of the DNA and also a change in the chemical and physical properties of the DNA–DNP complex that results in a decreased reactivity to the Feulgen–Schiff procedure and a decreased binding of intercalating fluorescent dyes like ethidium bromide and acriflavine. The fluorescence profile of the cells in an ejaculate sample can be obtained from analysis with microspectrophotofluorometry or flow cytometry.[18]

The technique has proven useful in monitoring the effects of mutagenic drugs in mice and in follow-up of patients with testicular carcinoma. Men taking sulphasalazine have a significant shift to the left in the DNA histograms, and there is also a clear difference between histograms for semen from fertile and infertile men, respectively.[7,16,18,19]

Lipids and Enzymes

The lipid composition of the sperm membranes and the occurrence or activity of acrosomal and other enzymes are variables that could reflect a biochemical maturation of the spermatozoa.[23,25] There are no reports on direct measurement of various lipids and/or enzymes in the spermatozoa, with reference to functional aspects of the male reproductive system.[9,27,37]

The resistance of membranes to lipid peroxidative attacks depends on their lipid composition, and measurements of the formation of lipid peroxides under standardized conditions could therefore give indirect information on the functional stability of the membranes. This methodologic approach has been applied by our group in studies on the in vitro effects of gossypol on spermatozoa from different species* but its usefulness for the study of in vivo effects of xenobiotic factors remains to be clarified.

Metabolism

Human spermatozoa have a very low oxygen consumption and the seminal plasma an unusually high oxygen consumption. Determination of the sperm respiration therefore requires that the sample is divided into two parts, one of which is centrifuged to obtain seminal plasma. From simultaneous measurements of the oxygen consumption in seminal plasma and whole semen, the respiration of the spermatozoa can be calculated and expressed as

$$Z_{O_2} = \mu l \text{ oxygen} \times 10^{-8} \text{ spermatozoa} \times \text{hour}^{-1}$$

---

* Eliasson R et al: Unpublished data, 1985.

The basal oxygen consumption is characteristic for a given man and may in longitudinal studies give information of importance with regard to xenobiotic factors. We recently noted that the spermatozoa in semen with biochemical signs of a germinal cell dysfunction (*i.e.*, high LDH-C_4 to sperm ratio) had a significantly higher oxygen consumption than do spermatozoa from semen with a normal LDH-C_4 to sperm ratio.[41]

Succinate is known to have an insignificant effect on sperm respiration when added to whole semen but can increase oxygen consumption with a factor of 2 to 8 if the membranes have been damaged (*e.g.*, by a detergent or by washing.)[26] The degree of succinate stimulation of sperm respiration in whole semen or under strictly standardized conditions could therefore be an indicator of membrane integrity, and as such be of interest in studies on potential male chemical contraceptives.

SEMINAL PLASMA

Biochemical analysis of the seminal plasma can give information on the secretory function of the organs contributing to this fluid, if organ- or cell-specific markers are known. The relative contribution from each organ is fairly constant in the healthy man but the variations between individuals are very large. Studies related to the function can therefore be meaningful only when the results are related to one organ or one cell type. To do this, one must use units that are relevant (*e.g.*, *zinc content* in the ejaculate is a marker of prostate function but *zinc concentration* [M] in seminal plasma is not). The lactate dehydrogenase isoenzyme C_4 (LDH-C_4) is specific for germinal cells after meiosis, and the relevant unit is therefore in relation to the number of spermatozoa (*e.g.*, nanokat/10^8 spermatozoa), but LDH-C_4 activity per ml seminal plasma (or per ejaculate) is not an informative variable.[12,40]

During emission and ejaculation, the organs contributing to the semen discharge their products in a strictly controlled way. If the ejaculate is collected in three or more fractions (split ejaculate), and each of the fractions is analyzed for organ-specific compounds, the emission pattern can be assessed. This technique opens a possibility to study the effect of drugs on the autonomic nerves regulating emission and to clarify the pattern of drug excretion into the seminal plasma. Information from the later type of study will assist in designing drugs with a desired excretion profile. Most of the available data have been obtained from experiments on animals with completely different accessory genital organs.[12,26]

Specific markers are known for the prostate (*e.g.*, zinc, citric acid, acid phosphatases, and some proteolytic enzymes), seminal vesicles (*e.g.*, fructose and prostaglandins), and epididymides (*e.g.*, free L-carnitine). It is important, however, to realize that each of these glandular systems is functionally multiglandular. The secretory function of an organ therefore cannot be fully assessed from analysis of only one marker. A semen sample can have a very low fructose content and still have a normal content of prostaglandins and vesicular proteins, or have a low zinc content but a normal value for the acid phosphatase activity.

The seminal plasma is regarded by most research workers as a transport fluid without any significance for male fertility. Studies on biochemical or functional properties of the spermatozoa have provided evidence that several variables can be directly affected, however—in a positive or negative way—by the fluids from the accessory genital organs. In principle, fluid from the seminal vesicles has a different effect than prostatic fluid, and this is the reason why there can be a correlation between sperm function and the zinc-to-fructose ratio.[3,23,24]

CONCLUSION

In searching for a contraceptive drug that will induce infertility by altering the fertilizing properties of the human spermatozoa, we will have little help from the methods used today in standard semen analysis, the only exception being motility evaluation. With more refined techniques for assessment of sperm morphology, as well as with function-oriented analyses such as determination of LDH-C_4, testing the nuclear chromatin decondensation, analysis of the DNA–DNP complex, assessment of the lipid peroxidation potential, testing sperm penetration (cervical mucus, and heterologous and homologous ova), and identification of membrane-specific proteins, to mention a few, we will be able to find new means to regulate male fertility, to understand causes of "unexplained infertility" (an interesting biological model for studies of new ways of inducing infertility), and to prevent unwanted side-effects of xenobiotic factors on male reproductive organs.

REFERENCES

1. AITKEN JR, BEST FSM, RICHARDSON DW, DJAHANBAKHCH O, MORTIMER D, TEMPELTON AA, LEES MM: An analysis of sperm function in cases of unexplained infertility: Conventional criteria, movement characteristics, and fertilizing capacity. Fertil Steril 38:212–221, 1982
2. AMANN RP: A critical review of methods for evaluation of spermatogenesis from seminal characteristics. J Androl 2:37–58, 1981
3. ARVER S: Studies on zinc and calcium in human seminal plasma. Acta Physiol Scand [Suppl] 507:1982
4. BELSEY MA, ELIASSON R, GALLEGOS AJ, MOGHISSI KS, PAULSEN CA, PRASAD MRN: Laboratory manual for the examination of human semen and semen-cervical mucus interaction. Singapore, Press Concern, 1980
5. BLOM E: The ultrastructure of some characteristic sperm defects and a proposal for a new classification of the bull spermiogram. Nord Vet Med 25:383–391, 1973
6. BROWN-WODDMAN PDC, POST EJ, GASS GC, WHITE IG: The effect of a single sauna exposure on spermatozoa. Arch Androl 12:9–15, 1984
7. CLAUSEN OPF, KIRKHUA B, ÅBYHOLM T: DNA flow cytometry of human ejaculates in the investigation of male infertility. Infertility 5:71–85, 1982
8. COSENTINO MJ, CHEY WY, TAKIHARA H, COCKETT AT: The effects of sulfasalazine on human male fertility potential and seminal prostaglandins. J Urol 132:682–686, 1984
9. DEL RIO AG, DE SANCHEZ LZ, SIRENA A: Evaluation of epididymal function through specific protein on spermatozoa. Arch Androl 12:195–196, 1984
10. ELIASSON R: Analysis of semen. In BURGER H, DE KRESTER D (eds): The Testis, pp 381–399. New York, Raven Press, 1981
11. ELIASSON R: Sperm Count and Fertility: Facts and myths. In FRAJESE G, HAFEZ ESE, CONTI C, FABBRINI A (eds): Oligozoospermia: Recent Progress in Andrology, pp 1–7. New York, Raven Press, 1981
12. ELIASSON R: Biochemical analysis of human semen. Int J Androl (Suppl) 5:109–119, 1982
13. ELIASSON R: Morphological and chemical methods of semen analysis as a means of quantitating damage to male reproductive function. In VOUK VB, SHEEHAN PJ (eds): Methods for Assessing the Effects of Chemicals on Reproductive Functions, pp 263–275. London, J Wiley & Sons, 1982
14. ELIASSON R: Clinical effects of chemicals on male reproduction. In DIXON RL (ed): Repro-

ductive Toxicology, Target Organ Toxicology Series, pp 161–172. New York, Raven Press, 1985
15. ELIASSON R, VIRJI N: LDH-C₄ in human seminal plasma and testicular function. II. Clinical aspects. Int J Androl 8:201–214, 1985
16. EVENSON DP, KLEIN FA, WHITMORE WF, MELAMED M: Flow cytometric evaluation of sperm from patients with testicular carcinoma. J Urology 132:1220–1225, 1984
17. FREISCHEM CW, KNUTH UA, LANGER K, SCHNEIDER HPG, NIESCHLAG E: The lack of discriminant seminal and endocrine variables in the partners of fertile and infertile women. Arch Gynecol 236:1–12, 1984
18. GLEDHILL BL, LAKE S, DEAN PN: Flow cytometry and sorting of sperm and other male germ cells. In MELAMED MR, MULLANEY PF, MENDELSOHN ML (eds): Flow Cytometry and Sorting, pp 471–484. New York, John Wiley & Sons, 1979
19. GOLDBERG SD, DEITCH AD, SCHEVCHUCK M, NAGLER H, DEVERE WHITE R: Comparison of histologic and flow cytometric evaluation of cyclophosphamide-induced testicular damage. Urology 24:472–475, 1984
20. HALAMKA J, GREY JW, GLEDHILL BL, LAKE S, WYROBEK AJ: Estimation of the frequency of malformed sperm by slit scan flow cytometry. Cytometry 5:333–338, 1984
21. HARGREAVE TB, ELTON RA: Is conventional sperm analysis of any use? Br J Urol 55:774–779, 1983
22. HURET JL: Variability of the chromatin decondensation ability test on human sperm. Arch Androl 11:1–7, 1983
23. JOHNSEN Ø, ELIASSON R, SAMUELSSON U: Conditioning effect of seminal plasma on the lipid peroxide potential of washed human spermatozoa. Acta Physiol Scand 116:305–307, 1982
24. KVIST U: Sperm nuclear chromatin decondensation ability. Acta Physiol Scand (Suppl) 486, 1980
25. MACLEOD J: Human seminal cytology as a sensitive indicator of the germinal epithelium. Int J Fertil 9:281–295, 1964
26. MANN T, LUTWAK-MANN C: Male reproductive function and semen. New York, Springer Verlag, 1981
27. MARTIN HF, GUDZINOWICZ BJ, FANGER H: Normal values in clinical chemistry. New York, Marcel Dekker, 1975
28. MEISTRICH ML: Stage-specific sensitivity of spermatogonia to different chemotherapeutic drugs. Biomed Pharmacother 38:137–142, 1984
29. METTLER L, PAUL S, BAUKLOH V, FELLER AC: Monoclonal sperm antibodies: Their potential for investigation of sperm as target of immunological contraception. Am J Reprod Immunol 5:125–128, 1984
30. MILINGOS S, ELIASSON R: Prostatitis–epididymitis and sperm chromatin stability (abstr). J Androl 6 (Suppl): 1985
31. OSSER S, GENNSER G, LIEDHOLM P, RANSTAM J: Variation of semen parameters in fertile men. Arch Androl 10:127–133, 1983
32. OVERSTREET J: Laboratory tests for human male reproductive risk assessment. Teratogenesis Carcinogen Mutagen 4:67–82, 1984
33. PASTEUR X, LAGET B, AZEMA J, JOURLIN M, LAURENT JL: In vitro decondensation of the human spermatozoan nucleus and image analysis: Quantitative data on the kinetics of in vitro decondensation of the human spermatozoan nucleus. Acta Eur Fertil 15:185–193, 1984
34. PHILLIPS DM: Analysis of sperm motility. J Submicrosc Cytol 15:29–35, 1983
35. PRADER A: Testicular size: Assessment and clinical importance. Triangle 7:240–243, 1966
36. SCHWARTZ D, LAPLANCHE A, JOUANNET P, DAVID G: Within-subject variability of human semen in regard to sperm count, volume, total number of spermatozoa and length of abstinence. J Reprod Fertil 57:391–395, 1979
37. SETCHELL BP: The Mammalian Testis. Ithaca, NY, Cornell University Press, 1980
38. SHORT RV: Testis size, ovulation rate, and breast cancer. In RYDER OA, BYRD ML (eds): One Medicine, pp 32–44. Berlin, Springer–Verlag, 1984
39. VIERULA M, ALANKO M, REMES E, VANHA-PERTTULA T: Ultrastructure of a tail stump sperm defect in an Ayrshire bull. Andrologia 15:303–309, 1983
40. VIRJI N: LDH-C₄ in human seminal plasma and testicular function. I. Methodological aspects. Int J Androl 8:193–200, 1985
41. VIRJI N, ELIASSON R: LDH-C₄ in human seminal plasma and testicular function. III. Relation to other semen properties. Int J Androl 8:201–205, 1985

13

Longitudinal Studies of Semen Measures in Normal Men

MARILYN L. POLAND

KAMRAN S. MOGHISSI

PAUL T. GIBLIN

JOEL W. AGER

JANE M. OLSON

Substantial variation in sperm quality and density among men has been established.[2,8,10] However, variation within a particular subject has received less attention and generally is limited to data obtained from ongoing clinical programs.[11,12] Serial analyses of semen from the same man provide information for the study of the correlates of natural variation and may have significant clinical application in the diagnosis and treatment of male infertility. The present study was undertaken to address the following questions:

1. What is the variation in semen analysis measures within men over an extended period?
2. What is the effect of short-term abstinence on semen measures?
3. Are semen measures substantially related to each other?
4. How many semen samples are necessary to establish reliable parameters?

METHODS AND MATERIALS

Fifteen healthy men volunteered to participate in a 6-month, longitudinal study. None was azoospermic, although semen quality was not a limiting factor for inclusion. Subjects provided a semen specimen every 2 weeks (± 3 days) over the study period, yielding a total of 12 specimens per subject. The men were not asked to abstain from ejaculating before their scheduled date for donating. Subjects filled out a questionnaire each time, indicating number of days since they last ejaculated; average number of ejaculations over the previous 2 weeks; alcohol, coffee and cigarette consumption over the previous 2 days; and any illnesses, drug use (including recreational drugs), and other diagnostic or treatment procedures since the last donation.

Semen was collected by masturbation into a sterile plastic cup in the temperature-controlled environment of a clinical setting. Specimens were analyzed within 90 minutes of their collection by two trained technicians located in a nearby laboratory. Semen analysis was performed according to standard procedures recommended by the World Health Organization (WHO), with a phase-contrast microscope.[3] Volume (ml) was measured to the nearest one tenth in a calibrated chamber. Sperm count was measured by hemocytometer, using both sides of the Neubauer counter chamber and then averaging the counts from both sides. Motility was assessed under low power to scan for representative areas followed by assessment of motion in 25 high-power fields. Quality of motility was evaluated subjectively on a scale from 0 to 3, with 0 representing no motion and scores from 1 to 3 representing gradations of direction and degree of motion. A total motility score (%) represented means of active cells over all fields. The eosin–nigrosin stain distinguished live from dead cells.[2] The Papanicolaou stain was used to examine morphology.[2] Normal cells were characterized by oval heads of average size. Major abnormal head forms included macrocephaly, microcephaly, amorphous forms, and double and tapered heads. Most common abnormal tail forms consisted of round, double, or bent tails. Semen measures included count (million/ml), normal morphology (%), live cells (%), head abnormalities (%), tail abnormalities (%), volume (ml), and motility (%). Total sperm output was derived by multiplying count and volume.

Split-sample reliability from 9 nonstudy subjects was assessed for count, motility, and morphology. Split-sample reliability for count was 0.91; motility was 0.93 and morphology was 0.86, using Spearman–Brown split-half reliability.[7]

STATISTICAL ANALYSIS

The focus of this chapter is the analysis of within-subject variation and covariation of human semen characteristics. Therefore statistics were calculated on the basis of individual data and then averaged over subjects. Frequency distributions were calculated for all variables. Because of the skewness of the individual frequency distributions on which these scores are based, the mean coefficients of variation and the mean of the individual medians are presented along with average means and standard deviations. Further, relationships of these measures and abstinence is reported by average within-subject correlations. Correlations of selected semen characteristics over time within subjects are reported. Finally, intraclass correlations of semen measures were computed to determine reliability of semen measures.

RESULTS

SUBJECTS

The 15 subjects averaged 26.4 years of age; 11 were single, 2 were married, and 2 were divorced. Three had fathered one or two children. The men ejaculated an average of 2.5 times/week (SD = 1.5). Patterns of cigarette smoking as well as alcohol and coffee use were stable within individual men. None experienced major health problems over the study period, although 9

TABLE 13-1. Average Within-Subject Frequency Distributions of Semen Factors

FACTOR	AVERAGE MEANS	AVERAGE S.D.	AVERAGE MEDIANS	RANGE*	AVERAGE COEFFICIENT VARIABLE
Count (million/ml)	74.8	33.2	65.8	1–351	0.48
Volume (ml)	3.2	0.9	3.0	0.2–9.9	0.29
Live cells (%)	75.5	7.4	76.2	41–95	0.10
Motility (%)	51.0	4.2	51.8	30–65	0.09
Normal forms (%)	45.7	6.8	45.5	18–75	0.16
Output (million)	229.9	147.6	197.1	3–2702	0.57

From Poland M, Moghissi K, Giblin K, Ager J: Variation of semen measures within normal men. Fertil Steril 44:396–400, 1985
* Range reported for combined sample n = 172.

had flu symptoms for 2 to 4 days, and several reported headaches requiring aspirin.

SEMEN

Average within subject frequency distributions based on 172 samples from 15 men were calculated for semen count (density), semen volume; percent live cells, normal morphology and motility; and total sperm output (Table 13-1). All values fell within normal expected limits. Frequency distributions for abnormal forms is presented in Table 13-2. Profiles of four men based on average sperm densities that were above, below, and equal to the sample mean are represented in Figs. 13-1 to 13-4 to illustrate the variability in sperm quality over time. While one subject (see Fig. 13-2) shows little variation, the others present dramatic shifts.

TABLE 13-2. Average Within-Subject Frequency Distributions of Abnormal Forms

FACTOR	AVERAGE MEANS	AVERAGE S.D.	AVERAGE MEDIANS	RANGE*	AVERAGE COEFFICIENT VARIABLE
Macrocephaly	0.09	0.23	0	0–2	1.69
Microcephaly	10.80	3.20	10.70	2–20	0.29
Tapering head	12.98	4.03	12.87	0–27	0.33
Double head	0.13	0.26	0	0–3	1.23
Amorphous	1.87	1.52	1.47	0–9	0.86
Round tail	10.46	3.09	10.10	0–24	0.34
Double tail	0.51	0.64	0.27	0–3	1.82
Bent tail	15.11	3.71	14.70	3–29	0.25
Total head	25.94	4.81	26.10	9–45	0.19
Total tail	26.02	4.79	26.00	7–46	0.20

* Range reported for combined sample n = 172.

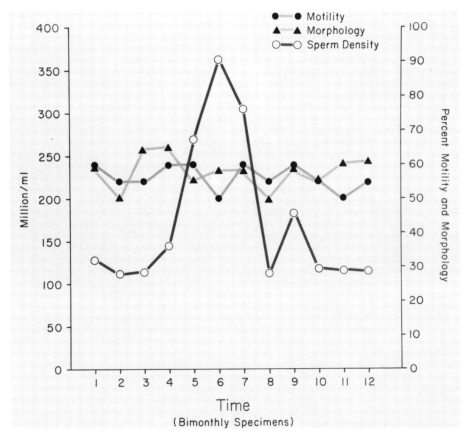

FIG. 13-1. Variation of sperm count (density), morphology, and motility in subject A. Note dramatic rise of sperm count between third and eighth samples.

Effects of abstinence on semen measures were assessed. Numbers of samples following 0, 1, 2, and 3 or more days of abstinence were 2, 28, 68, and 74, respectively.

All correlations in Tables 13-3 and 13-4 are based on within-subject correlations averaged over subjects. The procedures used for averaging are based on Fisher's r to z transformation.[7] A positive linear relationship between abstinence and selected semen measures is seen in Table 13-3. With increasing abstention, semen volume, sperm count, motility, and total sperm output were increased significantly, whereas morphology did not change.

Averaged within-subject correlations among means of selected semen measures are presented in Table 13-4. Notable is the absence of significant correlations among most semen measures. As a consequence of their definitions, percent live correlates with percent motile sperm, and total sperm output correlated with count and semen volume. Count and semen volume were moderately related.

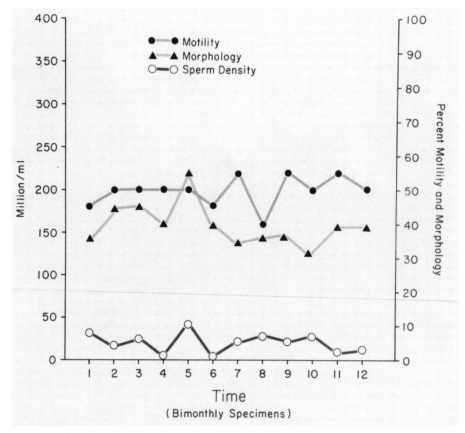

FIG. 13-2. Variation of sperm count (density), morphology, and motility in subject B. This man had a relatively low sperm count.

Intraclass correlations were performed to establish levels of reliability based on number of samples required. The first five intraclass correlations for sperm count, volume, motility, and morphology are seen in Table 13-5. Semen characteristics are fairly reliable ($r = 0.77 - 0.88$) after three specimens, with smaller increments noted after this number.

DISCUSSION

This study reports four findings. First, there is considerable variation within healthy men for semen measures, including count, volume, motility, and morphology. Second, short-term abstinence (0–3 or more days) affects the quality of semen, with a positive linear relationship for volume, motility, and count within the period studied. Only morphology was unaffected. Third, when semen characteristics were correlated within subjects (rather than between

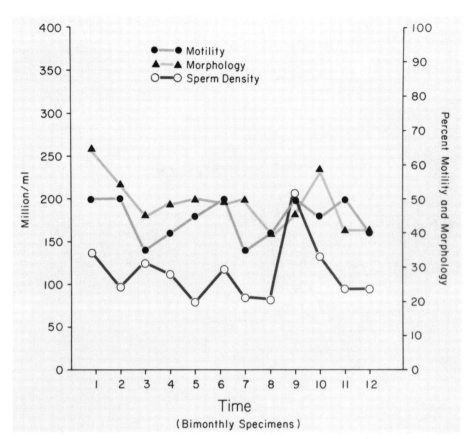

FIG. 13-3. Variation of sperm count (density), morphology, and motility in subject C.

subjects), the only clinically significant finding is the relationship between volume and sperm count (see Table 13-4). Finally, three semen samples are needed to determine reliable profiles of an individual's semen characteristics. Beyond that, little change was seen. One caveat is noted; the effects of abstinence in this study are limited to 0 to 3 or more days. Longer periods of specified abstinence are necessary to determine if further changes in semen measures might occur.

The present study is unique in its attention to collection and analysis of semen samples; namely, 2 weeks apart over a 6-month period. This methodology allowed us to examine within-subject variation of all semen measures and to measure the possible effects of abstinence.

A few studies of within-subject variation are available for comparison, although populations studied and methodologies employed differed somewhat from ours. Our findings of within-subject variation on all semen measures are supported by the reports of others.[5,11] Table 13-6 compares within-subject

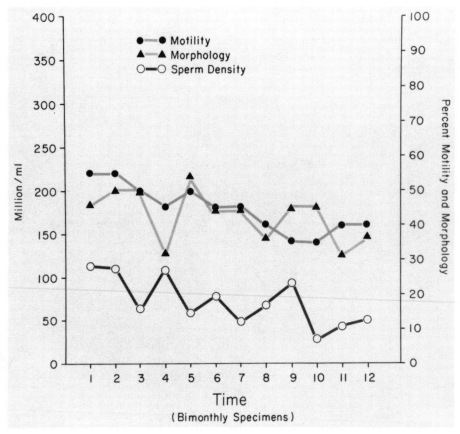

FIG. 13-4. Variation of sperm count (density), morphology, and motility in subject D. Note gradually declining levels and sperm count, motility, and morphology over 6 months.

coefficients of variation in the present study with the findings of several previous reports on human semen. Unfortunately, not all studies included variations for all semen measures. The findings of our study are similar to these values. Differences among laboratories, the subjectivity of estimates of motility and morphology, changes in semen analysis technique, and differences among populations studied all may contribute to the interstudy variations.[1,2,4,6]

This study is the first to report within-subject variation for abnormal forms (see Table 13-2). The most common head abnormalities in the sperm of our population were microcephalic and tapering forms; round and bent tails were the most frequently observed sperm tail anomalies. The wide ranges seen for the rare abnormal forms (macrocephalic, double heads, amorphous forms, and double tails) are reflected in their high average coefficients of variation. Interestingly, total head and tail anomalies were similar in occurrence and variation.

TABLE 13-3. Linear Relationship Between Abstinence and Selected Semen Factors*

FACTOR	$\bar{z}_r$	r	z
Volume	0.42	0.39	4.51†
Count	0.36	0.35	2.60†
Motility	0.24	0.24	2.60†
Morphology	−0.004	0.004	−0.05
Output	0.48	0.45	5.12†

* Conversion of average z_r to r.
† $p < 0.01$

TABLE 13-4. Average Within-Subject Correlations of Selected Semen Factors*

	NORMAL	MOTILE	ALIVE	COUNT	VOLUME	OUTPUT
Normal		0.150	0.146	−0.018	−0.084	−0.044
Motile			0.851†	0.130	0.026	0.095
Alive				0.164	−0.050	0.999
Count					0.238†	0.893†
Volume						0.674†
Output						

(From Poland M, Moghissi K, Giblin P, Ager J: Variation of semen measures within normal men. Fertil Steril 44:396–400, 1985)
* Average z_r calculated and transformed to r units.
† $p < 0.01$

TABLE 13-5. Intraclass Correlations of Selected Semen Measures (1–5 Samples)

MEASURE	SAMPLE 1	SAMPLE 2	SAMPLE 3	SAMPLE 4	SAMPLE 5
Count	0.60	0.75	0.82	0.86	0.88
Normal (%)	0.72	0.84	0.88	0.91	0.92
Active (%)	0.51	0.69	0.77	0.82	0.85
Volume	0.67	0.80	0.86	0.89	0.91

Abstinence was found to affect all semen characteristics but morphology in the present study. Freund reported similar findings when emission frequency was increased from an average of 3.5 to 8.6 times per week. A positive linear relationship between abstinence of under 7 days and sperm count has been reported by others.[9,11]

The only significant within-subject correlations observed among semen parameters was the positive relationship between sperm count and semen volume. Spermatozoa and seminal fluid are produced separately and therefore may not be expected to be correlated biologically. Our finding of a significant positive correlation between count and volume also has been reported by Freund.[5] Intersubject correlations do not detect this relationship, however.[12]

TABLE 13-6. Comparisons of Within-Subject Coefficients of Variation in Human Semen

	HOTCHKISS* (8)	MACLEOD AND GOLD* (10)	FREUND* (5)	SCHWARTZ (11)	BAKER† (2)	THIS STUDY‡
Subjects	23	12	12	36	177	15
Specimens	640	919	140	220	838	172
Count	0.36	0.40	0.41	0.39	0.80	0.48
Volume	0.24		0.29	0.28	0.26	0.29
Motility			0.19		0.32	0.09
Morphology	0.02		0.08		0.19	0.16
Output	0.42		0.75	0.55	0.94	0.57

From Poland M, Moghissi K, Giblin P, Ager J: Variation of semen measures within normal men. Fertil Steril 44:396–400, 1985

* Recalculated

† 459 specimens were oligospermic.

‡ Utilized mean of the individual coefficients.

Finally, intraclass correlations of semen characteristics provide an empirical clinical guide to the number of specimens that are necessary to establish a reliable semen profile. Based on our findings, three samples provide sufficient reliability for all major semen parameters. The men we studied were healthy and few were oligospermic, however. Sherins and associates reported that men with very high and low initial sperm counts generally remain in that category when subsequent semen specimens are obtained.[12] He also found that three samples were necessary to determine stability for men rated initially as having equivocal semen quality. MacLeod and Gold demonstrated that sperm counts vary more for men with initial counts under 60 million/ml than for those with higher counts.[10]

This study has implications for both research and clinical practice. First, findings reported here indicate substantial variations in all semen parameters over an extended period in humans. Second, duration of abstinence has implications for the study of variation in semen quality among and within subjects and should be recorded with every research and clinical specimen. Third, the finding of a positive correlation between sperm count and volume within subjects needs to be investigated further to determine its biologic implications. Finally, three semen specimens are needed to determine a reliable measure of an individual man's semen profile.

REFERENCES

1. AMANN R: A critical review of methods for evaluation of spermatogenesis from seminal characteristics. J Androl 2:37–58, 1981

2. BAKER H, BURGER H, DEDRETSER D, LORDING D, MCGOWAN P, RENNIE G: Factors affecting the variability of semen analysis results in fertile men. Int J Androl 4:609–622, 1981

3. BELSEY M, ELIASSON R, GALLEGOS A, MOGHISSI K, PAULSEN C, PRASAD M (eds): Laboratory Manual for the Examination of Human Semen and Semen-Cervical Mucus Interaction. Geneva, Switzerland, World Health Organization, 1980

4. CHONG A, WALTERS C, WEINRIEB S: The neglected laboratory test: The semen analysis. J Androl 4:280–282, 1983

5. FREUND M: Interrelationships among the characteristics of human semen and factors affecting semen-specimen quality. J Reprod Fertil 4:143–159, 1962
6. FREUND M, CAROL B: Factors affecting haemocytometer counts of sperm concentration in human semen. J Reprod Fertil 8:149–155, 1964
7. HAYES W (ed): Statistics for the Social Sciences, 2nd ed, pp 662–663. New York, Holt, Rinehart & Winston, 1973
8. HOTCHKISS R: Factors in stability and variability of semen specimens. J Urology 45:875–888, 1941
9. MACLEOD J, GOLD R: The male factor in fertility and infertility. VII. Semen quality in relation to age and sexual activity. Fertil Steril 4:194–209, 1953
10. MACLEOD J, GOLD R: The male factor in fertility and infertility. VIII. A study of variation in semen quality. Fertil Steril 7:387–410, 1956
11. SCHWARTZ D, LAPLANCHE A, JOUANNET P, DAVID G: Within-subject variability of human semen in regard to sperm count, volume, total number of spermatozoa and length of abstinence. J Reprod Fertil 57:391–395, 1979
12. SHERINS R, BRIGHTWELL D, STERNTHAL P: Longitudinal analysis of semen of fertile and infertile men. In TROEN P, NANKIN H (eds): The Testis in Normal and Infertile Men, pp 473–488. New York, Raven Press, 1977

14

Sperm–Mucus Interaction and Cervical Mucus Penetration Test

ERIK ODEBLAD

Sperm–cervical mucus interactions are biochemical, biophysical, immunological, and antibiotic. The purpose of this chapter is to describe biophysical interactions between sperm and cervical mucus and to discuss various tests for sperm penetration in cervical mucus.

Observations of sperm penetration in vitro show that 1) a few spermatozoa swim significantly faster than the bulk population; 2) the faster-moving sperm follow a special progression pattern; and 3) sperm cells that swim slowly and/ or have abnormal morphology tend to accumulate to the sides of the lanes used for rapid progression.

The widely accepted model for the structure of the ovulatory cervical mucus consists of three main mucus types, called S, L and G (Fig. 14-1A). (Previously S + L was called type E.)[7–10] About 65% of the ovulatory mucus consists of type L. This mucus has intermediate viscosity and is present in small units called loafs, of ovoid shape, about $0.5 \times 1 \times 2$ mm in size. The loafs come from secreting units (crypt regions) in the mucosa. Crypts in the lowest part of the cervical canal produce a still more viscid mucus, type G, making up 1% to 2% of the total amount of ovulatory cervical mucus. The remaining 30% to 35% of mucus is of the S type. It comes from crypts located mainly in the upper part of the cervical canal. It is the normal sperm-conducting mucus, very fluid and present in stringlike formations, 50 μm to 100 μm wide and 10 mm to 25 mm long. It flows continuously like "brooks" between "pebbles" of L mucus. The S mucus contains long filaments or micelles (Fig. 14-1B) made up of several hundred chains of mucin molecules. Each micelle is about 3 mm long and 500 nm wide. Sperm swim between micelles. The proximal end of a micelle is attached to the wall (L mucus); the distal end is free-floating. Due to the continuous streaming in the string, the micelle is directed downward, nearly parallel with the string direction.

Already in 1962, Odeblad postulated a sperm–mucus interaction involving quanta of vibrations or undulations (phonons) that aid in sperm transport.[6] Our study of such phenomena over the past 20 years has led us to the following conclusions:

When sperm swim, part of the energy released is transferred to the micelle, which comes into high-frequency vibration. In other cells, cleavage of ATP is known to release vibrational energy. Sosa and associates have shown that the sperm head also exhibits ATP-ase activity. The energy probably is transferred to the micelle when the sperm collides with a micelle or molecular chain. The

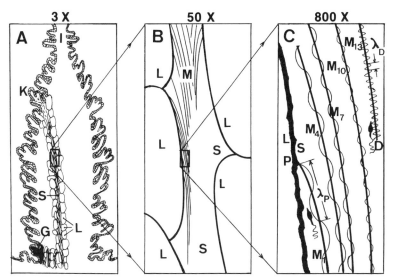

FIG. 14-1. Increasing magnifications of cervix at ovulation and the cervical mucus in vivo and biophysical sperm–mucus interactions. The S–L–G structure in vivo (*A*); the S mucus probably is secreted continuously from a crypt (*K*); the principal arrangement of micelles in the S mucus (*B*); the proximal ends of the micelles adhere to the loafs of L mucus. Phonon vibrations in micelles and sperm–micelle interactions (*C*).

S, L, and G stand for the three types of mucus, respectively. *I* equals isthmus of the uterus. *P* equals proximal end of a micelle, M_1. Every third micelle (M_4, M_7, M_{10}, and M_{13}) lying in the plane of the picture is shown in part C. λ_p and λ_D equal phonon wavelengths in the proximal and distal part of micelles at the same frequency (assumed to be about 30 MHz). The sperm cell near the proximal end of micelle M_1 is exposed to a long-wave vibration and the cell near the distal end of micelle M_{13} is exposed to short-wave vibrations. This phenomenon is exaggerated for long waves if the frequency is lower and for short waves if the frequency becomes higher. Cells interacting with shorter waves tend to cross the micelles and propagate rapidly, whereas cells interacting with long waves tend to follow the micelle path, come into the loaf of L mucus, and become captured.

energy of the evoked vibration is quantized in phonons of definite energy and frequency. Several phonons can exist simultaneously with the same energy, frequency, and phase (phonon condensation). Phonons can travel along the molecular chain or micelle with speeds to be discussed below.

In liquids and solids, phonons travel at the speed of sound, a characteristic parameter for each material. In a molecular chain or micelle in the S mucus, however, the speed depends on two factors: 1) the intrinsic elasticity, and 2) the tension due to hydrodynamic drag of mucus flow. Both factors add up to the restoring force essential for the speed of the waves. Data from our department indicate that the elastic modulus for transverse acoustic modes should be about 10^7 N/m² , corresponding to a speed of 30 m/sec.[11,16,17] The speed increment due to hydrodynamic drag is about 0.05 to 5 m/sec from distal to proximal end for a micelle, and 5 to 500 m/sec for a single molecular chain. Figure 14-1C indicates different phonon speeds in different sections of the micelles.

Biologic evidence suggests that the rapidly swimming sperm (see Fig. 14-1C) are attracted to micelle regions with short phonon waves (below 2 μm–3 μm), and slow swimmers and malformed sperm are attracted to phonon waves longer than 2 μm to 3 μm. In that way the phonons seem to regulate the selection of the best swimmers for upward transport, and other cells for capture in L mucus. Phonon mechanisms also explain the intercellular peak distribution of the rapid sperm collection,[10] initiated by uterine contraction phenomena.[14]

The phonon frequency border between long and short waves is about 30 MHz, corresponding to a quantum energy of 0.1 μeV (micron electron volts), or wave number of 0.001 cm^{-1}. The sperm sensitivity to different phonon wavelengths therefore can be alternatively given as follows: The rapidly swimming sperm are attracted by phonon energies above 0.1 μeV, and the slow or malformed sperm by phonon energies lower than 0.1 μeV. In both cases there is an excess number of phonons over the thermal distribution. Research is presently underway to elucidate the response of sperm to excess phonons of different energies.

Clearly, sperm progress and selection is a rather complicated phenomenon that requires a specific mucus structure during ovulation to be effective. Both L and S mucus are required. Sperm penetration tests not taking this fact into account cannot fully elucidate the normal processes going on in the cervical mucus. Unfortunately, most of the tests used today for routine application do not fulfill these criteria. In the slide tests,[4,5,12] the L–S structure can be partially maintained, as indicated by the phalanx phenomenon.[10] In the capillary tests,[1-3,13] artificial alignment of mucin molecules may occur in both L and S mucus, obscuring their borderlines. Thus, capillary tests seem more destructive to the mucus than does a properly performed slide test.

Attempts have been made to remove the entire mucus plug with its structure preserved in special glass tubes for in vitro penetration tests, but this technique works only when the canal is nearly circular and has a straight axis.[10] In addition, the continuous monitoring of sperm movement presents special optical problems. Even if these problems can be overcome, the cessation of mucus flow in the strings in vitro continues to vex investigators. The flow orientation of micelles in the living organism will be lost. The time before the micellar orientation becomes ineffective is equal to the relaxation time, which can be calculated from physical laws. Both calculations and measurements indicate that this period is approximately one half hour to an hour. Reliable in vitro penetration tests are unlikely.

Tests are necessary, however, even if the in vivo conditions cannot be duplicated. When applying the results from destructive tests such as the capillary tests, the investigator must identify the sources of error (*e.g.*, the artificial alignment of mucin molecules, which does not have any correspondence in the living state). This leads to an overestimation of the sperm progression rate. Furthermore, the natural selection mechanisms are completely destroyed in the capillary tests. In various slide tests, other factors come into play, but on the whole, the slide tests seem to be the least destructive for the mucus. Factors other than the biophysical ones discussed here exist, but are beyond the scope of this discussion.

SUMMARY

Biophysical sperm–cervical mucus interaction points to new mechanisms of sperm propagation and selection in cervical mucus. The mucin aggregates (micelles) in the sperm-conducting S mucus are forced into vibrations by energy released from the spermatozoa, and these vibrations (phonons) seem to be important for selection of the most suitable sperm for rapid transport upward.

REFERENCES

1. CARLBORG L: Determination of sperm migration rate in small samples of cervical mucus. Acta Endocrinol 59:636–643, 1968
2. KREMER J: A simple sperm penetration test. Int J Fertil 10:201–215, 1965
3. LAMAR J, SHETTLES L, DELFS E: Cyclic penetrability of human cervical mucus to spermatozoa *in vitro.* Am J Physiol 129:234–241, 1940
4. MILLER EG, KURZROK R: Biochemical studies on human semen. III. Factors affecting migration of sperm through the cervix. Am J Obstet Gynecol 24:19–26, 1932
5. MOGHISSI KS, DABICH D, LEVINE J, NEUHAUS OW: Mechanism of sperm migration. Fertil Steril 15:15–23, 1964
6. ODEBLAD E: Undulations of macromolecules in cervical mucus. Int J Fertil 7:313–319, 1962
7. ODEBLAD E: Physical properties of cervical mucus. In ELSTEIN M, PARKE DV (eds): Mucus in Health and Disease. Adv Exp Med Biol 89:217–225, 1977
8. ODEBLAD E: Cervical factors. Contr Gynecol Obstet 4:132–142, 1978
9. ODEBLAD E, HÖGLUND A: Sperm penetration in cervical mucus: A biophysical and group-theoretical approach. In INSLER V, BETTENDORF G (eds): The Uterine Cervix in Reproduction, pp 129–134. Stuttgart, Thieme Publication, 1977
10. ODEBLAD E, INGELMAN-SUNDBERG A, HALLSTRÖM L, HÖGLUND A, LEPPANEN U, LISSPERS K, PERENYI E, RUDOLFSSON-ÅSBERG K, SAHLIN K, LINDSTRÖM-SJÖGREN C, SJÖSTRÖM C, STRANDBERG-BERGSTRÖM L, WIKSTRÖM L, WIKSTRÖM M: The biophysical properties of the cervical–vaginal secretions. Int Rev Nat Family Plann 7:1–56, 1983
11. ODEBLAD E, PERENYI E: Studies on the Spinnbarkeit test. Unpublished data, 1985
12. PERLOFF WH, STEINBERGER E: *In vivo* penetration of cervical mucus by spermatozoa. Fertil Steril 14:231–236, 1963
13. SCHWARTZ R, ZISSNER H: Sperm motility: A simple method for analysis. Am J Med 17:124–126, 1954
14. SJÖSTRÖM C: Sperm distribution patterns in the S type of cervical mucus. Unpublished data, 1985
15. SOSA A, CALZADA L, ALVA S, GONZÁLEZ-ANGULO A: Distribution of ATPase in isolated human spermatozoa nuclei: A high-resolution cytochemical study. Int J Fertil 24:125–129, 1979
16. STRANDBERG-BERGSTRÖM L: A simple method for identification of cervical mucus, type S (the tilting test). Unpublished data, 1985
17. WOLF D, BLASCO L, KAHN M, LITT M: Human cervical mucus. I. Rheologic characteristics. Fertil Steril 28:41–46, 1977

15

Predictive Value of In Vitro Sperm Function Tests

R. JOHN AITKEN

STEWART IRVINE

JANE S. CLARKSON

DAVID WILLIAM RICHARDSON

The traditional basis of male fertility diagnosis is a conventional semen profile describing the number of spermatozoa present in the ejaculate, their morphology, and their capacity for movement. The assumption underlying this analysis is that conception is possible only if there are more than a certain critical number of motile, morphologically normal spermatozoa present in the ejaculate. The limitations of this concept are illustrated by the fact that around 20% of normal fertile men have sperm counts in the pathologic range ($<20 \times 10^6$ spermatozoa/ml),[21,23] whereas between 25% and 52% of men exhibiting idiopathic oligozoospermia are able to produce a pregnancy in their partner without treatment.[14,28,33] Such results emphasize that the number of spermatozoa in the ejaculate is not as important as the functional competence of the spermatozoa. Consequently, if we are to improve the accuracy of male fertility diagnosis, supplementing the traditional descriptive methods of semen analysis with bioassays designed to assess specific aspects of sperm function is critical. A variety of in vitro and in vivo tests are presently available for examining the biologic properties of human spermatozoa, particularly with respect to capacity for transport to the site of fertilization and to the act of fertilization itself. In this review, we shall consider the nature of these tests and assess the contribution they might make in both the infertility clinic and the development of new approaches to male contraception.

MEASUREMENT OF FERTILIZING POTENTIAL

PROPERTIES ASSESSED BY TRANS-SPECIES, IN VITRO FERTILIZATION

To fertilize the ovum, human spermatozoa must achieve a state of capacitation during their ascent of the female reproductive tract, bind to receptor sites on the surface of the zona pellucida, undergo the acrosome reaction, penetrate the zona, and finally fuse with the vitelline membrane of the oocyte.

Bioassays have been developed to examine several of these properties and interactions, including homologous and trans-species in vitro fertilization techniques, incorporating human ova and zona-free hamster oocytes respectively.

Although the in vitro fertilization of human ova might generate the most complete information on this aspect of sperm function, it is not a practical proposition in a routine diagnostic context for a variety of ethical and logistical reasons. Attention therefore has turned to an alternative system introduced in 1976 by Yanagimachi and associates that exploits the unique susceptibility of zona-free hamster oocytes to fusion with the spermatozoa of other eutherian mammals, including humans.[35] The biologic significance of the sperm–egg fusions detected by this system is indicated by the fact that it can occur only if the spermatozoa have capacitated and undergone the acrosome reaction previously, just as if human ova had been the target.[34] Furthermore, the ultrastructural details of the fusion process are identical to the homologous situation, in that contact between the gametes is initiated by the plasma membrane overlying the equatorial segment of the acrosome-reacted sperm head.[18]

The ability of human spermatozoa to generate a fusogenic equatorial segment is probably the most significant property assessed by the zona-free hamster oocyte penetration test. Although claims have been made that this system is also capable of assessing the ability of spermatozoa to capacitate and undergo the acrosome reaction, these conclusions are valid only with respect to the in vitro situation. Whether the ability of spermatozoa to capacitate and complete the acrosome reaction after prolonged incubation in simple media such as BWW[10] reflects their capacity to undergo these changes in vivo, is unknown. This uncertainty is largely a reflection of our poor understanding concerning the molecular nature of capacitation and the interactions within the female reproductive tract that lead to its induction. A similar degree of uncertainty surrounds our comprehension of the factors involved in the induction of the acrosome reaction. The evidence suggests that the acrosome reaction is induced normally at the surface of the zona pellucida by a glycoprotein component of the zona itself.[13] If this is the case, it further underlines the caution that should be exercised in interpreting the results of an in vitro fertilization system that is zona-free by definition.

Although we do not yet understand the biochemical nature of capacitation, the purpose of this change clearly is to permit the influx of calcium ions across the sperm plasma membrane.[32] Therefore the capacitation process may be bypassed by adding components to the medium that artificially stimulate calcium uptake. One such agent is the divalent cation ionophore. A23187, which in the presence of extracellular calcium raises the intracellular cytosolic concentration of this cation from 100 nM to about 400 nM in human spermatozoa.[5] This change in free calcium levels readily precipitates the acrosome reaction in uncapacitated spermatozoa, with the result that very high levels of hamster oocyte penetration are observed in the response to A23187 when normal, fertile semen donors are used.[5] Intriguingly, such high levels of fertilization are not achieved when the spermatozoa of infertile men exhibiting idiopathic oligozoospermia are exposed to A23187.[5] These and other findings suggest that the spermatozoa of oligozoospermic men are defective in their ability to respond to calcium, whether the influx of this ion is induced artificially by A23187,[5] or by allowing the spermatozoa to capacitate for several hours in calcium-containing media.[3] Similar findings have been recorded for other groups of infertile men, including those possessing varicoceles or exhibiting conditions such as asthenozoospermia and idiopathic infertility.

In the light of these considerations, we may conclude that the primary purpose of the zona-free hamster oocyte penetration test is to assess the ability of human spermatozoa to respond to the influx of calcium, by generating a fusogenic equatorial segment capable of interacting with the vitelline membrane of the oocyte. Since the capacitation observed following the prolonged incubation of spermatozoa in vitro is probably not physiologic, it seems reasonable to induce the calcium entry artificially and efficiently with calcium ionophores such as A23187. Through the use of this compound, very rapid, sensitive assays of the ability of human spermatozoa to respond to calcium can be obtained.[5]

The limited nature of the properties assessed by this test deserve emphasizing, particularly in the context of male fertility diagnosis. It is unreasonable to assume that all male infertility involves defects in the ability of the spermatozoa to generate a fusogenic equatorial segment, secondary to the influx of calcium across the sperm plasma membrane. There are, of course, many reasons for defective sperm function and the zona-free hamster oocyte penetration test is capable of assessing only one potential cause. This point is well illustrated by the positive fusions recorded between zona-free hamster oocytes and the spermatozoa of patients exhibiting Kartagener's syndrome.[6] The success of this interaction is surprising, because the spermatozoa of such patients are completely immotile owing to the congenital absence of ATP-ase activity in the axonemal complex of the sperm tails. An adequate degree of sperm motility is obviously critical for achieving ascent of the female reproductive tract, as well as penetration of the egg investments. For this reason, men presenting with Kartagener's syndrome are infertile. The fact that the spermatozoa from these patients nevertheless can fuse with zona-free hamster oocytes emphasizes the limitations of this diagnostic system and its susceptibility to generating false-positive results.

A related example of the limitations of the hamster egg test concerns the inability of this system to detect defects in the capacity of human spermatozoa to bind to and penetrate the zona pellucida.[34] The success of zona penetration depends on a number of properties that must be exhibited by the spermatozoon. To begin with, capacitated spermatozoa must be competent to recognize receptor sites on the zona surface and then respond to the zona pellucida by undergoing the acrosome reaction.[13] The latter then should result in the release and activation of proteases, particularly acrosin, to digest a path through the zona pellucida, which the spermatozoa then penetrate by virtue of the shearing forces generated by the vigorous beating of the sperm tail. This rather complex sequence of interactions constitutes an essential component of the fertilization process that cannot be examined by the zona-free hamster oocyte penetration test. This shortcoming of the test is a significant one because cases have been cited in the literature indicating that the failure of sperm–zona interaction can be a component in the etiology of human infertility.[25]

In summary, the zona-free hamster egg penetration test essentially provides specific information on the ability of human spermatozoa to fuse with the vitelline membrane of the oocyte. It cannot assess several other properties that are necessary for fertilization to occur, and, for this reason, the test should be expected to generate occasional false-positive results, as in the case of Kartagener's syndrome. In contrast, low or negative results with the test should be expected to show a strong correlation with infertility because sperm–oocyte fusion is an essential component of conception.

RELATIONSHIP BETWEEN HAMSTER OOCYTE PENETRATION AND FERTILITY

The first indication that the zona-free hamster oocyte penetration test might be of value in the diagnosis of fertility came from retrospective studies in which the fertilization values obtained from normal fertile men were compared with the results produced by patients exhibiting recognized types of male infertility. For example, an analysis of 35 men of proven fertility, using a hamster oocyte system incorporating a 7-hour capacitation period, gave a mean ($\pm$SE) penetration rate of $44.0 \pm 3.4\%$ with a range of 14% to 90%.[2] In contrast, when an identical system was used to investigate the functional competence of 27 severely oligozoospermic patients, the equivalent figures were $2.8 \pm 1.5\%$, with only 2 samples (7.4%) scoring more than 10%.[3] Even more intriguing were the results of a similar study on 85 patients with unexplained infertility. All of these patients exhibited normal semen profiles in the conventional sense, and yet the mean penetration rate of $30.8 \pm 3.4\%$ was significantly lower ($p < 0.05$) than the results obtained with normal fertile men. Of particular interest was the fact that just over one third of these patients (34.1%) exhibited penetration rates below the normal fertile range. These findings suggested that an important attribute of the hamster oocyte penetration test was that it could detect defects of sperm function in patients who would have been diagnosed as normal by traditional methods.

Whether such results have any clinical value can only be determined reliably by prospective studies. Such a prospective analysis of 68 couples exhibiting 5.1 ± 0.3 years of unexplained infertility, involved a follow-up period of 2.3 ± 0.06 years, during which time 25 (37%) of the women spontaneously achieved a pregnancy.[4] Because the female partner of each couple was normal by history and examination (including a diagnostic laparoscopy) and the couples had received no treatment during the follow-up period, an analysis was possible of the relationship between spontaneous conception and various criteria of semen quality measured at the beginning of the study. In terms of the zona-free hamster egg penetration test, none of the 4 men exhibiting 0% penetration scores managed to achieve a pregnancy during the follow-up period, supporting the suggestion that severe defects detected with this system should correlate with infertility. Subnormal penetration rates of <10%, on the other hand, were compatible with fertility, although the conception rate observed for these patients was significantly lower than that recorded for the remainder of the study population scoring >10% in the assay. With penetration rates above 10%, the frequency of conception rose to a maximum of approximately 60% for patients exhibiting scores of 25% to 75% but then fell to 36.4% for subjects scoring from 75.1% to 100%.[4]

In general, these results confirmed our expectations in indicating that a correlation exists between low or subnormal fertilization rates in the hamster oocyte assay and clinical infertility. The fall in pregnancy rates observed for subjects scoring over 75% in the assay may represent the emergence of the female factor in the etiology of unexplained fertility. Despite our efforts to recruit only couples in which the female partner was normal, there must be a female component to unexplained infertility, and the influence of this factor should be most apparent when the male partners are highly fertile.

A similar prospective study involving a 4.2 ± 1.1 year follow-up of 27 oligozoospermic patients married to normal female partners did not yield such promising results.[1] In this study, 70.4% of patients scored 0% in the hamster oocyte assay during the recruitment phase of the project. If the results obtained with the unexplained infertility group had been extrapolated to these oligozoospermic men, none of the patients scoring 0% in the assay would have been expected to achieve a spontaneous pregnancy on follow-up. In fact, of the seven patients successfully initiating a pregnancy during the follow-up period, four had previously scored 0% in the hamster oocyte assay.

A possible reason for the discrepancy between the penetration test results and the fertility of these oligozoospermic men may lie in the suboptimal nature of the technique used to induce capacitation, which in this case was a 7-hour incubation in normo-osmotic BWW. It is possible that recent modifications of this assay to increase its sensitivity,[5,8] using the ionophore A23187 in particular, might have improved the correlation with fertility. In this context, it may be significant that in a recent analysis of the influence of A23187 on the penetration rates observed with oligozoospermic men, this compound induced a fall in the proportion of patients scoring 0% penetration from 68.6% to 48.6%.[5]

The clinical value of the A23187-stimulated system has already been demonstrated in the context of an artificial insemination by donor (AID) service. In this study, hamster oocyte penetration rates were recorded in the presence of A23187 for semen samples that had either been successful or, on at least four occasions, unsuccessful in the initiation of a pregnancy. Using a multivariate discriminant analysis technique, it was not possible to discriminate the fertile from the infertile samples on the basis of the conventional semen profile alone. When the A23187-stimulated penetration rates were added to the analysis, however, a significant classification of the fertile and infertile semen samples was possible (p = 0.03). This discrimination was obtained on the basis of three criteria (Table 15-1), all of which were positively correlated with fertility, that described the concentration of motile spermatozoa inseminated, the proportion of motile spermatozoa remaining after a 3-hour incubation with A23187, and the results of the hamster egg penetration test. On the basis of these criteria, 74.1% of the fertile samples and 76.2% of the infertile samples were identified correctly, giving an overall correct classification of 75%.

TABLE 15-1. Analysis of the Ability of the Conventional Semen Profile and A23187-stimulated Hamster Egg Penetration Rates to Discriminate Fertile from Infertile Samples in an AID Service*

VARIABLE	DISCRIMINANT FUNCTION COEFFICIENT
Concentration of motile spermatozoa inseminated (10^6/ml)	0.54776
Percentage of motile cells after a 3-hr incubation with A23187	0.66146
Hamster oocyte penetration test expressed as mean number of spermatozoa/oocyte	0.55898

* Movement characteristics assessed following the isolation of motile spermatozoa on 7.5% albumin columns.

SPERM MOVEMENT CHARACTERISTICS

Several of the shortcomings of the hamster oocyte penetration test relate to its inability to assess aspects of sperm function that are heavily dependent on the vigorous motility of the spermatozoa, particularly zona penetration and sperm transport to the site of fertilization. A more accurate description of the fertilizing potential of human spermatozoa might therefore be possible, if the hamster oocyte test were supplemented with objective measurements of the quality of sperm motility. The importance of making separate assessments of sperm motility has recently been emphasized in several studies, indicating that the quality of sperm movement and the capacity for hamster oocyte penetration are quite separate entities that may be independently affected in male infertility.[9] Hence it is possible to record cases where the spermatozoa exhibited a normal potential for fertilization but an impaired capacity for movement, as in Kartagener's syndrome,[6] or, conversely, cases of impaired fertilizing potential but perfectly normal patterns of motility, as in some idiopathic infertility.[9]

Objective techniques that are currently available for analyzing the movement of human spermatozoa include the deployment of ultraviolet (UV)[22] and laser[20] light scattering, cinemicrography,[12] videomicrography,[16] and time-exposure photomicrography.[24] The advantage of the last three techniques is that they provide information on specific aspects of sperm movement, such as the linear velocity of progression or the amplitude of lateral sperm head displacement, which we now know to be critical for certain biologic functions, such as cervical mucus penetration.[7] In contrast, the UV or laser light scattering techniques provide information only on the overall movement exhibited by the sample.

In our laboratory, we have found the time exposure photomicrography technique to be simple, inexpensive, and informative (Fig. 15-1). Furthermore, our expectations have been borne out, in that the additional data describing the movement characteristics of the spermatozoa have been a valuable supplement to the hamster oocyte penetration test in the diagnosis of male fertility.

In the assessment of the fertilizing potential of semen samples in an AID clinic, for example, the addition of sperm movement characteristics to the

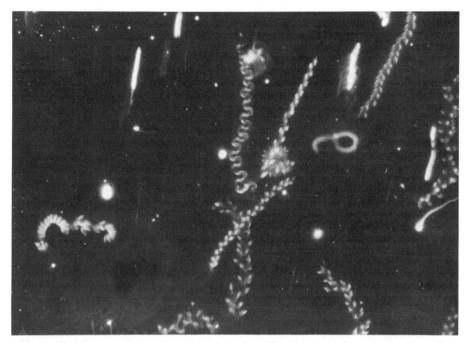

FIG. 15-1. Time exposure photomicrography of human spermatozoa; each motile spermatozoon leaves a track across the photographic print that then can be examined to obtain objective measurements of the various attributes of sperm motility (From Aitken RJ, Best FSM, Richardson DW, Djahanbakhch O, Lees MM: The correlations of fertilizing capacity in normal fertile men. Fertil Steril 38:68–76, 1982)

information provided by the conventional semen profile and hamster oocyte penetration test increased the power of the discriminant analysis from 75% to 81.3%. This discrimination of the fertile from the infertile samples was based on the data provided by the six variables recorded in Table 15-2. The movement characteristics included the linear velocity of progression, which was positively correlated with fertility, and the frequency of rotation of the progressively motile spermatozoa (moving at speeds in excess of 25 μm/sec), which was negatively associated with fertilizing potential. These data suggest that there is an optimal range of velocities compatible with fertility and that samples moving at inadequate or excessive speeds are correspondingly infertile.

The impaired fertility of spermatozoa exhibiting excessive forward velocities has also been emphasized in a prospective study of patients exhibiting idiopathic infertility. In this analysis, the identity of those patients spontaneously achieving a pregnancy during a follow-up period of 2.3 ± 0.06 years could be established, with an overall accuracy of 76.5%, using a combination

TABLE 15-2. Analysis of the Ability of the Conventional Semen Profile and A23187-stimulated Hamster Egg Penetration Rates and Sperm Movement Characteristics to Discriminate Fertile from Infertile Samples in an AID Service*

VARIABLE	DISCRIMINANT FUNCTION COEFFICIENT
Concentration of motile spermatozoa inseminated (10^6/ml)	0.45806
Percentage of motile cells after a 3-hr incubation with A23187	0.78173
Hamster oocyte penetration test expressed as mean number of spermatozoa/oocyte	0.54942
Total mean velocity (μm/sec)	0.88963
Percentage of yawing† spermatozoa	0.50769
Frequency of rotation of progressive (>25 μm/sec) spermatozoa (per sec)	−1.16133

* Movement characteristics assessed following the isolation of motile spermatozoa on 7.5% albumin columns.

† "Yawing" spermatozoa as defined by Overstreet and associates (24).

of data describing the hamster oocyte penetration rates and the movement characteristics of the spermatozoa. Once again, hamster oocyte penetration, percentage motility following incubation in vitro, and total mean velocity were all positively correlated with fertility, while the presence of spermatozoa exhibiting extremely high velocities (expressed as the mean progressive velocity) was negatively associated with fertilizing potential.

The importance of an optimal speed of progression has its counterpart in the need for an optimal amplitude of lateral sperm head displacement. As we shall discuss later, the amplitude of lateral sperm head displacement is positively correlated with the ability of human spermatozoa to penetrate cervical mucus. Samples possessing an inadequate degree of lateral displacement exhibit a poor capacity for mucus penetration. Conversely, samples exhibiting an excessive amplitude of displacement (>10 μm) possess a diminished capacity for fertilization in vitro[2] and an impaired potential for establishing a pregnancy in vivo.[4]

This requirement for an optimal degree of lateral displacement has been demonstrated in an analysis of the relationship between sperm quality and the success of AID therapy. If the discrimination of fertile and infertile specimens was attempted on the basis of the conventional semen profile and movement characteristics alone, a statistically significant (p = 0.04) classification was achieved that was, overall, 73% accurate. This discrimination was obtained on the basis of the five variables listed in Table 15-3. The concentration of motile spermatozoa in the inseminate and the total mean velocity of the spermatozoa were, again, positively correlated with fertility, whereas the remaining criteria, particularly the incidence of a small amplitude of lateral sperm head displacement, were negatively associated with the potential for establishing a pregnancy. The degree of discrimination achieved with these movement characteristics (73%) was approximately equal to that obtained with the conventional semen profile and hamster oocyte penetration (75%) but less than

TABLE 15-3. Analysis of the Ability of the Conventional Semen Profile and Movement Characteristics to Discriminate Fertile from Infertile Samples in an AID Service*

VARIABLE	DISCRIMINANT FUNCTION COEFFICIENT
Concentration of motile spermatozoa inseminated (10^6/ml)	0.56024
Total mean velocity (μm/sec)	0.64552
Amplitude of lateral head displacement of <4.5μm (%)	−4.50812
Frequency of rotation of progressive (>25μm/sec) spermatozoa (per sec)	−1.02452
Percentage of progressive (>25μm/sec) rolling† spermatozoa	−4.39228
Percentage of progressive (>25μm/sec) yawing† spermatozoa	−0.51156

* Movement characteristics assessed following the isolation of motile spermatozoa on 7.5% albumin columns.

† "Rolling" and "yawing" spermatozoa as defined by Overstreet and associates (24).

that recorded when the conventional criteria of hamster oocyte penetration and movement characteristics were used in combination (81%).

The prospective analysis of oligozoospermic patients also revealed that a significant prediction of fertility was possible if the data generated by the hamster oocyte penetration test were supplemented with data describing the movement characteristics exhibited by the spermatozoa. In keeping with the results presented above, this analysis emphasized the positive correlation between fertility and the total mean velocity of the spermatozoa and the negative contribution of an inadequate amplitude of lateral head displacement (Table 15-4).

In conclusion, the objective assessment of sperm movement does contribute significant information on the fertilizing potential of human spermatozoa, presumably because of the importance of sperm motility in achieving both penetration of the zona pellucida and transport to the site of fertilization.

BIOCHEMICAL INDICES OF FERTILIZING POTENTIAL

Despite the apparent value of the above techniques for measuring the fertilizing potential and movement characteristics of human spermatozoa, it is doubtful whether these procedures could be used in a routine diagnostic context, because they are either too complex or too time-consuming. As a result, some efforts have been made to identify biochemical markers for these activities that might be suitable for the rapid screening of large numbers of samples. The proposed role of cAMP in the control of sperm function has, for example, led to the investigation of this compound as a possible index of the fertilizing potential of human spermatozoa. Unfortunately, however, no change in the cAMP content of human spermatozoa has been detected during capacitation, and no significant relationship has been established between cyclic adenosine monophosphate (cAMP) and the performance of human spermatozoa in the zona-free hamster oocyte penetration test.[26]

TABLE 15-4. Analysis of the Ability of the Conventional Semen Profile, Movement Characteristics, and Hamster Oocyte Penetration Rates to Discriminate Fertile from Infertile Oligozoospermic Patients*

VARIABLE	DISCRIMINANT FUNCTION COEFFICIENT
Normal morphology (%)	0.37461
Total mean velocity (μm/sec)	0.70075
Amplitude of lateral head displacement <10μm (%)	−1.24570
Hamster oocyte penetration (%)	0.67765
Percentage of progressive (>25μm/sec) straight-swimming spermatozoa	0.52427
Log of progressive (>25μm/sec) spermatozoa exhibiting an amplitude of lateral head displacement of <10μm	−0.37791
Log concentration of spermatozoa in semen (10^6/ml)	−0.46905

* Movement characteristics measured after separation of the spermatozoa from seminal plasma and incubation in vitro for 7 hours.

A second possible biochemical marker for human sperm function is adenosine triphosphate (ATP), the presence of which has been shown to correlate with both the relative fertility of semen samples in an AID clinic and the results of the penetration assay.[11] We have been able to confirm both of these findings, although a detailed consideration of the results suggests that ATP levels are not of major significance in the diagnosis of male fertility. Thus the correlation between fertility and ATP levels in the context of an AID service is only of significance in determining the relative effectiveness of *fertile* samples; ATP determinations do not appear to be of value in separating fertile from infertile donors. Hence, in our own studies of AID donors, no significant discrimination of the fertile and infertile samples could be achieved when ATP assessments were added to the data describing the conventional semen profile. Similarly, addition of ATP data to the results of the hamster egg penetration test did not increase the ability of the latter to separate the fertile from the infertile samples.

The correlation observed between the outcome of the zona-free hamster oocyte penetration test and ATP levels may also be of little practical consequence. Although we have detected similar correlations within our own data set (r = 0.66), this association appears to be due largely to the relationship between seminal ATP levels and the concentration of motile spermatozoa in the ejaculate. If the ATP levels in semen are expressed as a function of the number of spermatozoa, the correlation with the outcome of the penetration assay disappears.

In conclusion, neither cAMP nor ATP determinations appear to be capable of replacing the direct measurement of sperm fertilizing ability and movement. Nevertheless, the more we investigate the biochemical basis of normal sperm function and understand the molecular nature of the lesions present in the spermatozoa of infertile men, the more likely it is that appropriate biochemical markers will be found of diagnostic significance.

MEASUREMENT OF SPERM TRANSPORT

The fertility of a semen sample depends not only on the fertilizing potential of the spermatozoa, but also on the capacity of these cells to ascend the reproductive tract to the site of fertilization. The diagnosis of male fertility should therefore include tests designed to assess the competence of human spermatozoa to achieve transport to the ampullae of the fallopian tubes. The most definitive test of this aspect of sperm function is an in vivo procedure involving the laparoscopic recovery of spermatozoa from the pelvic cavity, 12 to 24 hours after natural or artificial insemination.[30,31] The results obtained with this procedure have been shown to correlate with the subsequent incidence of spontaneous pregnancy in prospective studies,[31] although the technique itself is time-consuming and frequently impractical because the laparoscopy must be timed to coincide with the ovulatory stage of the menstrual cycle.

Alternative in vitro procedures therefore have been developed that focus on that aspect of sperm transport most clearly involving active participation by the spermatozoa, namely, penetration of the cervical barrier. The conventional system for measuring sperm–cervical mucus interaction is the Kremer technique,[19] in which measurements are taken of the distance traveled by spermatozoa through a column of cervical mucus. Expressing the results in this way is bound to be inaccurate, however, because the performance of an individual semen sample clearly will depend on the number of collisions between spermatozoa and the cervical mucus interface, and the collision frequency will, in turn, be a function of the number of motile sperm cells in the sample and their total mean velocity. A marked improvement on the Kremer test has therefore been introduced by Katz and associates,[17] in which the ability of spermatozoa to penetrate cervical mucus is expressed in terms of the concentration and velocity of motile cells in each semen specimen. The end result of this procedure is a percentage successful collisions (PSC) value, which describes the ratio between the number of spermatozoa colliding with the cervical mucus interface and the total number of successful entries into the mucus.

In our first studies with this test, we examined 20 patients exhibiting unexplained infertility for defects of sperm–cervical mucus interaction.[27] The results from these subjects revealed a wide range of PSC values (6.3–77.3), the magnitude of which appeared to be correlated with the quality of the spermatozoa rather than the properties of the cervical mucus. Of the seminal characteristics measured, the proportion of motile spermatozoa in the ejaculate and the ability of the spermatozoa to penetrate zona-free hamster oocytes showed the most significant correlations with cervical mucus penetration.[27] Intriguingly, this correlation between cervical mucus penetration and the fertilizing ability of human spermatozoa has been confirmed in independent studies employing both zona-free hamster oocytes[29] and intact human ova.[15] It is difficult to explain this association except in terms of the importance of sperm motility in fulfilling both aspects of sperm function.

In this context, we have examined the relationship between the movement characteristics of human spermatozoa and their capacity for cervical mucus penetration in both fertile donors and couples with unexplained infertility.[7] The concentration of motile spermatozoa and their total mean velocity were found to be important criteria regulating the frequency of collisions between the spermatozoa and the cervical mucus interface. Whether such collisions resulted in penetration of the mucus was significantly dependent on the amplitude of lateral sperm head displacement; the smaller the displacement, the smaller the probability of penetration. This association may be due to the fact that the amplitude of lateral sperm head displacement is an indirect reflection of the amplitude of the flagellar beat pattern. For spermatozoa colliding with the cervical mucus interface, the maximum forward thrust would be generated by flagellar beats of large amplitude. Spermatozoa with a small amplitude of lateral sperm head displacement may possess a pattern of flagellar activity with insufficient propulsive force to penetrate the mucus interface.

The clinical significance of these observations is indicated by the fact that couples have now been identified who are infertile because the spermatozoa of the male partner cannot penetrate cervical mucus. The only detectable defect in the semen profile of these patients is an inadequate amplitude of lateral sperm head displacement.[7] It is intriguing that such a subtle defect in the movement characteristics of the spermatozoa can lead to infertility, and discovery of this defect emphasizes the value of using high resolution objective techniques for the diagnosis of male fertility.

CONCLUSION

Prospective studies have emphasized the importance of both the zona-free hamster oocyte penetration test and the objective assessment of sperm movement in the diagnosis of male fertility. These procedures should find application in the evaluation of new approaches to male contraception. They do not examine all aspects of sperm function, however, and there is still a need to develop additional techniques to investigate factors such as sperm–zona recognition and to elucidate the normal physiologic mechanisms by which capacitation and the acrosome reaction are induced. Ultimately, such improvements in our fundamental knowledge of the processess regulating normal sperm function should permit the development of simple biochemical assays better suited to routine diagnosis of male fertility.

REFERENCES

1. AITKEN RJ, WARNER PE: Diagnostic value of the zona-free hamster oocyte penetration test and sperm movement characteristics in oligozoospermia. Int J Androl (in press)
2. AITKEN RJ, BEST FSM, RICHARDSON DW, DJAHANBAKHCH O, LEES MM: The correlations of fertilizing capacity in normal fertile men. Fertil Steril 38:68–76, 1982
3. AITKEN RJ, BEST FSM, RICHARDSON DW, DJAHANBAKHCH O, TEMPLETON AA, LEES MM: An analysis of semen quality and sperm function in cases of oligozoospermia. Fertil Steril 38:705–714, 1982
4. AITKEN RJ, BEST FSM, WARNER PE, TEMPLETON AA: A prospective study of the relationship between semen quality and fertility in cases of unexplained infertility. J Androl 5:297–303, 1984

5. AITKEN RJ, ROSS A, HARGREAVE T, RICHARDSON DW, BEST FSM: Analysis of human sperm function following exposure to the ionophore A23187: comparison of normospermic and oligozoospermic men. J Androl 5:321–329, 1984
6. AITKEN RJ, ROSS A, LEES MM: Analysis of sperm function in Kartagener's syndrome. Fertil Steril 40:696–698, 1983
7. AITKEN RJ, SUTTON M, WARNER PE, RICHARDSON DW: Relationships between the movement characteristics of human spermatozoa and their ability to penetrate cervical mucus and zona-free hamster oocytes. J Reprod Fertil 73:441–449, 1985
8. AITKEN RJ, WANG Y-F, LUI J, BEST FSM, RICHARDSON DW: The influence of medium composition, osmolarity and albumin content on the acrosome reaction and fertilizing capacity of human spermatozoa: Development of an improved zona-free hamster egg penetration test. Int J Androl 6:180–193, 1983
9. AITKEN RJ, WARNER PE, BEST FSM, TEMPLETON AA, DJAHANBAKHCH O, MORTIMER D, LEES MM: The predictability of subnormal penetrating capacity in cases of unexplained infertility. Int J Androl 6:212–220, 1983
10. BIGGERS JD, WHITTEN WK, WHITTINGHAM DG: The culture of mouse embryos *in vitro*. In DANIEL JC (ed): Methods in Mammalian Embryology, pp 86–96. San Francisco, Freeman, 1971
11. COMHAIRE F, VERMEULEN L, GHEDIRA K, MAS J, IRVINE S, CALLIPOLITIS G: Adenosine triphosphate in human semen: A quantitative estimate of fertilizing potential. Fertil Steril 40:500–504, 1983
12. DAVID G, SERRES C, JOUANNET P: Kinematics of human spermatozoa. Gamete Res 4:83–96, 1981
13. FLORMAN HM, STOREY BT: Mouse gamete interactions: The zona pellucida is the site of the acrosome reaction leading to fertilization *in vitro*. Dev Biol 91:121–130, 1982
14. GLASS RH, ERICSSON RJ: Spontaneous cure of male infertility. Fertil Steril 31:305–308, 1979
15. HULL MGR, MCLEOD FN, JOYCE DN, RAY BD, MCDERMOTT A: Human *in vitro* fertilization, *in vivo* sperm penetration of cervical mucus and unexplained infertility. Lancet iv:245–246, 1984
16. KATZ DF, OVERSTREET JW: Sperm motility assessment by videomicrography. Fertil Steril 35:188–193
17. KATZ DF, OVERSTREET JW, HANSON FW: A new quantitative test for sperm penetration into cervical mucus. Fertil Steril 33:179–186, 1980
18. KOEHLER JK, DE CURTIS I, STENCHEVER MA, SMITH D: Interaction of human sperm with zona-free hamster eggs: A freeze fracture study. Gamete Res 6:371–386, 1982
19. KREMER J: A simple penetration test. Int J Fertil 10:209–215, 1965
20. LEE WI, GADDUM-ROSSE P, SMITH D, STENCHEVER M, BLANDAU RJ: Laser light-scattering study of the effect of washing on sperm motility. Fertil Steril 38:62–67, 1982
21. MACLEOD J, GOLD RZ: The male factor in fertility and infertility. II. Spermatozoon counts in 1000 cases of known infertile marriage. J Urol 66:436–440, 1951
22. MAYEVSKY A, DAFNA BS, BARTOOV B: A multi-channel system for the measurement of spermatozoon collective motility. Int J Androl 3:436–446, 1980
23. NELSON CMK, BUNGE RG: Semen analysis: Evidence for changing parameters of male fertility potential. Fertil Steril 25:503–507, 1974
24. OVERSTREET JW, KATZ DF, HANSON FW, FONESCA JR: A simple inexpensive method for objective assessment of human sperm movement characteristics. Fertil Steril 31:162–172, 1979
25. OVERSTREET JW, YANAGIMACHI R, KATZ DF, HAYASHI K, HANSON FW: Penetration of human spermatozoa into the human zona pellucida and the zona-free hamster egg: a study of fertile donors and infertile patients. Fertil Steril 33:534–542, 1980
26. PERREAULT SD, ROGERS BJ: Relationship between fertilizing ability and cAMP in human spermatozoa. J Androl 3:396–401, 1982
27. SCHATS R, AITKEN RJ, TEMPLETON AA, DJAHANBAKHCH O: The role of cervical mucus-semen interaction in infertility of unknown aetiology. Br J Obstet Gynaecol 91:371–376, 1984
28. SMITH D, RODRIGUEZ-RIGAU ZJ, STEINBERGER E: Relation between indices of semen analysis and pregnancy rate in infertile couples. Fertil Steril 28:1314–1319, 1977

29. TEMPLETON AA, AITKEN RJ, MORTIMER D, BEST FSM: Sperm function in patients with unexplained infertility. Br J Obstet Gynaecol 89:550–554, 1982
30. TEMPLETON AA, MORTIMER D: Laparoscopic sperm recovery in infertile patients Br J Obstet Gynaecol 87:1128–1131, 1980
31. TEMPLETON AA, MORTIMER D: The development of a clinical test of sperm migration to the site of fertilization. Fertil Steril 37:410–415, 1982
32. TRIANA LR, BABCOCK DF, LORTON SP, FIRST N, LARDY HA: Release of acrosomal hyaluronidase follows increased membrane permeability to calcium in the presumptive capacitation sequence for spermatozoa of the bovine and other mammalian species. Biol Reprod 23:47–59, 1980
33. VAN ZYL JA, MENKVELD R, VAN KOTZE W, RETIEF AE, VAN NIEKERK WA: Oligozoospermia: A seven-year survey of the incidence, chromosomal aberrations, treatment and pregnancy rate. Int J Fertil 20:129–132, 1975
34. YANAGIMACHI R: Zona-free hamster eggs: Their use in assessing fertilizing capacity and examining chromosomes of human spermatozoa. Gamete Res 10:187–232, 1984
35. YANAGIMACHI R, YANAGIMACHI H, ROGERS BJ: The use of zona-free animal ova as a test system for the assessment of fertilizing capacity of human spermatozoa. Biol Reprod 15:471–476, 1976

16

Discussion: Assessment of Sperm Function

MODERATOR: EMIL STEINBERGER

IN THE HAMSTER IN VITRO FERTILIZATION TEST, WAS THE INCREASE IN THE PRECISION OF PREDICTABILITY USEFUL?

There was a difference in predictability; successful discrimination with the hamster oocyte penetration test alone was 75%; with the addition of the movement characteristics of the sperm, successful discrimination rose to 82%. It could be argued, however, that adding the movement characteristic study to add only a 7% increase in discrimination may not be useful.

WHAT IS THE IMPORTANCE OF WITHIN-ASSAY AND BETWEEN-ASSAY VARIABILITY AMONG SPERM SAMPLES FROM THE SAME MAN?

It is often difficult to ascertain from the way frequency distributions of ova penetration by normal spermatozoa are given, whether the frequency distribution is related to the performance of the bioassay system or is related to some inherent property of a particular subject. The within-assay coefficient of variation can be easily determined and it is about 7%. It is very difficult, however, to determine between-assay variability. The coefficient of variation for repeated ejaculates from the same man in a normal, fertile population is about 15%. Thus in the same man there is variation of sperm from sample to sample. The difference between a frequency distribution for an oligozoospermic population, in which 70% of the samples score zero, and the frequency distribution of a normal fertile population or a population treated with A23187, in which a majority of the samples score from 50% to 100%, are differences that would exist despite the variation between samples from the same man. So, if the coefficient of variation of a man who scores 10% on an individual assay is 15%, that means that on some assays the man will score as high as 30%. Although frequency distribution is described as normal, whether variations between samples from the same subjects have a normal distribution remains to be seen.

Panelists: R. John Aitken, Rune Eliasson, Kamran S. Moghissi, Eric Odeblad, Lourens J. D. Zaneveld. *Participants:* C. Wayne Bardin, B. Norman Barwin, Blaise Bourrit, Eric N. Chantler, Jean Cohen, Timothy Farley, Erwin Goldberg, Michel Thiery

IS IT PERHAPS TIME TO FOCUS ON THE REAPPLICATION OF BIOASSAY STATISTICS TO A CLINICAL BIOASSAY?

Statistics for bioassays have been available since the 1930s, when vitamin assays were first devised, yet today probably only a handful of people consider appropriate statistical analysis of the hamster oocyte penetration test. Possibly it is time to apply bioassay statistics to a clinical bioassay, although that is almost never done. It is probably useful to use the zona-free hamster oocyte penetration test to do that.

As reinforcement of this concept, the variation among men over time can be significant in terms of fertility. Frequently, it is assumed that every sample that a man produces must be a normal, fertile sample, and a zero penetration rate in some samples is considered a false-negative rate. That may be a wrong interpretation of what goes on among samples from the same man. It is important to remember when presenting data on populations that there are significant variations in the quality of individual ejaculates.

Bringing the criteria devised for standard statistical bioassays to the zona-free hamster oocyte penetration test is extremely important. One of the important points is the concept of sensitivity, a concept that exists in assays for hormones, and should be introduced for the hamster oocyte test, because one has to be sure that a significant number of "particles" exist in the form of gametes to make those assays viable.

DID THE FUNCTIONALLY INFERTILE PATIENTS UNDERGO ALL CLINICAL TESTS, INCLUDING SPERM–CERVICAL MUCUS INTERACTION?

No, they did not. The male partners underwent conventional semen analysis studies; the females underwent a normal history, examination, evaluation of menstrual cycles, and diagnostic laparoscopy. Postcoital tests to look at sperm–cervical mucus interaction usually were done, but in prospective studies it was noted that the results of those assays bore no relationship to fertility, so they subsequently were dropped.

IN PREDICTING FERTILIZATION, WAS THE SURVIVAL SPERM TEST USED?

The survival sperm test was the best criterion for one group of investigators, who looked at the survival of the sperm after 16 hours in the culture medium. If they saw 15% of survival sperms it gave 80% also of prediction of fertilization. One of the functions used to obtain those discriminations was motility of the sperm 3 hours after isolation on ovum in columns. The A23187 tests are much more rapid than a conventional hamster oocyte assay. Instead a 12- or 16-hour capacitation period, a 3-hour period is used. The motility after 3 hours was a discriminating variable in that analysis, but whether survival for longer periods of time would also be a discriminating variable is not known. Possibly it would depend to a large extent on how the spermatozoa were prepared. As they were prepared in the present study, they stayed motile for at least 48 hours. If the spermatozoa are prepared by repeated centrifugation, their survival times probably will be much shorter.

WHAT IS THE ROLE OF VISCOSITY OR CLUMPING OF THE SEMEN AS ONE OF THE PARAMETERS FOR FERTILIZING CAPACITY?

Viscosity changes are seen in patients with inflammatory situations or adnexitis, but these will disappear when the patient is treated. A few patients, for unknown reasons, have a very high viscosity and infertility, and in those cases the viscosity is probably part of the infertility problem, but what the biochemical background is we do not know.

It is stating the obvious to note that pregnancy is sum total of many favorable factors; it is difficult to isolate any factor such as a male, tubal, or cervical factor, and relate it to pregnancy outcome. It is hazardous to do this kind of study unless adequate allowance has been made for all other factors involved. Poor liquefaction, however, appears to be a serious drawback for adequate sperm function. Such sperm do not fertilize well in the in vitro fertilization systems, and they do not respond to A23187. Various proteolytic agents have been tested, trying to break up these clumps, and although some are effective in breaking up the poor liquefaction status, the sperms are no longer functional.

WHAT IS THE RATIONALE BEHIND THE STATEMENT THAT THREE SEMEN SAMPLES ARE REQUIRED TO ASSESS THE SEMEN QUALITY RELIABLY?

When the variables were subjected to frequency distribution valuation and analyzed, it appeared that to reach a mean level of the several variables in the semen, three semen samples would be required to reflect that mean. With only one sample, reliability was only about 70%. With three samples, reliability was almost 85%. With four or five samples, there was a modest increase in reliability determination but that increase was not significant.

HAVE SEASONAL CHANGES BEEN OBSERVED IN THE LONGITUDINAL STUDY OF SEMEN ANALYSIS?

One investigator has made a transectional study of 5000 sperm analyses and observed a nadir in August (perhaps because of the temperature). There are some seasonal changes, but these are not statistically significant. As part of this study, investigators also looked at the effect of various factors (*e.g.*, psychologic factors, smoking, examinations, and a host of other conditions on semen analysis). One interesting finding is that about 2 or 3 days after a stressful experience, many semen characteristics actually improve; there is an increase in the sperm density, an improvement in motility, and then it becomes depressed a few weeks later. The explanation for this change is really unclear, except perhaps that it results from the release of catecholemines, which have been shown to improve the semen qualities temporarily.

DOES SECRETION OF G, L, AND S TYPE OF MUCUS CONTINUE THROUGH THE MENSTRUAL CYCLE? WHAT CONTROL MECHANISM AT THE CELLULAR LEVEL ALLOWS LOCAL CONTROL?

The model with G, L, and S cervical mucus implies that adjacent parts of the cervical epithelium secrete cervical mucus with different viscoelastic properties, suggesting some kind of morphologic basis for the various types. It seems difficult to understand how different areas on a continuous epithelium can secrete mucus that has obviously different rheologic properties, so there must be local control. This question has been under consideration for a long time, and so far there is no obvious difference under electron microscopy of these different areas. Other factors seem to be involved, however.

DOES THE SECRETORY PATTERN CHANGE?

As far as we know, the G mucus is constantly produced by the same area in all parts of the cervix, but as regards the L and S mucus, we are less certain about the constancy of the producing areas. There seems to be some persistence in time from one month to the next in this secretory behavior. We do know that the cervix undergoes a number of changes over time. When the same woman is observed year after year, the constant remodeling of the microanatomy of the cervix can be documented by colpophotography.

When a patient begins taking the pill, the S and L secretions are more or less inactivated in the cervix; then, when the patient ceases taking the pill, it will take some time before the S and L functions are restored. There seems to be some kind of functional atrophy in the upper part of the cervix in these patients, and it takes a few months or a year or longer in some patients before the secretory areas are activated again. This shows that the cervical mucosa is dynamic, changing more or less continuously; it is not a static organ.

WHAT IS KNOWN ABOUT THE INFLUENCE OF PROSTAGLANDIN SYNTHESIS INHIBITORS ON THE FERTILITY OF MEN?

The literature on that subject is rather controversial. Some investigators claim that there is an enhancement of fertilization if prostaglandin inhibitors are given to the male; others claim there is not. In the female, prostaglandin inhibitors can suppress fertility by preventing ovulation and may have some other effects on the female genital tract as well.

Experimental Approaches for Male Contraception

17

Experimental Studies in the Development of Male Contraceptives

ANDRZEJ BARTKE

DO WON HAHN

ROBIN G. FOLDESY

JOHN L. MCGUIRE

Whereas considerable progress has been made in the development of highly effective, acceptable and reversible methods of birth control for women, progress for the male has been slow. The ancient method of coitus interruptus (withdrawal) and the use of condoms (prophylactics) continue to be widely practiced but are not highly popular, apparently because of the improved contraceptive methods for the female. Nonetheless, vasectomy has become commonplace in many countries, including the United States, and its acceptance indicates a willingness by many men to assume responsibility for family planning.

Considerable research into male contraception has been conducted during the last several decades. Three central issues that commonly appear in the literature demonstrate the difficulty in this field. The first is the issue of whether drug-induced azoospermia is a prerequisite for a male contraceptive or whether low level oligospermia is adequate. This issue is still under study, but unless azoospermia is attained, the clinical efficacy of a male contraceptive, the efficacy of which is related to reduced sperm levels, always will be questioned. One issue that must be addressed by workers in this field is whether the objective is a male contraceptive that is essentially as effective as the female oral contraceptive (*i.e.*, protection for the individual person) or whether the objective is a male contraceptive that may be less efficacious for the man than are other products but is effective in lowering the overall fertility rate within a population. If it is the former, either azoospermia must be achieved or clinical data must show that drug-induced oligospermia can protect a fertile couple from pregnancy.

The second issue relates to safety. The intended consumer of a male contraceptive normally will be a healthy, fertile male. As with female contraceptives, the risk versus benefit considerations of a male contraceptive will require that safety standards be greater than are those often accepted for therapeutic agents for the treatment of clinical disorders.

The third issue relates to the nature of the male reproductive system and our current lack of existing male contraceptive products. In reality, there is a great deal of knowledge to be learned about the male reproductive system. We do not know how to interdict the production of sperm safely and reversibly. This is true for many other pharmacologic classes of drugs, but in the field of male contraception, we also have no existing products. The result of this dilemma is that we do not know the adequacy or extrapolatability of our experimental models to humans. We do not even know, for example, the exact requirements of androgens for maintenance of normal libido.

The lack of existing male contraceptive drugs and knowledge about the male reproductive system should not cause pessimism. The same analogous situation existed with female oral contraceptives prior to the time of Pincus, Garcia, Chang, and Rock.[81] Increased interest in male contraception has been generated in recent years by work with gossypol and LHRH agonists.[83,84] There is reason to believe that future research will lead to a better understanding of male reproductive physiology and to the discovery of male antifertility agents.

The purpose of this chapter is to describe experimental studies related to research on male contraceptives. We first describe various test systems used for studying potential male antifertility agents and then highlight the general strategies used and their relationship to our understanding of male reproductive physiology. Experiments by most investigators in this area are based either on hormonal approaches or on pharmacologic approaches. The former have been tested substantially in men and hence are reviewed from a clinical standpoint. On the other hand, very few pharmacologic compounds have been evaluated clinically, and the review of this area focuses on animal studies.

TEST SYSTEMS FOR EVALUATING MALE ANTIFERTILITY AGENTS

In devising a male contraceptive, the basic objective is to prevent the release of fertile spermatozoa at the time of ejaculation. There are three ways to accomplish this task: 1) to prevent the formation of spermatozoa in the testes; 2) to prevent the maturation of spermatozoa in the epididymis; and 3) to alter the integrity of stored spermatozoa. The first concept deals with testicular processes and the latter two with post-testicular events. Each requires animal models capable of evaluating these sites of action.

Generally, the method of evaluating compounds for male antifertility activity consists of administering a compound to an animal and assessing its fertility level by the number of offspring produced from cohabitations with fertile females. Ancillary information, such as testicular, epididymal, or prostatic organ weights or histologic appearances, often is obtained on autopsy at the end of the experiment.

One typical test method commonly used for evaluating compounds that may have an effect on spermatogenesis consists of administering compounds to male rats under a prolonged dosing regimen. This regimen must be maintained long enough to cover the period required for spermatogenesis (approximately 8 weeks). The compounds would be administered daily and each male would be cohabited individually with a proestrus female whose estrous cycle had been monitored previously. The first cohabitation would occur 1 or 2 weeks after initiation of treatment and at 1- to 2-week intervals thereafter. To establish each compound's efficacy, the females are autopsied approximately 2 weeks after mating and the number of fetuses recorded. The doses used on initial evaluation are generally large and then lowered on retesting if the compound shows activity.

Compounds to be tested for post-testicular activity are evaluated in a manner similar to that described above. The dosing regimen is generally shortened to 2 weeks, however, because the time for sperm passage through the epididymis is under 14 days.

As discussed above, one problem that all investigators in this field face is lack of knowledge about which species or test systems extrapolate to humans, because no male antifertility compounds have yet been developed. We do know, however, that species differences do exist. For example, if one looks at male antifertility agents thus far identified, mice, which would seem ideal because of their small size and relatively short spermatogenic cycle, respond poorly or not at all to some antifertility agents, such as gossypol,[36] LHRH agonists,[101] and chlorosugars.[52] Conversely, 5-thio-D-glucose is effective in mice. Such insensitivities to potential drug effects can result in valid pharmacologic activities going undetected. Rabbits would seem to be ideal animals to study male antifertility agents because of the ease with which semen samples can be obtained. Androgens are effective male antifertility agents in rabbits, but the rabbit has failed to respond to other antifertility agents, (*e.g.*, α-chlorohydrin).[3] Hamsters are often used for screening male antifertility compounds. Gossypol is an effective male antifertility agent in the hamster, but α-chlorohydrin is less effective in the hamster than in other species. Conversely, to our knowledge, all the compounds that have been reported to have male antifertility activity are active in the rat. For this reason, and because of its well-defined male reproductive system, this species often is used as the primary test system.

HORMONAL REGULATION OF MALE FERTILITY

STEROID HORMONES

One strategy for controlling male fertility is to suppress production of the hormones that support spermatogenesis. Perhaps the biggest obstacle to this approach is that testosterone supports several physiologic functions, including not only maintenance of sperm production, but also of libido and potency, external male characteristics, and physical strength. Every compound that blocks sperm production by suppressing testosterone synthesis potentially produces unacceptable symptoms of hypogonadism, and many investigators believe that practical application of such compounds would require suitable androgen replacement therapy.

The impact of suppressing endogenous androgen production and of androgen replacement on libido and potency in men is very difficult to predict because of very limited understanding of the hormonal control of male sexual behavior. Early studies in Young's laboratory indicated that testicular androgens are necessary for male sexual behavior to be expressed, but individual differences in copulatory activity do not reflect differences in peripheral androgen levels.[34] Thus, genetically and/or developmentally encoded differences in the response of the central nervous system (CNS) to stimulation by adult androgen levels would appear to be more important than the androgen levels per se. This concept was strengthened by subsequent demonstration that in castrated rats implanted with testosterone in Silastic capsules normal sexual behavior can be maintained by serum testosterone levels corresponding to less than $\frac{1}{3}$ of values measured in intact control animals.[18] Testosterone levels in peripheral circulation of intact animals fluctuate within a rather wide range due to the episodic pattern of testicular secretion, however. It is not known how meaningful it is to compare the average levels resulting from constant release implants to those resulting from the physiologic pattern of secretion. Thus Michael and his colleagues obtained some evidence that sexual behavior of male rhesus monkeys is related to the lower limit of daily fluctuations in plasma testosterone levels rather than to average levels or to the number or amplitude of secretory pulses.[72] The complex nature of relationships between circulating androgen levels and male sexual behavior is emphasized further by demonstrations that presence of a female can cause marked acute elevations in plasma testosterone levels,[54,56,64] that absence of these "surges" correlates with deficiencies of sexual behavior in male rats,[54*] and that injections of testosterone administered to normal intact males can stimulate copulatory behavior.[66] Understanding of these relationships in the human male is complicated by the paucity of carefully controlled, quantitative studies of sexual behavior in men; by placebo effects; and by the multitude of psychologic, cultural, environmental, and occupational factors that may affect libido and potency. There is also some evidence that the impact of modest decreases in plasma androgen levels on libido and potency in men may be related significantly to the age of experimental subjects.[11]

Progestogens, estrogens and androgens, LHRH-analogue treatment, and suppression of gonadotropins such as follicle-stimulating hormone (FSH) all have been attempted as approaches to regulation of male fertility.

Progesterone,[41] and several synthetic progestogens and different estrogenic preparations[1,39,41] have been shown to induce reversible azoospermia in men; however, these studies also demonstrated the adverse effects of suppressing testosterone in terms of male libido and potency.

The demonstration that normal concentrations of serum testosterone can be chronically maintained in castrated animals by subcutaneous implantation of crystalline testosterone enclosed in Silastic capsules raised the possibility that blood testosterone levels could be maintained in men treated with contraceptive steroids, thus compensating for the drug-induced loss of endogenous testosterone. This was tested clinically in pilot studies sponsored by the International Committee for Contraception Research of the Population Council in the early 1970s. These studies involved a total of 38 volunteers and were conducted in 3 different laboratories.[15,30,53] Synthetic progestins (megestrol acetate, norethindrone, norgestrienone, or R2323) were administered as either subcutaneous Silastic implants, oral preparations, or a combination

---

* Sellers, Bartke: Unpublished data, 1985

of both. All men also received subcutaneous Silastic capsules containing testosterone. The treatment period varied from 3 to 24 weeks, and the response was assessed by sperm count or testicular biopsy. Azoospermia was produced in 14 men, whereas other subjects experienced various degrees of suppression of spermatogenesis, ranging from a modest reduction in sperm count to extreme oligozoospermia. Examination of biopsy material in 13 patients treated with norethindrone plus testosterone revealed Leydig cell atrophy.[26] Patients reported no change in libido or potency, and there was no change in ejaculate volume. Some patients experienced weight gain, and one developed gynecomastia. In a few patients who were monitored after the study, recovery of pretreatment sperm counts was recorded 5 to 13 weeks after treatment was discontinued. This approach was limited, however, by the failure to achieve azoospermia in over half of the treated men.

The potential of progestin and testosterone combinations for induction of reversible azoospermia was reinvestigated more recently using monthly intramuscular injections of depot medroxyprogesterone acetate (Depo-Provera) and either testosterone enanthate, a long-acting ester of testosterone, or Silastic implants of testosterone propionate. These investigations were conducted in four centers and reported in a series of papers in 1977.[2,8,31,32,71] A total of 99 men were treated for 6 weeks to 16 months. Because of differences in the length of treatment and in the design of the studies, it is difficult to determine the exact incidence of azoospermia, but sperm counts in the majority of the subjects were clearly reduced to below 1×10^6/ml. Serum levels of gonadotropins and testosterone were reduced, but in some patients these hormonal changes were either transient or not evident. In one segment of these studies, 41 patients of Frick and colleagues experienced a transient decrease in libido.[31,32] Of the remaining 58 men, 2 reported a decrease and 4 an increase in libido. In none of these studies were any detectable changes in the size of testes, prostate, or breast tissue reported, except for one case of gynecomastia. In some of the studies, weight gain was noted either throughout or during the initial treatment period. In one study in which the reversibility of this treatment was examined in 14 men,[8] sperm counts reached pretreatment values within 16 to 41 weeks after the treatment was discontinued. In contrast to these generally encouraging results, Alvarez-Sanchez and his collaborators noted that with continued treatment, the suppressed blood levels of testosterone, LH, and FSH began to increase and spermatogenesis to recover (the latter evidenced by small but detectable increases in sperm count).[2]

The possibility of developing a hormonal male contraceptive based on an estrogen rather than a progestin was tested by Briggs and Briggs.[9] These investigators succeeded in producing azoospermia in each of five volunteers with an oral regimen of ethinyl estradiol plus methyltestosterone. Libido did not seem affected, with some participants reporting a decrease and others an increase. No pregnancies occurred when the men were advised of their sterility after 18 weeks of treatment and were asked to use no other methods of birth control during the following 16 weeks. In spite of these encouraging preliminary results, the development of a male contraceptive containing estrogenic preparations appears very unlikely. Chronic treatment of prostatic cancer patients with estrogens reveals a variety of unacceptable side-effects, and prolonged exposure of a normal male population to estrogenic substances would be difficult to advocate.

Antifertility effects of cyproterone acetate, a progestogenic antiandrogen, in experimental animals stimulated interest in this compound as a potential male contraceptive. Petry and co-workers reported reversible suppression of spermatogenesis in five men treated with cyproterone acetate for 11 to 16 weeks without any apparent effects on libido,[82] whereas treatment with higher doses was shown in other studies to lead to loss of libido and potency.[73] More recent studies, however, indicated that significant suppression of serum gonadotropin and testosterone levels with low doses was accompanied by only a modest decline in sperm count.[25,102] The limited success in suppressing sperm production, the occurrence of two unplanned pregnancies in one of these studies,[25] and untoward side-effects in some of the participating volunteers lead to the conclusion that cyproterone acetate would be unsuitable as a single-entity agent for long-term male contraception.[102]

Another compound that attracted considerable attention as a possible male contraceptive is danazol, a synthetic analogue of ethinyl testosterone that has been referred to as an "incomplete androgen" owing to its unique profile of biologic effects. Skoglund and Paulsen reported that treatment with danazol alone led to only a modest reduction in sperm count, but in combination with testosterone esters (propionate or enanthate), it produced severe oligozoospermia and, in some instances, azoospermia.[93] The same laboratory subsequently reported that 6 months of oral danazol treatment combined with monthly intramuscular injections of testosterone enanthate[100] reduced sperm counts to less than 10×10^6/ml in men treated with 400 mg daily, and to below 5×10^6/ml in those given 600 mg daily. This was accompanied by a significant increase in the percentage of morphologically abnormal spermatozoa and immature forms in the ejaculate. Three months after the treatment was discontinued, sperm counts returned to normal. There were no changes in libido or ejaculate volume and no evidence of changes in liver function. The relatively high doses required for these effects, in addition to the lack of a uniform response in all subjects, impeded the further development of danazol as a male contraceptive.

The ability of exogenous androgens to suppress spermatogenesis in men has been known for over 40 years, but the contraceptive use of exogenous androgens appeared not to have been contemplated until very much later. Because testosterone can suppress gonadotropin release, and the concentration of testosterone in the testes normally is much higher than in the peripheral circulation, it was postulated by several investigators that treatment with testosterone should maintain serum testosterone concentration at a level that is sufficient for suppressing pituitary function, endogenous testosterone production, and spermatogenesis, and for maintaining libido and potency, but too low for exerting direct stimulatory effects on sperm production. This assumption was based on a considerable amount of evidence from animal studies.[6,20,23,98]

Reddy and Rao reported that men receiving daily injections of testosterone propionate for 2 months experienced azoospermia that was fully reversible and not accompanied by changes in libido or seminal volume.[81] Testicular size was reduced, but returned to normal when the treatment was discontinued.

The availability of testosterone enanthate, a long-acting ester of testosterone, overcame the necessity for daily intramuscular injections. The ability of testosterone enanthate to induce azoospermia had been reported in 1970 by Heller and his coinvestigators.[42] Subsequently, Mauss and his collaborators reported that injections of testosterone enanthate once a week for 21 weeks induced severe oligozoospermia in men as well as a reduction in sperm motility and the percent of normal forms, without affecting libido or ejaculate volume.[68,69] Plasma testosterone levels were increased approximately twofold, whereas LH and FSH levels were significantly depressed. Normal sperm counts were restored within 13 weeks after discontinuation of the treatment.

Although these results demonstrated unequivocally that reversible suppression of spermatogenesis in men can be achieved by treatment with testosterone alone, a number of important questions remained unanswered. These included the effectiveness of a less frequent (and thus presumably more acceptable) injection regimen, the ability of this type of treatment to maintain azoospermia or extreme oligozoospermia for prolonged periods of time and, in particular, the necessity for chronically maintaining elevated peripheral testosterone levels. The latter issue was considered to be of paramount importance because of possible untoward effects of chronic supraphysiologic levels of testosterone. There is little reason to believe that modest elevation of serum testosterone levels would have any undesirable effects, but pathologic changes in liver function have been described in men treated with high doses of various androgenic preparations.[104] There is also some concern over the possible effects on the prostate. There is no evidence that testosterone treatment can induce prostatic hypertrophy or cancer, but it is well established that testicular androgens can stimulate the growth of an existing carcinoma. Because the contraceptive use of testosterone would expose a segment of the male population to long-term testosterone therapy, even the most vague concerns about hepatic toxicity or development of prostatic cancer assume obvious significance.

In an attempt to overcome some of these potential problems, Steinberger and Smith devised a schedule of treatment with testosterone enanthate consisting of two phases: "induction" by administering 200-mg doses of testosterone enanthate twice weekly for 2 weeks, followed by "maintenance" with less frequent injections.[96] The intent of this regimen was to suppress LH and FSH release from the pituitary by significantly increasing peripheral testosterone levels during the induction phase, and subsequently to maintain this suppression with much lower doses of testosterone enanthate. Preliminary results were encouraging. Even though serum testosterone levels declined to normal during the maintenance phase, LH and FSH levels remained suppressed and the sperm count was reduced. In five men injected with testosterone enanthate every 10 to 12 days during the maintenance phase, serum LH levels were severely suppressed, and the sperm count was below 0.1 $\times$ 10^6/ml, with only occasional spermatozoa being detected in some of the ejaculates; the men were described as "essentially azoospermic." Most of the participants were recruited from patients who requested a vasectomy and underwent this procedure after completing the testosterone enanthate treatment. In those who later decided against vasectomy, there was good recovery of sperm count and motility, with a known return of fertility in two cases.[97] Similar results were reported by Swerdloff and associates.[99]

The relatively mild side-effects of injectable testosterone enanthate include transient weight gain, increase in skin oiliness and acne in some men, and the expected reversible reduction in testes size. Prostate size does not appear to be affected by this form of treatment and there is no evidence of changes in liver function or "blood chemistry."[17,97,99]

From the foregoing sections of this review, it is evident that steroid treatment can produce reversible suppression of sperm production in men without adverse effects on libido or potency, and with minimal side-effects. Administration of testosterone esters alone appears to be particularly promising. Much of the original skepticism toward the use of steroids for male contraception has not been dispelled completely, however. Complete azoospermia is difficult to achieve in all treated subjects, and the possibility of fertility with oligozoospermia has already been discussed. Furthermore, the possibility that chronic steroid treatment of men could affect their progeny was addressed in a literature survey conducted by Ketchell.[57] No increase in the incidence of spontaneous abortions or congenital abnormalities was reported in 1000 pregnancies resulting from conceptions during or after androgen treatment of the male. In those cases in which child development was followed, it was found to be entirely normal.

The side-effects of contraceptive steroid therapy do not appear severe or life-threatening, but most of the studies conducted involved relatively short treatment periods and few subjects. More extensive studies will be required before the concerns about safety and efficacy can be fully answered. Guidelines for conducting such studies were recently developed by the Food and Drug Administration.[88]

LHRH AND ITS ANALOGUES

Elucidation of the structure of hypothalamic luteinizing hormone-releasing hormone (LHRH) permitted routine synthesis of this peptide and opened new possibilities for experimental and clinical manipulation of reproductive functions. The potential for practical use of LHRH was advanced further by development of analogues that either degrade in vivo more slowly than the parent compound or bind to target cell receptors with greater affinity and therefore exhibit enhanced biologic potency. When LHRH agonists are given chronically to humans, the function of the pituitary–testicular axis is suppressed.[5,13,16,59,87,89] In men, progressive loss of pituitary responsiveness to LHRH appears to be the predominant mechanism of testicular suppression.[5]

The excellent responses in women treated with LHRH agonist in the form of intranasal spray indicate that injections could probably be circumvented.[78] Suppression of testicular function by LHRH agonist in a boy with precocious puberty,[37] and in patients with prostatic cancer[24] further attests to its potential for inducing infertility.

These findings suggested that LHRH agonists could be useful as a male contraceptive, and different regimens of LHRH-agonist administration have been tested for their ability to suppress spermatogenesis in men. The results demonstrated that daily subcutaneous self-administration of 50 μg doses of LHRH agonists produce a significant reduction in sperm count within a few weeks.[84] This effect was evident in each of eight participants and appeared readily reversible. Chronic treatment with LHRH agonist alone, however, is unsuitable as a male contraceptive because it should induce a precipitous decline in peripheral testosterone levels, with a consequent loss of libido and potency. Indeed, subjects have reported the occurrence of "hot flashes."[84] On the other hand, it is reasonable to expect that simultaneous testosterone replacement may prevent this from occurring. The recent demonstration of synergistic effects of testosterone and LHRH agonists on the inhibition of spermatogenesis in adult male rats[38] further emphasizes the contraceptive potential of treating men with a combination of LHRH agonists and an androgen. In this context, it is of interest that in laboratory animals LHRH can potentiate the effects of gonadal steroids on sexual behavior in male and female rats.[74] Extrapolating the sexual behavior in rats to libido in men is not clear, but these data suggest that, in men treated with LHRH agonists, it may be possible to maintain libido with modest doses of exogenous testosterone.

Extensive structure and activity studies with LHRH analogues also has led to the discovery of competitive LHRH antagonists. These compounds also interfere with the ability of endogenous LHRH to stimulate LH and FSH release, apparently by interacting with LHRH receptors present in gonadotropin-producing anterior pituitary cells. Gonzales-Barcena and associates reported that an LHRH antagonist attenuated the LH and FSH responses to exogenous LHRH in men.[33] Zarate and colleagues demonstrated the ability of LHRH antagonists to prevent ovulation in women by blocking the midcycle ovulatory surge of LH.[107] Chronic treatment of men with LHRH antagonists would seem almost certain to interfere with androgen biosynthesis, lead to loss of libido, and require testosterone substitution, as discussed above for LHRH agonists.

An interesting possibility of developing formulations of LHRH analogues suitable for oral treatment was suggested by studies of Nekola and her collaborators in the rat.[76]

CONTROL OF FSH SECRETION

The only fully documented effect of FSH is to maintain the Sertoli cells in a functional state necessary for the normal progression of spermatogenesis. In addition, FSH apparently contributes to the testicular responsiveness to LH, but it is unlikely that its deficiency in an adult male would compromise testosterone production significantly. Thus, on purely theoretical grounds, the release of FSH from the pituitary or its actions in the testes would appear to provide ideal targets for fertility suppression. In support of this possibility, Madwa, Raj, and Dym produced pronounced degenerative changes in the seminiferous tubules of immature rats by treatment with anti-FSH antibodies, without affecting Leydig cell structure, plasma testosterone levels, or weights of accessory reproductive glands.[65] Identical treatment of adult rats had little, if any, effect on spermatogenesis, however. Recent progress in isolation and purification of inhibin holds promise of developing a method for selective suppression of FSH release without resorting to active or passive immunization.

Inhibin, a substance produced by Sertoli cells and granulosa cells, suppresses FSH synthesis and release. Fractions enriched in inhibin activity have been prepared from testes, rete testes fluid, seminal plasma, and follicular fluid and have been partially characterized. Development of a radioimmunoassay for inhibin has also been reported.[91] However, the results obtained in different laboratories vary widely, particularly with respect to the estimates of molecular weight of the presumably purified inhibin.[4,85]

More importantly, recent studies raised significant doubts whether suppression of FSH release or its biologic activity could produce azoospermia in adult males. Treatment with human chorionic gonadotropin (hCG) can stimulate sperm production in men in whom endogenous gonadotropin secretion was suppressed by hCG, or by administration of testosterone enanthate.[7,55] Modest doses of human LH are also capable of stimulating spermatogenesis in men rendered azoospermic or severely oligospermic by testosterone administration.[67] Thus, although FSH is almost certainly involved in the control of seminiferous tubule function in normal men, suppression of peripheral FSH levels below the limit of detectability does not preclude continued production of spermatozoa.

PHARMACOLOGIC CONTROL OF MALE FERTILITY

COMPOUNDS WITH PHARMACOLOGIC ACTIONS ON TESTICULAR PHYSIOLOGY

One of the first compounds to be studied extensively as a male antifertility agent was the tumor-inhibiting substance, tretamine or TEM.[47] This and several chemically related compounds, including triethylenephosphoramide (TEPA), hexamethylphosphoramide (HMPA), and hexamethylmelamine (HMM), induced reversible sterility in male rats (Fig. 17-1). TEM and TEPA are potent alkylating agents that act presumably by binding to sperm nucleoproteins. Although they do not prevent the formation of spermatozoa, they apparently damage the genetic material so that embryonic development is arrested after fertilization occurs. HMPA produces the same result. When a single intraperitoneal dose of 0.2 mg/kg of TEM is given to adult male rats, transient sterility develops 4 weeks later. If this dose is given daily for 5 days, infertility develops immediately and persists for 35 days. Fertility returns if the treatment is not repeated. HMPA and HMM, as well as TEM, can also disrupt spermatogonial division and thereby prevent the completion of spermatogenesis. This causes infertility, beginning 60 to 70 days after the initial treatment.[48] The toxicity of these compounds, however, together with the possible conception of a genetically defective fetus following an inadequate dose, has discouraged further study of these agents.[61]

Shortly after the initial experiments with TEM,[47] it was observed that another alkylating agent, busulphan, also exhibited antifertility activity in male rats (Fig. 17-2). Busulphan, developed initially as a possible tumor inhibitor,

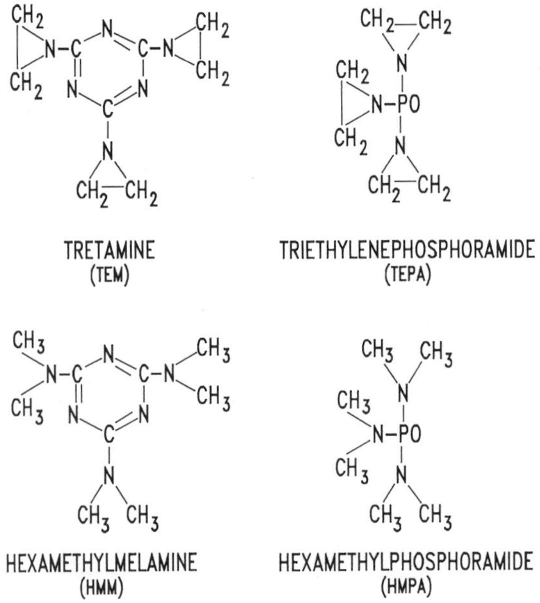

TRETAMINE
(TEM)

TRIETHYLENEPHOSPHORAMIDE
(TEPA)

HEXAMETHYLMELAMINE
(HMM)

HEXAMETHYLPHOSPHORAMIDE
(HMPA)

FIG. 17-1. Early tumor-inhibiting compounds possessing reversible antifertility effects in male rats.

did not possess as broad a cytotoxic effect as TEM. It interfered specifically with the development of spermatogonia but not with that of other germinal cells. Its antifertility effects therefore were not apparent until 7 weeks after administration.[49] Extending these studies, an attempt was made to explore structure and activity relationships of alkylating agents and to separate tumor-inhibiting properties from antifertility effects. A number of simple

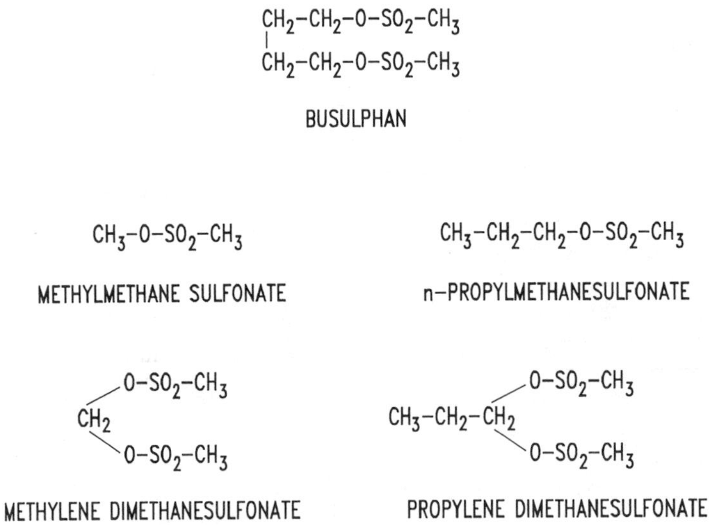

$$CH_2-CH_2-O-SO_2-CH_3$$
$$CH_2-CH_2-O-SO_2-CH_3$$

BUSULPHAN

$$CH_3-O-SO_2-CH_3$$

METHYLMETHANE SULFONATE

$$CH_3-CH_2-CH_2-O-SO_2-CH_3$$

n−PROPYLMETHANESULFONATE

$$CH_2 \begin{matrix} O-SO_2-CH_3 \\ O-SO_2-CH_3 \end{matrix}$$

METHYLENE DIMETHANESULFONATE

$$CH_3-CH_2-CH_2 \begin{matrix} O-SO_2-CH_3 \\ O-SO_2-CH_3 \end{matrix}$$

PROPYLENE DIMETHANESULFONATE

FIG. 17-2. Alkane sulfonic esters with reversible male antifertility activity.

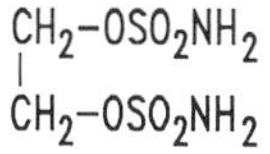

$$CH_2-OSO_2NH_2$$
$$CH_2-OSO_2NH_2$$

1,2-BIS-O-SULFAMYL-1,2-ETHANEDIOL

(ORF 11083)

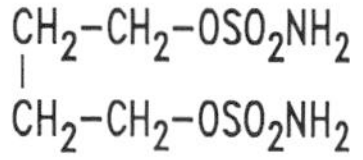

$$CH_2-CH_2-OSO_2NH_2$$
$$CH_2-CH_2-OSO_2NH_2$$

1,4-BIS-O-SULFAMYL-1,4-BUTANEDIOL

(ORF 11803)

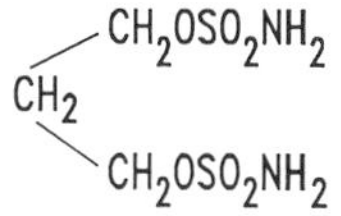

$$CH_2 \begin{array}{l} CH_2OSO_2NH_2 \\ \\ CH_2OSO_2NH_2 \end{array}$$

1,3-BIS-O-SULFAMYL-1,3-PROPANEDIOL

(ORF 11804)

FIG. 17-3. Three N-unsubstituted sulfamates found to be active in male antifertility laboratory studies.

alkane sulfonic esters were synthesized (Fig. 17-2) and their activities were comparable to those of TEM and busulphan.[12,49] Attempts also have been made to find more potent and less toxic derivatives of these compounds. A large number of N-unsubstituted sulfamates were synthesized and evaluated. Three were found to be active in male rats: ORF 11083, ORF 11803, and ORF 11804 (Fig. 17-3). Despite the structural similarity between the analogues, there were differences in their pharmacologic actions. When male rats were treated for 2 weeks with a dose of approximately 0.4 mMol/kg (80 mg/kg, ORF 11083; 100 mg/kg, ORF 11803, and ORF 11804) and then cohabited with females, ORF 11083 had no effect on the number of implants per female but did cause resorption of nearly all implants. Conversely, ORF 11803 totally prevented implantation whereas ORF 11804 reduced the number of normal implants and increased nonviable implants.[43] Further study with ORF 11083 revealed different pharmacologic actions in different species. Although the compound was active in rats, mice, and hamsters, its effect on fertility was greatest in the rat. Furthermore, moderate doses were extremely toxic to rabbits. ORF 11083 did not inhibit spermatogenesis but did affect spermatids and epididymal spermatozoa. This supported the concept first proposed by Jackson and associates that synthesis of compounds with selective effects on spermatozoa only, rather than on spermatogenesis as a whole, could be achieved.[49] This particular compound, however, displayed undesirable toxicity at higher doses, which precluded its further development.

Through the 1950s and early 1960s, a number of heterocyclic compounds were investigated for their ability to inhibit spermatogenesis. Four classes in

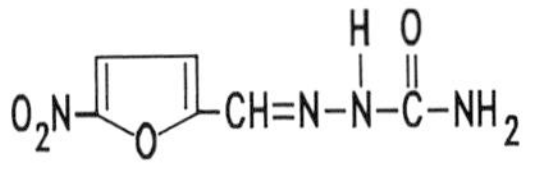

O₂N–[furan]–CH=N–N–C–NH₂ (with H and O above)

FURACIN

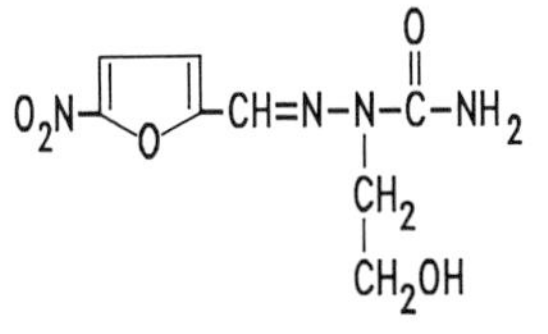

O₂N–[furan]–CH=N–N–C–NH₂
with CH₂ and CH₂OH below

FURADROXYL

O₂N–[furan]–CH=N–N with ring C—NH, CH₂–C=O

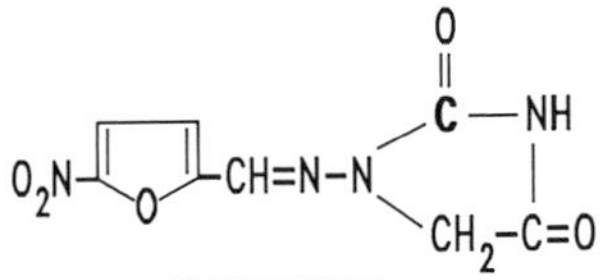

FURADANTIN

FIG. 17-4. Nitrofurans with reversible antifertility effects on spermatogenesis.

particular, nitrofurans, thiophenes, *bis*(dichloroacetyl)diamines, and dinitropyrroles, showed strong male antifertility activity that was reversible when treatment was withdrawn.

The antifertility activity of three nitrofurans (Fig. 17-4) in male rats was reported by Nelson and Steinberger.[77] All induced sterility, although there was a 30-fold difference in the potency of nitrofurazone (Furacin) over nitrofurantoin (Furadantin). Although the possibility of a hormonal involvement was never excluded completely, these compounds appeared to affect spermatogenesis directly, especially at the stage of the primary spermatocytes. The infertility was reversible on cessation of treatment. However, a limited study with nitrofurantoin (Furadantin) in human volunteers revealed gastrointestinal side-effects at the doses necessary for achieving antifertility effects.[94]

Of the class of compounds known as the thiophens, one in particular, 5-chlor-2-acetylthiophen (Ba 1044), shown in Fig. 17-5, was found to induce reversible sterility in male rats when given in the diet. Thirty days after treatment, all seminiferous tubules lacked spermatids and several were depleted of primary spermatocytes as well.[95] Because the treatment reduced the size of accessory reproductive glands, an effect on the endocrine system apparently was involved.[94] No further studies of this compound were conducted.

One of the few male antifertility compounds to have been evaluated in humans belongs to the class known as the *bis*(dichloroacetyl)diamines. These

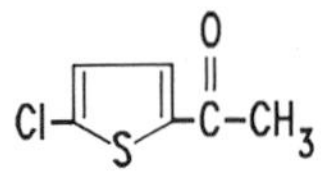

Cl–[thiophene]–C–CH₃ (with O above)

FIG. 17-5. Ba 1044, a thiophen, with antireproductive effects in male rats.

5–CHLOR–2–ACETYL–THIOPHEN

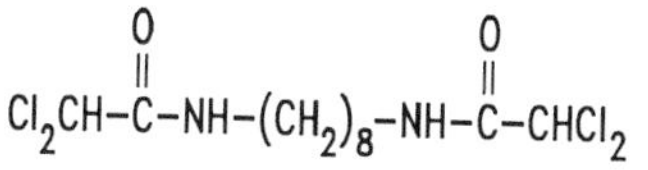

$$Cl_2CH-\overset{\overset{\displaystyle O}{\|}}{C}-NH-(CH_2)_8-NH-\overset{\overset{\displaystyle O}{\|}}{C}-CHCl_2$$

N,N'-BIS(DICHLOROACETYL)-1,8-OCTANEDIAMINE

(WIN 18446)

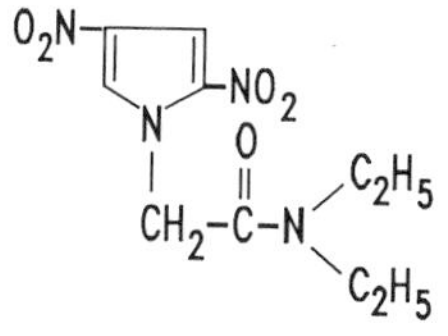

1-(N,N-DIETHYCARBAMYLMETHYL)-2,4-DINITROPYRROLE

(ORF 1616)

FIG. 17-6. Two antispermatogenic compounds, WIN 18446, a *bis*(dichloroacetyl)diamine, and ORF 1616, a dinitropyrrole.

compounds were intended originally for use as amebicidal agents. It was discovered, however, that some also possessed antispermatogenic activity and that a separation of their activities could be achieved.[79] Because of its potency and low toxicity, N,N'-*bis*(dichloroacetyl)-1,8-octanediamine or WIN 18446 (Fig. 17-6) appeared quite promising. When given to normal male volunteers twice daily, it produced a marked decline in sperm production within 12 weeks. The absence of changes in Leydig cell cytology as well as in the maintenance of secondary sex characteristics suggested no interference with androgen production.[40] Serum gonadotropin levels were elevated, but this may have been because of germ cell depletion.[19] The antifertility effects of the drug were reversible, and normal sperm production returned within 9 to 23 weeks. Nonetheless, WIN 18446 did not progress beyond the early clinical stages because of acute cardiovascular and CNS reactions, the so-called Antabuse effect, that results from increased concentrations of acetaldehyde in the body when alcohol is consumed during drug treatment.

The final class of heterocyclic compounds that showed promise as male antifertility drugs is that known as the dinitropyrroles. The most studied compound in this group was ORF 1616 (Fig. 17-6). Doses as low as 20 mg/kg/day in the diet induced functional sterility in rats within 12 weeks. A single dose of 500 mg/kg administered by gavage rendered rats sterile in about 3 weeks. Sterility lasted for about 4 weeks and could be maintained with monthly doses. After cessation of treatment, recovery was complete, even in animals that had been treated for 1 year. Partial recovery required about 1 month and full recovery, about 2 months. Spermatocytes and spermatids seemed most affected, whereas Leydig and Sertoli cells appeared unchanged as evaluated by light microscopy. ORF 1616 appeared to have little impact on serum androgens or gonadotropins. Although this drug induced similar alterations in the testes of guinea pigs and rabbits, the problem of its general toxicity prevented testing in humans.[80]

More recently, several other compounds with antispermatogenic effects have been investigated. One is 5-thio-D-glucose (Fig. 17-7), which was re-

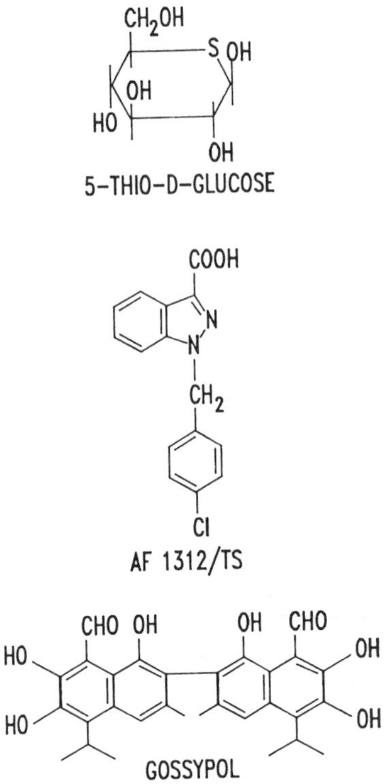

FIG. 17-7. Three compounds recently investigated for their male antifertility activities.

ported to produce reversible sterility in male mice.[108] The antifertility effects were evident after drug administration for 3 weeks in mice[108] and 5 weeks in rats.[46] Although the mechanism of action is not entirely clear, the compound has antispermatogenic effects, possibly through interference with testicular carbohydrate metabolism. After 5 weeks of daily treatment with a dose of 50 mg/kg, early testicular degeneration appeared with the presence of spermatidial giant cells, spermatogonia, and a few primary spermatocytes. The Leydig cells did not appear affected. The relative weights of the accessory reproductive organs and the endocrine glands were unchanged, and histopathologic examination of these and several other organs failed to detect any abnormalities.[46] The persistence of sterility in some animals long after cessation of treatment (Table 17-1), however, terminated pharmaceutical interest in this compound as a possible male contraceptive.[46,63]

The 1-halobenzyl-1H-indazole-3-carboxylic acids compose another class of recently discovered antispermatogenic compounds. The original compound in the series was 1-p-chlorobenzyl-1H-indazole-3-carboxylic acid (Fig. 17-7), referred to as AF 1312/TS.[92] It induced mainly a loss of spermatocytes and spermatids, probably through its effects on the Sertoli cell. Synthesis and evaluation of several related structures revealed two potent analogues, lonidamine and tolnidamine. Activity could be attained with high single doses or lower multiple doses. Furthermore, no loss in body weight was observed at antispermatogenic doses and no effects on the accessory reproductive organs

TABLE 17-1. Persistence of Antifertility Effects Following Oral Administration of 5-thio-D-glucose to Male Rats

DAILY DOSE* (mg/kg)	DURATION OF TREATMENT (wk)	WEEKS REQUIRED FOR COMPLETE INFERTILITY	MALES PERMANENTLY STERILE (%)†
12.5	15	14	60
25	8	6	100
50	8	5	100

* Each group contained 5 rats.

† Sterility was determined by weekly matings for a period of 9–12 months after cessation of drug treatment.

Adapted from Homm RE, Rusticus C, Hahn DW: The antispermatogenic effects of 5-thio-D-glucose to male rats. Biol Reprod 17:697–700, 1977)

were apparent.[14] The infertility, however, was not always reversible. In one study, fertility did not return in 60% of the rats receiving 50 mg/kg lonidamine weekly or monthly, and all rats receiving a single dose of 500 mg/kg were permanently sterile.[60] Another potential problem with these compounds was some evidence of renal toxicity.[60] Studies on this class of compounds continue.

Wiebe and Barr recently reported that a single intratesticular administration of 1,2,3-trihydroxypropane (glycerol) to adult rats leads to depletion of seminiferous tubules of germinal cells and sterility without affecting testicular production of androgenic steroids or suppressing sex behavior.[105] This may represent a possible new development in the search for a male contraceptive. The effects of glycerol on testicular function and fertility are discussed by Wiebe and co-authors in more detail in Chapter 24.

Gossypol, a naturally occurring substance derived from cottonseeds, was recently demonstrated to exhibit antispermatogenic activity (see Fig. 17-7). In studies conducted in China, gossypol has been tested in human volunteers. Significantly, the number of persons involved in these studies, nearly 9000 men, was far larger than that of any other male contraceptive study.[83] It is important also to note that three different forms—gossypol, gossypol acetic acid, and gossypol formic acid—have been used in the many clinical and laboratory studies, and that gossypol also exists as two optically active isomers. Its pharmacologic action has been studied in rats, hamsters, mice, dogs, rabbits, monkeys, and humans. Significant species differences exist, with the hamster being perhaps the most sensitive and the rabbit, the least (reviewed in 83 and in 106). Daily doses of 15 to 40 mg/kg for 2 to 4 weeks rendered male rats infertile, with the onset of infertility appearing to be dose related. The effects of gossypol on the testes were progressive and more pronounced with continued drug treatment. Initially, only spermatids displayed nuclear abnormalities, but these and other effects also involved spermatocytes with continued administration. After prolonged treatment, the seminiferous tubules became atrophic and almost completely devoid of cells.[75] Some investigators reported that gossypol lowers serum androgen concentrations in laboratory animals,[35] but others failed to detect any changes.[75,90]

TABLE 17-2. Recovery of Fertility in Hamsters and Rats Following Oral Administration of Gossypol Acetic Acid for 8 Weeks (20 mg/kg/day)

| | PERCENT OF FERTILE ANIMALS | | | |
| | WEEK OF RECOVERY | | | |
SPECIES	1	3	5	9
Hamster	0	0	33	50
Rat	0	75	100	NT

NT = Not tested.

Adapted from Hahn DW, Rusticus C, Probst A, Homm R, Johnson AN: Antifertility and endocrine activities of gossypol on rodents. Contraception 24:97–105, 1981

Despite these promising results with gossypol, side-effects have become a concern. First, in animals, gossypol appears to be relatively toxic. In rats, low doses of gossypol acetic acid failed to induce complete infertility, but a higher dose of 20 mg/kg/day killed seven of ten rats by the eighth week of treatment. Mice showed a similar type of response.[36] In human subjects, nausea and fatigue were not uncommon symptoms, and there was a nearly 1% incidence of hypokalemic paralysis.[83] The hypokalemia could be relieved in some cases with daily supplements of potassium chloride, but in others, problems persisted even after gossypol treatment was discontinued. In laboratory animals, infertility persists after cessation of treatment (Table 17-2). This appears to be related to the duration of treatment and the completeness of azoospermia achieved. In men, a similar effect appears to occur, and it has been estimated that as many as 25% of the men receiving long-term treatment with gossypol fail to regain fertility.[83] These findings are preliminary, of course, but occurrence of side-effects will be monitored carefully in future clinical studies with gossypol before we can know the potential clinical utility of the compound. (More recent studies with gossypol are discussed in Chap. 18).

COMPOUNDS WITH PHARMACOLOGIC ACTIONS ON POST-TESTICULAR PHYSIOLOGY

In the late 1960s, investigators at the Upjohn Company tested a number of compounds for antifertility activity in male rats. Because each animal was tested for only 8 days, only compounds directed at a post-testicular site (presumably the epididymis or the spermatozoa contained within) would be detected.[22] Thus, the concept of an agent directed at a specific site in the male was advanced further by these experiments.

This effort resulted in the discovery of several orally active compounds, the best-known and most-studied being 3-chloro-1,2-propanediol or α-chlorohydrin (Fig. 17-8). The minimal effective dose in rats was approximately 7 mg/kg. Infertility occurred within 8 days and, at higher doses (*e.g.*, 30 mg per rat), within 2 days. High doses, however, induced lesions in the epididymis that blocked normal fluid flow, causing testicular complications.[21,45] The mechanism by which lower doses produced infertility is not entirely clear.

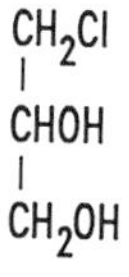

CH$_2$Cl
|
CHOH
|
CH$_2$OH

α-CHLOROHYDRIN

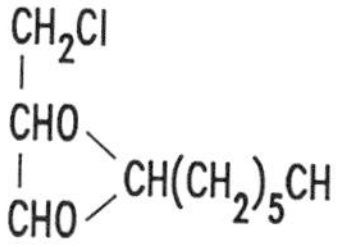

CH$_2$Cl
|
CHO
| CH(CH$_2$)$_5$CH
CHO

2-HEXYL-4-CHLOROMETHYL-1,3-DIOXOLANE
(ORF 8201)

FIG. 17-8. Two compounds with reversible antifertility effects at post-testicular sites.

Although α-chlorohydrin is known to inhibit several glycolytic enzymes of the spermatozoon,[10,27] short-term, low-dose treatment produces infertility without affecting the morphology, number, or motility of spermatozoa in the epididymis or in the female reproductive tract.[21,58] Nonetheless, with a therapeutic index (the ratio of the maximal tolerated dose to the effective dose) of less than ten[50] the development of α-chlorohydrin as a male contraceptive was never attempted. The possibility of finding a more potent, less toxic analogue was explored, however. Although none with potency greater than that of α-chlorohydrin was ever reported, potent compounds with reduced toxicity were synthesized. For example, 2-hexyl-4-chloromethyl-1,3-dioxolane (ORF 8201), shown in Fig. 17-8, had antifertility potency approximately equal to that of α-chlorohydrin with no apparent toxic side-effects at doses as high as 50 mg/kg. Furthermore, the LD$_{50}$ values in mice for ORF 8201 were nearly 20 times greater than those for α-chlorohydrin.[44] Despite this significant increase in the therapeutic index, the margin of safety still fell far short of that needed to warrant further development of this compound as a male contraceptive.

Because of the structural similarity of α-chlorohydrin and glycolytic metabolites, the possible antifertility activity of chloro-derivatives of six carbon sugars was explored. The first chlorosugars to be tested were derivatives of sucrose, shown in Figure 17-9.[28] More than 60 since have been evaluated for antifertility activity in male laboratory animals. Generally, a chlorine substitution on carbon number six is required for activity. Other halogens when substituted are generally inactive, although fluorine at the six position has antispermatogenic effects.[26] One of the most potent chlorosugars examined is 6-deoxy-6-chloroglucose (see Fig. 17-9). An oral dose of 24 mg/kg/day induced sterility in male rats within 7 days, and the effect could be sustained with continued treatment.[28] It was reported that dividing a single daily dose into two treatments per day increased its potency.[103] This finding, however, could not be duplicated in our laboratory (Table 17-3). The infertility caused

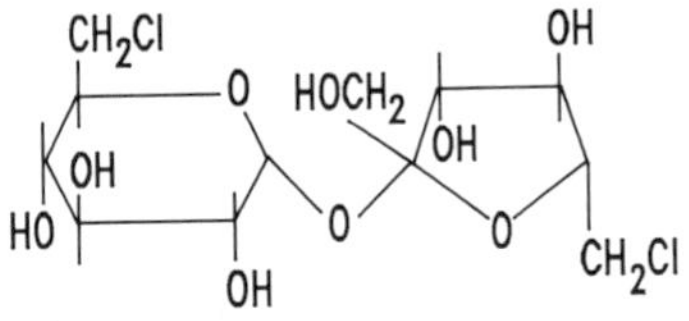

6,6'-DICHLORO-6,6'-DIDEOXY-SUCROSE

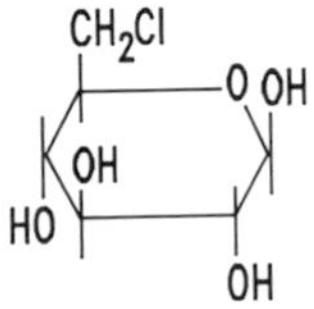

6-CHLORO-6-DEOXY-D-GLUCOSE

FIG. 17-9. Two chlorosugars recently investigated for their post-testicular antifertility activity.

by this compound was readily reversible and reportedly due to an impairment of sperm glucose oxidation.[29] Treatment for as long as 8 weeks had no apparent detrimental effect on the reproductive system or the hypophyseal–gonadal axis (Table 17-4), and doses insufficient for complete infertility did not appear to affect development. The LD_{50} for 6-chloroglucose, greater than 16 g/kg, is quite high.[28] Despite these promising results, it was subsequently shown that high doses given to marmosets caused hind limb paralysis and other CNS changes.[51] Subsequently, a detailed study in mice showed that 480 mg/kg daily for 8 days induced physical disabilities that were attributed to vacuolated lesions in the CNS.[52] The interest in chlorosugars as male antifertility agents since has declined.

TABLE 17-3. Comparison of Antifertility Effects of 6-chloro-glucose when Administered Orally to Male Rats Once or Twice a Day

NUMBER OF TREATMENTS PER DAY*	TREATMENT PERIOD (DAYS)	NUMBER OF MALES MATED	NUMBER OF FEMALES PREGNANT	NUMBER OF IMPLANTS PER PREGNANCY
None	3	6	6	11.0
	7	5	5	11.4
	14	6	6	13.7
1	3	6	6	12.0
	7	5	4	7.0
	14	6	2	1.5
2	3	4	4	12.5
	7	6	6	8.0
	14	6	5	1.6

* Total daily dose was 20 mg/kg.

Hahn DW: Unpublished data, 1980

TABLE 17-4. Relative Organ Weights of Rats Treated Orally with 6-chloro-6-deoxy-glucose at a Daily Dose of 30 mg/kg for 8 Weeks (Mean ± SE)

ORGAN*	RELATIVE WEIGHTS (mg/100 g BW)	
	CONTROL n = 4	TREATED n = 4
Epididymis	220.0 ± 7.7	224.8 ± 10.2
Testis	661.6 ± 25.7	674.6 ± 9.9
Ventral prostate	101.8 ± 9.1	129.9 ± 11.6
Seminal vesicle	107.8 ± 10.2	103.4 ± 2.2
Adrenal	5.5 ± 0.8	6.0 ± 0.2
Thyroid	3.0 ± 0.5	3.4 ± 0.5
Pituitary	3.3 ± 0.5	3.4 ± 0.7

* Histologic examination of the reproductive organs revealed no abnormalities. Mean body weights did not differ significantly between treated and control rats.

Hahn DW: Unpublished data, 1980

SUMMARY

The search for drugs with antifertility activity in the male has spanned several decades, but progress in this area of research has been slow. Part of this is due to the nature of the male reproductive system; part, interestingly, is due to the lack of drugs in this area. Had drugs been available, mechanism studies would have led normally to significant new knowledge about the pharmacologic control of the male reproductive system and the advent of new types of male contraceptives. Although a number of approaches have been proposed and many compounds exhibiting promising activity in vitro or in animals have been identified, few have been safe enough to study clinically and none thus far appear to be potential products. With more knowledge of the male reproductive system, improved screening methods, and good medicinal chemistry, we believe that a safe, acceptable male contraceptive will be found.

REFERENCES

1. ALBERT A: The mammalian testis. In YOUNG WC (ed): Sex and Internal Secretions, Vol 1, pp 305–365. Baltimore, Williams & Wilkins, 1961
2. ALVAREZ-SANCHEZ F, FAUNDES A, BRACHE V, LEON P: Attainment and maintenance of azoospermia with combined monthly injections of depomedroxyprogesterone acetate and testosterone enanthate. Contraception 15:635–648, 1977
3. BACK DJ, GLOVER TD, SHENTON JC, BOYD GP: The effects of α-chlorohydrin on the composition of rat and rabbit epididymal plasma: a possible explanation of species difference. J Reprod Fertil 45:117–128, 1975
4. BAKER HWG, EDDIE LW, HIGGINSON RE, HUDSON B, NIALL HD: Studies on the purification of ovine inhibin. Ann NY Acad Sci 383:329–342, 1982

5. BERGQUIST C, NILLIUS SJ, BERGH T, SKARIN G, WIDE L: Inhibitory effects on gonadotrophin secretion and gonadal function in men during chronic treatment with a potent stimulatory luteinizing hormone-releasing hormone analogue. Acta Endocrinol 91:601–608, 1979

6. BERNDTSON WE, DESJARDINS C, EWING LL: Inhibition and maintenance of spermatogenesis in rats with polydimethylsiloxane capsules containing various androgens. J Endocrinol 62:125–135, 1975

7. BREMNER WJ, MATSUMOTO AM, SUSSMAN AM, PAULSEN CA: Follicle-stimulating hormone and human spermatogenesis. J Clin Invest 68:1044, 1981

8. BRENNER PF, MISHELL DR JR, BERNSTEIN GS, ORTIZ A: Study of medroxyprogesterone acetate and testosterone enanthate as a male contraceptive. Contraception 15:679, 1977

9. BRIGGS M, BRIGGS M: Oral contraceptive for men. Nature 252:585–587, 1974

10. BROWN-WOODMAN PDC, MOHRI H, MOHRI T, SUTER D, WHITE IG: Mode of action of α-chlorohydrin as a male antifertility agent. Biochem J 170:23–37, 1978

11. COMHAIRE F, VERMEULEN A: Plasma testosterone in patients with varicocele and sexual inadequacy. J Clin Endocrinol Metab 40:824–829, 1975

12. COOPER ERA, JACKSON H: Comparative effects of methylene, ethylene, and propylene dimethanesulphonates on the male rat reproductive system. J Reprod Fertil 23:103–108, 1970

13. CORBIN A, BEX FJ: Inhibition of male reproductive processes with an LH–RH agonist. In CUNNINGHAM GR, SCHILL WB, HAFEZ ESE (eds): Regulation of Male Fertility, pp 55–63. Boston, Martinus Nijhoff, 1980

14. CORSI G, PALAZZO G, GERMANI C, BARCELLONA PS, SILVESTRINI B: 1-Halobenzyl-1H-indazole-3-carboxylic acids: A new class of antispermatogenic agents. J Med Chem 19:778–783, 1976

15. COUTINHO EM, MELO JF: Successful inhibition of spermatogenesis in man without loss of libido: A potential new approach to male contraception. Contraception 8:207–217, 1973

16. CROWLEY WF JR, BEITINS IZ, VALE W, KLIMAN B, RIVIER J, RIVIER C, MCARTHUR JW: The biologic activity of a potent analogue of gonadotropin-releasing hormone in normal and hypogonadotropic men. N Engl J Med 302:1052, 1980

17. CUNNINGHAM GR, SILVERMAN VE, THORNBY J, KOHLER PO: The potential for an androgen male contraceptive. J Clin Endocrinol Metab 49:520–526, 1979

18. DAMASSA DA, SMITH ER, TENNENT B, DAVIDSON JM: The relationship between circulating testosterone levels and male sexual behavior in rats. Horm Behav 8:275–288, 1977

19. DEBELJUK L: Serum follicle-stimulating hormone and lutenizing hormone levels in male rats with experimentally induced damage of the germinal epithelium. J Endocrinol 66:53–60, 1975

20. DESJARDINS C, EWING LL, IRBY DC: Response of the rabbit seminiferous epithelium to testosterone administered via polydimethylsiloxane capsules. Endocrinology 93:450–460, 1973

21. ERICSSON RJ, BAKER VF: Male antifertility compounds: Biological properties of U-5897 and U-15,646. J Reprod Fertil 21:267–273, 1970

22. ERICSSON RJ, YOUNGDALE GA: Male antifertility compounds: Structure and activity relationships of U-5897, U-15,646 and related substances. J Reprod Fertil 21:263–266, 1970

23. EWING LL, STRATTON LG, DESJARDINS C: Effect of testosterone polydimethylsiloxane implants upon sperm production, libido and accessory sex organ function in rabbits. J Reprod Fertil 35:245–253, 1973

24. FAURE N, LEMAY A, BELANGER A, LABRIE F: Inhibition of androgen biosynthesis in the human male by chronic administration of [D-Ser(TBU)⁶-des-Gly-NH₂¹⁰]-LHRH ethylamide (Buserelin). In ZATUCHNI GI, SHELTON JD, SCIARRA JJ (eds): LHRH Peptides as Female and Male Contraceptives. Harper & Row, Philadelphia, 307–320

25. FOGH M, CORKER CS, HUNTER WM, MCLEAN H, PHILIP J, SCHOU G, SKAKKEBAEK NE: The effects of low doses of cyproterone acetate. Acta Endocrinol 91:545–552, 1979

26. FORD WCL: The effect of 6-deoxy-6-fluoroglucose on the fertility of male rats and mice. Contraception 25:535–545, 1982

27. FORD WCL, HARRISON A: Effect of α-chlorohydrin on glucose metabolism by spermatozoa from the cauda epididymidis of the rhesus monkey (*Macaca mulatta*). J Reprod Fertil 60:59–64, 1980

28. FORD WCL, WAITES GMH: Chlorinated sugars: A biochemical approach to the control of male fertility. Int J Androl (Suppl) 2:541–564, 1978

29. FORD WCL, HARRISON A, WAITES GMH: Effects of 6-chloro-6-deoxysugars on glucose oxidation in rat spermatozoa. J Reprod Fertil 63:67–73, 1981

30. FRICK J: Control of spermatogenesis in men by combined administration of progestin and androgen. Contraception 8:191–206, 1973

31. FRICK J, BARTSCH G, WEISKE WH: The effect of monthly depot medroxyprogesterone acetate and testosterone on human spermatogenesis. I. Uniform dosage levels. Contraception 15:649, 1977

32. FRICK J, BARTSCH G, WEISKE WH: The effect of monthly depot medroxyprogesterone acetate and testosterone on human spermatogenesis. II. High initial dose. Contraception 15:669–677, 1977

33. GONZALEZ-BARCENA D, KASTIN AJ, COY DH, NIKOLICS K, SCHALLY AV: Suppression of gonadotrophin release in man by an inhibitory analogue of LH-releasing hormone. Lancet ii:997–998, 1977

34. GRUNT JA, YOUNG WC: Consistency of sexual behavior pattern in individual male guinea pigs following castration and androgen therapy. J Comp Physiol Psychol 46:138–144, 1953

35. HADLEY MA, LIN YC, DYM M: Effects of gossypol on the reproductive system of male rats. J Androl 2:190–199, 1981

36. HAHN DW, RUSTICUS C, PROBST A, HOMM R, JOHNSON AN: Antifertility and endocrine activities of gossypol in rodents. Contraception 24:97–105, 1981

37. HAPP J, SENNERICH T, KRAUSE U, BEYER J: Pernasal gonadorelin (GNRH) analog therapy in a boy with early puberty. Neuroendocrinology (Letter) 3:255–260, 1981

38. HEBER D, SWERDLOFF RS: Gonadotropin-releasing hormone analog and testosterone synergistically inhibit spermatogenesis. Endocrinology 108:2019–2021, 1981

39. HELLER CG, LAIDLAW WM, HARVEY HT, NELSON WO: Effects of progestational compounds on the reproductive processes of the human male. Ann NY Acad Sci 71:649–665, 1958

40. HELLER CG, MOORE DJ, PAULSEN CA: Suppression of spermatogenesis and chronic toxicity in men by a new series of *bis*(dichloroacetyl) diamines. Toxicol Appl Pharmacol 3:1–11, 1961

41. HELLER CG, MOORE DJ, PAULSEN A, NELSON WO, LAIDLAW WM: Effects of progesterone and synthetic progestins on the reproductive physiology of normal men. Fed Proc 18:1057–1065, 1959

42. HELLER CG, MORSE HC, SU M, ROWLEY MJ: The role of FSH, ICSH, and endogenous testosterone during testicular suppression of exogenous testosterone in normal men. In: The Human Testis: Advances in Experimental Medicine and Biology, pp 249–259. Vol 10. New York, Plenum Press

43. HIRSCH AF, KASULANIS C, KRAFT L, MALLORY RA, POWELL G, WONG B: Synthesis and evaluation of the male antifertility properties of a series of N-unsubstituted sulfamates. J Med Chem 24:901–903, 1981

44. HIRSCH AF, KOLWYCK KC, KRAFT LA, HOMM RE, HAHN DW: Antifertility effects of chlorine-substituted dioxolanes, dithiolanes, and dithianes in male rats. J Med Chem 18:116–117, 1975

45. HOFFER AP, HAMILTON DW, FAWCETT DW: The ultrastructural pathology of the rat epididymis after administration of α-chlorohydrin (U-5897). I. Effects of a single high dose. Anat Rec 175:203–230, 1973

46. HOMM RE, RUSTICUS C, HAHN DW: The antispermatogenic effects of 5-thio-D-glucose in male rats. Biol Reprod 17:697–700, 1977

47. JACKSON H, BOCK M: Effect of triethylene melamine on the fertility of rats. Nature 175:1037–1038, 1955

48. JACKSON H, FOX BW, CRAIG AW: The effect of alkylating agents on male rat fertility. Br J Pharmacol 14:149–157, 1959

49. JACKSON H, FOX BW, CRAIG AW: Antifertility substances and their assessment in the male rodent. J Reprod Fertil 2:447–465, 1961

50. JACKSON H, ROONEY FR, FITZPATRICK RW: Characterization and antifertility activity in rats of S(+)−α-chlorohydrin. Chem Biol Interactions 17:117–120, 1977

51. JACOBS JM, DUCHEN LW: Effects of 6-chloro-6-deoxyglucose on the nervous system of the marmoset. Neuropath Appl Neurobiol 6:236–237, 1980

52. JACOBS JM, FORD WCL: The neurotoxicity and antifertility properties of 6-chloro-6-deoxyglucose in the mouse. Neurotoxicology 2:405–417, 1981

53. JOHANSSON EDB, NYGREN K-G: Depression of plasma testosterone levels in men with norethindrone. Contraception 8:219–226, 1973

54. KAMEL F, FRANKEL AL: Hormone release during mating in the male rat: Time course, relation to sexual behavior, and interaction with handling procedures. Endocrinology 103:2172–2179, 1978

55. KARPAS AE, MATSUMOTO AM, PAULSEN CA, BREMNER WJ: Effect of selective FSH deficiency induced by chronic hCG administration on spermatogenesis in normal men. Proc. 64th Annual Meeting of The Endocrine Society, San Francisco, p 198. June 16–18, A473

56. KATONGOLE CB, NAFTOLIN F, SHORT RV: Relationship between blood levels of luteinizing hormone and testosterone in bulls, and the effects of sexual stimulation. J Endocrinol 50:457–466, 1971

57. KETCHEL MM: Available clinical data concerning effects of androgen treatment of men on outcome of subsequent pregnancies. In PATANELLI DJ (ed): Hormonal control of Male Fertility DHEW Publication No. (NIH) 78-1097, 1977

58. KIRTON KT, ERICSSON RJ, RAY JA, FORBES AD: Male antifertility compounds: Efficacy of U-5897 in primates (*macca mulatta*). J Reprod Fertil 21:275–278, 1970

59. LARON Z, DICKERMAN Z, ZEEV ZB, PRAGER-LEWIN R, COMARU-SCHALLY AM, SCHALLY AV: Long-term effect of D-Trp^6-luteinizing hormone-releasing hormone on testicular size and luteinizing hormone, follicle-stimulating hormone, and testosterone levels in hypothalamic hypogonadotropic males. Fertil Steril 35:328–331, 1981

60. LOBL TJ: 1-(2,4-dichlorobenzyl)-1H-indazoles-3-carboxylic acid (DICA), an exfoliative antispermatogenic agent in the rat. Arch Androl 2:353–363, 1979

61. LOBL TJ, BARDIN CW, CHANG CC: Pharmacologic agents producing infertility by indirect action on the male reproductive tract. In Zatuchni GI, Labbok MJ, Sciarra JJ (eds): Research Frontiers in Fertility Regulation, pp. 146–168. Hagerstown, Harper & Row, 1980

62. LOBL TJ, FORBES AD, KIRTON KT, WILKS JW: Characterization of the exfoliative antispermatogenic agent 1-(2,4-dichlorobenzyl)-1H-indazole-3-carboxylic acid in the rhesus monkey. Arch Androl 3:67–77, 1979

63. LOBL TJ, PORTEUS SE: Antifertility activities of 5-theo-D-glucose in mice and rats. Contraception 17:123–130, 1978

64. MACRIDES F, BARTKE A, DALTERO S: Strange females increase plasma testosterone levels in male mice. Science 189:1104–1106, 1975

65. MADHWA RAJ HG, DYM M: The effects of selective withdrawal of FSH or LH on spermatogenesis in the immature rat. Biol Reprod 14:489–494, 1976

66. MALMNAS CO: Short-latency effect of testosterone on copulatory behavior and ejaculation in sexually experienced intact male rats. J Reprod Fertil 51:351–354, 1977

67. MATSUMOTO AM, PAULSEN CA, BREMNER WJ: Stimulation of sperm production by human lutenizing hormone in gonadotropin-suppressed normal men. J Clin Endocrinol Metab 59:882–887, 1984

68. MAUSS J, BÖRSCH G: Investigations on the use of testosterone oenanthate as a male contraceptive agent. Contraception 10:281–289, 1974

69. MAUSS J, BÖRSCH G, BORMACHER K, RICHTER E, LEYENDECKER G, NOCKE W: Effect of long-term testosterone oenanthate administration on male reproductive function: Clinical evaluation, serum FSH, LH, testosterone, and seminal fluid analyses in normal men. Acta Endocrinol 78:373–384, 1975

70. MEISTRICH ML: Quantitative correlation between testicular stem cell survival, sperm production, and fertility in the mouse after treatment with different toxic agents. J Androl 3:58–68, 1982

71. MELO JF, COUTINHO EM: Inhibition of spermatogenesis in men with monthly injections of medroxyprogesterone acetate and testosterone enanthate. Contraception 15:627, 1977

72. MICHAEL RP, ZUMPE D, BONSALL RW: Sexual behavior correlates with diurnal plasma testosterone range in intact male rhesus monkeys. Biol Reprod 30:652–657, 1984

73. MORSE HC, LEACH DR, ROWLEY MJ, HELLER CG: Effect of cyproterone acetate on sperm concentration, seminal fluid volume, testicular cytology and levels of plasma and urinary ICSH, FSH and testosterone in normal men. J Reprod Fertil 32:365–378, 1973

74. MOSS RL, DUDLEY CA, FOREMAN MM, MCCANN SM: Synthetic LRF: A potentiator of sexual behavior in the rat. In MOTTA M, CROSIGNANI PG, MARTINI L (eds): Hypothalamic Hormones, pp 269–278. New York, Academic Press, 1975

75. National Coordinating Group on Male Antifertility Agents (China): Gossypol: A new antifertility agent for males. Gynecol Obstet Invest 10:163–176, 1979

76. NEKOLA MV, MOZVATH A, GE L-J, COY DH, SCHALLY AV: Suppression of ovulation in the rat by an orally active antagonist of luteninzing hormone-releasing hormone. Science 218:160–162, 1982

77. NELSON WO, STEINBERGER E: Effects of nitrofuran compounds on the testis of the rat. Fed Proc 12:103, 1953

78. NILLIUS SJ, BERGQUIST C, WIDE L: Chronic treatment with the gonadotropin-releasing hormone agonist D-Ser(TBU)^6-EA^{10}-LRH for contraception in women and men. Int J Fertil 25:239–246, 1980

79. PATANELLI DJ: Suppression of fertility in the male. In HAMILTON DW, GREEP RO (eds): The Handbook of Physiology, Sec 7, Vol V, pp 245–258. Washington, DC, American Physiological Society, 1975

80. PATANELLI DJ, NELSON WO: A qualitative study of inhibition and recovery of spermatogenesis. In PINCUS G (ed): Recent Progress in Hormone Research, Vol. XX, pp 491–543. New York, Academic Press, 1964

81. PINCUS G: Some effects of progesterone and related compounds upon reproduction and early development in mammals. Acta Endocrinol (Suppl) 28:18–36, 1956

82. PETRY R, MAUSS J, RAUSCH-STROOMANN R, VERMEULEN A: Reversible inhibition of spermatogenesis in men. Horm Metab Res 4:386–388, 1972

83. PRASAD MRN, DICZFALUSY E: Gossypol. Int J Androl (Suppl) 5:53–67, 1982

84. RABIN D, LINDA R, DOELLE G, ALEXANDER N: Experience with a potent gonadotropin releasing hormone agonist in normal men: An approach to the development of a male contraceptive. In ZATUCHNI GI, SHELTON JD, SCIARRA JJ (eds): LHRH Peptides as Female and Male Contraceptives, pp 296–306. Philadelphia, Harper & Row, 1981

85. RAMASHARMA K, SAIRAM MR: Isolation and characterization of inhibin from human seminal plasma. In BARDIN CW, SHERINS RJ (eds): Cell Biology of the Testis. Ann NY Acad Sci 383:307–328, 1982

86. REDDY PRK, RAO JM: Reversible antifertility action of testosterone propionate in human males. Contraception 5:295–301, 1972

87. RIVIER C, RIVIER J, VALE W: Chronic effect of [D-Trp^6,Pro^9-NET] luteinizing hormone-releasing factor on reproductive processes in the male rat. Endocrinology 105:1191–1201, 1979

88. SCHAFFENBURG CA, GREGOIRE AT, GUERIGUIAN JL: Guidelines for clinical testing of male contraceptive drugs. J Androl 2:225–228, 1981

89. SEGUIN C, BELANGER A, ANSO L, PELLETIER G, REEVES JJ, LEFEBVRE F-A, KELLY PA, LABRIE F: Relative importance of the adenohypophyseal and gonadal sites of inhibitory action of LHRH agonists. Biol Reprod 24:889–901, 1981

90. SHANDILYA L, CLARKSON TB, ADAMS MR, LEWIS JC: Effects of gossypol on reproductive and endocrine functions of male cynomolgus monkeys (Macaca fascicularis). Biol Reprod 27:241–252, 1982

91. SHETH AR, VAZE AY, THAKUR AN: Development of RIA for inhibin of human seminal plasma and its application for physiological studies, pp 233–240. Proc International Symposium for Recent Advances in Reproduction and Fertility. New Delhi, October, 1978

92. SILVESTRINI B, BURBERI S, CATANESE B, CIOLI V, COULSTON F, LISCIANI R, BARCELLONA PS: Antispermatogenic activity of 1-p-chlorobenzyl-1H-indazol-3-carboxylic acid (AF 1312/TS) in rats. I. Trials of single and short-term administrations with study of pharmacologic and toxicologic effects. Exp Mol Pathol 23:288–307, 1975

93. SKOGLUND RD, PAULSEN CA: Danazol-testosterone combination: A potentially effective means for reversible male contraception. A preliminary report. Contraception 7:357–365, 1973

94. STEINBERGER E: Recent advances in regulation of male fertility. In MOGHISSI KS, EVANS TN (eds): Regulation of Human Fertility, pp 274–290. Detroit, Wayne State University Press, 1976

95. STEINBERGER E, BOCCABELLA A, NELSON WO: Cytotoxic effects of 5-chlor-2-acetyl thiophen (Ba 11044, Ciba) on the testis of the rat. Anat Rec 125:312, 1956

96. STEINBERGER E, SMITH KD: Effect of chronic administration of testosterone enanthate on sperm production and plasma testosterone, follicle-stimulating hormone, and luteinizing hormone levels: A preliminary evaluation of a possible male contraceptive. Fertil Steril 28:1320–1328, 1977

97. STEINBERGER E, SMITH KD, RODRIGUEZ-RIGAU LJ: Suppression and recovery of sperm production in men treated with testosterone enanthate for one year: A study of a possible reversible male contraceptive. Int J Androl (Suppl) 2:748–760, 1978

98. STRATTON LG, EWING LL, DESJARDINS C: Efficacy of testosterone-filled polydimethylsiloxane implants in maintaining plasma testosterone in rabbits. J Reprod Fertil 35:235–244, 1973

99. SWERDLOFF RS, CAMPFIELD LA, PALACIOS A, MCCLURE RD: Supression of human spermatogenesis by depot androgen: Potential for male contraception. J Steroid Biochem 11:663–670, 1979

100. ULSTEIN M, NETTO N, LEONARD J, PAULSEN CA: Changes in sperm morphology in normal men treated with Danazol and testosterone. Contraception 12:437, 1975

101. WANG N-G, SUNDARAM K, PAVLOU S, RIVIER J, VALE W, BARDIN CW: Mice are insensitive to the antitesticular effects of luteinizing hormone-releasing hormone agonists. Endocrinology 112:331–335, 1983

102. WANG C, YEUNG KK: Use of low-dosage oral cyproterone acetate as a male contraceptive. Contraception 21:245–272, 1980

103. WARREN LA, MCRAE G, VICKERY B: Antifertility efficacy of twice daily oral administration of 6-chloro-6-deoxy-D-glucose (6CDG) in male rats. Contraception 20:275–289, 1979

104. WESTABY D, OGLE SJ, PARADINAS FJ, RANDELL JB, MURRAY-LYON JM: Liver damage from long-term methyltestosterone. Lancet ii:261, 1977

105. WIEBE JP, BARR KJ: Suppression of spermatogenesis without inhibition of steroidogenesis by a 1,2,3-trihydroxypropane solution. Life Sci 34:1747–1754, 1984

106. ZATUCHNI GI, OSBORN CK: Gossypol: A possible male antifertility agent: Report of a workshop. In ZATUCHNI GI, OSBORN K (eds): Research Frontiers in Fertility Regulation, pp 1–15. Chicago, Northwestern University, 1981

107. ZARATE A, CANALES ES, SCHALLY AV, COY DH, COUMARU-SCHALLY AM: The use of LHRH agonists and antagonists as antifertility agents in the human female. In ZATUCHNI GI, SHELTON JD, SCIARRA JJ (eds): LHRH Peptides as Female and Male Contraceptives, pp 227–236. Philadelphia, Harper & Row, 1981

108. ZYSK JR, BUSHWAY AA, WHISTERLER RL, CARLTON WW: Temporary sterility produced in male mice by 5-thio-D-glucose. J Reprod Fertil 45:69–72, 1975

18

Toxicology and Mechanism of Action of Gossypol

DONALD P. WALLER

XIN-YI NIU

INCHULL KIM

Gossypol has been a focal point of male contraceptive research for the past several years. The ability of gossypol to exert antifertility effects in several species of animals and reduce sperm counts in humans has been clearly demonstrated. Several reviews have been written on the antifertility actions of gossypol.[15,33,34,35,49] The enthusiasm of scientists for gossypol as a new male contraceptive has been somewhat tempered, however, because of the lack of safety of gossypol demonstrated in early toxicologic studies. These studies focused on gossypol as the primary cause of intoxication in farm animals fed cotton seed meal as a food supplement.[2] The demonstration of not only the efficacy of gossypol, but also a large therapeutic index, will be necessary before gossypol is accepted generally as an oral contraceptive for men.

The growing body of information on the interactions of gossypol with biochemical model systems are sometimes conflicting and difficult to interpret. The chemical properties of gossypol probably contribute to this confusion. The presence of six phenolic hydroxyl groups results in a highly reactive chemical. The hydroxyl groups are strongly acidic and readily react to form esters and ethers. They also can form Schiff bases with free amine groups such as those found in lysine residues of proteins. Gossypol is an antioxidant and a good chelator of cations, especially iron. These chemical properties can lead to nonspecific interactions during in vitro biochemical evaluations. Appropriate controls always should be included in biochemical investigations of gossypol to ensure that specific interactions with gossypol are being observed and not just artifacts due to the chemical reactivity of gossypol.

Gossypol is very insoluble in water and must be suspended or solubilized before it can be added to biochemical preparations or administered to an animal. There are several different ways in which gossypol has been solubilized. Investigators use short-chain alcohols and high pH to solubilize gossypol. Unfortunately, gossypol is not stable in some polar solvents, such as the short-chain alcohols [30, 13], nor in basic solutions. Gossypol dissolved in acetic acid will form a gossypol–acetic acid complex. This form of gossypol appears to be somewhat more stable than gossypol and also has been used for some studies. It is unfortunate that most biologic studies have little information on the purity of the gossypol being used because this can have significant effects on antifertility actions.[47] Studies or assays of gossypol must be designed carefully to minimize artifacts resulting from the degradation of gossypol or the presence of impurities.

Several different dosage forms of gossypol, including gum acacia suspensions and polyvinylpyrollidone (PVP) coprecipitates, have been used in antifertility studies and could account for inconsistencies in gossypol effects. Studies in our laboratory have demonstrated a decreased bioavailability of an orally administered gossypol gum acacia suspension compared to an oral dose of a gossypol–PVP coprecipitate. The bioavailability of the gum acacia suspension compared to a gossypol PVP–coprecipitate was 28% less in the rat and 45% less in the hamster for a 20 mg/kg dose of gossypol.[29] Caution must be observed when extrapolating data from experiments using different suspending agents.

Most chemical and biologic studies have used optically inactive gossypol; however, gossypol can exist as two optical isomers because of the restricted rotation around the binaphthalene C—C bridge (Fig. 18-1). The (+) isomer was first isolated from the plant Thespesia populnea.[22] Little work has been performed on its chemical and biologic properties, even though this isomer of gossypol has been available for many years. It is known, however, that the (+) isomer of gossypol is not an effective male antifertility agent when administered orally to rats[50,53] and hamsters.[46] In addition, the toxicity of the (+) isomer, as assessed by weight loss, was less than that observed with the administration of racemic gossypol (Table 18-1).

The (+) optical isomer of gossypol appears to be quite different from racemic gossypol in its antifertility activity and toxicity. Unfortunately the (−) optical isomer has not been readily available for study. Only recently the

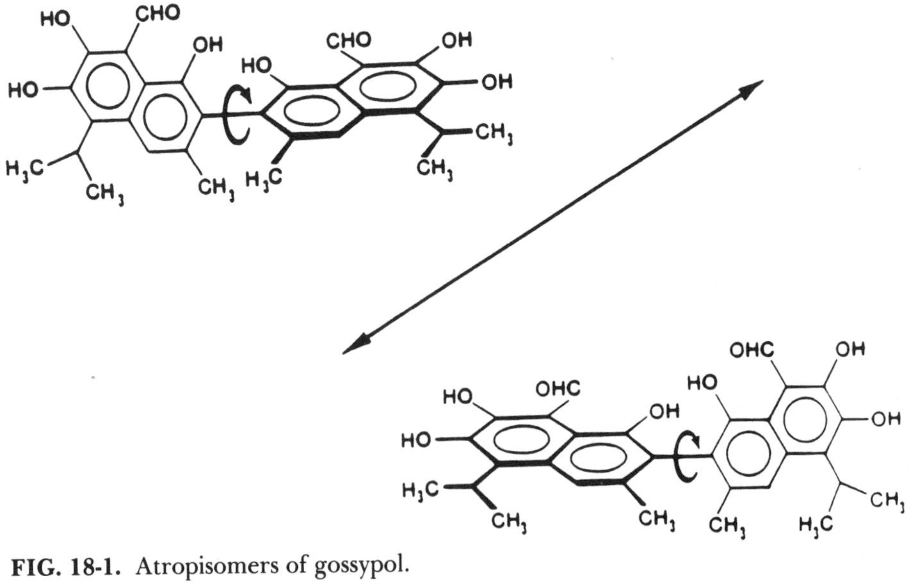

FIG. 18-1. Atropisomers of gossypol.

TABLE 18-1. Effects of Gossypol on Body Weight of Male Hamsters (g)*

TREATMENT GROUP	DAYS OF TREATMENT			
	1	*21*	*42*	*54*
Control	127 + 9	133.0 + 11.3	137.2 + 10.6	141.0 + 11.4
(+)−Gossypol	124 + 9	127.7 + 6.8	127.6 + 7.7	128.1 + 9.3†
Racemic Gossypol	124 + 11	123.7 + 11.1‡	118.7 + 12.8‡	113.4 + 13.9§

* Oral dose of 40 mg/kg
† Significantly different from control at $p < 0.01$
‡ Significantly different from control at $p < 0.05$
§ Significantly different from control at $p < 0.02$
Waller DP, Bunyapraphatsara N, Martin A, Vournazos CJ, Ahmed MS, Soejarto DD, Cordell GA, Fong HHS: Effect of (+)−gossypol on fertility in male hamsters. J Androl 4:276–279, 1983

existence of (−) gossypol was confirmed when the (+) and (−) optical isomers were resolved as Schiff bases using chromatographic techniques.[26,39] Techniques for the isolation of adequate quantities for biologic studies of the (−) optical isomer are now in progress. The availability of both optical isomers should lead to chemical and biologic studies that will result in a better understanding of the specific and nonspecific interactions of gossypol.

TOXICOLOGY

ANIMAL TOXICITY

The symptoms and pathologic events following gossypol intoxication in animals are well documented and described in earlier reviews.[40,52] These studies clearly demonstrated the large variation in the response of different species to acute (Table 18-2) and chronic exposure to gossypol.

The pig, dog, guinea pig, and rabbit appear most susceptible to gossypol intoxication; the rat and hamster are more resistant. Daily oral doses as low as 1.5 mg/kg for 28 days can cause death in swine.[42] Exposure of dogs for more than 7 days to 5 mg/kg also can lead to severe toxicity and death.[10] The cause of death in the two species, however, appears to be from completely different mechanisms. Respiratory distress is the primary cause of death in swine whereas dogs respond with cachexia and myocardial damage. Rats and hamsters show impaired fertility at doses that result in few symptoms of toxicity, however, mice and rabbits, the latter especially, exhibit severe toxicity close or prior to the dose that causes reproductive effects.

Gossypol appears to also have anticholinergic properties.[25] Anticholinergic blockade of sweating was the probable cause of several deaths attributed to heat prostration after accidental exposure to gossypol.

The large species and even strain differences in target organ toxicity with gossypol will reduce the confidence of extrapolating animal experiments to humans. Little is known about the mechanism of gossypol toxicity. The mon-

TABLE 18-2. Gossypol: Single Dose, LD_{50} (in mg/kg body weight) in Animals*

SPECIES	LD_{50}
Rat	2400–3340
Mouse	500–1000
Rabbit	350–600
Guinea pig	280–300
Pig	550

* The compounds were administered as an aqueous suspension. The same effect was seen with at least 10% less of gossypol, when administered in oil. The dose of gossypol administered in the clinical studies carried out in the People's Republic of China was usually 20 mg daily for 60–70 days followed by a maintenance dose of 60 mg weekly.

Prasad MRN, Diczfaluszy E: Gossypol. In Harrison RF, Bonnar, Thompson W (eds): Fertility and Sterility, pp 255–268. Lancaster, England, MTP Press, 1984

itoring of liver enzymes and other blood components in animals administered gossypol, including rats, rabbits, dogs and monkeys, demonstrate inconsistent and nonconclusive data.[35] Pathologic examination of tissues such as liver, kidney, and heart have not provided definitive answers on the mechanism of gossypol toxicity.

The liver is a consistent target organ for gossypol toxicity in most species. Some work implicated increased oxygen-free radical generation as a possible mechanism of gossypol toxicity in the liver,[8] but subsequent studies point to an inhibition of adenosine triphosphate (ATP) generation as the primary mechanism of an in vitro damage of hepatocytes.[9] Other studies implicate gossypol-induced membrane perturbations as a mediator of gossypol toxicity.[38]

There is little doubt in the Western scientific community that a low therapeutic index and a lack of understanding of gossypol toxicity will prevent gossypol from becoming an accepted antifertility agent in the future.

HUMAN TOXICITY

Although gossypol is recognized as a toxic substance, the results of several clinical studies of gossypol in men have provided some encouragement for continued study.[5,6,12,24] Few side-effects were reported, and most were minor in nature. Recovery of reproductive function was usually complete on cessation of treatment. The incidence of nonrecovery of reproductive function appears to be related directly to the duration and amount of gossypol administered. Only the appearance of hypokalemic-induced paralysis in a small number of treated men has caused concern. Currently no animal has developed hypokalemia following gossypol administration. Thus, it is impossible to use animal models to study this toxic response observed in humans. This points out the difficulty in studying gossypol toxicity and extrapolating data across species.

TABLE 18-3. The Pharmacokinetic Parameters of
Gossypol-PVP in the Rat

AGENT	DOSAGE	
	IV 20 mg/kg	PO 20 mg/kg
AUC (µg hr/ml)	622.4	112.3
AUMC (µg hr/ml)	3063.9	1640.5
T 1/2 terminal (hr)	8.8	8.6
CL (ml/hr/kg)	31.8	
Vss (ml/kg)	158	
Bioavailability (%)		18.0

Human exposure to gossypol has not been limited to males in antifertility studies. Recently, gossypol was used on a limited basis to treat endometriosis and leiomyoma.[35] Human exposures to gossypol also have occurred in the practice of traditional medicine.[35] No reports of toxic responses to gossypol for the above uses have been published, which does not necessarily mean that toxicity was not observed.

TOXICOKINETICS

Early studies clearly demonstrated that orally administered gossypol accumulates in the liver, spleen, and intestinal tract. Only small amounts of gossypol gain access to the general circulation for distribution to peripheral compartments, such as the testes.[1,16] It is surprising that the very small amounts of gossypol that reach the testes, as calculated from previous work on the distribution of gossypol,[16] would be able to cause any effect on the function of the testes. Further studies are needed to establish the apparent selectivity of gossypol for effects on the testes. It is not at all surprising that toxicologists are most concerned about chronic toxicity to organs such as the liver, spleen, and intestinal tract, where large amounts of gossypol accumulate. Further studies are needed to establish the apparent selectivity of gossypol for effects on the testes. Increased access of gossypol to the testes with decreased systemic exposure should increase the safety of gossypol greatly.

Pharmacokinetic parameters must be established to characterize and monitor tissue exposure to gossypol. Previous studies used radiolabeled gossypol to determine tissue concentrations and pharmacokinetic parameters of several species. In some species, there is a good correlation between the accumulation of gossypol and the primary site of gossypol toxicity. High concentrations of gossypol were observed in heart tissue following the administration of gossypol to dogs.

The pharmacokinetic parameters of a single intravenous or oral dose of 20 mg/kg of gossypol–PVP to rats (Table 18-3) and hamsters (Table 18-4) were determined using an HPLC method to quantitate gossypol. These data were needed to establish a correlation between the blood plasma levels and the toxicity and antifertility effects of gossypol (Table 18-3).

The area under the curve (AUC) for an oral dose of 20 mg/kg of gossy-

TABLE 18-4. The Pharmacokinetic Parameters of
Gossypol-PVP in the Hamster

	DOSAGEe	
AGENT	*IV 20 mg/kg*	*PO 20 mg/kg*
AUC (μg hr/ml)	242.4	16.8
AUMC (μg hr/ml)	415.1	126.3
T 1/2 terminal (hr)	5.6	5.7
CL (ml/hr/kg)	82.5	
Vss (ml/kg)	140.9	
Bioavailability (%)		6.9

pol–PVP in the rat was 112 μg/hr/ml. The terminal half life was 8.6 hours
and bioavailability was 18%. Peak blood values occurred about 6 hours after
administration (Fig. 18-2). The AUC for an oral dose of 20 mg/kg of gossypol–PVP in the hamster was 16.8 μg/hr/ml. The terminal half-life was 5.7
hours, and bioavailability was 6.9%. Peak blood values occurred about 2 hours
after administration (Fig. 18-3). These data are most interesting because the
hamster is more sensitive to the toxic and antifertility effects of gossypol than
the rat. This is in spite of the greater bioavailability, larger amounts of gossypol, and higher peak blood values found in the rat. The pharmacokinetic
parameters determined from the blood compartment cannot explain the

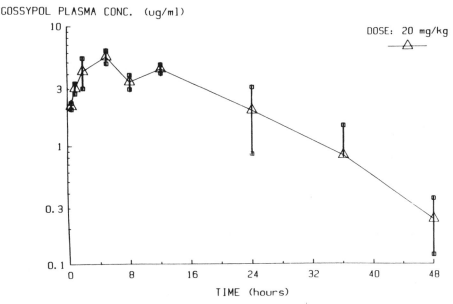

FIG. 18-2. Blood plasma levels of gossypol in the rat following administration of 20
mg/kg gossypol–PVP by oral gavage. At selected time points following
administration, a minimum of three animals were sacrificed and blood plasma
obtained. Analysis for gossypol was by HPLC.

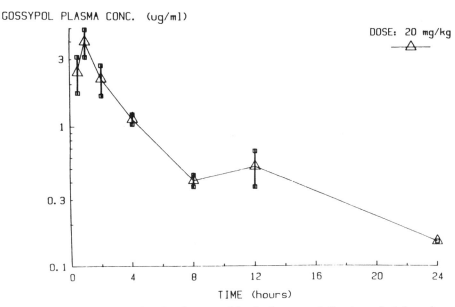

GOSSYPOL PLASMA CONC. (ug/ml)

FIG. 18-3. Blood plasma levels of gossypol in the hamster following administration of 20 mg/kg gossypol–PVP by oral gavage. At selected time points following administration, a minimum of three animals were sacrificed and blood plasma obtained. Analysis for gossypol was by HPLC.

greater sensitivity of the hamster to toxicity and the male antifertility effects of gossypol compared to the rat.

Preliminary studies in our laboratories on the pharmacokinetics of the (+) optical isomer of gossypol indicate a difference in the pharmacokinetic parameters of the different optical isomers of gossypol. The differences may explain the decreased toxicity of the (+) isomer but not the lack of antifertility effects for (+) gossypol.

OTHER FACTORS INFLUENCING TOXICITY

The toxicity and variability of animal responses to gossypol may involve interactions with important nutrients in the body. Past experiments have demonstrated the ability of metal ions such as iron to decrease or prevent the toxicity of gossypol.[7] It may be involved directly in gossypol toxicity. Selenium is an essential micronutrient involved in many biochemical processes in the body. Dietary intake of selenium varies greatly in different geographic locations around the world. Both a dietary deficiency (Keshan's disease) and an excess of selenium have resulted in toxicity.[4] Glutathione peroxidase is a selenium-requiring enzyme that has important protective functions in organs such as the liver, kidney, and spleen.[37] Gossypol is an inhibitor of glutathione peroxidase.[27]

We recently studied the interaction of gossypol with selenium in male hamsters, using weight gain as a primary indicator of gossypol toxicity. Control

TABLE 18-5. Effects of Gossypol, Selenium, and
Concurrent Gossypol/Selenium Weight
Gain (%) of Male Hamsters*

	DAYS OF TREATMENT (% GAIN)	
	14	*27*
Control	+4.8	+9.9
Selenium (selenous acid)	+0.5	+1.0
Gossypol	−2.4	−5.6
Gossypol + selenous acid	−6.8	−17.0

* (N = 8 per group)

animals gained weight throughout the 27-day treatment period. Compared with controls, animals treated with selenium (intraperitoneally as selenous acid, 500 μg/kg) for 27 days gained only a small amount of weight, whereas male hamsters administered gossypol (40 mg/kg PO) lost weight during the 27-day treatment period. In animals treated concurrently with gossypol (40 mg/kg PO) and selenium (500 μg/kg intraperitoneally) a 6.8% decrease in weight at 14 days and a 17% decrease at 27 days of treatment were observed (Table 18-5).

Gross observations confirmed the poor health status of animals treated with the combination of gossypol and selenium when compared to the other treatment groups. It appears that the toxicity of gossypol is enhanced by selenium. The large variations of dietary selenium observed around the world may be an important factor in the toxic effects of gossypol.

MECHANISM OF GOSSYPOL ACTION

STEREOSELECTIVITY OF GOSSYPOL ACTION

A large body of information has been generated in the search for the mechanism of action of gossypol. Most of this research used the readily available racemic gossypol. Gossypol was added to numerous preparations to determine if it inhibited specific enzymes or processes in the reproductive tract. Many cellular, subcellular, and enzyme preparations responded to the addition of gossypol. This is not surprising in view of the chemical reactivity of gossypol and its potential to interact in a nonspecific manner with biologic preparations. A recent study claims the (−) isomer of gossypol is an effective antifertility agent and may be even more potent than the racemic form.[26] The results of this study must be considered as preliminary due to the limited number of animals tested.

The very low amounts of gossypol found in the testicular compartment and the difference in antifertility activity of its stereoisomers provide evidence of a very specific stereoselective mechanism of action. Pharmacokinetic differences in the two isomers may account for the observed differences in antifer-

TABLE 18-6. Antimotility Effects of (±) Gossypol, (+) Gossypol, (−) Gossypol, and Gossypolone As the PVP Complexes

	CONCENTRATION OF TEST COMPOUNDS (mg/ml)*							
	(±) GOSSYPOL		*(+) GOSSYPOL*		*(−) GOSSYPOL*		*GOSSYPOLONE*	
TEST SPECIES	*20 sec*	*3 min*	*20 sec*	*3 min*	*20 sec*	*3 min*	*20 sec*	*3 min*
Human†	40	5	40	5	40	5	40	15
Monkey†	20	5	20	5	NT§	NT§	20	15
Rabbit†	15	5	15	5	NT§	NT§	15	5
Rat‡	5	1	5	1	NT§	NT§	5	1
Hamster‡	5	1	5	1	5	1	5	1
Mouse‡	5	1	5	1	NT§	NT§	5	1

* Minimum concentration of test compound to observed the total immobilization of sperm.

† Ejaculated semen

‡ Caudal epididymal sperm

§ Not tested because of the shortage of material

From Kim IC, Waller DP, Marcelle GB, Cordell GA, Fong HHS, Pirkle WH, Pilla L, Matlin SA: Comparative in vitro spermicidal effects of (+) −gossypol, (+) gossypol, (−) −gossypol, and gossypolone. Contraception 30:253–259, 1984

tility action, but this is unlikely because there is no correlation between the blood levels of gossypol and species sensitivity to the antifertility effects of gossypol in the rat and hamster.

The availability of the two optical isomers provides a powerful tool in the study of gossypol actions in the reproductive tract. Studies of subcellular fractions and purified enzyme preparations can be used to compare the effects of the different optical isomers of gossypol. These results will assist in the determination of whether the effect of gossypol in a particular biochemical model system is mediated in a stereoselective manner.

We have investigated the effects of the optical isomers of gossypol on several proposed sites of gossypol action; sperm motility, the mitochondrial respiratory chain, and on the testes-specific lactate dehydrogenase (LDH) isozyme, LDH C-4.

EFFECTS ON MOTILITY

Loss of motility is one of the earliest changes that appears in the male reproductive tract of infertile animals treated with gossypol. The possibility of a direct effect of gossypol on spermatozoa led to investigations on gossypol action on spermatozoal motility.[32] Gossypol was shown to be spermicidal and even was proposed as a potential vaginal spermicide.[47] We recently compared the spermicidal effects of the different optical isomers of gossypol on spermatozoa from several species of animals (Table 18-6).[21]

There was no difference between the spermicidal activity of the different gossypol optical isomers in the specimens tested. Both ejaculated (human, primate, rabbit) and epididymal (rat, mouse, hamster) spermatozoa responded in a similar manner (Table 18-6). A higher amount of gossypol was required for the inhibition of the ejaculated samples. This probably was due to the presence of the secretions of the sex accessory organs that protect the spermatozoa. Gossypolone, a proposed biotransformation product of gossypol, also was shown to be spermicidal. These data demonstrate the ability of gossypol to act in a nonspecific manner with spermatozoa. Compounds possessing naphthoquinone moieties are known to inhibit the respiratory chain[3] and may explain the actions of gossypol and related compounds on motility. Gossypol also has been shown to interfere with other enzyme systems vital to the maintenance of motility, such as glycolysis[41] and the generation of ATP.[45,51] Other studies have demonstrated the ability of gossypol to disrupt membrane function.[36] The study of direct effects of gossypol on spermatozoa may lead to the mechanism(s) that mediate spermicidal activity; however, these mechanisms may have little involvement in the in vivo antifertility actions of gossypol in the male.

POTENTIAL SUBCELLULAR SITES FOR GOSSYPOL ACTION

Histologic observations of the testes and the onset of infertility indicate the site of gossypol action is not a direct effect on mature spermatozoa but probably on the spermatid stage of spermatogenesis. The circulating blood levels of testosterone and other reproductive hormones during gossypol administration are relatively unchanged and probably do not mediate the effects of gossypol.

Gossypol inhibition of the testicular and spermatozoal mitochondrial respiratory chain has been subjected to investigation by several laboratories.[17,43] The specificity of the inhibition for the mitochondrial respiratory chain isolated from the testes has been demonstrated.[19] Concentrations of gossypol up to 300 μM did not suppress succinate-mediated reduction of the mitochondrial respiratory chain derived from the liver of either the rat or hamster (Fig. 18-4). In contrast, reduction by succinate of the mitochondrial respiratory chain preparations from the testes of the rat and hamster were completely suppressed with 75 μM concentrations of gossypol (see Fig. 18-4). Similar effects were observed when the (+) optical isomer of gossypol was added to the system (Fig. 18-5). Chemical reduction of the mitochondrial respiratory chain by sodium dithionite was not inhibited in any of the preparations. This provides some evidence that the actions of gossypol on the mitochondrial respiratory chain, although somewhat organ specific, may be only a general chemical interaction and not directly related to the in vivo antifertility effects of gossypol because no difference was observed between the actions of the (+) optical isomer of gossypol and racemic gossypol.

One of the most widely studied interactions of gossypol is its effects on the testes-specific enzyme, LDH-X. Several studies on both crude testes preparations[11,14,44] and isolated enzymes[23,31] demonstrated a high sensitivity of this testes-specific enzyme to gossypol. Studies in our laboratory have evaluated the ability of both the (+) and (−) optical isomers of gossypol to inhibit cytosolic preparations containing LDH-X.[20] Rat and hamster testicular cytosolic LDH-X were prepared and incubated with different concentrations of gossy-

LIVER

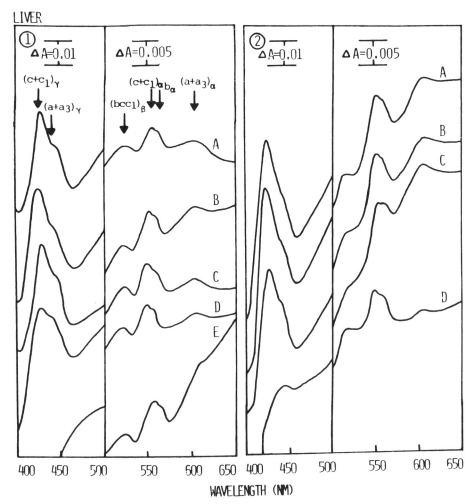

FIG. 18-4. Effects of racemic gossypol on the difference spectra of liver mitochondria from the hamster (*Panel 1*) and rat (*Panel 2*). Suspensions of hamster and rat mitochondria (2 mg protein/ml in 0.1 M phosphate buffer, pH 7.4, containing 5 mM $MgCl_2$ and 20 mM KCL) were treated with various amounts of racemic gossypol (A:0, B:75 μM, C:150 μM, D:300 μM, respectively). After addition of 1 mM ADP and 19.4 mM succinate to sample cuvettes, both sample and reference cuvettes were incubated at 25°C for 17 minutes prior to recording the difference spectra (sample cuvettes were closed during experiments.) (Kim IC, Waller DP: Specific inhibition of the testicular mitochondrial respiratory chain in vitro by gossypol. J Androl 5:426–430, 1983)

pol. Both racemic gossypol and its optical isomers inhibited testicular cytosolic LDH-X activity in preparations from the rat and the hamster (Fig. 18-6). The proposed active isomer (−) gossypol was actually less effective in inhibiting the LDH-X enzyme. Preliminary investigations with purified preparations of the

TESTIS

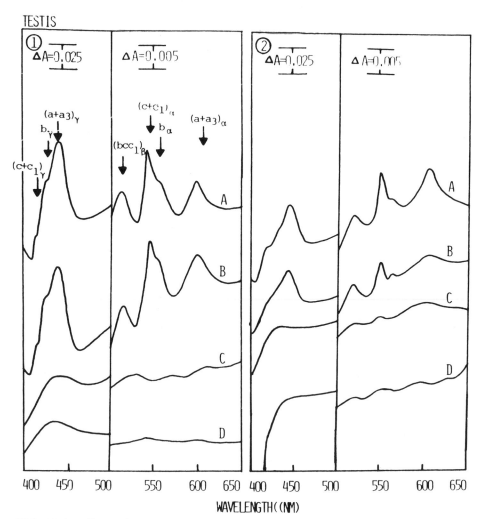

WAVELENGTH((NM)

FIG. 18-5. Effects of racemic gossypol on the difference spectra of testes mitochondria from the hamster (*Panel 1*) and rat (*Panel 2*). A:0, B:75 μM, C:150 μM, D:300 μM of racemic gossypol were added to the suspensions of testes mitochondria. The procedures were the same as described for Figure 18-4. (Kim IC, Waller DP: Specific inhibition of the testicular mitochondrial respiratory chain in vitro by gossypol. J Androl 5:426–430, 1983)

different LDH isozymes from the mouse also exhibit equal inhibition with the addition of either gossypol or its optical isomers. There is no apparent stereoselectivity of action nor selectivity for the testes form of LDH. These data do not support the testes-specific LDH-X enzyme as the primary target of gossypol.

LIVER

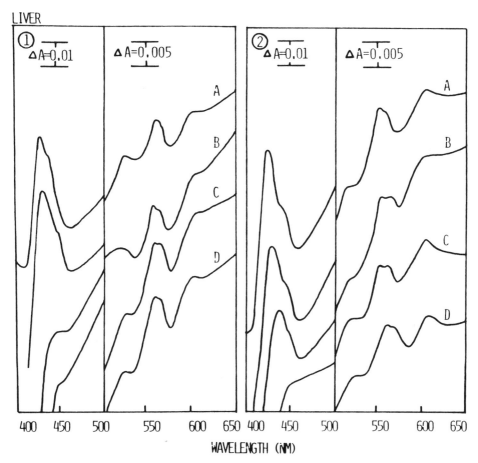

FIG. 18-6. Effects of (+) gossypol on the difference spectra of hamster and rat liver mitochondria. Panel 1, hamster; Panel 2, rat. A = 0, B = 30 μM, C = 75 μM, D = 150 μM of (+) gossypol were added to the suspensions of liver mitochondria, respectively. The procedures were the same as those described in Figure 18-4. (Kim IC et al: J Androl 5:426–430, 1983)

OTHER INFLUENCES ON FERTILITY EFFECTS

Data presented previously in this chapter demonstrated a toxic interaction between gossypol and selenium.[18] In addition to its important role in protective mechanisms in the liver and other organs, it is extremely important in the maintenance of spermatogenesis.[28] Selenium is incorporated into an essential structural protein in the testes at the late spermatocyte/early spermatid stage of spermatogenesis, just preceding the period of major disruption of spermatogenesis observed in gossypol-treated animals. In recently completed ex-

TESTIS

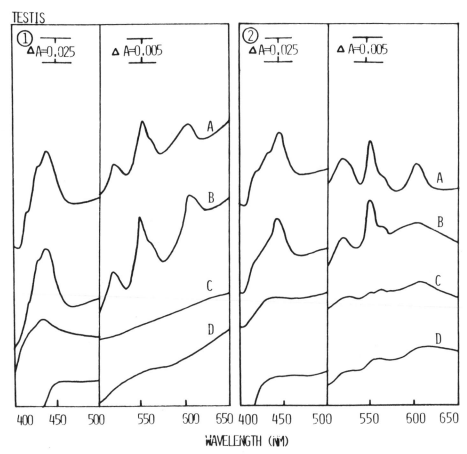

FIG. 18-7. Effects of (+)−gossypol on the difference spectra of hamster and rat testicular mitochondria. Panel 1, hamster; Panel 2, rat. A-0, B-30 μM, C-75 μM, D-150 μM of (+)−gossypol were added to the suspensions of testicular mitochondria, respectively. The procedures were the same as described for Figure 18-4. (Kim IC et al: J Androl 5:426–430, 1983)

periments, selenium was administered concurrently with gossypol and the fertility of the animals evaluated. Control (10/11 pregnant) and selenium-treated (9/12)* groups did not differ in fertility. Both gossypol (3/10)* and gossypol with selenium-treated (3/11) groups had significant reductions in fertility. Many more spermatozoa were observed in vaginal smears of the females mated with the gossypol-only treated group than with the gossypol with selenium-treated group, however. Studies are in progress to characterize

---

* Number of animals pregnant/number of animals mated.

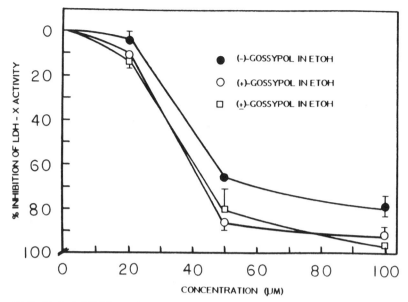

FIG. 18-8. Inhibition of rat testicular cytosolic LDH-X activity by racemic gossypol, (+)−gossypol, and (−)−gossypol. Gossypol isomers (20 μM, 50 μM and 100 μM) were incubated with enzyme for 15 minutes at 37°C before adding the substrate α-ketoglutarate and NADH). The activity measured with an equivalent amount of 95% ethanol added to the reaction mixture was used as the control to calculate the inhibition of LDH-X for each concentration of gossypol isomer. The bar represents the standard deviations of duplicate measurements from four different preparations. (Kim IC et al: J Androl. Submitted for publication)

more carefully the interactions of gossypol with selenium in the male reproductive tract.

CONCLUSION

Gossypol in its present form is unsuitable and will not be approved by western drug regulatory agencies as a male contraceptive agent. There is great concern that the therapeutic index of gossypol is too small. This is a major problem, considering the interaction of gossypol with several components of dietary intake that may greatly alter its bioavailability (iron) or its toxicity (selenium). The nature of toxic interactions of gossypol following chronic administration have not been well characterized. The poor distribution of gossypol to its reproductive system target organ (testes), and high concentrations in organs such as the liver, lead to significant exposures of tissues not involved in the primary desired effect of gossypol and increase the potential for toxicity. If the distribution problems can be solved by using compounds or

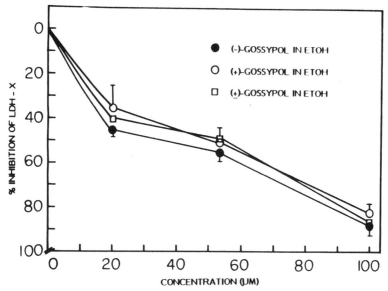

FIG. 18-9. Inhibition of hamster testicular cytosolic LDH-X activity by racemic gossypol, (+)−gossypol, and (−)−gossypol. Twenty, 50, and 100 μM gossypol isomers (20 μM, 50 μM, and 100 μM) were incubated with enzyme for 15 minutes at 37°C before adding the substrate (α-ketoglutarate and NADH). The bar represents the standard deviations of duplicate measurements from four different preparations. (Kim IC et al: J Androl. Submitted for publication)

delivery systems with similar actions on the testes only, these compounds may be developed eventually as safe male contraceptives. It would be a long hard fight to have the "toxin" gossypol accepted as a safe male contraceptive.

Gossypol may prove to be a very important compound even if it is never widely used as an antifertility agent. It may lead to a new site in the male reproductive tract for exploitation as a mechanism for the development of future male antifertility agents. It may also lead to a better understanding of the processes involved in male fertility. The excitement and interest in the male reproductive tract and male contraception caused by gossypol has encouraged investigators and funding agencies to increase activities in the field. This alone has been of great benefit to those who attempt to understand the complex processes of the male reproductive tract with the hopes of developing a safe, acceptable and effective method of contraception for the male.

REFERENCES

1. ABOU-DONIA MB: Physiological effects and metabolism of gossypol. Res Rev 61:124–159, 1976
2. BERNARDI LC, GOLDBLATT LA: Gossypol. In LENIER E (ed): Food Science and Technology of Toxic Constituents of Plant Foodstuffs, pp 211–267. New York, Academic Press, 1969
3. BRAGINI RE, FILKA MA, PARDINI RS: The inhibition by a series of potentially bioreductive

naphthoquinone of rat liver mitochondria and sarcoma 180 tumor cell respiration. Res Comm Chem Pathol Pharmacol 33:293–304, 1981

4. CHEN X, CHEN X, YANG G, WEN Z, CHEN J, GE K: Relation of selenium deficiency to the occurrence of Keshan disease. In SPALLHOLZ JE, MARTIN JL, GANTHER HE (eds): Selenium in Biology and Medicine, pp 171–191. Westport, CT, AVI Publishing, 1981

5. COUTINHO EM: Clinical studies with gossypol. Arch Androl 3:37–38, 1982

6. COUTINHO EM, MELO JF, BARBOSA I, SEGAL SJ: Antispermatogenic action of gossypol in man. Fertil Steril 42:424–430, 1984

7. DANEKE RJ, TILLMAN AD: Effect of free gossypol and supplemental dietary iron on blood constituents of rats. J Nutrition 17:493–498, 1965

8. DEPEYSTER A, QUINTANILHA A, PACKER L, SMITH NP: Biochem Biophys Res Commun 118:573–579, 1984

9. DEPEYSTER A, SANDY M, SMITH MT: Mechanisms involved in the acute toxicity of gossypol to isolated hepatocytes. Toxicologist 5:149, 1985

10. EAGLE E: Effect of repeated doses of gossypol on the dog. Arch Biochem 26:68, 1950

11. ELIASSON R, VIRJT N: Effects of gossypol acetic acid on the activity of CDH-C_4 from human and rabbit spermatozoa. Int J Androl 66:109–112, 1983

12. FRICK J, DANNER C, KOHLE R, KUMIT G: Male fertility regulation. In CORTES-PRIETO J, COMPOS-DA-PAZ A, NEVES-E-CASTRO M (eds): Research on Fertility and Sterility, pp 300–302. Lancaster, England, MTP Press, 1981

13. FONG HHS: Current status of gossypol, zoapatanol, and other plant-derived fertility regulating agents. In KROGSGAARD-LARSEN P, BROGGER CHRISTENSEN S, KOFOD H (eds): Natural Products and Drug Development, Alfred Benzon Symposium 20, pp 355–373. Copenhagen, Munksgaard, 1984

14. GIRIDHARAN N, BAMJI MS, SANKARAN AVB: Inhibition of rat testis LDH-X activity by gossypol. Contraception 26:607–615, 1982

15. GU ZHIPING: Present status on studies of gossypol. Yu Biyun 3:8–10, 1983

16. JENSEN DR, TONE RH, SORENSEN RH, BOZEK SA: Deposition pattern of the antifertility agent gossypol in selected organs of male rats. Toxicology 24:65–72, 1982

17. KALLA NP, WEI JFT: Effect of gossypol acetic acid on respiratory enzymes in vitro. IRCS Med Sci 9:792, 1981

18. KIM IC, MARTIN AM, PATEL P, FAKRODDIN C, WALLER DP: Changes in the reproductive tract of the male hamster following treatment with a combination of gossypol and selenium. J Androl 6:49, 1985

19. KIM IC, WALLER DP: Specific inhibition of the testicular mitochondrial respiratory chain in vitro by gossypol. J Androl 5:426–430, 1984

20. KIM IC, WALLER DP, FONG HHS: LDH-X inhibition by gossypol optical isomers. J Androl 6:344–347, 1985

21. KIM IC, WALLER DP, MARCELLE GB, CORDELL GA, FONG HHS, PIRKLE WH, PILLA L, MATLIN SA: Comparative in vitro spermicidal effects of (+)−gossypol, (+)gossypol, (−)−gossypol, and gossypolone. Contraception 30:253–259, 1984

22. KING TJ, DE SILVA LB: Optically active gossypol from Thespesia populnea. Tetrahedron Lett 3:261–263, 1968

23. LEE CYG, MOON YS, YUAN JH, CHEN AF: Enzyme inactivation and inhibition by gossypol. Mol Cell Biochem 47:65–70, 1982

24. LIU ZQ, LIU GZ, HEI LS, ZHANG RA, YU CZ: Clinical trials of gossypol as a male antifertility agent. In FEN CC, GRIFFIN D, WOLLMAN A (eds): Recent Advances in Fertility Regulation, pp 160–163. 1980

25. MA RH, JIANG CS, WU XR: Effect of gossypol on some functions of autonomic nervous system. Acta Acad Med Wuhan 1:65–67, 1980

26. MATLIN SA, ZHOU R, BIALY G, BLYE RP, NAQVI RH, LINDBERG MC: (−)−Gossypol: An active male antifertility agent. Contraception 31:141–149, 1985

27. MAUGH TH: Male "pill" blocks sperm enzyme. Science 212:314, 1981

28. MCCONNELL KP, BURTON RM: Selenium and spermatogenesis. In SPALLHOLZ JE, MARTIN JL, GANTHER HE (eds): Selenium in Biology and Medicine, pp 132–145. Westport, CT, AVI Publishing, 1981

29. NIU XY, WALLER DP, FONG HHS: Pharmacokinetics of gossypol in rats and hamsters. Pharmacologist 26:167, 1984

30. NOMEIR AA, ABOU-DONIA MB: Gossypol: High performance liquid chromatographic analysis and stability in various solvents. J Am Oil Chem Soc 59:546–549, 1982

31. OLGIATI KL, HOFFER AP, TOSCANO WA: Gossypol modulation of nucleotide metabolizing enzymes in the reproductive tract of male rats. Biol Reprod 31:759–770, 1984
32. PÖSÖ H, WICHMANN K, JÄNNE J, LUUKKAINEN T: Gossypol, a powerful inhibitor of human spermatozoal metabolism. Lancet i:885–886, 1980
33. PRASAD MRN, DICZFALUSY E: Gossypol. In Benagiano G, Diczfalusi E (eds): Endocrinological Mechanisms of Fertility Regulation, pp 233–48. Paris, CNRS, 1983
34. PRASAD MRN, DICZFALUSY E: Gossypol. In HARRISON RF, BONNAR J, THOMPSON W (eds): Fertility and Sterility, pp 255–268. Lancaster, England, MTP Press, 1984
35. QIAN SZ, WANG SG: Gossypol: A potential antifertility agent for males. Ann Rev Pharmacol Toxicol 24:329–60, 1984
36. REYES J, ALLEN J, TANPHAICHITR N, BELLVE AR, BEMOS DJ: Molecular mechanism of gossypol action on lipid membranes. J Biol Chem 259:9607–9615, 1984
37. ROTRUCK JT: Selenium: Biochemical role as a component of glutathione peroxidase. Science 179:588–590, 1973
38. SAUERHEBER RD, HYSLOP PA, DEPEYSTER A: Membrane structural/functional perturbations induced by gossypol. Toxicologist 5:201, 1985
39. SI Y, ZHOU J, HUANG L: Resolution of racemic gossypol. Kexue Tongbao 28:1574, 1983
40. SMITH HA: The pathology of gossypol poisoning. Am J Pathol 33:353, 1957
41. STEPHENS DT, GRITCHLOW LM, HOSKINS DD: Mechanism of inhibition by gossypol of blycolysis and motility of monkey spermatozoa in vitro. J Reprod Fertil 69:447–452, 1983
42. TOLLET JT, STEPPHENSON EL, DIGGS BG: Histopathology of gossypol poisoning in young pigs. J Anim Sci 16:1081, 1957
43. TSO WW, LEE CS: Variation of gossypol selectivity in boar spermatozoal electron transport chain segments. Contraception 24:569–570, 1981
44. TSO WW, LEE CS: Lactate dehydrogenase-X: An isozyme particularly sensitive to gossypol inhibition. Int J Androl 5:205–209, 1982
45. TSO WW, LEE CS, TSO MYW: Effect of gossypol on boar spermatozoal adenosine triphosphate metabolism. Arch Androl 9:319–331, 1982
46. WALLER DP, BUNYAPRAPHATSARA N, MARTIN A, VOURNAZOS CJ, AHMED MS, SOEJARTO DD, CORDELL GA, FONG HHS: Effect of (+)−gossypol on fertility in male hamsters. J Androl 4:276–279, 1983
47. WALLER DP, FONG HHS, CORDELL GA, SOEJARTO DD: Antifertility effects of gossypol and its impurities on male hamsters. Contraception 23:653, 1981
48. WALLER DP, ZANEVELD LJD, FONG HHS: In vitro spermicidal activity of gossypol. Contraception 22:183–187, 1980
49. WALLER DP, ZANEVELD LJD, FARNSWORTH NR: Gossypol: Pharmacology and Current Status of Gossypol As a Male Contraceptive. San Diego, CA, Academic Press, 1985
50. WANG NG, LEI HP: Antifertility effect of gossypol acetic acid on male rats. Chung-hua I Hseuh Tso Chih 59:402–405, 1979
51. WICHMANN K, KAPYAHO K, SINERVIRTA R, JÄNNE J: Effect of gossypol on motility and metabolism of human spermatozoa. J Reprod Fertil 69:259–314, 1983
52. WITHERS WA, CARRUTH FE: Gossypol, the toxic substance in cotton seed meal. J Agric Res 5:261, 1915
53. YAO X-Y: Studies on the isolation and the antifertility effect of (+)−gossypol. Reprod Contracep China 2:51–52, 1981

19

Development of a New Reversible Vas Deferens Occlusion Device

LOURENS J. D. ZANEVELD

JAMES W. BURNS

STAN A. BEYLER

WILLIAM A. DEPEL

SEYMOUR W. SHAPIRO

During the past two decades, several investigators have attempted to develop reversible techniques of vas occlusion or diversion in the hope that such methodology would be more attractive to men than the more permanent technique of vasectomy. Although vasectomy can be reversed through vaso-vasostomy, this technique requires microsurgery, and only a few clinicians report a high degree of success. Additionally, vasovasostomy is complicated and expensive and is not readily applied to a large number of men. The increasing requests for vasovasostomy indicate that even those men who were convinced that they desired no additional children may change their minds. Presumably a much larger number of men would undergo vas obstruction if they had reasonable assurance that the procedure would be reversible.

The reversible devices that have been tested can be divided into occlusive and nonocclusive devices. Occlusive devices are those that reversibly block sperm transport and can be subdivided into extravasal and intravasal occlusive devices. Extravasal devices are those that surround the vas deferens and occlude flow by applying pressure on the vas wall. Reversal is accomplished surgically by removal of the device. An example of these are the vas clips.[14] Problems with the extravasal devices arose when tissue necrosis was found to be induced if the pressure of the device was large enough to obstruct sperm transport.

The intravasal devices can be divided somewhat arbitrarily into intraluminal and extraluminal devices.[5] Intraluminal devices are located entirely within the vas lumen and are implanted through a small incision in the vas,

Research support for the development of the Shug (PARFR- 339) was provided by the Program for Applied Research on Fertility Regulation, Northwestern University, under a Cooperative Agreement with the United States Agency for International Development (AID) (DPE-0546-A-00-1003-00). The views expressed by the authors do not necessarily reflect the views of AID.

after which the vas either is closed with a few sutures or allowed to heal spontaneously. Such devices often are held in place by a small suture or other device located outside the vas and frequently surrounding it. The device is removed surgically after a small incision is made in the vas deferens. Various intraluminal devices have been tested in laboratory animals and men, including silicone injectables, cylindrical plugs, spherical beads, and threads of silicone or suture material,[10,13,15,16,18,21,22] or polypropylene devices consisting of a series of connected, progressively smaller spheres (Brodie devices).[9] Although some initial successes were reported with the intravasal thread in humans,[17,19] none of the devices ultimately found clinical application because 1) they did not sufficiently prevent sperm passage owing to the dilation of the vas lumen around the device; 2) they were not adequately reversible, most commonly because of fibrosis and perforation; or 3) they were never evaluated adequately.

The extraluminal device is located partially within and partially outside the vas lumen. The primary example of this type of device is the valve. The first device of this type was the gold valve developed by Davis.[8] Other metal devices (with or without ceramic coating) also were tested until the conclusion was reached that such rigid devices had the tendency to erode through the vas.[3] The rigid devices appeared to work well when they were implanted intra-abdominally in some animal species. In animal models such as the dog, however, which has pendulous testes like men, the motion and external pressures on the scrotum could not be accommodated by the rigid devices, and the vas was perforated.

The subsequent generation of extraluminal devices was flexible. One such device, the SPACER, consisted almost entirely of silicone, with an internal valve mechanism of stainless steel located between hollow silicone tubes in each end of the vas.[4,6,7] The device possessed Dacron velour on its outer surface or on suture rings, which encouraged tissue implantation to such an extent that the strength required to pull the vas from the device was almost the same as that required to pull apart an intact vas. The SPACER was tested extensively in dogs. The results were very encouraging, but the project was discontinued when it became clear that significant bioengineering efforts still were required to improve the valve mechanism of the flexible device, and funding was no longer available for the project. Another flexible device, the reversible intravasal occlusive device (RIOD), basically consisted of hollow tubes inserted into two ends of the vas, which could either be connected, allowing sperm passage, or plugged, preventing sperm transport.[11,12] The Bionyx control valve (PHASER) was tested as a reversible valve device in men, but problems were noted with obstruction and sperm bypass.[20]

Nonocclusive devices do not block sperm transport when infertility is desired but cause deviation of their course so that the sperm are voided in urine or destroyed. Such a shunt may either direct the spermatozoa to the bladder or pass them into or through a spermicidal vessel.[23] Alternately, devices that are connected to the vas lumen can be implanted in the scrotum and will release a spermicidal solution into the vas. An example of this is the copper coil that was placed around the vas and said to be contraceptive owing to the release of copper into the vas.

Although several of these approaches seemed to have clinical potential, most research on vas device methodology was halted some time ago for two reasons: 1) reversible device methodology was considered unnecessary because vasovasostomy could be accomplished surgically; and 2) vasectomy as a whole received careful scrutiny because sperm antibodies, produced as a consequence of this procedure, might cause health problems. It is now clear that neither is applicable. Vasovasostomies have the drawbacks described previously, and it has been established that in a regular human population, no side-effects are associated with vasectomy, in spite of the sperm antibody buildup (see Chap. 4). The sperm antibodies are still of concern from a reversibility standpoint, however, because such antibodies may interfere with fertilizing capacity of the spermatozoa after their passage through the vas is no longer hindered.[1] Indeed, although vasovasostomies have been successful in allowing sperm transport, the fertility rate in patients undergoing such reversal is relatively low (see Chap. 6). This may be due to other factors besides sperm antibodies, however, such as altered epididymal and testicular function and the formation of a constriction in the vas at the site of reversal. This constriction may partially block sperm passage, causing sperm to pool and possibly age before ejaculation. If the lumen of the vas becomes normally patent on reversal, sperm antibody formation may cease, and this problem may be avoided. In addition, correctly designed devices are much less likely to alter vas physiology after reversal than is a vasovasostomy because the latter requires the suturing together of the vas, from which a major section has been removed. For these reasons, development of the reversible obstruction of the vas by use of devices is sought again. The following is a summary of our experience with a new intraluminal device developed for this purpose.

INITIAL EXPERIMENTATION

After considering all the possible alternatives, we decided that the simplest method was the best as a start. For this reason, it was decided to give the vas plug, that is, an intraluminal device, again serious consideration. It was known that a single silicone plug or thread in the vas was insufficient to cause complete vas obstruction, however, primarily because of the expansion of the vas at the site of implantation. It was therefore decided to wrap Dacron sheeting around the vas at the site of the plug to prevent vasal expansion. The sheet was applied so loosely that no pressure necrosis should occur. The intraluminal plug and the extraluminal sheet were held together by a suture thread.

The device, called the Shug, was tested first in rabbits and proved successful in occluding sperm passage and generally allowing sperm output again after removal.[24] When the same device was tested in primates, however, necrosis of the vas wall occurred invariably, even if the sheet was applied so loosely that it was freely movable. Fibrous tissue invariably was found to surround the sheet, and it was suggested that this fibrous tissue caused enough pressure on the sheet surrounding the vas that necrosis occurred. Thus, it became clear that artificial wrapping could not be applied to the primate and probably not to the human. As these conclusions were reached, Beheri in Cairo, Egypt, related his experience in placing a tissue wrap around the vas consisting of a portion of the spermatic sheath; he proposed that this would be tested instead of the artificial wrap. Beheri came to Chicago and demonstrated his tissue-wrap technique in the primate. When the tissue wrap was applied in the absence of the plug, no obstruction of sperm passage took place.

Problems also were encountered in inserting the plug into the vas deferens of the primate. The vas of the primate, in contrast to that of the rabbit, is very muscular, so that the soft silicone had a tendency to be pulled apart on implantation. For this reason, instead of using silicone, #2 prolene was employed. To keep the prolene in place, its first portion was inserted into the proximal lumen of the scrotal vas and the final portion into the distal lumen, with the middle portion extending outside the vas. This plug successfully obstructed sperm passage but tended to move entirely into and farther down the vas deferens so that it was very difficult to remove. In addition, prolene is probably too rigid for practical purposes. The design appeared useful, however, and the subsequent series of devices consisted of silicone plugs held together by a small suture thread.[2] The plugs were placed inside the vas lumen and held together by a suture thread that passed from one plug, through the vas wall, extended for about 1 cm on the outside of the vas, and then passed back through the vas wall to the other plug. In this fashion, the plugs were freely movable for some distance but could not be dislodged. The movability of the plug, as well as the construction (*i.e.*, of soft silicone), should prevent the perforation problems seen with more rigid, immovable devices.

METHODOLOGY

The new device, still called the Shug (Fig. 19-1), consists of two silicone (medical grade) plugs held together by a nylon (Ethicon) suture (4-0). The plugs are hollow except at their tips, where the ends of the suture are encapsulated with silicone. The diameter of the plugs is either 0.7 mm or 1 mm so that they can be easily inserted into the vas and does not distend the vas lumen significantly; that is, they fit snugly but do not apply excessive pressure on the wall. A small metal stylus in the lumen of each plug gives it rigidity when the device is being implanted. After implantation, the stylus is removed.

In our laboratory, to implant the plugs, the vas was exposed and two small puncture holes were made in the vas, approximately 1 cm apart, with a 16- or 18-gauge needle. Each plug was pushed through one of the openings. The plug that was inserted into the puncture hole closest to the epididymis was pushed toward that organ, whereas the plug that was inserted into the puncture hole farthest from the epididymis was pushed distally. In this fashion, both plugs were inserted in opposite directions and the connecting thread remained outside the vas except for the ends that were attached to the plugs (Fig. 19-1). The metal stylus gave the plugs sufficient rigidity that they could be inserted through the puncture holes. After placement of the plugs, the styluses were removed. No sutures were necessary to close the puncture holes. Smooth muscle contractions closed them spontaneously.

During the first series of experiments, a tissue wrap was placed around the vas where the plugs were located (with one exception). During the second

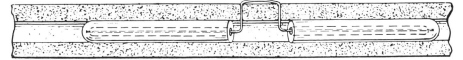

FIG. 19-1. Schematic representation of the Shug in the vas deferens.

series of the experiments, the tissue wrap was omitted. To wrap the tissue around the vas, a portion of the spermatic sheath was looped around the vas (at some distance from its cut ends) and sutured into place. Subsequently the cut ends were sutured together as usual to enclose the vas, pampiniform plexus, and so forth. The result was a small loop of sheath around the vas, which was in turn surrounded by the spermatic cord contents encased by the rest of the sheath.

To remove the plugs, the vas again was exposed, the tissue wrap incised, and small incisions made in the vas at the entries of the connecting thread into the vas. The plugs were removed from the vas by pulling on the thread. The incisions were closed with two 5-0 Dexon sutures. At times, it was not possible to identify exactly where the connecting thread entered the vas wall. In that case, the incisions were made as close as possible to the first portion of each plug. All the experiments were performed in mature rhesus macaques (*Macaca mulatta*).

OBSERVATIONS AND DISCUSSION

During the first series of experiments, six rhesus macaques were implanted with the devices; five also received the tissue wrap. The devices were implanted in both sides of the vasa deferentia of each animal. The Shugs remained for 7 months in all the primates except two, in which a device was inserted in one of the vasa for 11–12 months. These were the first experimental implants, after which some further device modifications were made (see above) that were finally tested. Semen samples were obtained from all the animals every 2 weeks before, during, and after implant. In 5 of the animals, 0.7 mm diameter devices were implanted, whereas the sixth animal received 1 mm devices. Although the 1 mm device is probably the one that will be applied to the human, these generally were too large for the primate. The length of the proximal plugs was adjusted at surgery by removing the first portion to correct the length for the particular primate. The lengths varied from 17.5 to 35 mm, generally measuring from 20 mm to 25 mm.

Before implantation, semen samples were collected over a 2-month period. The average sperm concentration for all the animals was 151×10^6/ml, with 77% sperm motility and a forward progression of 3 (on a scale of 0 to 4). None of the primates ejaculated spermatozoa at any time while the Shugs were implanted over the 7-month period, with the exception of one animal, the third ejaculate of which contained some immotile spermatozoa (10^5/ml). Spermatozoa were not ejaculated at any other time by this primate.

At the time of device removal, milky white, sperm-containing fluid could be seen to exude after the proximal (closest to the epididymis) plug was removed but not after removal of the distal plug. None of the vasa showed any signs of necrosis on visual inspection. Five of the six primates possessed spermatozoa in the first ejaculate obtained after device removal. The sixth primate ejaculated spermatozoa after the second ejaculate. Sperm concentrations and motility were initially lower than preimplantation values but increased after some ejaculates have been obtained to the point at which the sperm concentrations became higher than before the implant, with one exception. The last five ejaculates obtained from the primates averaged as a group 353×10^6 sperm/ml, with a motility of 74% and a forward progression of 3. The primate whose sperm concentration decreased went from 160×10^6 sperm/ml to 95×10^6 sperm/ml. The increased overall sperm concentration probably was because of the animals' having become used to the ejaculation procedure and/or to the fact that a newly constructed electroejaculator was used.

The results obtained with the one animal in whom the tissue wrap was omitted were identical to that of others; therefore, a second series of experiments in the rhesus macaque was performed to determine if the tissue wrap was necessary to prevent sperm passage. Six more primates were implanted with the devices, but no tissue wrap was applied. The preimplantation sperm concentrations for the group averaged 56×10^6/ml, with a sperm motility of 76%, of which 78% had forward progression. The devices again were implanted for a 7-month period. After implantation, the first ejaculate of several of the primates possessed some immotile spermatozoa, but no spermatozoa were ejaculated thereafter, with one exception. This primate continued to ejaculate spermatozoa, and an exploratory surgery was performed. One of the plugs had been implanted incorrectly and was outside the vas. The device was removed and a vasectomy was performed on that side; that is, the other side was kept intact with a Shug in place.

Thereafter, all ejaculates of this animal were azoospermic. These results show that the tissue wrap is not necessary to prevent sperm passage by the plugs. Wrapping the vas in tissue also increased the time required for implantation and for device removal, so that it did not seem useful to continue this technique.

The devices were removed from three of the primates, and the animals were studied for the resumption of sperm output. The vasa of the other animals were removed for histologic evaluation. The procedure again was 100% reversible. The average sperm concentration of the last five ejaculates of these three primates was 48×10^6/ml, with a motility of 68% and a forward progression of 75% (compared to their preimplantation values of 47×10^6/ml, 82% motility, and 85% forward progression). Two of the animals showed increased sperm concentrations, whereas the third showed a decreased concentration (from 130×10^6/ml to 57×10^6/ml).

CONCLUSIONS

The reason that the present design of the plug is more successful than previous designs in preventing sperm passage is at best speculative. The Shug consists of two plugs that are snugly situated in the vas but do not apply excessive pressure on the vas wall. As such, the vas physiology is unaltered, as indicated by the sperm passage that occurs after removal of the Shug. During device removal, it was noted that milky white fluid containing spermatozoa was present at the epididymal end of the proximal plug and some fluid was found in between the two plugs, but none thereafter. Possibly the first plug is the primary block to sperm passage, but sperm can pass around this plug, as has been reported by other investigators. Pressure applied at the beginning of the first plug probably accounts for some vas distention and the passage of the sperm. Because only a relatively small space is present between the two plugs, however, it is possible that not enough pressure can be built up at the beginning of the second plug for the sperm to pass around this device. Thus, the space between the plugs may act as a trap for the spermatozoa. Further research is needed to evaluate these suggestions, however.

The data show that at least in the primate, the Shug is completely successful in preventing sperm passage while the device is in place, and that sperm passage occurs again in 100% of the primates on removal of the device. The implantation procedure is simple and requires time equivalent to or less than that required by a regular vasectomy. The Shug has the disadvantage that it needs to be surgically removed, but this is a simple procedure and should not require much more time than a regular vasectomy. The simplicity of the technique makes it practical for clinicians who are not experienced in microsurgery. It appears to be a worthwhile technique for further exploration, and clinical trials are planned as soon as approval is obtained from the U.S. Food and Drug Administration (FDA).

REFERENCES

1. ALEXANDER NJ: Vasectomy and vasovasostomy in rhesus monkeys: The effect of circulating antisperm antibodies on fertility. Fertil Steril 28:562–569, 1977
2. BURNS JW, BEYLER SA, ZANEVELD LJD, SHAPIRO S, DEPEL W: Design and evaluation of a reversible vas deferens occlusion device. Third International Congress on Andrology, 1985
3. BRUESCHKE EE, ZANEVELD LJD, BURNS M, RODZEN R, WINGFIELD JR, MANESS JH: Development of a reversible vas deferens occlusive device. IV. Rigid prosthetic devices. Fertil Steril 26:269, 1975
4. BRUESCHKE EE, ZANEVELD LJD, RODZEN R, MAYERHOFER K, BURNS M, MANESS JH, WINGFIELD JR: Development of a reversible vas deferens occlusive device. V. Flexible prosthetic devices. Fertil Steril 26:40, 1975
5. BRUESCHKE EE, ZANEVELD LJD, FREE M, WINGFIELD JR: Vas deferens contraceptive methodology. In HAFEZ ESE (ed): Human Semen and Fertility Regulation in Men, pp 543–555. St. Louis, CV Mosby, 1976
6. BRUESCHKE EE, ZANEVELD LJD, KALECKAS RA, WINGFIELD JR: Development of a reversible vas deferens occlusive device. VI. Long term evaluation of flexible prosthetic devices. Fertil Steril 31:575, 1979
7. BRUESCHKE EE, KALECKAS RA, WINGFIELD JR, WELSH TJ, ZANEVELD LJD: Development of a reversible vas deferens occlusive device. VII. Physical and microscopic observations after long-term implantation of flexible prosthetic devices. Fertil Steril 33:167, 1980
8. DAVIS JE: Vas occlusion and obstruction. Contraception 5:329, 1972
9. DERRICK FC, FRENSELLI FJ: Experience with a reversible vas device. J Urol 111:523, 1974
10. FARCON E, HOTCHKISS RS, NUWAYSER ES: An absorbable intravasal stent and a silicone intravasal plug. Invest Urol 13:108–112, 1975
11. FREE MJ: Development of a reversible intravasal occlusive device (RIOD). In SCIARRA JJ, MARKLAND C, SPEIDEL JJ (eds): Control of Male Fertility. New York, Harper & Row, 1975
12. FREE MJ: Reversible intravasal devices: State of the art. In SCIARRA JJ, ZATUCHNI GI, SPEIDEL JJ (eds): Reversal of Sterilization, p 68. Hagerstown, Harper & Row, 1977

13. HRDLICKA JM, SCHWARTZMAN WH, HASEL K, ZINSSER HH: New approach to reversible seminal diversion. Fertil Steril 18:289–296, 1967
14. JHAVER PS, DAVIS JE, LEE H, HULKA JE, LEIGHT G: Reversibility of sterilization produced by vas occlusion clip. Fertil Steril 22:263, 1971
15. KAR AB, KAMBOJ VP: Spermatozoa disintegration in rats with an intravas deferens device. Indian J Exp Biol 2:240–244, 1964
16. KLAPPROTH HJ, YOUNG IS: Vasectomy, vas ligation and vas occlusion. Urology 1:292, 1973
17. KOTHARI MM, PARDANANI DS: Temporary sterilization of the male by intravasal contraceptive device: A preliminary communication. Indian J Surg 29:357–363, 1967
18. LEE HY: Experimental studies on reversible vas occlusion by intravasal thread. Fertil Steril 20:735, 1969
19. LEE HY: Studies on vasectomy. IX. Current status of reversible vas occlusion method. Korean J Urol 13:17–25, 1972
20. LYNN CM, POLITANO V: Early experience with the Bionyx control valve (Phaser). In SCIARRA JJ, ZATUCHNI GI, SPEIDEL JJ (eds): Reversal of Sterilization, p 91. Hagerstown, Harper & Row, 1977
21. MOHR KL, JOHNSON PT: Vasovasostomy and vas occlusion: Preliminary observations using artificial devices in guinea pigs. Fertil Steril 30:696–701, 1978
22. MOON KH, BUNGE RG: Temporary occlusion of the vas deferens. Invest Urol 8:292–298, 1970
23. SWARTWOUT JR, ZANEVELD LJD: Research on nonocclusive devices. In SCIARRA JJ, MARKLAND C, SPEIDEL JJ (eds): Control of Male Fertility, p 150. Hagerstown, Harper & Row, 1975
24. ZANEVELD LJD, BEYLER SA, PRINS G, TAFT F, GOODPASTURE JC, REDDY JM, ANDERSON RA, ANDERSON C: Reversible vas deferens occlusion: A new device. In SCIARRA JJ, ZATUCHNI GI, SPEIDEL JJ (eds): Reversal of sterilization, p 81. Hagerstown, Harper & Row, 1977

20

Capacitation and Fertilization: Acrosin Inhibitors (Aryl 4-Guanidinobenzoates) As Vaginal Contraceptives

LOURENS J. D. ZANEVELD

JOANNE KAMINSKI

DONALD P. WALLER

LUDWIG BAUER

This chapter presents a brief review of the capacitation and fertilization processes and a summary of our recent work to develop inhibitors of the sperm enzyme acrosin as vaginal contraceptives. As any other physiological event, the fertilization process is under enzymatic control. By interference with one or more of these enzyme systems, one can prevent a particular step essential to fertilization and, thus, prevent conception.[14,15] Several of the enzymes involved in the fertilization process are specific to the male or female genital tract or gametes, so that it should ultimately be possible to develop an inhibitor that is specific for the reproductive tract. With the exception of antibodies, no specific inhibitor is as yet available. For this reason, delivery of the inhibitors has thus far been local, i.e., into the vagina or uterus.

THE SPERM CELL

The spermatozoon consists of a head and a flagellum (tail). As any other flagellum, the tail contains contractile fibers and is capable of motion, propelling the spermatozoon forward. Sperm motility appears to be particularly

Because of the brevity of this review, it is not possible to quote even a small proportion of the articles on the subjects of capacitation and fertilization and do justice to all the investigators who have contributed to the presented information. Therefore, specific references have been omitted and the reader is referred to more detailed books and book chapters written on the subject matter (*e.g.*, 5, 6, 8, 11, 12, 13, 14).

Support for the development of aryl 4-guanidinobenzoates as contraceptives and the kinetic studies (PARFR- 338) was in part provided by the Program for Applied Research on Fertility Regulation, Northwestern University, under a Cooperative Agreement with the United States Agency for International Development (AID) (DPE-0546-A-00-1003-00). The views expressed by the authors do not necessarily reflect the views of AID. Support was also provided by NIH grant HD19555.

important for the penetration of the spermatozoon through cervical mucus and the layers surrounding the egg but may be less important for passage of the spermatozoon through the uterus and fallopian tube. In these organs, the ciliated surface of the lumen and the myometrial contractions can cause migration of particles, even if they are not motile.

Approximately 65% of the human sperm head consists of the nucleus. The nucleus contains DNA and nucleoproteins that are packed so tightly that the nucleus appears essentially homogeneous on electron microscopy, although occasionally it may be coarsely granular. The haploid chromatids of the nucleus carry the genetic information of the male.

The anterior portion of the nucleus is surrounded by the acrosome, and the posterior portion by the postnuclear cap. The acrosome and postnuclear cap overlap at the equatorial segment. The entire surface of both the sperm head and tail is covered by a plasma membrane. The acrosome is a saclike, lysosomal structure limited by two bilayered membranes. The membrane closest to the nucleus is the inner acrosomal membrane, and the one farthest away is the outer acrosomal membrane. The acrosome proper, probably consisting of compartmentalized material, is located between the inner and outer acrosomal membranes. The acrosome has a particularly important function in the capacitation and fertilization process.

Similar to a lysosome, the acrosome contains a number of lytic enzymes, some of which have been shown to play a role in the fertilization process. Typical enzymes are hyaluronidase, a proteinase called acrosin, an esterase called corona penetrating enzyme (CPE), a neuraminidase, acid and alkaline phosphatase, aspartylamidase, and several glycosidases such as β-glucuronidase and N-acetylglucosaminidase.[1] For the present discussion, acrosin is of particular interest (see Section on acrosin inhibitors as vaginal contraceptives). Human acrosin has certain properties in common with trypsin but differs from this enzyme as well as other proteinases by its molecular weight and structure as well as by its kinetic properties, including the interaction with inhibitors. No immunologic cross-reactions occur between human trypsin and acrosin. Similar to trypsin, acrosin is primarily present on the ejaculated spermatozoon in an inactive zymogen form called proacrosin. At least one inhibitor of acrosin (acrostatin) is also associated with the spermatozoon. The presence of the natural inhibitor prevents fertilization, and it has to be at least partially removed before the spermatozoon can penetrate successfully into the oocyte.

CAPACITATION

After being deposited into the vagina, spermatozoa need to pass through the cervix to reach the uterus. Cervical passage occurs primarily at midcycle when the mucus within the estrogen-stimulated cervix undergoes rheologic changes that allow sperm penetration. Even at midcycle, it is estimated that only about 0.1% to 1% of the vaginal spermatozoa arrive in the uterus. Of these, fewer than 10,000 spermatozoa reach the egg.

Ejaculated or cauda epididymal spermatozoa, even though fully mature, cannot fertilize an egg until certain biochemical and morphologic changes take place. Spermatozoa normally undergo an activation process (called capacitation) in the uterus and/or fallopian tubes. Capacitated spermatozoa can change morphologically (called the acrosome reaction) when they contact the egg (see further). In vitro, spermatozoa become capacitated on addition of follicular fluid, blood serum, or serum albumin. Not until these capacitation techniques were used was the in vitro fertilization of human gametes very successful. Additional evidence that human spermatozoa require capacitation is the presence of antifertility factors on ejaculated spermatozoa that must be removed before fertilization can occur, the occurrence of the acrosome reaction when the spermatozoa come in contact with the egg, the removal of surface components when human spermatozoa are incubated in a foreign uterus, and the fact that capacitation occurs in all other mammalian species studied so far.

In animal species, capacitation requires from 2 to 6 hours (primates require 3 hrs). Based on in vitro data, the time period for the capacitation of human spermatozoa is estimated to be about 4 hours. The uterus and fallopian tube may work synergistically to induce capacitation. In the rabbit, spermatozoa normally require 6 hours for capacitation in the uterus, unless the uterotubal junction is ligated, in which case 15 hours are required. Capacitation is not required for sperm penetration through cervical mucus. Capacitation is under hormonal control. It requires estrogen stimulation and does not occur in the progesterone-dominated uterus.

Capacitation is a fairly species-specific process, although the major block to heterologous fertilization is the egg itself (see further). Some cross capacitation may occur in closely related species, and partial capacitation can take place in foreign uteri. The capacitation of spermatozoa by fluids in vitro is also quite species specific. For instance, hamster spermatozoa are capacitated much more readily by hamster follicular fluid and hamster serum than by those fluids from other species.

During capacitation, biochemical changes occur primarily in the plasma membrane and acrosome, but no morphologic changes are induced. The nature of these changes still is incompletely understood, but they appear to include an alteration of the lipid components of the membranes. Additionally, certain compounds are at least partially removed from the sperm surface, such as acrostatin (the acrosin inhibitor) and a glycoprotein often called decapacitation factor (DF). When added to capacitated spermatozoa, these two agents prevent fertilization by hindering their passage through the egg's investments. Their removal is essential if fertilization is to take place. They presumably act by inhibiting an acrosomal enzyme and/or stabilizing the membranes. Finally, during capacitation, an increase in metabolism and motility as well as a change in the pattern of movement of the spermatozoa may occur, although the latter may be associated mostly with the acrosome reaction. No change in the acrosomal enzyme content appears to be associated with capacitation, with the possible exception of some hyaluronidase release in a few species, no activation of proacrosin to acrosin takes place.

The physiologic factors that cause the biochemical changes during capacitation are not yet known. Contact with the endometrium does not appear to be required, at least in the rabbit, because spermatozoa from this species become capacitated inside a Millipore filter when this is placed in the uterus. Thus, one or more compounds in the female genital tract secretions appear to be the causative factor, but their identity is at present only speculative. Capacitated spermatozoa become penetrating cells capable of passing not only into the oocyte but also into other cells. One can speculate that the physiologic importance of capacitation is to prevent the penetrating activity of the spermatozoa until this is actually needed, that is, when they approach the egg, so that spermatozoa do not enter the tissues of the male genital tract or the vagina and cervix.

FERTILIZATION

Fertilization takes place in the ampulla of the fallopian tube in the neighborhood of the isthmic–ampullary junction. The egg (oocyte) remains optimally fertile for 12 to 24 hours after ovulation. The egg is ovulated as a secondary oocyte that contains one polar body and is surrounded by two or three layers, depending on the species. The innermost layer, the zona pellucida, is present in all species. The zona is acellular and contains mucopolysaccharides. The middle layer is the corona radiata (absent in species such as rodents, but present in humans) and the outermost layer is the cumulus oophorus. Both are cellular layers and together are called the follicle cell layer. The cumulus cells are held together by a glycoprotein matrix containing hyaluronic acid. The fertilizing spermatozoon rapidly penetrates the egg, with these layers intact. The notion is incorrect that many spermatozoa have to be around the egg, releasing their lytic enzymes and thus causing the dispersal of the external layers before the actual fertilizing spermatozoon can fuse with the ovum. Rather, the spermatozoon most likely uses its acrosomal enzymes sequentially to lyse a small path through these layers and then, probably by virtue of its motility, passes through the opening so generated. It is reasonably well established that hyaluronidase is used by spermatozoa to pass through the cumulus oophorus and acrosin to pass through the zona pellucida.

Noncapacitated spermatozoa readily pass through the cumulus oophorus but never pass through the zona pellucida. If the spermatozoon is adequately capacitated, the plasma membrane and the outer acrosomal membrane of the spermatozoon fuse, vesiculate, and disappear just before or after the spermatozoa bind to the zona. This is called the acrosome reaction. Little definitive information is as yet available regarding the biochemical aspects of the acrosome reaction. The process appears to require activation by calcium ions. Calcium channels and the membrane ATP-ase system are most likely involved in the transport of this ion across the membrane; receptors also may play a role in the activation. Evidence suggests that as one of the subsequent events, phospholipase hydrolyzes membrane lipids to lysophospholipids and arachidonic acid. The lysophospholipids can alter membrane stability and structure. Arachidonic acid is metabolized to prostaglandins, which in turn appear to increase the rate at which the morphologic changes occur. Leukotrienes also may influence the acrosome reaction. Acrosin inhibitors prevent the acrosome reaction, implying that acrosin is also essential for this process. During the acrosome reaction, acrosomal enzyme release occurs and about half of the proacrosin is activated and released. The proacrosin that remains associated with the inner acrosomal membrane is exposed and can now be used for the penetration of the spermatozoon through the zona.

Zona binding by spermatozoa may involve receptors that are, to a greater or lesser extent, species specific. Some evidence is also available that one and maybe more of the acrosomal enzymes (acrosin and/or a glycosidase) have a role in sperm's binding to the zona. The spermatozoon passes through the zona in a typical oval trajectory. Only spermatozoa from the same species as the egg can enter the zona. The zona pellucida is also the barrier to polyspermy because it allows only a single spermatozoon to penetrate. After that, it changes its properties, becoming harder, as indicated by the much greater difficulty in dispersing the zona with sulfhydryl-reducing agents or proteinases. The cause of this change is unknown. Some data suggest that the acrosomal neuraminidase may induce this, whereas other results imply that the material extruded by the cortical granules during the cortical reaction has a hardening effect on the zona. At any rate, the passage of other spermatozoa is prevented, and those that have already entered the zona are halted. Removal of the zona or an ineffective zona reaction leads to polyspermy and possibly polyploidy. Since polyploidy is lethal, the block to polyspermy is an important function of the zona pellucida.

When the spermatozoon enters the perivitelline space, the cortical reaction is induced. The cortical granules of the egg cytoplasm migrate to and fuse with the vitelline membrane and release their material into the perivitelline space. At the same time, the presence of the spermatozoon triggers the completion of the second meiotic division of the egg, which was halted at metaphase II just before ovulation. The double-stranded chromosomes undergo centromeric division, which proceeds to telophase and is completed with the extrusion of the second polar body. Because the completion of the meiotic division is much slower than the cortical reaction, the second polar body differs from the first in that it has few if any cortical granules. The haploid chromosomes of the egg coalesce, swell, and become surrounded by a nuclear envelope, forming the female pronucleus.

The spermatozoon attaches sideways (flat) to the vitelline membrane at the area of the postnuclear cap. The membranes of the two gametes fuse with each other, forming a cytoplasmic bridge. The entire spermatozoon enters the cytoplasm of the egg (ooplasm), where its membranes dissolve rapidly. The nuclear envelope of the spermatozoon and the nuclear proteins break down, exposing, releasing, and rehydrating the chromatin material. A pronuclear membrane is synthesized and surrounds the DNA, thus forming the male pronucleus. Up to eight nucleoli have been found in both the male and female pronuclei. The sperm tail disrupts first at the midpiece. The mitochondria are rapidly dispersed into the cytoplasm, where they either disappear or become part of the egg mitochrondria. The fibrous sheet and the nine outer dense fibers disperse next, followed finally by the axoneme.

The male pronucleus begins to develop at the site of its entry into the egg, that is, along the periphery. It moves toward the center of the egg, where the female pronucleus also becomes located. The nucleoli subsequently disappear, the chromosomes condense, the pronuclear membranes break down, and the chromosomes from each pronucleus become located on the equatorial plate of the cleavage spindle. The first cleavage follows immediately, thus concluding the fertilization process.

ACROSIN INHIBITORS (ARYL 4-GUANIDINOBENZOATES) AS VAGINAL CONTRACEPTIVES

This discussion focuses on the acrosin inhibitors synthesized and tested by the authors,[9,10] however other investigators[2,3,4,7,18] also have developed and tested acrosin inhibitors with encouraging results.*

One of the most active inhibitors of human acrosin is 4'-nitrophenyl 4-guanidinobenzoate (NPGB). Primate studies with this inhibitor have shown that on vaginal placement, the compound is equally as active as, or slightly more active than, nonoxynol-9, even at much lower concentrations. Nonoxynol-9 is the active ingredient (spermicide) used in most vaginal contraceptive preparations on the market today. These preparations have not proven sufficiently effective during clinical trials. Although this usually is blamed on use failure rather than the potency of the ingredients, several animal studies have shown that the formulations and active ingredients are much less potent contraceptively in vivo than could have been expected from in vitro data. Apparently, the in vitro potency of a spermicide is not necessarily related to its in vivo efficacy. Thus, preclinical (animal or human) testing is essential to determine the relative potency of a compound. Nonoxynol-9 is a surfactant that may have problems contacting spermatozoa, particularly when they are entrapped in the coagulum or if they rapidly enter cervical mucus. New sperm-directed agents that are either more spermicidal in vivo and/or inactivate spermatozoa by different mechanisms should be developed. Such new agents can be used either alone or in combination with nonoxynol-9. Inhibitors of acrosin and, more specifically, compounds that are similar to NPGB may be such agents.

When NPGB interacts with acrosin, it probably forms a stable, covalently linked acyl-enzyme intermediate with the serylhydroxy- group at the active site and releases 4-nitrophenol. The stable binding causes the enzyme-inhibitor complex to be pseudoirreversible, so that dissociation is slow. This is important because reversible inhibitors such as the natural inhibitors are removed from the spermatozoa as they migrate through the female genital tract.

The release of nitrophenol when NPGB reacts with acrosin is undesirable because of the potential toxic properties of the nitrophenol. Thus, a series of aryl 4-guanidinobenzoates were synthesized, with different substituents attached to the 2, 3, or 4 positions of the o-aryl portion. The resultant compounds consist of guanidinobenzoic acid and a phenol that is presently marketed in the U.S. and approved by the Food and Drug Administration for

---

* More detailed reviews summarizing the properties of acrosin and the use of enzyme inhibitors as contraceptive agents were published previously.[15-17]

human use. These compounds were expected to be of low toxicity, and further experimentation bore this out.

Synthesis of the aryl 4-guanidinobenzoates was accomplished by the dicyclohexylcarbodiimide (DCC) coupling procedure using anhydrous 4-toluenesulfonic acid as acid catalyst. Nine such FDA-approved phenol derivatives were synthesized. Their inhibitory properties toward human acrosin were compared to human trypsin by performing I_{50} determinations (the amount of compound required to inhibit enzyme activity by 50%). The compounds were potent inhibitors of acrosin with I_{50} values ranging from about 10^{-7} M to 10^{-10} M. Another 17 aryl 4-guanidinobenzoates also were synthesized and tested. No large differences in the inhibition of acrosin versus trypsin were observed, so that no clear leads were established by which more specific acrosin inhibitors could be synthesized. More detailed kinetic studies of the inhibitors with human acrosin were performed subsequently with some select aryl 4-guanidinobenzoates. At the concentrations employed (10^{-8} M–10^{-10} M), inhibition followed first-order kinetics. The inhibitors displayed both reversible and irreversible properties. Complex formation of the inhibitor and enzyme was initially reversible; thereafter irreversible inhibition, progressive with time, was observed. The rate of acylation was in the range of 10^{-2} sec^{-1} with a second-order rate constant of about 10^6 M^{-1} sec^{-1}. Thus, the synthesized compounds are potent and rapid inhibitors of human acrosin.

The vaginal contraceptive efficacy of the nine synthesized aryl 4-guanidinobenzoates (with phenol derivatives approved by the FDA for human use) was compared to nonoxynol-9, using the rabbit as animal model. At the concentration applied (0.1 mg/ml), the aryl 4-guanidinobenzoates were generally potent contraceptives. The 4-carbethoxyphenyl, the 4-acetamidophenyl, and the 2-carbomethoxyphenyl esters were very active, reducing the fertilization rates to 0.3%, 8.3%, and 10.1%, respectively. Nonoxynol-9 at 1 mg/ml and 10 mg/ml concentrations reduced fertilization to 32.4% and 16.3%, respectively. Thus, even at 100-fold lower concentrations, these three aryl 4-guanidinobenzoates are of equal potency or are slightly more potent than nonoxynol-9. Several of the aryl 4-guanidinobenzoates also were tested in the zona-free hamster assay with human spermatozoa and found to decrease penetration at 10^{-5} M to 10^{-6} M concentrations. Inhibition of sperm penetration presumably was due to the inhibition of the acrosome reaction because the zona pellucida was absent from the eggs.

Recent experiments have shown that the three aryl 4-guanidinobenzoates described in the previous paragraph can rapidly bind to the sperm membranes and inhibit acrosin. When these compounds were mixed with whole semen for 2 minutes or less and the spermatozoa separated from the seminal plasma and unbound aryl 4-guanidinobenzoates, only small amounts of acrosin could be detected after allowing proacrosin activation to take place. The amount of acrosin inhibition depended on the concentration of inhibitor. The ED_{50} (the concentration of inhibitor added to semen at which the sperm acrosin activity was decreased by 50%) in these experiments ranged from about 10^{-5} M to 10^{-6} M. It should be noted that the 10^{-5} M to 10^{-6} M concentrations are about 100 to 1000 times smaller than those we hope to apply vaginally to women.

The acute toxicity of the aryl 4-guanidinobenzoates was assessed by intraperitoneal injection of mice with the compounds and determining the LD_{50} (LD_{50} is the amount of compound that causes death in 50% of the mice). Comparisons with nonoxynol-9 were performed. All the aryl 4-guanidinobenzoates tested were less toxic than nonoxynol-9. The LD_{50}s of the inhibitors ranged from 235 mg/kg to more than 2000 mg/kg, whereas that of nonoxynol-9 was 180 mg/kg. Fairly long-term (50-day) preliminary toxicity studies with selected aryl 4-guanidinobenzoates in rats showed that these inhibitors also are less toxic than nonoxynol-9 on chronic intraperitoneal application. On chronic vaginal application to rats, none of the inhibitors showed toxicity as compared to the controls. Vaginal irritation studies in rabbits are presently in progress and the data so far indicate that these selected aryl 4-guanidinobenzoates are less irritating to the vagina than is nonoxynol-9, with one of them causing no vaginal irritation at all.

From these studies, it can be concluded that certain select aryl 4-guanidinobenzoates have potential in finding clinical application as vaginal contraceptives, if the results in the human are consistent with those obtained in animal species. This is likely because the inhibitors rapidly penetrate human spermatozoa and cause the inactivation of acrosin. It is particularly encouraging that several of the aryl 4-guanidinobenzoates appear to have much lower acute and chronic toxicity than nonoxynol-9 and are potent contraceptives on vaginal application to rabbits.

REFERENCES

1. BHATTACHARYYA AK, ZANEVELD LJD: The sperm head. In ZANEVELD LJD, CHATTERTON RT (eds): Biochemistry of Mammalian Reproduction, pp 119–151. New York, John Wiley & Sons, 1982
2. BURCK PJ, ZIMMERMAN RE: The inhibition of acrosin by sterol sulphates. J Reprod Fertil 58:121, 1980
3. BURCK PJ, THAKKAR AL, ZIMMERMAN RE: Antifertility action of a sterol sulphate in the rabbit. J Reprod Fertil 66:109, 1982
4. DREW JH, LOEFFLER LJ, HALL IH: Antifertility activity of N-protected glycine activated esters. J Pharm Sci 70:60, 1981
5. GREEP RO, ASTWOOD EB (eds): Handbook of Physiology, Sect 7, Vol V. Washington, American Physiology Society, 1975
6. HAFEZ ESE, EVANS TN (eds): Human Reproduction: Conception and Contraception. New York, Harper & Row, 1973
7. HALL IH, DREW JH, SAJADI Z, LOEFFLER L: Antifertility and antiproteolytic activity N-carbobenzoxy amino acid esters. J Pharm Sci 68:696, 1979
8. HAMMER CE (ed): Sperm Capacitation. New York, MSS Information, 1973
9. KAMINSKI J, BAUER L, ZANEVELD LJD, BHATTACHARYYA AK, NUZZO N, VAN DER VEN HH: Synthesis and evaluation of enzyme inhibitors with contraceptive potency. XIXth Annual Meeting Medicinal Chemistry, Iowa City, Iowa, 1981
10. KAMINSKI JM, ZANEVELD LJD, BAUER L: Aryl 4-guanidinobenzoates as inhibitors of human acrosin. National American Chemical Society Meeting, Kansas City, Missouri, 1982
11. MEIZEL S: The mammalian acrosome reaction, a biochemical approach. In JOHNSON MH (ed): Development in Mammals, Vol 3, pp 1–64. Amsterdam, Elsevier/North Holland, 1978
12. MOGHISSI KS, HAFEZ ESE (eds): Biology of Mammalian Fertilization and Implantation. Springfield, IL, Charles C Thomas, 1972
13. ROGERS BJ, BRENTWOOD BJ: Capacitation, acrosome reaction and fertilization. In ZANE-

VELD LJD, CHATTERTON RT (eds): Biochemistry of Mammalian Reproduction, pp 203–230. New York, John Wiley & Sons, 1982

14. YANAGIMACHI R: Mechanisms of fertilization in mammals. In MASTROIANNI L, BIGGERS JD (eds): Fertilization and Embryonic Development *In Vitro*, pp 81–182. New York, Plenum Press, 1981

15. ZANEVELD LJD: Sperm enzyme inhibitors as antifertility agents. In HAFEZ ESE (ed): Human Semen and Fertility Regulation in Men, pp 570–582. St. Louis, CV Mosby, 1976

16. ZANEVELD LJD: Sperm enzyme inhibitors for vaginal and other contraception. In ZATUCHNI GI (ed): Research Frontiers in Fertility Regulation, Vol 2, No. 3. Chicago, PARFR, 1982

17. ZANEVELD LJD: Sperm enzyme and fertilization: Development and testing of acrosin inhibitors as vaginal contraceptives. In SCIARRA JJ (ed): Gynecology and Obstetrics, Vol 6, Ch 18, pp 1–7, Philadelphia, Harper & Row, 1985

18. ZIMMERMAN RE, NARIN RS, ALLEN DJ, JONES CD, GOETTEL ME, BURCK PJ: Antifertility effects of tetradecyl sodium sulphate in rabbits. J Reprod Fertil 68:257, 1983

21

Prototype of a New Long-Acting Spermistatic Agent

DO WON HAHN

JOHN L. MCGUIRE

Most currently available vaginal contraceptives consist of various formulations containing spermicides such as nonoxynol-9, Triton X-100 or menfegol. These spermicides are ionic or nonionic surfactants that exert their action by disrupting sperm cell membranes, resulting in rapid immobilization and cell death.[9] Although these formulations are known to be effective and safe, research continues in many centers in an effort to find new and improved products. Areas for needed improvement include the desire to make vaginal contraceptives more esthetically pleasing and to increase the duration of action of the products to increase patient compliance and use-effectiveness.

We have had a program in place for many years attempting to identify new types of longer-acting vaginal contraceptive agents. One approach that we are following is a search for spermistatic agents, that is, intravaginally administered compounds that would alter cervical mucus and by this action inhibit sperm transport and exert an antifertility effect.

Cervical mucus plays an important role in human reproduction. The characteristic change in cervical mucus that occurs at midcycle and that has been used to predict ovulation is well known, but cervical mucus also plays a role in fertility. It is known that the secretory activity of the cervical epithelium is controlled by ovarian steroids, beginning about day 9 of the menstrual cycle and increasing gradually until time of ovulation. Increasing production of estrogens during the follicular phase stimulates the secretion of watery, acellular mucus within the vagina and cervix. This type of mucus is a favorable medium for sperm survival and for migration of sperm up the reproductive tract, leading to fertilization. Following ovulation, endogenous progesterone produced during the luteal phase of the cycle causes the cervical secretion to become scanty and viscous. This type of mucus inhibits ascent of sperm toward the uterus, with sperm being unable to penetrate in any appreciable number.

These changes in mucus can also be induced pharmacologically. For example, a single 100-mg injection of progesterone results in increased viscosity within 5 days, and mucus viscosity can be changed within 6 to 8 hours to the ovulatory type by administration of estradiol benzoate or ethinyl estradiol.[5] It

We would like to thank Dr. G. F. Kiplinger for his aid in the preparation of this manuscript.

is interesting that during pregnancy cervical secretions form a highly viscous gel that occludes the cervical canal, acting as an effective barrier against invasion of the uterine cavity by both sperm and bacteria.

It appeared to us and others[3,5] that cervical mucus could be a target for new antifertility drugs. Physiologically, abnormalities of cervical secretions in women are considered to be the responsible factor in approximately 15% of infertility cases.[7] This conclusion is based on two observations. First, the number of sperm in cervical mucus correlates well with the number of sperm found in the uterine cavity and oviducts. Second, the pregnancy rate in infertile women has been shown to be significantly higher in the presence of a favorable cervical mucus. A substance that would retard the transport of sperm by safely inducing reversible changes in cervical mucus could be an effective antifertility agent.

Cervical mucus is a complex and dynamic secretion. At the outset of our program, it was clear that although much was known about the physiology and biochemistry of cervical mucus and its interaction with sperm, much also was unknown. Theoretically, one might target compounds for development that would interfere with specific components of cervical mucus. In our judgment, the tremendous gaps in our knowledge of cervical mucus made the probability of success with a targeted approach somewhat remote. Therefore, we relied on a simple in vitro assay as our primary test procedure, followed by in vivo testing for antifertility activity. We also resorted to random screening of compounds for their effects on cervical mucus, to find pharmacophores that subsequently could be modified chemically to enhance specific characteristics of the compound.

TEST SYSTEMS

Three laboratory test systems were used as the basic screens in this research program. They included: 1) an in vitro test that measured the ability of sperm to migrate through cervical mucus, and the ability of test compounds to alter cervical mucus in such a way that sperm migration is retarded; 2) the well-known Sander–Cramer test was used to exclude the possibility that the test compound was acting as a spermicide;[8] 3) an in vivo animal model obviously was needed because one never can be certain whether compounds active in vitro will retain that activity in vivo. In this program, the rabbit model used previously was adopted. These three laboratory test systems are discussed below.

EFFECTS ON CERVICAL MUCUS

The ability of compounds to alter cervical mucus penetration by sperm in vitro was assessed by a modification of the Kremer test.[6] Compounds are incorporated at various concentrations into fresh bovine or human cervical mucus and drawn into flat, rectangular capillary tubes 50 mm in length with a 0.3 mm path length (Vitro Dynamics, Rockaway, NJ). The tubes then are placed on well slides with one end over the depression. A square glass cover containing a hanging drop of human semen along one edge is adjoined to the

SPERM PENETRATION TEST

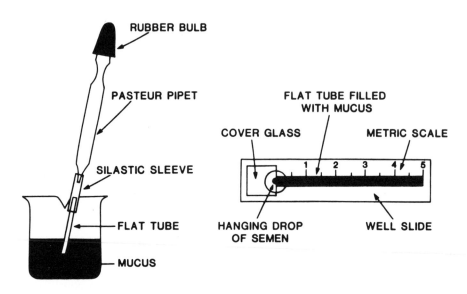

FLAT TUBE LOADING METHOD   SLIDE CONFIGURATION FOR ASSESSMENT

FIG. 21-1. Schematic of test system for sperm penetration in cervical mucus.

tubes so that semen and mucus interface, and penetration distance made by vanguard spermatozoa is observed microscopically at intervals thereafter (Fig. 21-1).

SANDER–CRAMER TEST

The Sander–Cramer test, which was developed in our laboratories in 1941,[8] remains the primary in vitro testing procedure used by investigators for evaluating the spermicidal activity and potency of vaginal contraceptives. It has been well documented previously.[5] This test basically involves the addition of 1.0 ml of diluted test compound to 0.2 ml of human semen at room temperature. The endpoint is the greatest dilution of the test material, which immobilizes all sperm within 20 seconds. If variables such as pH, semen age, temperature, and semen donor variation all are controlled, the Sander–Cramer test provides reliable quantitative potency data on spermicides.

IN VIVO TESTING METHOD

Several in vivo testing procedures for evaluation of vaginal contraceptive products have been reported.[3,10] In 1976, our laboratories proposed the use of the rabbit as a reliable animal model. Although the anatomy of the rabbit

TABLE 21-1. Inhibition of Human Sperm Penetration by ORF 13904 in Bovine or Human Cervical Mucus

MUCUS	ORF 13904 (μg/ml)	DISTANCE AT 30 min (mm, mean ± SE)
Bovine	0	50.0 ± 0.0
	10	46.7 ± 2.0
	25	39.7 ± 2.2
	50	12.3 ± 0.3
	100	12.3 ± 2.2
Human	0	50.0 ± 0.0
	5000	1.5 ± 0.5

vagina differs from that of the human, and extrapolation of animal data to clinical efficacy is questionable, the model has been used previously to measure accurately the contraceptive effectiveness of spermicidal vaginal contraceptives.

In actual studies, adult female New Zealand rabbits exhibiting both vaginal and behavioral signs of estrus are selected for use. An aliquot of test material is deposited at the cervix of each doe with a syringe attached to a slightly bent glass pipette 18 cm long with a 4-mm bore. Within 2 to 3 minutes following intravaginal administration of the test material, each doe is mated once to a fertile buck. A sham group serves as a control. The does are sacrificed on day 15 of gestation and the number of fetuses is recorded.

COMMENTS

Although this test program has been ongoing for only a relatively short time, preliminary results have been encouraging. Numerous compounds have been tested and shown to have no effect on sperm transport through cervical mucus. However, we have been able to identify a series of compounds, typified by ORF 13904,[4] which has at least some of the properties sought in this program. Data presented here demonstrate the kind of pharmacologic activity that a future nonspermicidal, long-acting vaginal contraceptive might possess.

ORF 13904 is a long-chain sulfonated polystyrene polymer, which, when incorporated at various concentrations into fresh bovine or human cervical mucus, impedes sperm penetration through the mucus in a dose-dependent manner (Table 21-1). At a concentration of 100 μg/ml, sperm penetration essentially was arrested in the first few millimeters, whereas sperm penetration through control cervical mucus was completed within 30 minutes.

Microscopic examination revealed that sperm tail movement appeared normal, but all of the cells had accumulated in large aggregates (Fig. 21-2). No freely swimming, forward-progressing spermatozoa were evident. When washed spermatozoa were incubated with ORF 13904, some agglutination of sperm occurred, but many freely swimming cells were observed.

When ORF 13904 was tested in the Sander–Cramer test versus nonoxynol-9, no effect on sperm motility could be demonstrated. Human sperm

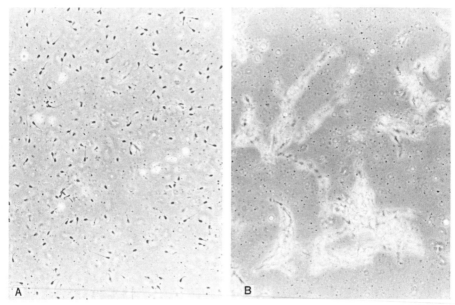

FIG. 21-2. Ejaculated rabbit spermatozoa in (*A*) PBS or in (*B*) PBS containing ORF 13904 at a final concentration of 1 mg/ml (phase contrast, 100×).

were obtained by masturbation from three different subjects, and 0.2-ml aliquots were rapidly mixed with each of several concentrations of ORF 13904, up to 10 mg/ml prepared in physiologic saline. When a drop of each mixture was examined microscopically for several hours, no remarkable effects on sperm motility were observed (Table 21-2), whereas nonoxynol-9 immobilized sperm motility at a concentration of 100 μg/ml. These data suggest that ORF 13904 is not a spermicide.

Contraceptive activity of ORF 13904 was tested in sexually receptive rabbits by the procedure described earlier. ORF 13904, or the control, nonoxynol-9, was dissolved in a gel at various concentrations and 1-ml aliquots were introduced intravaginally to female rabbits prior to mating with mature bucks of proven fertility. The does subsequently were sacrificed, and the number of fetuses recorded. ORF 13904 and nonoxynol-9 were both effective in reducing both the pregnancy rate and the mean number of implants per mated female (Fig. 21-3). In the vehicle-treated control animals, the gel itself had no

TABLE 21-2. Spermicidal Activity of ORF 13904 and Nonoxynol-9 in the Sander-Cramer Test

TREATMENT	(mg/ml)	DURATION OF SPERM MOTILITY (min)
Nonoxynol-9	0.10	0.3
ORF 13904	0.10	>150.0
	1.0	>150.0
	10.0	>150.0

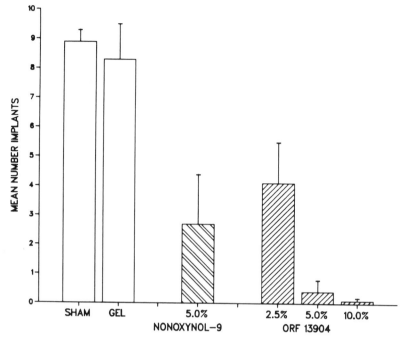

FIG. 21-3. Effect of immediate mating on the antifertility activity of nonoxynol-9 and ORF 13904 in gel formulations following vaginal delivery to rabbits.

effect because the fertility of this group was similar to that of the sham-manipulated group.

Of considerable interest was the fact that if mating was delayed up to 6 hours after intravaginal administration of this compound, good contraceptive efficacy in this model still could be demonstrated (Fig. 21-4). Even after 8 hours, ORF 13904 exerted a modest contraceptive effect. Labeling for existing contraceptive products recommends application of nonoxynol-9 formulations within an hour of use to ensure maximal protection against pregnancy. As would be expected, in these studies the contraceptive action of nonoxynol-9 diminished significantly between 2 and 4 hours after application. Of equal interest is the fact that the contraceptive activity of ORF 13904 is clearly reversible; by 24 hours after administration of the compound, fertility had returned.

When multiple matings occurred following only one treatment with ORF 13904, the fertility rate remained low (Table 21-3). Again, labeling for nonoxynol-9 containing products recommends the user reapply the product after coitus before any subsequent coital act. In these studies, the fertility rate did not remain as low when multiple matings occurred after only one treatment with nonoxynol-9.

Foldesy and associates have expanded these early studies in an attempt to better understand the mechanism by which ORF 13904 affects sperm.[1] The results of their studies suggest that the antifertility activity of ORF 13904 is

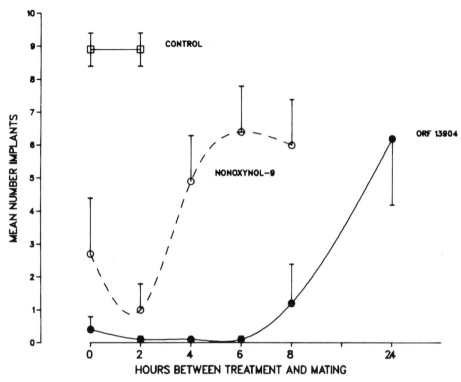

FIG. 21-4. Duration of the antifertility activity of nonoxynol-9 and ORF 13904 in 5% gel formulations when treated at 0 hour only and subsequently mated.

complex. In an interesting series of studies, these workers observed that if sperm treated with ORF 13904 in the absence of cervical mucus were inseminated into female rabbits, no ova were fertilized. Some freely swimming spermatozoa that presumably could have penetrated the cervix and fertilized ova still existed after treatment with ORF 13904. The fact that this did not occur suggests that effects on the spermatozoa may be as important as the agglutination of sperm within cervical mucus caused by treatment with ORF 13904. It is possible that ORF 13904 affected the cell surface of the spermatozoa, but Foldesy and his group also demonstrated that ORF 13904 has the

TABLE 21-3. Vaginal Contraceptive Activity of ORF 13904 Administered Prior to Multiple Mating in the Rabbit

MATING INTERVALS FOLLOWING A SINGLE TREATMENT*	NUMBER PREGNANT/ NUMBER TREATED	NUMBER IMPLANTS (Mean ± SE)
Initial mating and 2 hr later	1/5	1.4 ± 1.4
Initial mating and 4 hr later	2/5	3.4 ± 2.4

* Administration of 1 ml (50 mg/ml) prior to initial mating

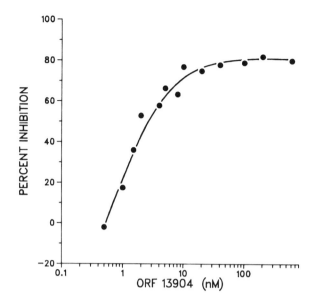

FIG. 21-5. Inhibition of acrosin enzyme activity by ORF 13904.

ability to inhibit human acrosin enzyme (Fig. 21-5), with a potency apparently greater than that of other acrosin inhibitors such as TLCK and nitrophenyl p-guanidinobenzoate.[2] Acrosin is believed to have a role in penetration of the zona pellucida by sperm, and one mechanism of action by which ORF 13904 exerts an antifertility effect may be by inhibiting acrosomal enzymes required for sperm penetration and fertilization of ova.

CONCLUSION

ORF 13904 appears to be a unique vaginal contraceptive agent in the experimental studies conducted to date. It lacks spermicidal activity, inhibits sperm penetration through cervical mucus, causes sperm agglutination, inhibits acrosin enzyme activity and prevents pregnancy in at least one animal model.

Studies designed to understand better the mechanisms by which ORF 13904 exerts its antifertility action and to extend these findings to other subhuman species are ongoing currently. It remains to be determined whether this compound will be effective in humans, but data presented above suggest the possibility that ORF 13904 may be the prototype for a new class of vaginal contraceptives.

REFERENCES

1. FOLDESY RG, HOMM RE, LEVINSON SL, HAHN DW: Multiple actions of a novel vaginal contraceptive compound, ORF 13904. Fertil Steril (in press)
2. GOODPASTURE JC, POLAKOSKI KL, ZANEVELD LJD: Acrosin, proacrosin, and acrosin inhibitor of human spermatozoa: Extraction, quantitation and stability. J Androl 1:16, 1980
3. HAHN DW, HOMM RE, MCKENZIE BE: Preclinical evaluation of new vaginal contraceptives. In SCIARRA JJ, ZATUCHNI GI, SPEIDEL JJ (eds): Vaginal Contraception: New Developments, p 234. Hagerstown, Harper & Row, 1979

4. HOMM RE, FOLDESY RG, HAHN DW: ORF 13904: A new long-acting vaginal contraceptive. Contraception 32:267–274, 1985
5. KESSERU E: Assessment of the rheology of cervical mucus. In ELSTEIN M, MOGHISSI KS, BORTH R (eds): Cervical Mucus in Human Reproduction, p 45. Copenhagen, Scriptor, 1973
6. KREMER J: A simple sperm penetration test. Int J Fertil 10:209–215, 1965
7. MOGHISSI KS: Sperm migration through the human cervix. In ELSTEIN M, MOGHISSI KS, BORTH R (eds): Cervical Mucus in Human Reproduction, p 128. Copenhagen, Scriptor, 1973
8. SANDER FV, CRAMER SD: A practical method for testing the spermicidal action of chemical contraceptives. Hum Fertil 6:134–138, 1941
9. WILBORN WH, HAHN DW, MCGUIRE, JL: Scanning electron microscopy of human spermatozoa after incubation with the spermicide nonoxynol-9. Fertil Steril 39:717, 1983
10. ZANEVELD LJ, ZATUCHNI B, HAHN DW: Animal testing and new vaginal contraceptive agents. In SCIARRA JJ, ZATUCHNI GI, SPEIDEL JJ (eds): Vaginal Contraception: New Developments, p 247. Hagerstown, Harper & Row, 1979

22

Sulfasalazine as a Male Contraceptive Agent

DAVID R. WHITE

R. JOHN AITKEN

Sulfasalazine (also known as salicylazosulfapyridine, salzopyrin, or azulfidine) is an antifertility drug that has been employed in the management of inflammatory bowel disease since the early 1940s.[2] Its use is now established for the treatment of ulcerative colitis, and more recently, it has been used against the effects of colonic Crohn's disease.[30] This drug had been in constant daily use for almost 40 years before two groups separately reported an association between sulfasalazine therapy and male infertility.[16,32] Chronic administration of the drug was documented to cause a reduction in sperm density and sperm motility, while increasing the numbers of morphologically abnormal spermatozoa present in the semen. Several independent studies subsequently have confirmed and enlarged upon these original observations.[4,12,20,31,33]

An analysis of the onset of seminal abnormalities in patients taking sulfasalazine indicated that sperm motility was impaired before density and morphology were affected.[31] Hence, seven men treated for less than 2 months presented semen samples in which only $30 \pm 1.5\%$ of the spermatozoa were progressively motile, significantly different from the normal range, which has a lower limit of 60%. In contrast, the concentration of spermatozoa in these semen samples ($82.5 \pm 21.9 \times 10^6$/ml) was within the normal range ($>40 \times 10^6$/ml) as was the sperm morphology (70% normal forms). When the duration of sulfasalazine treatment was extended for more than 2 months in 17 patients, however, there was a significant reduction in both the concentration of spermatozoa ($20.9 \pm 4.2 \times 10^6$/ml) and motility ($29.0 \pm 4.2\%$ progressively motile forms). Morphology also was affected significantly after 2 months of sulfasalazine therapy, with $39 \pm 4.5\%$ abnormal forms present.

All three seminal parameters measured tended to improve within 2 months of sulfasalazine withdrawal, although none of these changes was statistically significant. Thus 2 months after the cessation of treatment, 11 out of 14 patients possessed normal concentrations of spermatozoa in the ejaculates ($53.6 \pm 6.9 \times 10^6$/ml) and exhibited improvement in sperm motility ($45.08 \pm 2.5\%$ progressively motile), although defects in sperm morphology were still evident. Data from a number of centers[7,9,31] indicated that normal fertility

We gratefully acknowledge Family Health International for the financial support of this research.

returns to patients who have ceased sulfasalazine therapy before any seminal characteristics have reverted to normal levels. From this it would seem that the primary antifertility action of the drug is occurring late in spermatogenesis or during epididymal maturation of spermatozoa.

These findings also indicate that the actual mechanism of action that renders the spermatozoa infertile may be a much more subtle alteration of sperm function, as opposed to the gross changes detected in the conventional semen profile. In this context, one group has produced preliminary results indicating that spermatozoa from patients undergoing sulfasalazine treatment have a reduced capacity to bind to and fuse with the vitelline membrane of zona-free hamster oocytes.[13] In such instances, the disruption of sperm-fertilizing potential may reflect the inability of the spermatozoa to capacitate, acrosome react, or generate a fusogenic equatorial segment. Because the capacity of the spermatozoa to undergo these changes is conferred during the transit through the epididymis,[26] the latter clearly deserves attention as a possible site of action for sulfasalazine.

In contrast to the changes in both sperm function and the semen profile, the circulating levels of luteinizing hormone (LH), follicle-stimulating hormone (FSH), testosterone, 5-α-dihydrotestosterone, and prolactin show no changes before, during, and after sulfasalazine treatment,[31] suggesting that the antifertility action does not have an overt endocrinologic basis.

The side-effects produced by the drug are numerous and dose related, including nausea, vomiting, headaches, fever, reticulocytosis, arthralgia, blood dyscrasia, bronchospasm, pulmonary eosinophilia, and peripheral neuropathy.[32] Elucidation of the mechanism of action of sulfasalazine therefore is desirable to allow the development of a target-specific, nonhormonal male contraceptive, devoid of deleterious side-effects. In addition, such research may cast light on the etiology of idiopathic oligozoospermia, a condition that accounts for approximately one-third of male infertility and involves the presence of a semen profile very similar to that induced by sulfasalazine. Intriguingly, the male contraceptive agent gossypol also induces a condition similar to that observed in the presence of sulfasalazine, characterized by the presence of oligoasthenozoospermia and the absence of any obvious effects on testosterone or gonadotropin levels. The possibility therefore arises that gossypol and sulfasalazine share a common mechanism of action that might in turn reflect on the origins of idiopathic male infertility.

Investigations into the mechanism of action of sulfasalazine in ulcerative colitis have shown that this drug is a potent inhibitor of prostaglandin metabolism.[14] Prostaglandins (PGs) are cyclic derivatives of certain unsaturated fatty acids with 20 carbon atoms. They are found in many animal tissues and have a variety of profound hormonelike physiologic and pharmacologic properties. PG levels within tissues are governed by the rates of their production and degradation. They are not stored, and therefore their action within a certain organ is controlled as much by metabolism as by synthesis. Sulfasalazine is reported to inhibit the first enzyme of the PG metabolic pathway, namely, 15-hydroxyprostaglandin dehydrogenase (15-PGDH).[19] Inactivation of PG breakdown is postulated to invoke the cytoprotective and antiulcerative effects of PGs in the colonic mucosa.[14]

Since the influence of sulfasalazine on ulcerative colitis involves the inhibition of prostaglandin catabolism, a rational approach to the investigation of its antifertility action is to examine the role that prostaglandins play in the regulation of male reproductive function. Although very little is known about the levels of PGs present in the human testis and epididymis, endocrine functions of the testis and epididymis have been shown to include PG production.[6,8,11] The 15-PGDH enzyme is known to be present in rat testis[22–24] and has been shown to be under steroidal control.[24] Furthermore, PGs are thought to bind to human[18] and rabbit[3] spermatozoa and are known to have a profound effect on the fertilizing potential of human spermatozoa in vitro.[1] In light of these observations, it would seem reasonable to suppose that PGs are involved in some way in the regulation of male reproductive function, and that sulfasalazine and possibly gossypol exert their antifertility effects through the disruption of PG catabolism. We have therefore investigated this possibility by analyzing the activity of the 15-PGDH enzyme, as well as its regulation by sulfasalazine and gossypol, in the male reproductive tract of the rat and human.

METHODS

Human testicular and epididymal tissue was removed from cadavers in the postmortem room of the Royal Infirmary of Edinburgh while rat testicular and epididymal tissue was excised from freshly sacrificed rats. Both tissue types were treated identically. Tissue was placed in ice-cold (50 mM) Tris/glycerol (1:1), weighed, homogenized, and centrifuged at 1500 g for 10 minutes. The supernatant then was removed and stored at a tissue concentration of 100 mg/ml at $-18°C$. Prior to use, the partially purified enzyme was diluted to a concentration of 10 mg of tissue per ml with ice-cold Tris buffer. One milliliter of this enzyme preparation was then incubated at 35°C using 5 μM PGE$_2$ as the substrate and 1 mM NAD+ as cofactor. Enzyme, cofactor and, when appropriate, the test concentration of drug were preincubated for 5 minutes before the substrate was added.

After a final incubation time of 15 minutes, the reaction was terminated by the addition of 1 ml of methoxymating solution (0.12 mM methoxyamine hydrochloride in 1.0 M sodium acetate). Methoxymation of the prostaglandins present was achieved by heating the incubation at 60°C for 30 minutes. Two aliquots then were removed from each incubation and the concentration of 15-ketoprostaglandin E$_2$ present in each was determined by radioimmunoassay, using antisera raised against this compound. The inter- and intra-assay coefficients of variation were 8.4% and 3.5% respectively.

RESULTS

Appreciable quantities of 15-PGDH activity were recorded in the testis and epididymis of both the rat and the human. In the latter, the 15 PGDH activity (measured in terms of amount of the first metabolite of prostaglandin metabolism produced per mg protein per minute) was 4.1 ± 0.4 ng/mg/min in the

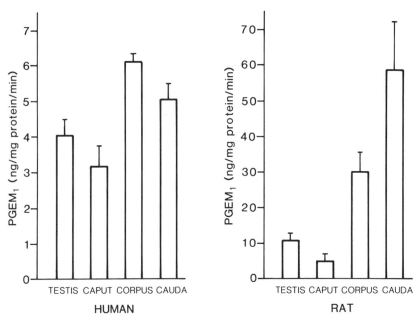

FIG. 22-1. 15-PGDH activity in the testis and caput, corpus and cauda epididymides of the rat and human.

testis and 3.2 ± 0.6 ng/mg/min in the caput region of the epididymis. Slightly higher levels of enzyme activity were detected in the more distal regions of the epididymis, giving 6.1 ± 0.3 ng/mg/min in the corpus and 5.1 ± 0.4 ng/mg/min in the cauda. In the rat the activity of the 15 PGDH enzyme was somewhat higher than in the human, although the relative distribution of activity was very similar. Hence in the rat testis and caput epididymis, the levels were 12.0 ± 2.0 ng/mg/min and 5.2 ± 1.5 ng/mg/min respectively, rising to 30.0 ± 5.5 and 58.8 ± 6.0 ng/mg/min in the corpus and cauda (Fig. 22-1).

The effect of sulfasalazine and its metabolites, sulfapyridine and 5-aminosalicylate, on 15-PGDH activity was assessed using enzyme obtained from homogenates of the rat epididymis. A dose-dependent study (Figs. 22-2 to 22-4) revealed in the case of sulfasalazine a biphasic response incorporating a stimulation of enzyme activity at low levels, around $0.5 \mu M$ to $1 \mu M$, followed by inhibition at doses in excess of $100 \mu M$. The stimulation of enzyme activity was found to be statistically significant ($p < 0.05$) and to represent a $30.0 \pm 2.3\%$ increase over control levels at a dose of $0.5 \mu M$. Sulfapyridine also tended to increase the activity of this enzyme over a wide range of doses, although in this case the stimulation was statistically insignificant. The second metabolite of sulfasalazine, 5-aminosalicylate, did induce a significant increase in the activity of this enzyme, equivalent to a rise of $64.2 \pm 4.2\%$ over control levels at a dose of $1 \mu M$ (Fig. 22-4). As shown in Fig. 22-5, gossypol produced a dose response curve that was very similar to sulfasalazine, incorporating the same stimulation of activity at low doses of $0.5 \mu M$ to $1 \mu M$, followed by an

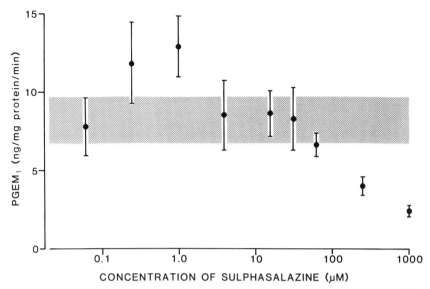

FIG. 22-2. Dose response curve for the effects of sulfasalazine on rat epididymal 15-PGDH activity.

inhibitory action at concentrations above 100 μM. Furthermore, this activity appeared to be confined largely to the optical enantiomer of gossypol, (−) gossypol, which is thought to be responsible for the contraceptive properties of this compound (Table 22-1).

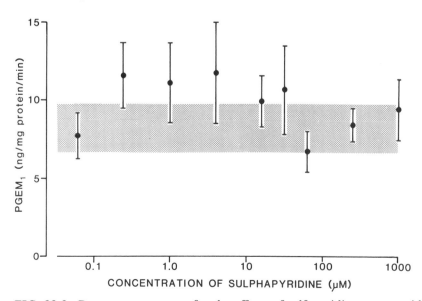

FIG. 22-3. Dose response curve for the effects of sulfapyridine on rat epididymal 15-PGDH activity.

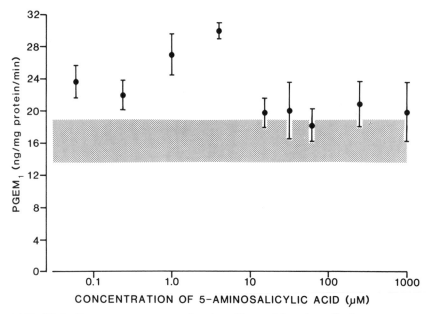

FIG. 22-4. Dose response curve for the effects of 5-aminosalicylate on rat epididymal 15-PGDH activity.

DISCUSSION

These studies have demonstrated that the enzyme targeted by sulfasalazine in the large intestine, 15-PGDH, is also present in the testis and epididymis of both the rat and human. In both species the activity of this enzyme increases in the distal portions of the epididymis paralleling, in the rat at least, the distribution of PGE_2, the concentration of which is four times higher in the cauda than in the caput epididymis. The biologic role of the PGE_2 detected in the epididymis is unknown, although PGs recently have been shown to exert direct effects on the motility of both rabbit and human spermatozoa.[1,28] Prostaglandins of the E series have also been shown to stimulate the fertilizing potential of human spermatozoa in a trans-species in vitro fertilization system.[1] The mechanism by which PGEs influence sperm motility and fertilizing potential appears to involve the induction of calcium influx, through the ionophorelike activity of these compounds, and the simultaneous increase in cAMP levels,[10] either through the direct activation of adenylate cyclase or secondarily, through the activation of this enzyme by calcium.

The influence of sulfasalazine on ulcerative colitis appears to involve the inhibition of prostaglandin catabolism and the cytoprotective action of prostaglandins; these subsequently build up in the intestine. Although the 15-PGDH activity in the testis and epididymis also was suppressed by high doses (>100 μM) of sulfasalazine, this action is probably irrelevant in a contraceptive context because although such levels may be achieved in the bowel, whether they would be attainable in the peripheral circulation is extremely doubtful.

Of greater interest in terms of male fertility control was the significant

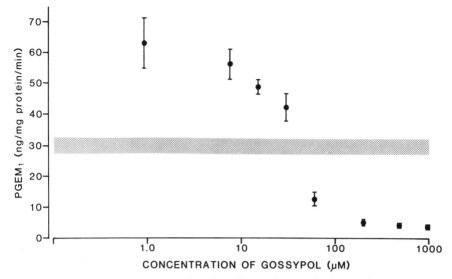

FIG. 22-5. Dose response curve for the effects of racemic gossypol on rat epididymal 15-PGDH activity.

increase in 15-PGDH activity observed with much lower doses (0.5 μM–1 μM) of sulfasalazine. Intriguingly similar concentrations of the male contraceptive agent gossypol also induced a similar increase in the activity of this prostaglandin catabolizing enzyme. Furthermore, when the resolved enantiomers of gossypol were examined for their influence on 15-PGDH activity, only (−) gossypol was found to possess stimulatory activity. This is of significance because it is only the (−) enantiomer that is thought to be capable of disrupting fertility.

Stimulation of 15-PGDH activity in vivo would be expected to lower the PG content of the epididymis and testis. Some evidence that such a reduction of PG levels within the male reproductive tract might disrupt fertility has been obtained from studies in which aspirin has been shown to exert a contraceptive action, presumably through its ability to disrupt PG synthetase activity.[5]

TABLE 22-1. Influence of the Resolved Enantiomers of Gossypol on the 15 PGDH Activity (n = 8)

TREATMENT	ACTIVITY (ng/mg/min)
CONTROL	7.17 ± 0.56
(−) Gossypol 0.5 μM*	9.71 ± 0.92
(−) Gossypol 1.0 μM	8.05 ± 0.58
(+) Gossypol 0.5 μM	7.45 ± 0.52
(+) Gossypol 1.0 μM	8.8 ± 0.62

* F = 4.52: p < 0.05 ((−) gossypol vs control)
Dunnetts t = 2.9: p < 0.01 (0.5 μM vs control)

Also, addition of exogenous 15-PGDH to rabbit seminal plasma has been shown to reduce sperm motility.[28] The latter is most sensitive to the disruptive effects of both sulfasalazine and gossypol, however, at present, direct evidence for a lowering of testicular or epididymal prostaglandin levels following treatment with sulfasalazine or gossypol is lacking. Analysis of seminal prostaglandin levels in patients receiving sulfasalazine treatment has not revealed any significant deviations from the normal pattern,[9] but the prostaglandin content of seminal plasma is largely a reflection of the synthetic capacity of the seminal vesicles[15] and is unlikely to reflect the levels obtaining in the testis and epididymis.

Additional studies on the influence of sulfasalazine on prostaglandin metabolism seem warranted, provided that a reliable animal model can be identified. To date the rat is the only animal model in which fertility can be reduced, but not blocked, through the administration of sulfasalazine.[17,25,27] The response of this species to sulfasalazine also involves a loss of libido and a limited decline in sperm density and motility, both of which contrast with the responses in the human, namely, severe oligoasthenozoospermia and no loss of libido. In view of the results obtained in this study, which suggest a common mechanism of action for both sulfasalazine and gossypol, it is possible that the hamster might be a useful model. This species already is known to be sensitive to gossypol. The identification of an adequate animal model also would facilitate the screening of drugs related to sulfasalazine for their contraceptive potential. For example, another sulfonamide, dapsone, has been reported to cause infertility in humans,[12] as have sulfatrimethaprim combinations containing the sulfonamide, sulfamethoxazole.[21]

The limited studies that have been carried out on the rat have suggested that one of the metabolites of sulfasalazine is the active antifertility agent. Sulfasalazine undergoes azoreduction to 5-aminosalicylic acid and sulfapyridine in the intestine, and only the latter appears to be capable of reducing fertility in the rat.[25,27] The 5-aminosalicylate is ineffective in the rat and also is known to have no effect on fertility in the human,[7,29] presumably because of a lack of bioavailability, because this metabolite can be largely recovered unchanged in the feces. Although the putative contraceptive component of sulfasalazine, sulfapyridine, reduces fertility in rats, it is not as efficient in this respect as an equivalent dose of sulfasalazine. This is difficult to equate with the claim that sulfapyridine is the active metabolite, unless the bioavailability of the latter in the rat is a problem. It is not known whether sulfapyridine causes infertility in humans. Further studies on the influence of sulfapyridine on male fertility are clearly important; if this compound is active it would obviously counteract the suggestion that stimulation of 15-PGDH activity is a significant factor in the contraceptive action of either sulfasalazine or gossypol, since our in vitro studies indicate that sulfapyridine does not exert a significant effect on this enzyme.

CONCLUSION

These studies have demonstrated the existence of a prostaglandin-catabolizing enzyme, 15-PGDH, in the testis and epididymis of the rat and human. The concentration of this enzyme was greater in the corpus and caudal regions of the epididymis, and its activity could be modulated by the male contraceptive agents sulfasalazine and (−) gossypol. The available data suggest an important role for prostaglandins in the control of male reproduction function; agents that disrupt the synthesis or catabolism of this group of compounds may have potential for male contraception.

REFERENCES

1. AITKEN RJ, KELLY RW: Analysis of the direct effects of prostaglandins on human sperm function. J Reprod Fertil 73:139–146, 1985
2. BARON JH, CONNEL AM, LENNARD-JONES JE, AVERY-JONES F: Sulphasalazine and salicylazo-sulphadimidine in ulcerative colitis. Lancet i:1094–1096, 1962
3. BARTOSZEWITCZ W, DANDEKAR P, GLASS RM, GORDON M: Localisation of prostaglandin in the plasmalemma of rabbit sperm. J Exp Zool 191:151–160, 1975
4. BIRNIE GG, MCLEOD TIF, WATKINSON G: Incidence of sulphasalazine-induced male infertility. Gut 22:452–455, 1981
5. BISWAS NM, SANYAL S, PATRA DB: Antispermatogenic effect of aspirin and its prevention by PGE₂. Andrologia 10:137–141, 1978
6. BUHRLEY LE, ELLIS LC: Contractility of rat testicular seminiferous tubules *in vitro:* prostaglandin F_1 and indomethacin. Prostaglandins 10:151–163, 1975
7. CANN PA, HOLDSWORTH CD: Reversal of male infertility on changing treatment from sulphasalazine to 5-aminosalicylic acid. Lancet i:119, 1984
8. CARPENTER MP, WISEMAN B: Prostaglandins of rat testis. Fed Proc 29:248, 1970
9. COSENTINO MJ, CHEY WY, TAKIHARA H, COCKETT ATK: The effects of sulphasalazine on human male fertility potential and seminal prostaglandins. J Urol 132:682–686, 1984
10. COSENTINO MJ, HASTINGS NE, ELLIS LE: Prostaglandins and cyclic nucleotides in the ram reproductive tract (abstr). J Androl 3:39, 1982
11. GEROZISSIS K, DRAY F: Selective and age-dependent changes of prostaglandin E-2 in the epididymis and vas deferens of the rat. J Reprod Fertil 50:113–115, 1977
12. GRIEVE J: Male infertility due to sulphasalazine (letter). Lancet ii:464, 1979
13. HALL JL, SESSIONS JP, FRIED FA: Sperm fertilizing deficiency in patients treated with sulphasalazine (abstract). Fertil Steril 35:245, 1981
14. HOULT JRS, MOORE PK: Effects of sulphasalazine and its metabolites on prostaglandin synthesis, inactivation, and actions on smooth muscle. Br J Pharmacol 68:719–730, 1980
15. KELLY RW: Prostaglandin synthesis in the male and female reproductive tract. J Reprod Fertil 62:293–304, 1981
16. LEVI AJ, FISHER AM, HUGHES L, HENDRY WF: Male infertility due to sulphasalazine. Lancet ii:276–278, 1979
17. LEVI AJ, TOOVEY S, SMETHURST P, ANDREWS B: Sulphasalazine and male infertility. In JEFFCOATE SL, SANDLER M (eds): Progress towards a male contraceptive, pp 209–219. London, John Wiley & Sons, 1982
18. MERCADO E, VALLALOBOS M, DOMINIGUEZ R, ROSADO A: Differential binding of PGE_1, and PGF_2 to the human spermatozoa membrane. Life Sci 22:429–436, 1978
19. MOORE PK, HOULT JRS, LAURIE AS: Prostaglandins and mechanism of action of sulphasalazine in ulcerative colitis. Lancet ii:98–99, 1978
20. MUDGE TJ: Semen and sulphasalazine. Clin Reprod Fertil 1:157–158, 1982
21. MURDIA A, MATHUR V, KOTHARI LK, SINGH KP: Sulpha-trimethoprin combinations and male infertility (letter). Lancet ii:375–376, 1978
22. NAKANO J, MONTAGUE B, DARROW B: Metabolism of prostaglandin E_1 in human plasma, uterus, and placenta in swine ovary and in rat testicle. Biochem Pharmacol 20:2512–2514, 1971
23. NAKANO J, PRANCAN AV: Metabolic degradation of prostaglandin E_1 in the rat plasma and in rat brain, heart, lung, kidney and testicle homogenates. J Pharm Pharmacol 23:231–232, 1971
24. OHUO-OBASIOLU CC, GROESBECK MD, ELLIS LC: Control of rat testicular prostaglandin dehydrogenase, Δ^{13} prostaglandin reductase, and total prostaglandin dehydrogenase activities. J Androl 3:329–336, 1982
25. O'MORAIN CA, SMETHURST P, HUDSON E, LEVI AJ: Further studies on sulphasalazine-induced infertility. Gastroenterology 82:1140, 1982

26. ORGEBIN-CRIST MC, FOURNIER-DELPECH S: Sperm–egg interaction: Evidence for maturational changes during epididymal transit. J Androl 3:429–433, 1982
27. PHOLPRAMOOL C, SRIKHAO A: Antifertility effect of sulphasalazine in the male rat. Contraception 28:273–279, 1983
28. SCHLEGEL W, FISCHER S, BEIER HM, SCHNEIDER HPG: Effects on fertilization of rabbits of insemination with ejaculates treated with PG-dehydrogenase and antisera to PGE_2 and PGF_2. J Reprod Fertil 68:45–50, 1983
29. SHAFFER JL, KERSHAW A, BERRISFORD MH: Sulphasalazine-induced infertility reversed on transfer to 5-aminosalicylic acid. Lancet i:1240, 1984
30. SUMMERS RW, SWITZ DM, SESSIONS JT, BECKTEL JM, BEST WR, KERN F, SINGLETON JW: National cooperative Crohn's disease study: Results of drug treatment. Gastroenterology 77:847–869, 1979
31. TOOVEY S, HUDSON E, HENDRY WF, LEVI AJ: Sulphasalazine and male infertility: reversibility and possible mechanism. Gut 22:445–451, 1981
32. TOTH A: Reversible toxic effect of salacylazosulfapyridine on semen quality. Fertil Steril 31:538–540, 1979
33. TRAUB AI, THOMPSON W, CARVILLE J: Male infertility due to sulphasalazine. Lancet ii:639–640, 1979

23

Tolnidamine in Male Contraception: A Survey of Preclinical Data

PATRIZIO SCORZA BARCELLONA

VALERIO CIOLI

CESARE DE MARTINO

C. WAYNE BARDIN

IRVING M. SPITZ

Tolnidamine, or 1-[(4-chloro-2-methylphenyl)methyl]-1H-indazole-3-carboxylic acid (Fig. 23-1), belongs to the chemical class of 1H-indazole-3-carboxylic acids. These agents exert antispermatogenic activity.[3] The initial investigations were focused mainly on AF 1312/TS, the monochlorinated, and lonidamine, the dichlorinated, compound. AF 1312/TS was the first compound studied for its antispermatogenic activity,[2,4-6,14,16] and the more potent lonidamine[11,17] was used to assess the mechanism of action[7,8,10] and the toxicologic profile[1,9,15] of this chemical class.

The experience acquired to date indicates that these drugs interfere directly with the spermatogenic process, blocking meiotic and postmeiotic cell maturation.[18] Unlike the majority of other antispermatogenic agents, the effects are evident even a few hours after a single oral administration.[18] Moreover, depending on the dosage used, the antispermatogenic activity appears to be reversible because spermatogonia are unaffected.[18]

Despite its strong antispermatogenic activity, lonidamine was discarded as a male contraceptive because of its nephrotoxicity in the monkey. However, this agent is currently in phase II human studies as an anticancer drug.

Tolnidamine is one of the most active compounds of the 1H-indazole-3-carboxylic acids on the seminiferous epithelium, and at the moment it seems a promising candidate as a "male pill."

This chapter presents the published and unpublished preclinical data currently available on this drug.

ANTISPERMATOGENIC ACTIVITY

The inhibitory activity of tolnidamine on the seminiferous epithelium was studied in sexually mature rats. A dose range between 25 and 200 mg/kg was administered as a single dose by the oral route, and the effects on the testis,

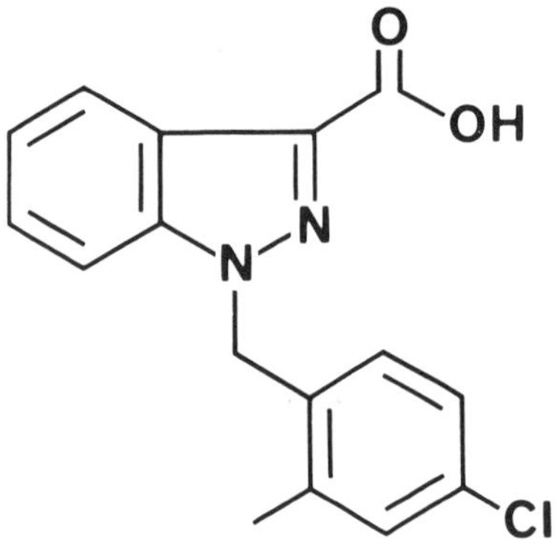

FIG. 23-1. Structure of tolnidamine.

epididymis, ventral prostate, and seminal vesicle weights were measured 20 days later. Single doses of 50, 70, 100, and 140 mg/kg produced a dose-dependent reduction in testis weight, although 25 or 35 mg/kg were ineffective (Fig. 23-2). Doses higher than 140 mg/kg did not produce further inhibition. In the same experiment, the epididymis also underwent a reduction in weight (Fig. 23-2).

In another experiment, doses of tolnidamine from 17.5 to 280 mg/kg were administered daily for 5 days, and the animals were sacrificed after 20 days. In this experiment, doses in a range of 35 to 100 mg/kg also produced a dose-dependent reduction in both testis and epididymal weights (Fig. 23-3). No further reduction was obtained with higher dosages. In neither of these experiments were alterations in ventral prostate and seminal vesicle weight observed.

The study of the time course of testicular inhibition after 250 mg/kg of tolnidamine showed a transient reduction in testis weight at 4 to 8 hours with subsequent recovery by 16 hours.[19] The most dramatic effects were seen at a later period with a 33% reduction in testis weight by 5 days and epididymal weight by 12 days.[19] Similar results were obtained by Lobl and associates who detected the first effects 24 hours after 500 mg/kg or 48 hours after 60 mg/kg of the drug.[12] The greatest inhibition occurred after 8 days with both doses. These investigators also confirmed the lack of effects on ventral prostate and seminal vesicle weights.

Histologic examination showed no alterations in paraffin sections of rat testes 24 hours after 50 mg/kg of tolnidamine. At the same time, semithin plastic sections showed only occasionally vacuolated Sertoli cells and swelling of the elongated spermatids. The most dramatic change was found in the lumina of the proximal portion of the caput epididymis, where exfoliated round spermatids were present in addition to mature spermatozoa (Fig. 23-4).

Two days after treatment, the seminiferous epithelium appeared disorganized, with reduced and altered round spermatids (Fig. 23-5), and reduction of normal elongated spermatids (Fig. 23-6). Electron microscopy of these elements showed severe alterations, consisting of dark hyaloplasm, swelling and whorling of the smooth endoplasmic reticulum, damage to the nuclear and acrosomic membranes, and modified mitochondria (Figs. 23-7 and 23-8). Moreover, several Sertoli cells had swollen and disrupted mitochondria (Fig.

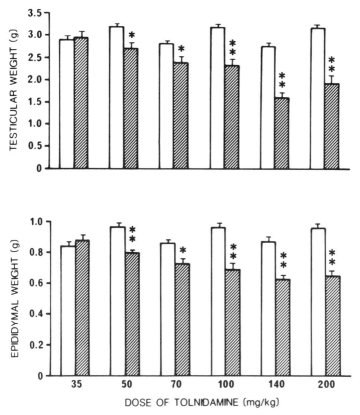

FIG. 23-2. Testicular and epididymal weights 20 days after a single administration of tolnidamine at different doses. Each column represents the mean ± SEM of control (*open*) or treated rats (*shaded*). Asterisks indicate significant differences from controls: *p < 0.01; **p < 0.001.

23-7). The lumina of the caput epididymis contained many exfoliated germ cells and only a few anomalous sperms (Fig. 23-9).

Five days after administration of tolnidamine, the seminiferous epithelium appeared severely affected: round spermatids had a large nuclear vacuole, spermatocytes were reduced in number and exfoliated in the tubular lumina, and no maturation phase spermatids were detected (Fig. 23-10). The epididymal lumina were filled with some exfoliated degenerated germ cells (Fig. 23-11).

HORMONAL EFFECTS

Spitz and associates evaluated Leydig and Sertoli cell function in rats for up to 12 days following the administration of tolnidamine (250 mg/kg) by oral gavage.[19] Serum follicle-stimulating hormone (FSH) levels did not change and

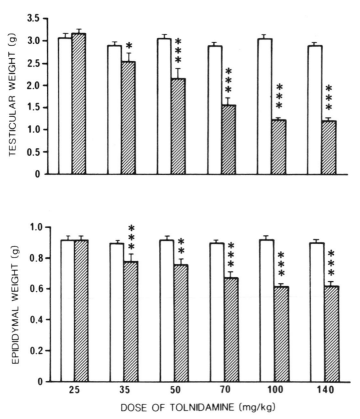

FIG. 23-3. Testicular and epididymal weights 20 days after 5 daily administrations of tolnidamine at different doses. Each column represents the mean ± SEM of control (*open*) or treated rats (*shaded*). Asterisks indicate significant differences from controls: *p < 0.05; **p < 0.01; ***p < 0.001.

luteinizing hormone (LH) levels showed a transient increase between 64 hours and 8 days. Except for an initial increase at 2 hours, there were no changes in serum testosterone (Fig. 23-12). In contrast to these observations, slight increases in FSH but not LH levels have been observed previously in the rat with large doses of tolnidamine.[12] It thus can be concluded that single doses of tolnidamine do not produce major alterations in gonadotropins or testosterone.

Androgen-binding protein (rABP) was used to study Sertoli cell function. In the intact animal, 80% of this protein is secreted from the apex of Sertoli cells into the tubular lumen, from where it is transported to the epididymis; the remainder is secreted from the base of Sertoli cells into the blood and lymphatics of the interstitial space.[13] According to these observations, rABP is secreted bidirectionally from Sertoli cells.

Following a single oral dose of 250 mg/kg of tolnidamine, epididymal

(*Text continues on p. 246*)

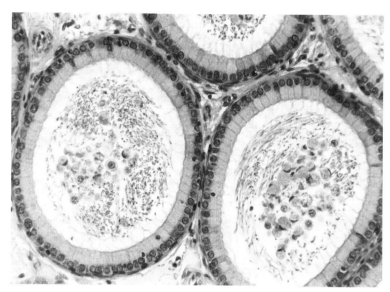

FIG. 23-4. Rat caput epididymis 1 day after 50 mg/kg of tolnidamine by oral gavage. Normal sperms, round spermatids, and eosinophilic droplets fill the tubular lumina (H and E, magnification × 270).

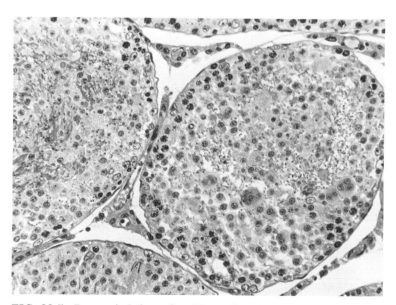

FIG. 23-5. Rat testis 2 days after 50 mg/kg of tolnidamine by oral gavage. Disorganization of the seminiferous epithelium with altered and fused round spermatids are noted (H and E, magnification × 270).

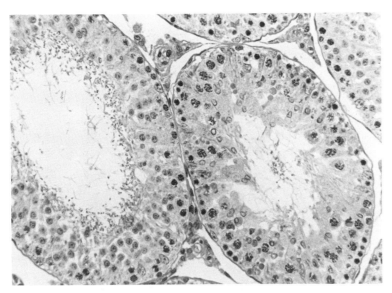

FIG. 23-6. Same testis of Figure 23-5. There is an absence of normal maturation-phase spermatids (H and E, magnification × 270).

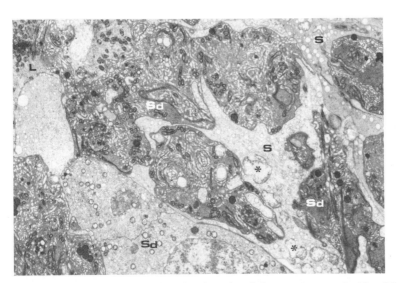

FIG. 23-7. Electron micrograph of testis of the same rat as in Fig. 23-5. Several maturation phase spermatids (white Sd) at stage I of seminiferous epithelium cycle, with swollen and whorled smooth endoplasmic reticulum, are observed. Many mitochondria appear elongated. Sertoli cell (S) mitochondria are swollen with disrupted cristae (*asterisks*). Tubular lumen (L); spermatid at Golgi phase (black Sd) (magnification × 3800).

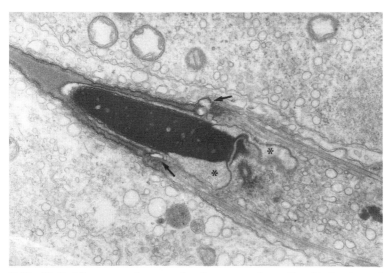

FIG. 23-8. Electron micrograph of same testis as Fig. 23-7. Note the maturation phase spermatid at stage V of the seminiferous epithelium cycle with widening of the space between posterior chromatin and redundant nuclear membranes (*asterisks*), and vacuolation of the postacrosomal cap membranes (*arrows*) (magnification × 8700).

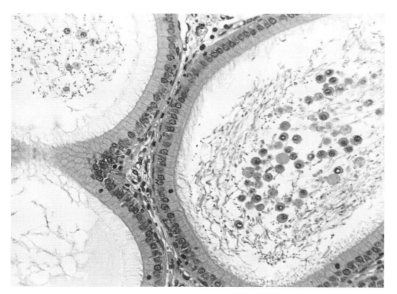

FIG. 23-9. Caput epididymis of the same rat as in Fig. 23-5. Degenerated round spermatids and abnormal sperms in the tubular lumina. (H and E, magnification × 270).

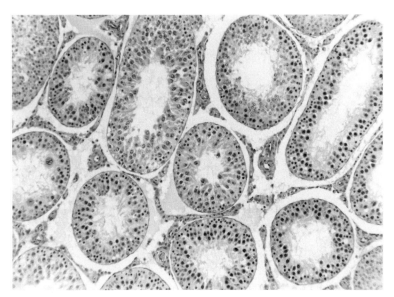

FIG. 23-10. Rat testis 5 days after 50 mg/kg of tolnidamine by oral gavage. Alterations of meiotic and postmeiotic germ cells, and lack of elongated spermatids are evident (H and E, magnification × 110).

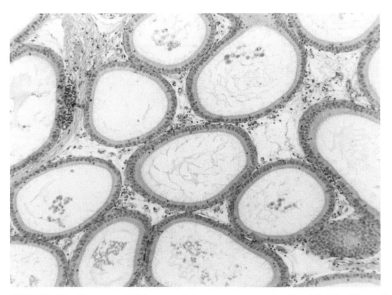

FIG. 23-11. Caput epididymis of the same rat as in Fig. 23-10. The tubular lumina contain only a few degenerated immature germ cells (H and E, magnification × 110).

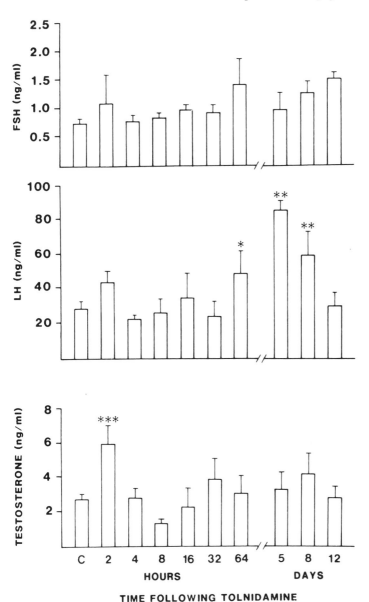

FIG. 23-12. The FSH, LH, and testosterone response to tolnidamine (250 mg/kg). Each bar represents the mean ± SEM of six rats. Twelve control rats were given vehicle alone: six were sacrificed at 4 hours and six at 32 hours. Because there were no differences between the two control groups, the results were pooled. Asterisks indicate significant differences from controls: *p < 0.05; **p < 0.01; ***p < 0.001.

rABP concentrations and content declined as early as 8 hours, with the lowest values occurring at 5 and 12 days. By 16 hours there was an increase in testicular rABP, which was also evident at 8 days and 12 days. Within 16 hours there was a rise in serum rABP, which persisted until the end of the experiment (Fig. 23-13). In a further experiment, single oral doses of tolnidamine (50, 100, 250, and 500 mg/kg) were administered to other groups of rats and the animals were sacrificed after 24 hours and 5 days. With increasing doses of tolnidamine there was reduction in epididymal rABP with increase in testis and serum rABP levels. In vitro experiments showed that tolnidamine had no effect on rABP secretion from Sertoli cells cultured from 20-day-old rats.

These results indicate that tolnidamine had a dramatic and rapid effect on seminiferous tubule function as manifest by disruption of the dynamics of rABP secretion. The reduction in epididymal rABP may best be explained by inhibition of passage of tubular fluid to the epididymis. The increase in testicular rABP was presumably related to accumulation secondary to reduced secretion into, or transport from, the seminiferous tubular lumen. The rise in serum rABP is best explained by the increased testicular rABP concentration. The failure to observe a change in rABP concentration during incubation of cultured Sertoli cells with increasing doses of tolnidamine implies a lack of a direct effect of tolnidamine on rABP synthesis and suggests that this drug primarily alters the kinetics of secretion from the intact tubule.

TOXICOLOGY

Acute toxicity was studied in mice and rats administering tolnidamine by the oral and intraperitoneal routes.[9] The LD_{50}s for mice were 515 mg/kg by the intraperitoneal route and 1250 mg/kg by the oral route. Rats appeared more resistant, and the corresponding LD_{50} values were 1120 mg/kg and greater than 4000 mg/kg, respectively. The reactions to treatment were generally characterized by initial prostration followed by tremors or jerks. Mortalities mainly occurred within a few days after treatment. Autopsy revealed occasional moderate irritative changes in the intestinal tract with both the oral and intraperitoneal routes. A marked reduction of the testes' size was observed in rats sacrificed at term.

Single administration of tolnidamine at doses of 400 mg/kg by the oral route, 200 mg/kg by the intraperitoneal route, or 10 mg/kg by the intravenous route (doses that exert a strong antispermatogenic activity), did not produce adrenolytic, antidopaminergic, antiserotoninergic, and anticholinergic effects either centrally or peripherally. The drug did not interfere with blood pressure and was devoid of blocking effects on vascular α and β receptors. Moreover, tolnidamine did not block serotonin and histamine effects on the bronchi.

Tolnidamine also was administered to rats by gavage at daily doses of 100, 200, 400, and 800 mg/kg for 4 weeks.[9] There were no deaths nor clinical signs related to compound administration. A statistically significant retardation in the rates of overall body weight gain for animals of the 800 mg/kg treated groups was observed. No adverse effects on serum urea concentrations were seen at the end of treatment. There was a marked reduction in the

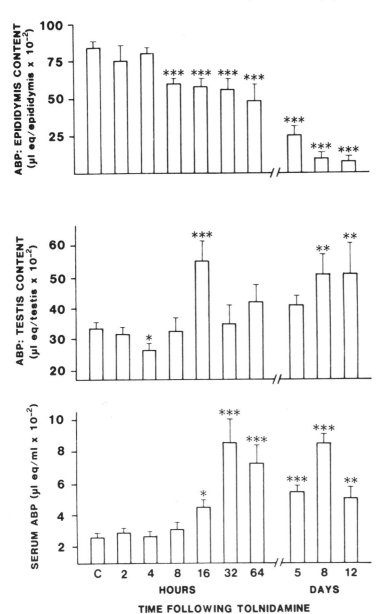

FIG. 23-13. The change in androgen-binding protein (rABP) after tolnidamine (250 mg/kg). (See legend for Fig. 23-12 for details.) Top graph shows epididymal rABP content (μl eq/epididymis $\times 10^{-2}$). Middle graph depicts testis rABP content (μl eq/testis $\times 10^{-2}$). Bottom graph shows serum rABP (μl eq/ml $\times 10^{-2}$). Asterisks indicate significant differences from controls: *p < 0.05; **p < 0.01; ***p < 0.001.

weight of testes, prostate, and seminal vesicles of all treated males. The effect on the accessory sex organs was due to the prepubertal age at which the treatments were started, as previously observed with the parent compound AF 1312/TS.[2] The pituitary weights of treated males were slightly increased, although there was considerable individual variation. Reduced ovarian and pituitary weights were apparent for females receiving the highest dosage of tolnidamine.

Microscopic examination, restricted to control groups and those receiving 800 mg/kg, revealed aplasia of the seminiferous epithelium, absence of spermatozoa in the epididymides, and reduced eosinophilia of prostate secretion in male rats. Reduced ovarian activity, characterized by an increase of atretic follicles and reduction in corpora lutea, and the presence of cysts were evident in female rats given tolnidamine at 800 mg/kg. These effects did not appear with lower dosages. No morphologic changes were detected in the liver, kidneys, and seminal vesicles.

A 4-week pilot study also was performed in Rhesus monkeys.[9] Tolnidamine was administered to four groups of two males at the doses of 25, 70, 200, or 400 mg/kg. Subdued behavior was noted on several occasions, and pale feces were noted throughout the dosing period in the animals receiving 400 mg/kg. There was a dose-related trend in suppression of body weight gain among the animals receiving tolnidamine at doses higher than 25 mg/kg. Laboratory investigations performed 2, 7, 14, and 28 days after starting treatment gave normal values at all times for monkeys dosed with 25 or 70 mg/kg of the compound. With higher dosages, abnormal renal function was evident. This was characterized by raised blood urea and creatinine values after day 7 with the 400 mg/kg dose and on day 28 with the 200 mg/kg dose. Moreover, reduced urinary concentrating ability, proteinuria, and hematuria were observed with these dosages.

No treatment-related macroscopic postmortem abnormalities were found in monkeys receiving 25, 70, or 200 mg/kg. Increased kidney weight was apparent for the 400 mg/kg treated group. Histologic abnormalities were found in the kidneys of animals receiving 200 or 400 mg/kg, and consisted of focal areas of minimally dilated renal cortical tubules showing increased basophilia. Some of these tubules contained colloid and/or necrotic debris. The histologic appearance of the testes varied. At dose levels of less than 200 mg/kg the seminiferous tubules showed spermatogenesis proceeding to at least the primary spermatocyte stage. One animal given 70 mg/kg of tolnidamine showed normal spermatogenesis. Morphologically abnormal spermatozoa were found in the urine of a monkey treated with 25 mg/kg. Dosages of 200 or 400 mg/kg of tolnidamine produced aplasia of the germinal epithelium with Sertoli cells only. These changes must be considered in view of the fact that the monkeys used were adolescent animals.

A possible mutagenic activity of tolnidamine was assessed by four in vitro tests; that is, the Ames test on *Salmonella typhimurium*, the forward mutation (methionine suppressors) in *Aspergillus nidulans*, the mitotic gene conversion in *Saccharomyces cerevisiae* and mitotic crossing-over in *Aspergillus nidulans*. All tests were performed both with and without metabolic activations (S-9 mix) and validated by using standard mutagens. All the results obtained in these experiments were negative, thus suggesting a lack of mutagenic activity of tolnidamine.

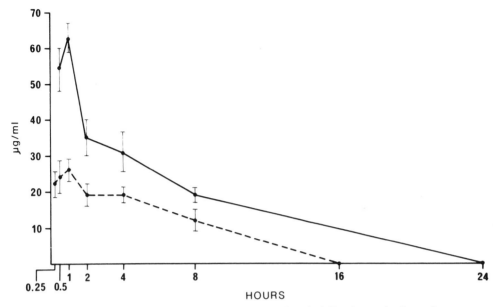

FIG. 23-14. Time course of serum tolnidamine levels following a single oral administration of 70 (*solid line*) or 35 (*broken line*) mg/kg of the drug by oral gavage to rats. Values shown are mean ± SEM.

PHARMACOKINETIC PARAMETERS

Preliminary experiments were performed in rats to study the time course of serum levels of tolnidamine and its excretion through the urine. Groups of five male rats were given a single dose of 35 or 70 mg/kg by the oral route, and the animals were exsanguinated at various time intervals. The urinary excretion of tolnidamine was measured in four rats dosed orally with 70 mg/kg 4 and 24 hours after treatment. A spectrophotofluorimetric method was used for both serum and urinary drug determination. Dose-related peaks of drug concentration occurred 1 hour after treatment and were 26 and 63 μg/ml after the low and the high dose. After 8 hours, tolnidamine decreased to 12 and 19 μg/ml respectively, and by 16 hours only traces were detected (Fig. 23-14).

The percentage of the administered dose found in urine after 4 hours ranged from 0.014% to 0.040%. After 24 hours it rose to cumulative values of 0.13% to 0.28%.

CONCLUSIONS

The data collected with tolnidamine may be summarized as follows:

In rats, tolnidamine exerts a strong antispermatogenic activity, which after repeated administration is of the same magnitude as that reported for lonidamine.[6] Tolnidamine also possesses an antispermatogenic activity in the monkey, but with a lower degree of both general and renal toxicity than that produced by lonidamine.

In the rat, tolnidamine profoundly alters seminiferous tubular function, as evidenced by the marked alterations in testicular weights, as well as rABP concentrations in serum, testis, and epididymides. In contrast, Leydig cell function was spared, because testosterone levels were unchanged and only minimal alterations were observed in LH levels. FSH levels also remained normal.

Acute toxicity studies in rats indicate that the drug was well tolerated. Repeated administration was not accompanied by untoward effects, even at doses exceeding those required for an antispermatogenic action. In monkeys, tolnidamine produced alterations of both renal function and morphology. Nevertheless, with an appropriate dosage schedule, antispermatogenic effects may be obtained without producing renal damage.

Considering the poor therapeutic index of other compounds acting directly on the seminiferous epithelium, there is a potential for the use of tolnidamine as a male contraceptive. Even if subsequent studies will preclude the use of this drug as a "male pill," tolnidamine will remain a valuable tool to probe male reproductive physiology.

REFERENCES

1. BARALE R, CAMPANA A, LOPRIENO N, MONACO M, MOSESSO P, ROSSI V, SCORZA BARCEL-LONA P: *In vitro* and *in vivo* mutagenicity studies on lonidamine. Mutat Res 113:230–231, 1983
2. BURBERI S, CATANESE B, CIOLI V, SCORZA BARCELLONA P, SILVESTRINI B: Antispermatogenic activity of 1-p-chlorobenzyl-1H-indazol-3-carboxylic acid (AF 1312/TS) in rats. II. A study of treatments of duration between 5 and 180 days. Exp Mol Pathol 23:308–320, 1975
3. CORSI G, PALAZZO G, GERMANI C, SCORZA BARCELLONA P, SILVESTRINI B: 1-halobenzyl-1H-indazole-3-carboxylic acids: A new class of antispermatogenic agents. J Med Chem 19:778–783, 1976
4. COULSTON F, DOUGHERTY WJ, LEFEVRE R, ABRAHAM R, SILVESTRINI B: Reversible inhibition of spermatogenesis in rats and monkeys with a new class of indazol-carboxylic acids. Exp Mol Pathol 23:357–366, 1975
5. DE MARTINO C, STEFANINI M, AGRESTINI A, COCCHIA D, MORELLI M, SCORZA BARCEL-LONA P: Antispermatogenic activity of 1-p-chloro-benzyl-1H-indazole-3-carboxylic acid (AF 1312/TS) in rats. III. A light and electron microscopic study after single oral doses. Exp Mol Pathol 23:321–356, 1975
6. DE MARTINO C, MALORNI W, BELLOCCI M, FLORIDI A, MARCANTE ML: Effects of AF 1312/TS and lonidamine on mammalian testis. A morphological study. In SILVESTRINI B, CAPUTO A (eds): Lonidamine—A New Pharmacological Approach to the Study and Control of Spermatogenesis and Tumors. Chemotherapy (Suppl 2) 27:27–42, 1981
7. FLORIDI A, DE MARTINO C, MARCANTE ML, APOLLONJ C, SCORZA BARCELLONA P, SILVES-TRINI B: Morphological and biochemical modifications of rat germ cell mitochondria induced by new antispermatogenic compounds. Studies *in vivo* and *in vitro*. Exp Mol Pathol 35:314–331, 1981
8. FLORIDI A, MARCANTE ML, D'ATRI S, FERIOZZI R, MENICHINI R, CITRO G, CIOLI V, DE MARTINO C: Energy metabolism of normal and lonidamine-treated Sertoli cells of rats. Exp Mol Pathol 38:137–147, 1983
9. HEYWOOD R, JAMES RW, SCORZA BARCELLONA P, CAMPANA A, CIOLI V: Toxicological studies on 1-substituted-indazole-3-carboxylic acids. In SILVESTRINI B, CAPUTO A (eds): Lonidamine—A New Pharmacological Approach to the Study and Control of Spermatogenesis and Tumors. Chemotherapy (Suppl 2) 27:91–97, 1981
10. HILDEBRANDT-STARK HE, MILLS SW, FAWCETT DW: Localization of tritiated 1-(2,4-dichlorobenzyl)-1H-indazole-3-carboxylic acid ([^{3}H]AF 1890) in rat testis using freeze-drying autoradiography. Biol Reprod 27:459–503, 1982

11. LOBL TJ: 1-(2,4-dichlorobenzyl)-1H-indazole-3-carboxylic acid (DICA), an exfoliative anti-spermatogenic agent in the rat. Arch Androl 2:353–363, 1979

12. LOBL TJ, BARDIN CW, GUNSALUS GL, MUSTO NA: Effects of lonidamine (AF1890) and its analogues on follicle-stimulating hormone, luteinizing hormone, testosterone, and rat androgen-binding protein concentrations in the rat and Rhesus monkey. In SILVESTRINI B, CAPUTO A (eds): Lonidamine—A New Pharmacological Approach to the Study and Control of Spermatogenesis and Tumors. Chemotherapy (Suppl 2) 27:61–76, 1981

13. MATHER JP, GUNSALUS GL, MUSTO NA, CHENG CY, PARVINEN M, WRIGHT W, PEREZ-INFANTE V, MARGIORIS A, LIOTTA A, BECKER R, KRIEGER DT, BARDIN CW: The hormonal and cellular control of Sertoli cell secretion. J Steroid Biochem 19:41–51, 1983

14. SCORZA BARCELLONA P, CIOLI V, BURBERI S, SILVESTRINI B: Effects of 1-p-chlorobenzyl-1H-indazol-3-carboxylic acid (AF 1312/TS) on the fertility of rats. J Reprod Fertil 50:159–161, 1977

15. SCORZA BARCELLONA P, CAMPANA A, SILVESTRINI B, DE MARTINO C: The embryotoxicity of a new class of antispermatogenic agents, the 3-indazole-carboxylic acids. Arch Toxicol (Suppl) 5:197–201, 1982

16. SILVESTRINI B, BURBERI S, CATANESE B, CIOLI V, COULSTON F, LISCIANI R, SCORZA BAR-CELLONA P: Antispermatogenic activity of 1-p-chlorobenzyl-1H-indazol-3-carboxylic acid (AF 1312/TS) in rats. I. Trials of single and short-term administrations with study of pharmacologic and toxicologic effects. Exp Mol Pathol 23:288–307, 1975

17. SILVESTRINI B, DE MARTINO C, CIOLI V, CAMPANA A, MALORNI W, SCORZA BARCELLONA P: Antispermatogenic activity of diclondazolic acid in rats. In FABBRINI A, STEINBERGER E (eds): Recent Progress in Andrology, Vol 14, pp 453–457. Proceedings of the Serono Symposia. New York, Academic Press, 1978

18. SILVESTRINI B, CIOLI V, DE MARTINO C, SCORZA BARCELLONA P: 3-Indazole-carboxylic acids as male antifertility agents. In HAFEZ ESE, LOBL TJ (eds): Male Fertility and its Regulation, pp 3–11. Lancaster, MTP Press Limited, 1985

19. SPITZ IM, GUNSALUS GL, MATHER JP, THAU R, BARDIN CW: The effects of the indazole carboxylic acid derivative, tolnidamine, on testicular function. I. Early changes in androgen binding protein secretion in the rat. J Androl 6:171–178, 1985

24

Prospects of a Male Contraceptive Based on the Selective Antispermatogenic Action of 1,2,3-Trihydroxypropane (THP, Glycerol)

JOHN P. WIEBE

KEVIN J. BARR

KEVIN D. BUCKINGHAM

P. DOUGLAS GEDDES

PATRICIA A. KUDO

An "ideal" contraceptive for the male would be one that effectively arrests the production of spermatozoa or blocks their fertilizing capacity, without inhibiting libido, accessory sex glands, production of male steroid hormones, and pituitary function. In addition, there should be an absence of toxic or untoward side-effects and the method should be easily administered. Such a contraceptive agent or procedure is currently unavailable, although a large number of compounds have been explored for the purpose of arresting spermatogenesis.[2,4,8]

Although many of the compounds tested possess some antispermatogenic or antifertilizing capacity, their potential contraceptive action is invariably overshadowed by observations that the compounds are toxic, result in undesirable side-effects, affect libido, sex accessory glands, or the male endocrine system, or require prolonged, continuous use to be effective.[4,8] Invariably, the treatment has been by the oral route (*e.g.*, gossypol[11] or medroxyprogesterone acetate[16]) or by repeated intramuscular injections,[14] subcutaneous implantations,[6] or by percutaneous applications,[16] (*e.g.*, the synthetic or natural steroids). The net result has been that the man's body is subjected to an exogenous chemical burden, while the targeted process, namely spermatogenesis or sperm maturation, may or may not be controlled effectively. In some instances, not only the treated man but also his sexual partner may be affected, as witnessed in hair growth and increased testosterone levels in women

These studies were supported by grants from NSERC of Canada and the Program for Applied Research on Fertility Regulation, Agency for International Development (PARFR-363).

partners of men using percutaneous androgen treatment.[5] Because of the variation in individual minimally effective dose, to ensure efficacy it is necessary to administer somewhat larger doses, so the long-term effects on various tissues of the continuously added synthetic or natural chemicals may be undesirable. For example, attempts at inhibiting pituitary and testicular function with LHRH analogues have in some instances resulted in involution of the prostate and marked decreases in serum testosterone and impotence or loss of libido without impairment of fertility.[13] A more desirable male contraceptive method would appear to be one in which a biologic, nontoxic, nonsteroidal antispermatogenic agent is targeted directly at the testes, without a systemic effect.

Our laboratory recently discovered that when 1,2,3-trihydroxypropane (THP, glycerol), an important component of living cells, is injected into the testes of rats, long-term cessation of spermatogenesis is observed without an apparent effect on Leydig cell steroidogenesis, libido, secondary sex characteristics, or serum hormone levels.[19,21–24] Our findings are summarized and results of some recent studies are described below. These findings suggest that an intratesticular injection of THP might serve as a nonhormonal, nontoxic, biologic contraceptive and/or sterilization technique for males.

MATERIALS AND METHODS

THP SOLUTIONS

Solutions were prepared using deionized, double-distilled water. Several brands of THP were employed: 1) Fisher (No. G-33, Lot 715489), 2) BDH Analar (No. B10118, Lot #94851/2537), 3) Baker Analyzed Reagent (No. 2136-1, Lot #417602), 4) Aldrich Spectrophotometric Grade (No. 19,161-2). Solutions of water/THP, or saline/THP, or water/THP/ethanol, or saline/THP/ethanol in various ratios (from 9% to 70% THP) were employed. The solutions were sterile filtered (0.2 micron Nalgene or Millipore sterilization filter units) and stored in sterile vials (4°C). Volumes of 50 μl to 200 μl were injected per rat testis; larger volumes were employed in rabbits and cynomolgus (*Macaca fascicularis*) monkeys.

METHODS OF ADMINISTERING THP SOLUTIONS

Injections were made with a 26- or 27-gauge needle, being careful to avoid peripheral blood vessels, efferent ducts, and epididymides. Rats were lightly anesthetized with ether, the scrotum was wiped with alcohol, and the solution was injected directly into the approximate center of a testis. Rabbits were placed on a blanket-covered bench, calmed, and then gently held by one person in an upright sitting position, to allow the testes to descend. The scrotum was wiped with alcohol and the testes injected into the central mediastinum by a second person. To date, several dozen injections have been performed in this manner on rabbits without anesthesia and none of the animals has struggled or shown signs of discomfort or pain as a result of the injection. Cynomolgus monkeys have been injected following anesthesia with ketamine.

SPERM COUNTS AND SEMEN SAMPLES

To estimate the number of sperm contained in rat epididymides, the tissue was finely minced with scissors and thoroughly dispersed in 5 ml to 10 ml phosphate-buffered saline (0.01 M; pH 7.0). Aliquots (10 μl–50 μl) of the fluid were then spread in 200 mm^2 areas on microscope slides. Slides were air-dried, fixed (10% buffered formalin), and stained (Ehrlich's hematoxylin). Sperm heads were counted in 20 ocular fields and the total number per epididymis was determined by correcting for sample area and the dilution factor.[21] Semen was collected from rabbits by means of an artificial vagina,[1,3] and sperm numbers and motility were determined by hemocytometer. Semen was incubated for 1 minute in a nigrosin–eosin mixture and dye exclusion was used as a measure of sperm viability.

MEASUREMENT OF LIBIDO AND FERTILITY

The measurements of sexual behavior, libido, and fertility in rats have been described.[21,22] Libido in rabbits was measured by their capacity to ejaculate, to experience orgasm with artificial does (rabbit fur), and their ability to mate with does.

TISSUE DISTRIBUTION AND METABOLISM OF ^{14}C-THP

To determine the distribution of THP to the rest of the body, ^{14}C-labeled THP solution (approximately 10^6 DPM/150 μl) was injected into each testis. At times 0, 5, 15, 30, and 45 min and 1, 2, 4, 8, and 24 hours, tissues (testes, epididymis, seminal vesicles, prostate, adrenal, blood, portions of liver and fat) were removed. Tissues were homogenized in 80% aqueous ethanol, centrifuged, and the radioactivity in the supernatants and pellets determined by liquid scintillation spectrometry. To estimate the conversion of THP to CO_2, each rat was injected intratesticularly with ^{14}C-THP and immediately placed inside a sealed dessicator equipped with controlled air flow into the chamber and a trap that forced all the vented air to pass through a KOH solution. The KOH solution was monitored for radioactivity at 1, 2, 3, 4, and 24 hours. To determine possible excretion of THP by means of the feces and urine, food was withheld from rats for 16 hours, and they were then injected intratesticularly with ^{14}C-THP, placed inside metabolic chambers, and the 24-hour feces and urine samples were measured for radioactivity.

MEASUREMENT OF SERUM HORMONE LEVELS AND HORMONE RECEPTORS

Serum levels of LH and FSH were measured by double antibody radioimmunoassays (RIA) as previously described.[21] Gonadotropin binding to receptors in the testes essentially was measured as described previously.[12,20]

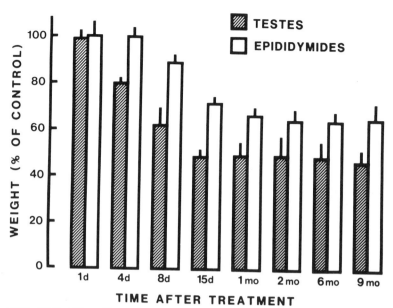

FIG. 24-1. The effect of a single intratesticular injection of THP solution (150 μl/ testis) on the weights of the testes and epididymides at various times following the treatment. Bars and lines represent means and SEM (n = 6–12).

Determinations of serum androgens, testicular steroidogenesis, steroid enzyme activities, histochemistry and histology, and statistical analyses have been described elsewhere.[21,22]

RESULTS AND DISCUSSION

EFFECT ON WEIGHTS OF REPRODUCTIVE TISSUES

An intratesticular injection of THP solution results in a rapid decrease in weights of testes to about 50% of those in controls by 15 days, and this decreased weight is still present 9 months after the injection (Fig. 24-1). A less pronounced, but similarly persistent decrease in weights of epididymides is evident (see Fig. 24-1). In none of the treatment regimens has the weight of prostates and seminal vesicles ever been significantly different from the controls (see also Table 24-3).[21,22]

Because the germinal cells compose the major bulk of the seminiferous tubules in a normal mature testis, any treatment that blocks spermatogenesis can be expected to result in a decrease in testicular size. Similarly, when no new spermatozoa enter the epididymides, they will decrease in size as the stored sperm are voided. Decreases in testis size (by about 50%) have been noted in human subjects following treatment with 19-nortestosterone for the purpose of testing its potential contraceptive action.[14] According to those

TABLE 24-1. The Effects of THP Concentration on Weights of Testes and Epididymides, and on Epididymal Sperm Number*

THP (%)	6 MONTHS			9 MONTHS		
	TESTES (g)	EPIDIDYMIDES (g)	SPERM NUMBER ($\times 10^{-7}$)	TESTES (g)	EPIDIDYMIDES (g)	SPERM NUMBER ($\times 10^{-7}$)
0	3.75 (0.11)	1.69 (0.10)	41.6 (10.4)	3.59 (0.12)	1.73 (0.10)	37.7 (6.7)
9	2.78 (0.35)†	1.41 (0.10)	25.9 (5.7)	2.37 (0.71)	1.37 (0.13)	28.5 (13.6)
18	2.36 (0.20)§	1.14 (0.07)‡	18.8 (3.3)	2.49 (0.14)‡	1.26 (0.08)†	29.7 (5.1)
35	1.71 (0.14)§	1.01 (0.05)§	0.97 (0.31)§	1.66 (0.15)§	1.10 (0.09)§	1.56 (0.56)§
70	1.80 (0.13)§	1.11 (0.05)§	1.02 (0.25)§	1.56 (0.08)§	1.14 (0.08)§	1.15 (0.51)§

* Sixty young adult rats (250 g) were injected intratesticularly with 150 µl of either saline or saline containing various concentrations of THP. Six months after the injection, 6 rats from each treatment group were sacrificed and the weights of the testes and epididymides and the number of sperm in the epididymides were determined. The rest of the rats were examined 9 months after the treatment. Values are the means; values in parentheses represent SEM.

† Significantly differernt from controls at $p < 0.05$.
‡ Significantly different from controls at $p < 0.01$.
§ Significantly different from controls at $p < 0.001$.

TABLE 24-2. Effects of the Volume Injected on the Weights of Testes and Epididymides, and on Epididymal Sperm Number*

VOLUME (μl)	TESTES (g)	EPIDIDYMIDES (g)	SPERM NUMBER ($\times 10^{-7}$)
0	3.25 (0.21)	1.55 (0.11)	49.8 (13.8)
100 H₂O	3.49 (0.25)	1.58 (0.11)	47.8 (15.5)
50 THP	2.39 (0.36)†	1.23 (0.09)†	31.2 (9.1)
100 THP	2.03 (0.23)§	1.19 (0.08)§	16.3 (7.5)‡
200 THP	1.86 (0.12)§	1.11 (0.06)§	0.29 (0.14)§

* Five mature male rats (400 g) were used per treatment group and received either no injection, an injection of distilled water, or 50 to 200 μl of a 70% THP solution. Ten months after the injection, the rats were sacrificed and the weights of the testes and epididymides and the number of sperm in the epididymides were determined.

Values are the means; values in parentheses represent SEM.

† Significantly different from controls at $p < 0.05$.

‡ Significantly different from controls at $p < 0.01$.

§ Significantly different from controls at $p < 0.001$.

investigators ". . . none of the subjects, nor their sexual partners, noticed the reduction in testicular size . . ." and they did not consider this unrecognized effect as an impeding side-effect.[14]

EFFECT OF THP CONCENTRATION AND VOLUME INJECTED

The dose-dependent effect of THP treatment on weights of testes and epididymides and on numbers of epididymal sperm is illustrated in Table 24-1. A single injection, into each testis, of 150 μl of solution, consisting of either 9%, 18%, 35%, or 70% THP, resulted in approximately progressive decreases in gonadal and epididymal weights and sperm numbers, the maximum effect occurring with solutions containing 35% to 70% THP. Table 24-1 also shows that this effect is still evident 9 months after the injection. The distribution of THP throughout the testis following injection appears to depend primarily on diffusion, and consequently treatment with 50 μl, 100 μl, or 200 μl of a 70% solution of THP indicates the most pronounced effect with the 200 μl injection (Table 24-2); this volume-related response still is in evidence 10 months after a single injection (Table 24-2).

EFFECT ON NUMBER OF STORED (EPIDIDYMAL) SPERM

An intratesticular injection of THP results in a decline in the number of sperm stored in the epididymides. In young adult rats, significantly fewer sperm result by 8 days following a treatment (Fig. 24-2), and, although the number of epididymal sperm in the controls continues to increase, there appear to be no further additions in the treated animals, so that by 51 days following an injection, there are over 90% fewer sperm (Fig. 24-2). The treatment has much the same effect in mature males; by 15 days after an injection, an 80% to 90% reduction in sperm numbers may be observed in the

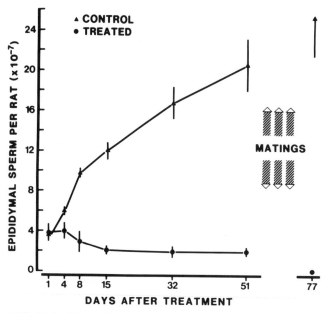

FIG. 24-2. The effect of an injection (150 μl/testis) of either saline (control) or THP solution (treated) on numbers of sperm in epididymides of young adult rats at various times (days) after the treatment. After three matings by each male, the epididymal sperm count continued to increase in the controls, but dropped to less than 0.01% in the THP-treated rats.

epididymides. Sperm may be stored in the epididymides for considerable periods, and a better measure of the treatment effect on sperm production is obtained after several matings.

When animals have been mated to rid the tissues of sperm stored before treatment, the number of sperm remaining in the epididymides of treated rats is reduced by 99.99% in relation to the number of sperm remaining in controls (Fig. 24-2).[21] This effect is easily observed with the unaided eye when epididymides are chopped in a saline solution (Fig. 24-3). A milky suspension results from the control tissues owing to the many spermatozoa, whereas the solution containing the tissues from the treated rats is clear.

EFFECT OF THP TREATMENT ON LIBIDO, SEXUAL BEHAVIOR, AND FERTILITY

Numerous experiments on rats, hamsters, and rabbits have shown that libido is not reduced by the THP treatment. The effect of THP treatment on sexual behavior and mating in rats is illustrated in Fig. 24-4, which shows the combined results from several separate experiments. The percentage of matings when males are caged with virgin females is essentially the same for treated and control rats. The behavioral observations indicate that the THP-treated

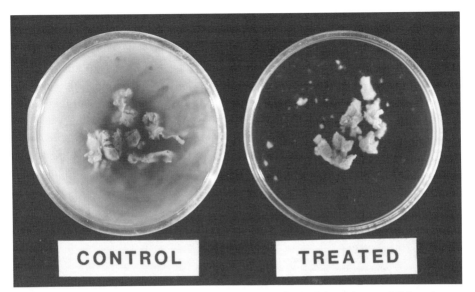

FIG. 24-3. The effect of a single THP treatment (200 μl/testis) on epididymal content of sperm. Rats were allowed to mate, and one week later epididymides were removed, chopped with scissors in 10 ml phosphate-buffered saline, and contents dispersed by gentle shaking. Note the milky appearance (due to approximately 4.5 $\times 10^8$ sperm) in the petri dish containing tissue from a control rat, whereas the saline in the dish containing tissue from a treated rat is essentially clear.

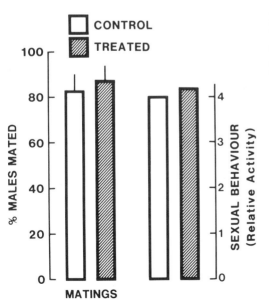

FIG. 24-4. The effect of THP treatment on mating frequency and sexual behavior during cohabitation with females. Sexual behavior was measured in relative terms, based on 10 minutes of observation at the time a virgin female was introduced and two 10-minute periods per day thereafter for 6 weeks. A different female was placed in the cage with a male every 7 days. Mating data are based on the presence of vaginal plugs and are the results from approximately 120 cohabitations for each group.

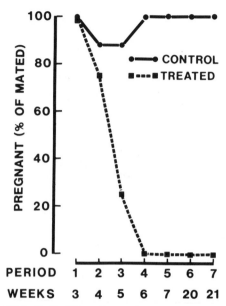

FIG. 24-5. The effect of a single treatment with THP on fertility. Rats received an injection in each testis of 200 μl THP solution (70%) or distilled water (control). Fourteen days later, a virgin female rat was placed with each male for a period of 5 days, or until the appearance of a vaginal plug. The appearance of a plug was taken as evidence that mating had occurred. The procedure was repeated with fresh virgin females on 5 consecutive weeks (periods 1–5) and again at 20 and 21 weeks after treatment (periods 6 and 7). Pregnancy and number of fetuses were assessed by examination of uteri 10 days after the end of each cohabitation. (Data adapted from Wiebe JP, Barr KJ: The control of male fertility by 1,2,3-trihydroxypropane[THP; glycerol]: rapid arrest of spermatogenesis without altering libido, accessory organs, gonadal steroidogenesis, and serum testosterone, LH, and FSH. Contraception 29:291, 1984)

males exhibit approximately the same number of sexual advances (*i.e.*, nosing, genital sniffing, chasing, and mounting attempts) as the control males (see Fig. 24-4). The lack of effect on libido is clearly important in considerations of any chemical contraceptive technique. The abolition of libido that may result from some treatments, for example, gonadotropin-releasing hormone agonists,[18] is of course unacceptable (although clearly a very effective contraceptive method). On the other hand, providing the male body with supplemental androgens when pituitary gonadotropin stimulation of testicular steroidogenesis has been suppressed,[6,16] might require more careful regulation and individual adjustment to maintain a normal level of sex drive without restoring fertility than has been emphasized.

The results from one experiment showing the effects of THP on fertility are presented in Figure 24-5. The THP treatment did not reduce the number of matings; in this experiment every treated male mated at least once during

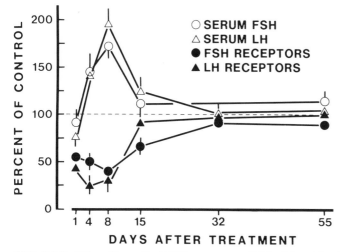

FIG. 24-6. The effect of a THP treatment (150 μl/testis) of a 70% THP solution on serum FSH and LH levels and on testicular FSH- and LH-receptor binding at various times after the treatment. Symbols and vertical lines represent the means and SEM (n = 8–11).

each period of cohabitation. The fertility of the THP-treated males declined markedly between the first and third mating, however all treated males were shown to be infertile by the fourth mating (Fig. 24-5), presumably because the stored sperm were not being replenished. The infertility was still evident 20 and 21 weeks after the injection (cohabitation periods 6 and 7, Fig. 24-5).

EFFECT OF THP TREATMENT ON SERUM GONADOTROPIN LEVELS AND ON GONADOTROPIN RECEPTORS

Previous measurements had shown that 9 weeks after an injection, the serum levels of LH and FSH did not differ significantly between control and THP-treated rats.[21,22] Figure 24-6 shows the results combined from three separate experiments, in which rats were injected with 150 μl (per testis) of either the control or a 70% solution of THP and then were sampled at 1, 4, 8, 15, 32, and 55 days after the injection. The THP treatment appears to result in increases in serum LH and FSH by 4 to 8 days after the treatment, and thereafter the levels appear to be the same as in the controls (see Fig. 24-6). On the other hand, the LH-receptor and FSH-receptor bindings are reduced significantly (p < 0.05) between days 1 and 8 after the THP treatment (Fig. 24-6). By 15 to 32 days after the treatment, the gonadotropin-receptor binding appears to have returned to the control values. No differences between control and treated tissues were observed 32 or 55 days after the treatment (Fig. 24-6).

These results suggest that there may be an initial effect on the pituitary gonadotropins that is reversed within 2 weeks of the treatment. The gonadotropin-receptor binding is almost a mirror image of the serum gonadotropin

TABLE 24-3. The Effect of THP Treatment on Androgen Production*

TIME† (months)	SERUM ANDROGEN‡		ANDROGEN-DEPENDENT TISSUES (g) PROSTATE (Seminal Vesicles)	
	CONTROL	*THP*	*CONTROL*	*THP*
0.5	2.14 + 1.04	2.86 + 0.85	0.63 + 0.05 (1.47 + 0.08)	0.55 + 0.03 (1.48 + 0.13)
1	2.12 + 0.77	2.31 + 1.19	0.87 + 0.06 (1.62 + 0.09)	0.87 + 0.13 (1.52 + 0.09)
6	2.03 + 0.76	1.96 + 0.64	1.25 + 0.06 (1.70 + 0.06)	1.29 + 0.11 (1.60 + 0.09)
9	2.08 + 1.14	1.89 + 0.56	1.42 + 0.23 (2.03 + 0.12)	1.39 + 0.19 (1.94 + 0.19)

* Sexually mature rats (n = 5–6) received one intratesticular injection (200 μl) of either saline (control) or THP (70%) solution, and serum androgen levels and weights of androgen-dependent secondary sex tissues were determined at the indicated times after the treatment.

Values represent mean + SEM.

† Time refers to time (in mo) after the intratesticular injection.

‡ Serum androgen was detemined by RIA and represents total testosterone, 5α-dihydrotestosterone, and 5α-androstane-$3\alpha(\beta)$,17β-diols in ng/ml of serum.

levels and may be a reflection of higher receptor occupancy during the first 2 weeks, when serum levels are high. Increases in serum gonadotropin levels could be due to decreased steroid feedback, although serum testosterone levels (days 1–54) of treated rats did not differ significantly from those of controls. The return to normal values is a desirable feature and is in contrast to methods involving continuous administration of exogenous steroids, which significantly lower LH and FSH levels[6,14,16] during the treatment period, and either increase[6,16] or decrease[14] androgen levels.

EFFECT OF THP TREATMENT ON SERUM TESTOSTERONE AND ON TESTICULAR STEROIDOGENESIS

Previous results have shown that serum testosterone levels, testicular steroidogenic enzyme activities, and in vitro steroidogenic capacity of the testes do not appear to be significantly altered by the THP treatments.[21,22] Table 24-3 compares the serum androgen (total of testosterone, dihydrotestosterone, and 5α-androstane-3α,17β-diol) level in control and THP-treated rats at 0.5, 1, 6, and 9 months after an injection. The results show that THP treatment does not cause any significant changes in serum androgen levels as measured by RIA. The lack of effect on the weights of the androgen-dependent accessory sex structures (prostate and seminal vesicles) confirms that androgenesis does not appear to be affected by the THP treatment (Table 24-3).

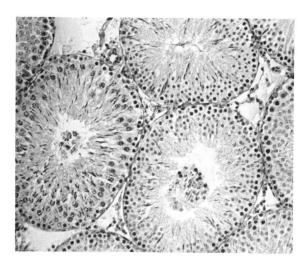

FIG. 24-7. Cross-section of a control rat testis, 9 months after an injection (150 μl) of distilled water (magnification × 180).

THE LONG-TERM EFFECTS OF THP TREATMENT

It is noteworthy that no tissue deterioration in the testes and accessory sex structures has been observed in rats as much as 9 months after an injection (see Figs. 24-7–24-9). Sertoli cells still fill many of the tubule cross-sections (Fig. 24-8), and their nuclei appear normal. The Leydig cells are similar in appearance to those of the control animals and no invasion of fibrous tissue or destruction of blood circulation has been observed (Fig. 24-8). The epididymal sperm numbers are still reduced at 9 to 10 months after a 150 μl to 200 μl injection with the 70% THP solution. Animals injected with lower concentrations or smaller volumes of THP, however, show a trend toward increased numbers of epididymal sperm between 6 and 9 months (see Table 24-1).

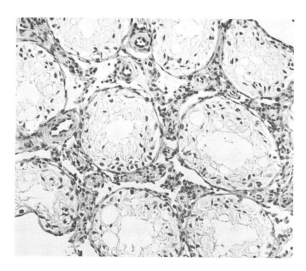

FIG. 24-8. Cross-section of an area of a treated testis, 9 months after an injection (150 μl) of THP solution. Note the Sertoli cell nuclei and the complete absence of spermatogenesis within the seminiferous tubules (magnification × 180).

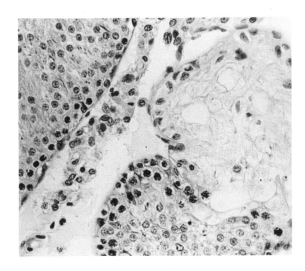

FIG. 24-9. Cross-section of another portion of the testis in Fig. 24-8 showing resumption of spermatogenesis in some tubular regions. Note normal appearing Leydig and Sertoli cell nuclei (magnification × 350).

Experiments are in progress to determine whether the sperm present at extended times following the treatment are due to regeneration of spermatogenic activity or whether spermatogenesis was not halted in every region following the treatment. In terms of histology, it appears that 9 months after a 150 μl injection (70% THP) there may be some regeneration of spermatogenic activity; in some areas of treated testes, active spermatogenesis can be observed adjacent to inactive areas (Fig. 24-9). In terms of behavior and libido, serum androgens, and gonadotropins, no differences have been noted between the treated and control animals up to 10 months after treatment.

THE DISTRIBUTION AND METABOLISM OF THP

To determine the extent to which THP is distributed to the rest of the body tissues, ^{14}C-THP was injected intratesticularly and tissues were examined for radioactivity at various periods from 5 minutes up to 7 days. The radioactivity within the testes rapidly decreased to about 25% by 1 hour, 13% by 2 hours, and 0.2% by 24 hours (Fig. 24-10). About 1.5% of the radioactivity was transferred to the epididymides, 0.2% to the prostate, and 0.4% to the seminal vesicles within 5 to 15 minutes of an injection, and the radioactivity in these tissues then gradually declined to less than 0.09% by 24 hours. An increase up to 13.6% of the injected radioactivity was observed in the blood during the first 30 minutes, followed by a rapid decline to 2.6% at 1 hour and 0.9% at 24 hours (Fig. 24-10). Small percentages of radioactivity were noted in other tissues, the peaks occurring at 30 minutes in the kidneys (0.6%), 45 minutes in the fat (1.9%), and at 60 minutes in the liver (1.7%).

That some of the THP injected intratesticularly may be metabolized is suggested by the radioactivity recovered from the expired air, the urine, and the feces. About 1.2% of the initial radioactivity was present in the CO_2 trapped in KOH during the first hour after an injection, and the total radioactivity recovered in the KOH in a 24-hour period following an injection

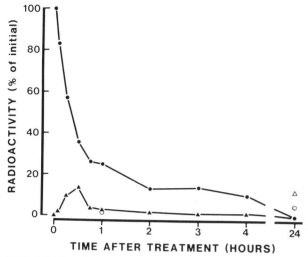

FIG. 24-10. The fate of radioactivity of 70% THP after intratesticular injections of ^{14}C-THP (150 μl/testis; approximately 1×10^6 dpm). Injections were made and at time 0, 5, 15, 30, 45, 60 minutes, and 2, 3, 4, and 24 hours, three rats were sacrificed, tissues removed and radioactivity determined. ($\bullet$——$\bullet$ testes; $\blacktriangle$——$\blacktriangle$ blood, assuming 12.5 ml total per rat). In other experiments, rats were placed in respiration or metabolic chambers to collect urine and feces ($\triangle$) and CO_2 ($\bigcirc$).

amounted to approximately 5%. In a 24-hour period, about 10% and 1.3% of the initial radioactivity was recovered in the urine and feces, respectively (Fig. 24-10).

THP (glycerol) is normally present in the serum of mammals.[9] In rats, it may vary from 0.4 mM shortly after birth to about 0.1 mM in the adult but may be markedly affected by starvation, exercise, and hormones.[9] The rate of utilization of serum THP by the tissues (principally the liver and kidney) is proportional to the serum concentration of the compound up to 1 mM. It is easily removed from the blood, and in humans the half-time of elimination following an intravenous infusion of 0.1 g of THP per kilogram of body weight is about 40 min. THP is highly gluconeogenic, and the liver is chiefly responsible for this process.[9] Other cells and tissues known to utilize THP at a significant rate are brain, intestine, leukocytes, lung, and spermatozoa.[9] Enzymes that metabolize THP, such as glycerol-kinase and glycerol-3-phosphate dehydrogenase, are distributed in many tissues. Interestingly, among the various rat tissues, the mitochondria of the testes have the highest glycerol-3-phosphate dehydrogenase activity per milligram of protein.[9]

TOXICITY OF THP

In none of the studies conducted in our laboratory have we observed any lesions or unusual morphology in body tissues other than the testes at dissection. Some animals have been held for nearly a year following treatment. Because of the normal ubiquitous distribution of THP in animal tissues, the fairly high circulating levels, and its involvement in cellular structures and in lipid and carbohydrate metabolic pathways, a toxic effect from a single local injection of a relatively small amount is not anticipated in other tissues in the body. In one study,[17] mild kidney damage was reported when rats were maintained for 6 months with 5% THP in their drinking water; at this dosage level the rats received about 6500 times as much THP as in the highest dose of our treatment. In humans, an oral dose of THP at 1 g/kg body weight once every 6 hours is considered safe,[9] and intravenous injections of 50 g of THP have not resulted in any adverse symptoms.[9]

THE MECHANISM OF THP ACTION IN THE TESTES

The mechanism whereby intratesticular administration of THP results in selective inhibition of spermatogenesis without any apparent adverse effects on other testicular functions remains unknown. Spermatogenesis occurs in a highly regulated and specialized environment resulting from the blood–testis barrier and the occluding junctions between adjacent Sertoli cells.[10] This unique environment appears to be essential for the successful progression of spermatogenesis,[10] and a disruption of the barrier might be expected to interfere with the normal sequence of cell divisions and maturations. Our first effort at explaining the mechanisms of antispermatogenic action of THP has therefore been directed at an examination of the occluding junctions.

Figure 24-11 is an electron micrograph showing the junctional region between two Sertoli cells from a testis that was treated with THP 9 days previously. At a higher magnification (Fig. 24-11, upper inset) it is apparent that there is no disruption or separation of the complexes and the appearance is essentially identical to that of junctional complexes from control testes. Figure 24-11 also shows normal appearing spermatogonia in the basal compartment. Because in this treated tissue, spermatogenic stages beyond spermatogonia are highly disrupted (Fig. 24-11, lower inset), the histologic picture suggests that the THP treatment specifically affects the germinal cells in the adluminal compartment without an apparent effect on cells in the basal and interstitial compartments and without disrupting the Sertoli–Sertoli cell junctions.

Additional experiments are needed to determine if the THP action is by way of changes in the basal lamina, membrane permeability, Sertoli and/or germinal cell metabolism, or some other mechanism specifically affecting the intratubular environment.

EFFECT ON OTHER SPECIES

The results summarized above were obtained from experiments employing rats, and tests are in progress to determine if the antispermatogenic effect is species specific. Preliminary data show that intratesticular injections of THP results in significant decreases in hamster testis weights and epididymal sperm number. In a pilot experiment New Zealand rabbits received several injections of either saline or 70% THP solution. The ejaculates showed no significant decrease in volume but a 99.99% reduction in sperm number and a highly significant ($p < 0.001$) reduction in motility and viability of those sperm still present (Table 24-4). Libido was not reduced. All the control animals

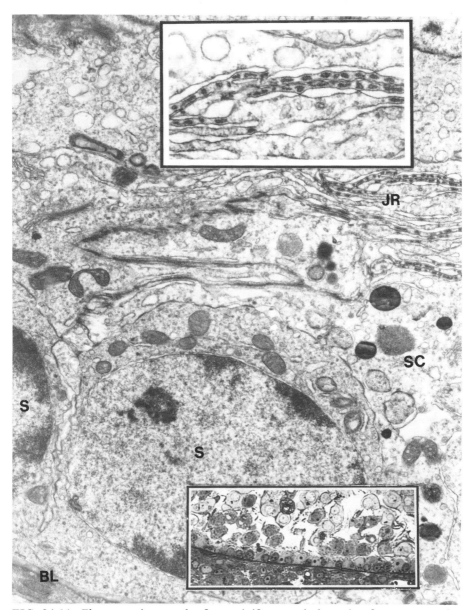

FIG. 24-11. Electron micrograph of a seminiferous tubule region from a rat testis that was treated with 150 μl THP solution (70%) 9 days prior to perfusion fixation. Note the basal lamina (*BL*) at the lower left, primary spermatogonium (*S*), Sertoli cell (*SC*) cytoplasm and Sertoli–Sertoli cell junctional region (*JR*). The spermatogonia appear normal and are still enclosed within the basal compartment formed by the occluding junctions (*JR*) between Sertoli cells (magnification × 19,000). The upper inset, at higher magnification (magnification × 41,500), shows that the junctional complex is normal in appearance. The lower inset shows interstitial, basal, and adluminal regions in a semithin section (magnification × 700); note the organized basal layer of cells (*BC*) and the disrupted adluminal compartment (*AL*).

TABLE 24-4. The Antifertility Action of THP in the Rabbit*

TREATMENT	EJACULATIONS/ RABBIT	EJACULATE VOLUME (ml)	SPERM NO./ EJACULATE (×10⁻⁶)	SPERM MOTILITY† (0–4)	SPERM VIABILITY‡ (%)	FERTILITY (litters/mating)
Control	11.3 + 1.3	0.78 + 0.07	500 + 187	3.50 + 0.22	69 + 2	6/6
THP	14.8 + 1.9	0.68 + 0.91	0.06 + 0.04	0.36 + 0.28	0.02 + 0.02	0/6

* Twelve sexually mature New Zealand rabbits of similar age were used in this pilot experiment. Six were injected intratesticularly with saline (control) and six with THP solution (70%). Each rabbit received 0.2 ml solution per testis about every 2 months. After the 4th injection the sperm count in the THP-treated bucks was reduced by about 90%. The rabbits then received 0.8 to 1.0 ml solution per testis and the ejaculates were collected by an artificial vagina over a 2-month period. Then each male was allowed to copulate (2 copulations each) with a receptive doe.

† Sperm motility was evaluated microscopically and was rated on a scale of 0 to 4, 0 being motionless and 4 showing rapid directional motion.

‡ Sperm viability was determined by the ability to exclude nigrosin–eosin stain.

sired litters while none of the THP-treated males was fertile (Table 24-4). The testes and epididymides of the treated rabbits were reduced in size, but the weight of the prostate was not altered by the treatment. Histologic preparations of treated monkey testes show suppression of spermatogenesis in the region of treatment similar to that observed in the rat testis.

CONCLUSION

Recent studies in our laboratory have presented the first evidence that the nonhormonal, biologic substance, 1,2,3-trihydroxypropane (THP, glycerol) acts as a selective and potent antispermatogenic agent in rats, without any apparent toxic or endocrine side-effects.[21,22] These studies have been extended. Laboratory rats were injected intratesticularly (50 μl–200 μl) with either control solution (distilled water or saline with 5% ethanol) or THP (9%, 18%, 35%, or 70%) solution and histologic, biochemical, hormonal, libido, and fertility determinations were made for up to 10 months after a single injection. A dose-related response was noted. At the higher concentrations of THP, the testis and epididymis weights and the number of epididymal sperm declined rapidly and remained reduced for at least 10 months following a single injection. Initial matings produced normal offspring but after the third copulation, the epididymal sperm number declined by 99.99% and succeeding matings were infertile. There was no change in the serum androgen levels and in testicular steroidogenesis and no decline in libido or sexual activity. Following a slight perturbation in serum gonadotropin levels and gonadotropin-receptor binding during the first few days after an injection, these values returned to normal and remained the same as the controls until termination of the experiments. Histologically, the Leydig and Sertoli cells appeared normal 9 months after a treatment. Although most of the seminiferous tubules were devoid of spermatogenic activity, some regions in the testis had begun to show germinal cell activity after 9 months. Ultrastructural studies indicate that the primary action of THP on the seminiferous tubules is not by means of a disruption of the Sertoli–Sertoli cell junctional complexes. Metabolic studies indicate that by 24 hours after an injection, more than 99% of the THP has disappeared from the testis. Preliminary tests on hamsters, rabbits, and monkeys indicate that intratesticular injection of THP arrests spermatogenesis in these species. The results from these studies show that a direct injection of THP acts as a potent inhibitor of spermatogenesis, resulting in long-term infertility without affecting steroidogenesis, libido, secondary sex characteristics, mating behavior, serum hormone levels, and without any apparent untoward side-effects. Further studies are required to demonstrate whether THP injections could provide an "ideal" contraceptive for the human male.

REFERENCES

1. ADAMS CE: Artificial insemination in the rabbit: the technique and application to practice. J Appl Rabbit Res 4:10, 1981
2. BENNETT JP: Chemical Contraception, p 133. New York, Columbia University Press, 1974
3. BREDDERMAN PJ, FOOTE RH, YASSEN AM: Improved artificial vagina for collecting rabbit semen. J Reprod Fertil 7:401, 1964

4. DAVIES AG: Effects of Hormones, Drugs and Chemicals on Testicular Function, Vol 1. Westmount, Eden Press, 1980
5. DELANE D, FOUGEYROLLAS B, MEYER L, THONNEAU P: Androgenisation of female partners of men on medroxyprogesterone acetate/percutaneous testosterone contraception. Lancet 1:276, 1984
6. EWING LL, COCHRAN RC, ADAMS RJ, DARNEY KJ, BERRY SJ, BORDY MJ, DESJARDINS C: Testis function in rhesus monkeys treated with a contraceptive steroid formulation. Contraception 27:347, 1983
7. EWING LL, HUBER AC, STRANDBERG JD, ADAMS RJ, COCHRAN RC, DESJARDINS C: Somatic tissue responses of male rhesus monkeys treated with a contraceptive steroid formulation. Contraception 27:363, 1983
8. JEFFCOTE SL, SANDLER M (eds): Progress Towards a Male Contraceptive. Chichester, England, John Wiley & Sons, 1982
9. LIN ECC: Glycerol utilization and its regulation in mammals. Ann Rev Biochem. 46:765, 1977
10. NEAVES WB: The blood–testis barrier. In JOHNSON AD, GOMES WR (eds): The Testis, Vol 4, p 126. New York, Academic Press, 1977
11. QIAN SZ, WANG ZG: Gossypol: A potential antifertility agent for males. Ann Rev Pharmacol Toxicol 24:329, 1984
12. SALHANICK AI, WIEBE JP: FSH receptors in isolated Sertoli cells: Changes in concentration of binding sites at the onset of sexual maturation. Life Sci 26:2281, 1980
13. SANDOW J: Inhibition of pituitary and testicular function by LHRH analogues. In JEFFCOTE SL, SANDLER M (eds): Progress Towards a Male Contraceptive, p 19. Chichester, England, John Wiley & Sons, 1982
14. SCHÜRMEYER T, BELKIEN L, KNUTH UA, NIESCHLAG E: Reversible azoospermia induced by the anabolic steroid 19-nortestosterone. Lancet i:417, 1984
15. SESTOFT L, FLERON P: Kinetics of glycerol uptake by the perfused rat liver: Membrane transport, phosphorylation and effect on NAD redox level. Biochim Biophys Acta 375:462, 1975
16. SOUFIR J, JOUANNET P, MARSON J, SOUMAH A: Reversible inhibition of sperm production and gonadotrophin secretion in men following combined oral medroxyprogesterone acetate and percutaneous testosterone treatment. Acta Endocrinol 102:625, 1983
17. TOURTELLOTTE WW, REINGLASS JL, NEWKIRK TA: Cerebral dehydration action of glycerol. 1. Historical aspects with emphasis on the toxicity and intravenous administration. Clin Pharmacol Ther 13:159, 1972
18. TREMBLAY Y, BELANGER A: Reversible inhibition of gonadal functions by a potent gonadotropin-releasing hormone agonist in adult dog. Contraception 30:483, 1984
19. WIEBE JP, BARR KJ: Suppression of spermatogenesis without inhibition of steroidogenesis by a trihydroxypropane (glycerol) solution. Biol Reprod 28:256, 1983
20. WIEBE JP, SALHANICK AI, MYERS KI: On the mechanism of action of lead in the testis: In vitro suppression of FSH receptors, cyclic AMP and steroidogenesis. Life Sci 32:1997, 1983
21. WIEBE JP, BARR KJ: The control of male fertility by 1,2,3-trihydroxypropane (THP; glycerol): rapid arrest of spermatogenesis without altering libido, accessory organs, gonadal steroidogenesis, and serum testosterone, LH and FSH. Contraception 29:291, 1984
22. WIEBE JP, BARR KJ: Suppression of spermatogenesis without inhibition of steroidogenesis by a 1,2,3-trihydroxypropane solution. Life Sci 34:1747, 1984
23. WIEBE JP, BARR KJ: Male antifertility action of 1,2,3-trihydroxypropane (THP, glycerol). Biol Reprod 30:147, 1984
24. WIEBE JP, BARR KJ: Control of male fertility by 1,2,3-trihydroxypropane: Rapid arrest of spermatogenesis without altering libido, accessory sex organs, gonadal steroidogenesis, and serum testosterone, LH and FSH. Seventh International Congress of Endocrinology, Quebec, Abstract No. 2525, 1984

25

Toward a Same-Day, Orally Administered Male Contraceptive

BRIAN H. VICKERY

MARTHA B. GRIGG

JESSIE C. GOODPASTURE

KAREN K. BERGSTRÖM

KEITH A. M. WALKER

Attempts at chemical control of male fertility stretch back over four decades (Table 25-1). The earliest report of this approach concerned use of the male hormone itself and was based on the observation that administration of testosterone to male rats was antispermatogenic, an example of capitalization upon negative feedback control of pituitary gonadotropins.[21] This study was succeeded by investigations of a variety of nonhormonal agents with testicular action,[3,28,30,41,47,53] some of which, notably the nitrofurans and the *bis*(dichloroacetyl)diamines, reached clinical testing before being abandoned.[26,37] From time to time in the intervening years, hormonal negative feedback was reevaluated. For example, with the advent of the oral contraceptives for women, the effect of the new progestogens was assessed in men.[24,25,34] A nonsteroidal inhibitor of pituitary function, methallibure, also reached clinical trials.[61] More recently, the effects of androgenic steroids, such as danazol or progestational steroids, and the testosterone esters, either alone or in various combinations, have been studied.[15,33,42]

Apart from the problems of efficacy, side-effects, and tolerance to these agents, the major drawbacks to the use of antispermatogenic agents appear to be the long latent period to interference with fertility, latency to reversal of effect, and possible mutagenicity. In 1969, the first post-testicular candidate, α-chlorohydrin, was identified in two laboratories.[2,10] For the first time, an interval-to-onset of antifertility as short as 7 days was noted,[56] suggesting the effects to be exerted on the fully formed sperm at the level of the epididymis.[12,29,52] The finding of induction of epididymal spermatoceles and back

We are grateful to J. Burns and L. J. D. Zaneveld for helping with some of the early in vivo studies with ketoconazole; to A. Bajka for performing testosterone radioimmunoassays; to K. Wu for performing rat Leydig cell testosterone production assays; to B. Lewis, B. Berkoz, and G. Cooper for their synthesis of the compounds studied; to H. Parnes for supplying radiolabeled RS-68287; and to M. Chaplin, S. Smith, and B. Rice for performing the in vivo metabolism assay with [³H]-RS-68287.

TABLE 25-1. Chronology of Male Chemical Contraception

AGENT	YEARS STUDIED
Testosterone	1949–1952
Nitrofurans	1950–1957
Alkylating agents	1952–1965
Thiophenes	1956
Progestins	1958–1959
Bis-diamines	1960–1963
Methallibure	1961–1965
Dinitropyrroles	1963–1967
Cyproterone acetate	1965–1970
α-Chlorohydrin	1969–1972
Gossypol	1970–Present
Testosterone enanthate combinations	1975–1980
Lonidamine	1976–Present
6-halo-6-deoxy-D-sugars	1978–1980
LHRH analogues	1978–Present

pressure effects at the testis from high doses,[13] together with frank toxicity of these suspect alkylating agents in monkeys,[31] signaled their demise as candidates for human use, although α-chlorohydrin presently is marketed as a rodenticide.[11]

Interference with the hormonal control of epididymal function was reported with a steroid, cyproterone acetate.[46] This claim did not stand up to further studies, however.[48,49]

A new class of compounds, the 6-deoxy-6-halosugars, again exerting their effect at the epididymal level and interfering with metabolism of the sperm so they become immotile after ejaculation, was widely heralded.[16,17,23,62] Unfortunately, the block to glucose metabolism, useful at the level of the epididymis, led to neurotoxicity centrally.

Most recently, a factor from cotton seed oil, gossypol, is under clinical evaluation.[14,32] Gossypol appears to have multiple sites of action[1,19,20,60] and may cause antifertility as rapidly as 2 to 3 weeks, but its antispermatogenic effects are not always reversible.

These compounds, together with others working by means of chemical interference with the ejaculatory process,[27,43,51] constitute the range of male contraceptive drug candidates so far.

In the search for alternative possibilities, we were intrigued by reports that a wide variety of drugs, ranging from antimicrobials to methadone, have been detected in human semen.[5,7,8,36,54] The nitroimidazoles, in particular metronidazole, were detected in microgram quantities in human and dog seminal plasma within 1 hour of oral administration.[6,38] We had been evaluating a series of 1-substituted imidazoles for spermicidal activity when admixed with semen either in vitro or when placed intravaginally in female monkeys.[57,58,63] These observations, taken together, suggested the possible existence of compounds that could be administered orally to the male, be accumulated in the accessory organ secretions, and on ejaculation, be mixed with the sperm to exert a spermicidal or spermatostatic effect.

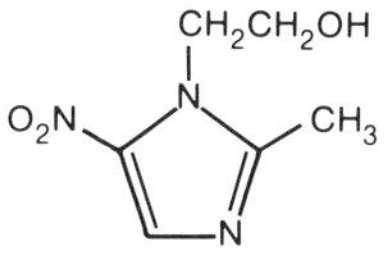

Metronidazole

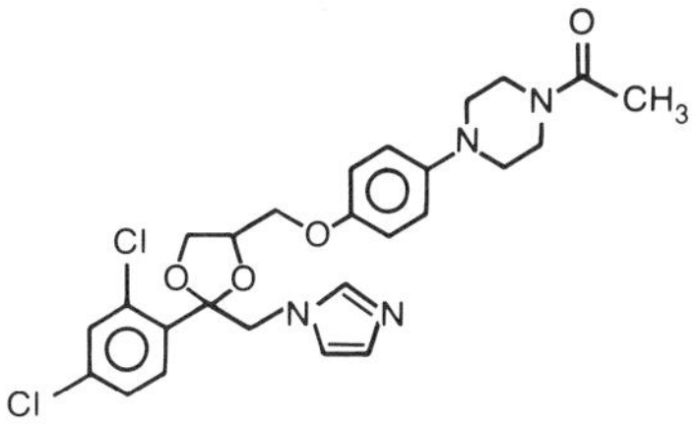

Ketoconazole

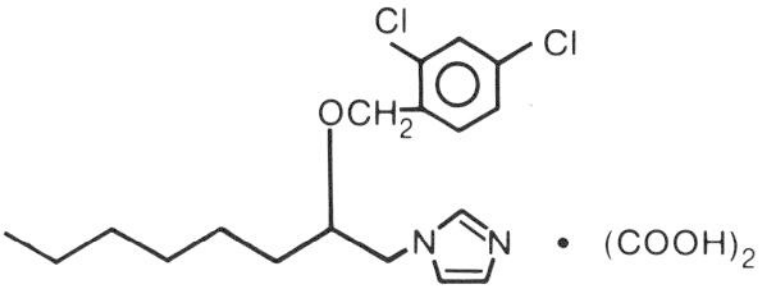

RS-37367

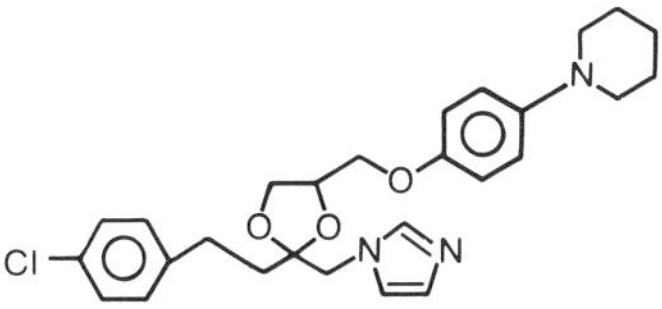

RS-29984

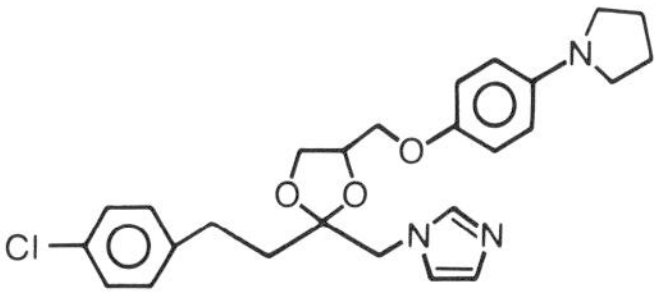

RS-29636

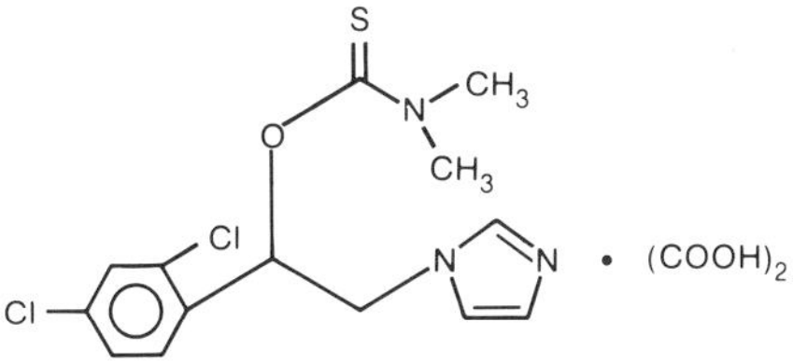

RS-90847

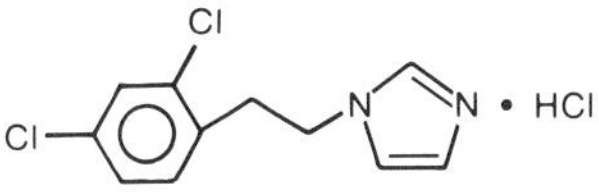

RS-41353

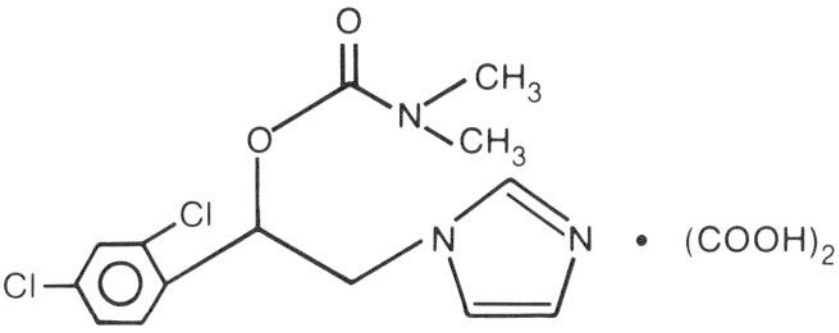

RS-68287

FIG. 25-1. Structures of compounds evaluated for in vivo spermicidal activity.

EARLY STUDIES

The relevance to eventual human use of secretory findings after oral administration in the dog was already noted for metronidazole.[6,38] Previously, we had demonstrated the sensitivity of dog sperm to spermicidal activity of the 1-substituted imidazoles and the correlation of those findings to effects on human spermatozoa.[18,40,57] The dog was therefore chosen as preliminary model for our studies.

It was quickly established that metronidazole (Fig. 25-1) is not spermicidal against dog spermatozoa, showing no effect at final in vitro concentrations of

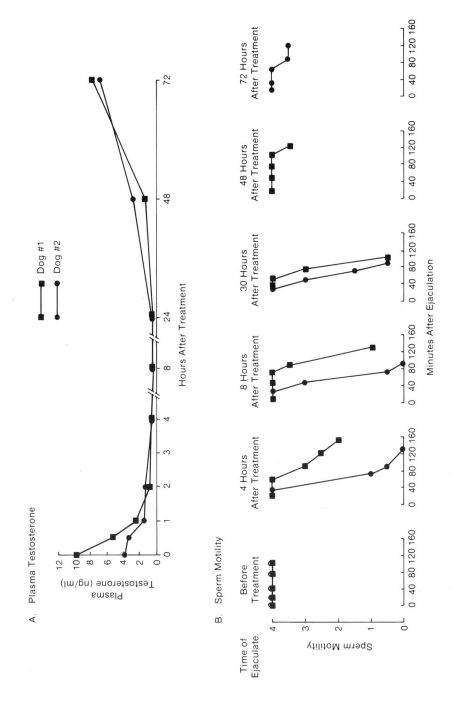

A. Plasma Testosterone

Dog #1
Dog #2

Plasma Testosterone (ng/ml)

Hours After Treatment

B. Sperm Motility

Sperm Motility

Time of Ejaculate:

Before Treatment

4 Hours After Treatment

8 Hours After Treatment

30 Hours After Treatment

48 Hours After Treatment

72 Hours After Treatment

Minutes After Ejaculation

FIG. 25-2. Effect of single oral administration of 1 g of ketoconazole to male beagle dogs on (A) plasma testosterone levels and (B) motility of ejaculated spermatozoa. Ejaculates were obtained sequentially after dosing, at the times indicated above each panel. Motility was scored on an increasing scale of 0 through 4 on aliquots of the ejaculate kept at 37°C in a closed humid system.

←――――――――――――――――――――――――――――――――――――

100 µg/ml. RS-37367, as previously noted, is highly spermicidal to dog sperm in vitro (Table 25-2). RS-37367 was tested by oral administration to male beagles from which ejaculates were obtained at various times after dosing. As in control animals, the motility of the sperm in these ejaculates was maintained at a high level for at least 2 hours after ejaculation. Following oral administration of ^{14}C-RS-37367, radioactivity could be detected in both plasma and ejaculated semen, demonstrating systemic absorption. No intact compound could be measured by HPLC assay of these samples, however. We concluded that RS-37367 is metabolized extensively and rapidly, probably by a "first-pass effect" known to be shared by other members of this class of compound.

Before mounting an extensive synthetic effort, we elected to prove the concept of this type of rapid-onset, reversible, orally active male contraception with a known and available compound, even if it had low potency or undesirable characteristics. Ketoconazole was determined to be such a compound. Assay of in vitro spermicidal activity against dog spermatozoa showed immobilization of sperm in 15 minutes at ketoconazole concentrations of 100 µg/ml. In addition, ketoconazole is known to be well absorbed following oral administration and resistant to metabolism; high maintained blood levels can be achieved.[4,35]

EFFECTS OF KETOCONAZOLE

Initial in vivo studies were performed in two male beagles.[59] Ejaculates obtained from the study dogs demonstrated, that before treatment, the ejaculated sperm retained excellent motility for at least 100 minutes. Each dog then was administered 1 g of ketoconazole orally in a capsule. Ejaculates were obtained sequentially at 4, 8, 30, 48, and 72 hours after dosing. In the first of this series of ejaculates, a dramatic decline in sperm motility was observed with time after ejaculation (Fig. 25-2). A similar effect was noted for the 8- and

TABLE 25-2. Comparison of the Effects of RS-37367 and Ketoconazole on Dog Spermatozoa In Vitro

COMPOUND	CONCENTRATION (µg/ml)	TIME TO COMPLETE IMMOBILIZATION (min)
Vehicle		>60
RS-37367	5.0	<1
	2.5	<15
	1.2	<15
	0.6	~60
Ketoconazole	100.0	<15
	10.0	>60

TABLE 25-3. Concentrations of Ketoconazole in Semen
Collected Sequentially from Dogs at Different Times
after Oral Administration of 1 g

DOG	TIME FROM DOSE (hr)	CONCENTRATION (μg/ml)
IPS3	4	1.011
	8	0.837
	31	0.691
IQP4	4	0.492
	8	0.380
	30	0.216
IGS4	4	0.697
	32	<0.2

30-hour ejaculates, but not for the 48-hour or later ejaculates. Radioimmunoassay of testosterone levels in blood samples obtained from these treated dogs over this same period also demonstrated the known antisteroidogenic effect of the compound.[45,55]

Although we acknowledge that withdrawal of testosterone might interfere with epididymal function and influence maturation and motility of sperm, we think it unlikely that such effects would be so acutely manifest. HPLC assay of the ejaculates from these dogs revealed intact ketoconazole in the seminal plasma (Table 25-3).

The observation of apparent increased potency of ketoconazole in vivo versus in vitro cannot be explained at this time. Possibilities include 1) exposure of the sperm to ketoconazole within the male reproductive tract potentiates the effect after ejaculation; 2) ketoconazole is metabolized into a molecule that is more spermicidal than ketoconazole; and/or 3) a (more potent) metabolite is accumulated preferentially in the accessory glands.

We also evaluated ketoconazole in male rabbits. Again it was established that, prior to dosing, ejaculated sperm retained good motility, albeit with some loss in progressivity over a period of hours following ejaculation (Table 25-4). After a dose of 1 g of ketoconazole was administered to each rabbit, the

TABLE 25-4. Effect of Oral Administration of 1 g
of Ketoconazole to Rabbits on the Motility
of Sperm Ejaculated 4 Days Later

	PREDOSING		POSTDOSING
	TIME AFTER EJACULATION (min)		
RABBIT	*60*	*120*	*120*
1	85/2.5*	80/2.5	42/0
2	80/2.5	50/1.0	52/0
3	90/3.5	80/1.5	85/1.0

* Percentage motility/forward progressivity score (scale of 0–4).

animals appeared lethargic, and no ejaculates could be obtained until the fourth day after dosing. Two hours after ejaculations on this fourth day, however, forward motility of the sperm from two of three animals was abolished.

In a further study, 1 g of ketoconazole was administered to each of four rhesus monkeys and the effect followed after electroejaculation of the anesthetized animals, using a rectal probe. There was clear inhibition of sperm motility after dosing (Fig. 25-3). The inhibition of progressive, forwardly directed motility in particular was rapid and complete. We believe, on the basis of in vitro observations, that the first effect of low concentrations of these compounds is the disruption of coordinated movement of the sperm. Higher concentrations abolish all movement and have a pronounced effect on membranes and mitochondria.

HPLC assay of a limited number of semen samples from human volunteers following oral ingestion of 800 mg of ketoconazole established the presence of only very low levels of the compound. With ketoconazole, however, we felt that we had established the possibility of rapid-onset, reversible, orally administered male contraception. The noted effects of ketoconazole on steroidogenesis, behavior, and the concerns over idiosyncratic hepatotoxicity[22] militated against pursuit of higher doses of this compound, however.

SCREENING STUDIES

Many imidazole compounds (399) were screened for in vitro spermicidal activity against dog and human spermatozoa, and 124 of these were tested in vivo in the beagle dog. In general, the in vitro potency showed relatively little correlation with the structure of the imidazole side chain, being dependent more on the overall lipophilicity of the molecule. Previous studies with 1-substituted imidazoles also had shown the most spermicidal compounds in vitro to be lipophilic molecules.* On the other hand, optimum in vivo potency was now found with more lipophobic compounds.

The lead compound in this search was ketoconazole (Fig. 25-1). The synthesis and biologic testing of new compounds led to a gradual simplification of the structure, until even RS-41353 was shown to be among the most potent agents in vivo. For good oral activity, the imidazole group is necessary, other heterocycles being marginally potent or inactive in vivo, even though in vitro spermicidal activity was present. As would be anticipated, the best compounds had structural features that were consistent with metabolic stability, for example, a carbamate group or compounds related to ketoconazole, which is long-acting orally. Within the above constraints, lipophilicity seemed to be the overriding feature. Although spermicidal potency in vitro was related directly to lipophilicity, oral potency required greater hydrophilicity, presumably because of enhanced distribution and serum levels. Although further decreasing the lipophilicity might have enhanced uptake into seminal fluid (*e.g.*, metronidazole), apparently the drop in spermicidal activity reduced and eventually abol-

---

* Lewis B, Walker KAM: Unpublished data, 1984

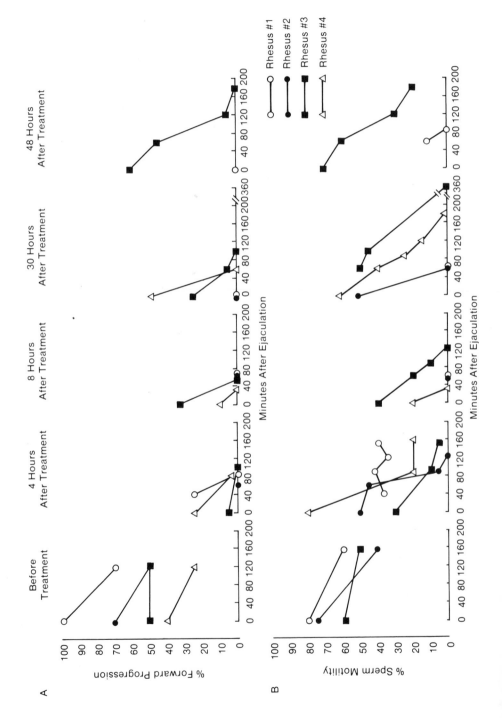

FIG. 25-3. Effect of single oral administration of 1 g of ketoconazole to male monkeys on (*A*) the degree of progressive motility and (*B*) the percentage of ejaculated spermatozoa that were motile with time in ejaculates obtained by electroejaculation at various times after dosing.

←——————————————————————————————————————

ished oral activity in even more hydrophobic molecules. Systemic activity thus seems to depend on a balance between spermicidal potency per se and efficient transport of the compound into the seminal fluid. It was not possible to identify structural features that had a profound effect on spermicidal potency in vitro.

In general, two classes of compounds were found to be effective in vivo: those represented by RS-90847 and RS-68287, and those represented by RS-29984 and RS-29636. The in vitro potency of these compounds is shown in Table 25-5.

Because of the undesirable effects of ketoconazole on steroidogenesis, some of these compounds were screened for effect on hCG-stimulated production of testosterone by rat Leydig cells in vitro, using a modification of a published method.[9] In keeping with reports in the literature,[44] ketoconazole caused a dose-related inhibition of testosterone production (Fig. 25-4). Both RS-29984 and RS-29636 had low potency as inhibitors of testosterone production in vitro, suggesting a favorable therapeutic ratio (Table 25-6). RS-90847 was assessed in vivo by oral administration to the dog, followed by measurement of circulating levels of testosterone, and also appeared to have a favorable ratio of desired to undesired activity (Table 25-7).

IN VIVO CHARACTERIZATION

All animals were ejaculated 2 days prior to dosing to standardize time of depletion of accessory gland contents, and thus perhaps their secretory activity (with respect to the oral dosing), and to obtain pretreatment control data for the animals.

Compounds of particular interest were RS-29984, RS-29636, RS-90847, and RS-68287. Figures 25-5 and 25-6 show the effect of the compounds, when given as a single oral dose to dogs, on the motility of subsequently ejaculated spermatozoa. RS-29984 caused a dramatic suppression of sperm

TABLE 25-5. Comparison of the Effects on Dog Sperm Motility of 25 μg/ml of RS-90847, RS-68287, RS-29984 and RS-29636 Added In Vitro

COMPOUND	APPROXIMATE TIME TO COMPLETE IMMOBILIZATION (min)
RS-90847	5
RS-68287	60
RS-29984	5
RS-29636	5

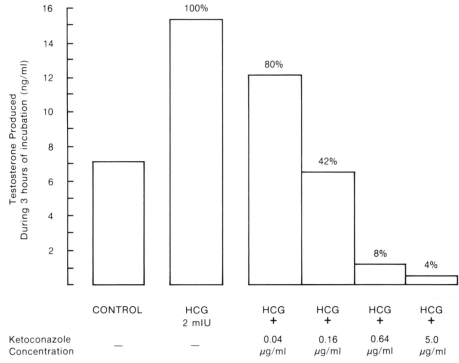

FIG. 25-4. Effect of ketoconazole on in vitro testosterone production by hCG-stimulated dispersed rat Leydig cells.

motility in the first ejaculate taken (4 hr after treatment). A similar inhibition was noted in sequential ejaculates collected up to 48 hours after dosing, although at the latter time the rate of decrease of motility was less than in the earlier ejaculates. At 72 hours after dosing no inhibition was noted. Similar effects were noted for RS-29636, although the suppression of sperm motility first was observed in the ejaculate obtained 8 hours after dosing and was still evident in the ejaculate obtained at 72 hours after dosing. The profile of activity of RS-90847 and RS-68287 more closely resembled that of RS-29984. Sperm motility was inhibited in ejaculates obtained up to 48 hours after administration of RS-90847, but reduction in sperm motility was only noted in the 4-hour ejaculate of the dog receiving RS-68287.

TABLE 25-6. Comparison of Relative Spermicidal and Testosterone Suppressive Effects of Candidate Compounds

COMPOUNDS	TESTOSTERONE-SUPPRESSING POTENCY (A)	IN VITRO SPERMICIDAL POTENCY (B)	A/B
Ketoconazole	1	1	1
RS-29984	0.17	>50	<0.003
RS-29636	0.12	>10	<0.012

TABLE 25-7. Comparison of Relative In Vivo Spermicidal and Testosterone Suppressive Effects of Ketoconazole and RS-90847

COMPOUND	DOSE (mg/kg)	TESTOSTERONE-SUPPRESSING POTENCY (A)	IN VIVO SPERMICIDAL POTENCY (B)	A/B
Ketoconazole	97	1	1	1
RS-90847	90	1	11	0.09

No compound was effective in all animals at an oral dose of 10 mg/kg. Further testing of the compounds by either subcutaneous or intravenous routes showed no increase in activity, suggesting that absorption from the gastrointestinal tract was not a limiting factor.

RS-68287 had rather greater potency in vivo than would have been predicted on the basis of its in vitro potency, by comparison with the other compounds (see Table 25-5, Fig. 25-6), and this suggested that either metabolic activation or enhanced uptake of a metabolite could be taking place. To check these possibilities, a dog was administered a single oral dose of 30 mg/kg of [³H]-RS-68287, and the plasma and semen were monitored for total radioactivity and major products. Plasma concentrations of total radioactivity, RS-68287 and the major metabolite, identified as RS-68287–free alcohol (RS-51801), are shown in Table 25-8. RS-68287 appeared to be absorbed rapidly and efficiently, inasmuch as the peak concentration of total ³H was about 25 μg/ml within 3 hours of dosing. Without further studies, however (intravenous and/or excretion experiments), the actual efficiency of gastrointestinal absorption cannot be stated. There was little metabolic degradation of RS-68287 during the absorption process, and over the 0- to 24-hour time span, RS-68287 was the major compound circulating in the plasma. The terminal plasma $T_{\frac{1}{2}}$ of RS-68287 calculated over the 24-hour period was approximately 6 hours. Conversion of RS-68287 to RS-51801 does not occur in plasma because when RS-68287 was incubated in vitro with dog plasma at 37°C for 2 hours, no RS-51801 was detected. At 4 and 24 hours after dosing, concentrations of both RS-68287 and RS-51801 were lower in semen than in plasma (Table 25-9). The semen-to-plasma ratios indicate that neither compound is concentrated in semen after oral administration of a single, 30 mg/kg dose of RS-68287. As in blood, the major compound in the seminal plasma was RS-68287, presumably the agent responsible for decrease in sperm motility after ejaculation.

One variable that could be controlled in vitro but not in the in vivo studies was sperm number. Three dogs were given a single oral dose of 60 mg/kg of RS-29984 and ejaculates collected 4 hours later. Efficacy, judged by time to immobilization of the spermatozoa, appeared to be affected by both sperm concentration and total sperm numbers (Fig. 25-7).

Following ejaculation, at least in intravaginal inseminators, sperm presumably are separated rapidly from the seminal plasma as they enter the cervix and ascend the female tract. It was therefore felt essential to discover whether the antimotility effect of a compound would persist if spermatozoa were removed from the seminal plasma of treated dogs. The ejaculate of a dog treated with 60 mg/kg of RS-29984 and collected 4 hours after dosing was

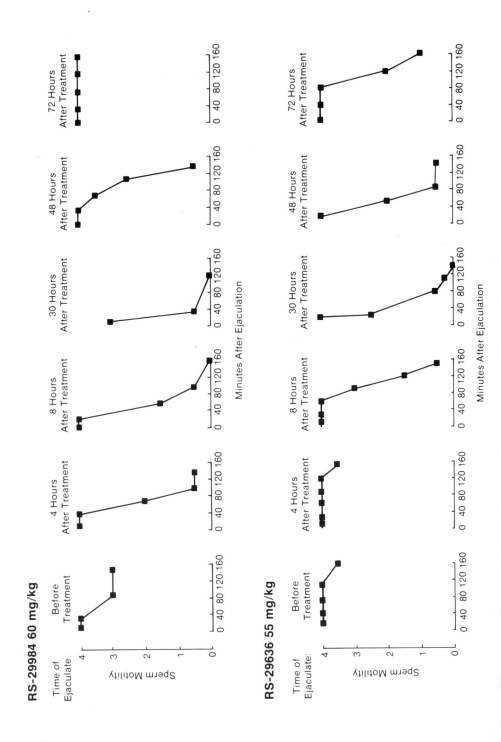

RS-29984 60 mg/kg

RS-29636 55 mg/kg

282

FIG. 25-5. Effect of single oral administration of RS-29984 and RS-29636 to male beagle dogs on motility of spermatozoa with time from ejaculation in ejaculates obtained sequentially at various times after dosing. Motility was scored on an increasing scale of 0 through 4 on aliquots of the ejaculate kept at 37°C in a closed humid system.

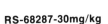

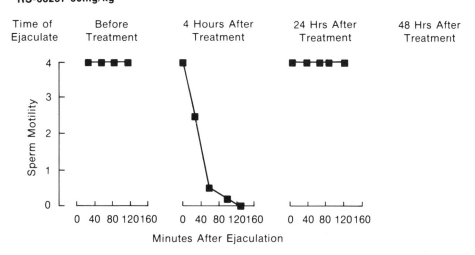

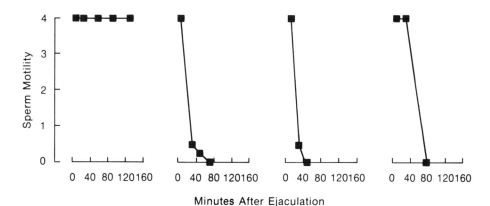

FIG. 25-6. Effect of single oral administration of RS-68287 and RS-90847 to male beagle dogs on motility of spermatozoa with time from ejaculation in ejaculates obtained sequentially at various times after dosing. Motility was scored on an increasing scale of 0 through 4 on aliquots of the ejaculate kept at 37°C in a closed humid system.

TABLE 25-8. Plasma Concentrations of Total Radioactivity (^{3}H),
RS-68287, and RS-51801 in a Male Dog
Following a 30 mg/kg Single Oral Dose of [^{3}H]-
RS-68287

	PLASMA CONCENTRATION (μg/ml)		
TIME (hr)	TOTAL ^{3}H	RS-68287	RS-51801
0.5	11.1	9.4	0.4
1	21.7	18.8	1.1
2	24.9	20.9	2.6
3	26.7	20.5	3.4
5	23.1	16.5	4.4
7	19.2	11.5	5.7
24	7.8	1.7	5.4

divided into three aliquots (Fig. 25-8). An ejaculate also was obtained from an untreated dog. The spermatozoa and seminal plasma were separated, recombined, and the resulting sperm motility over time compared with motility of the spermatozoa in the original (homologous) seminal plasma. No loss of sperm motility was seen over 2 hours after ejaculation for the spermatozoa of the untreated dog in homologous seminal plasma. The spermatozoa of the treated dog lost motility in the characteristic fashion. Control spermatozoa, when mixed with seminal plasma from the treated dog, however, lost motility at the same rate as did the spermatozoa in seminal plasma from the treated dog. Most important, spermatozoa removed from the semen of the treated dog also lost motility, even though mixed with seminal plasma from the control dog. These results indicate that the compound or some form of the compound was present in the ejaculate of the treated dog, where it adversely affected sperm motility, and the effect was not reversible, at least under these conditions.

In the hope of attaining higher concentrations of compound in the accessory gland fluid, the effect of administering compound on several consecutive days was investigated. RS-29984 was administered at 60 mg/kg for 3 consecutive days and ejaculates were obtained 4 hours following each dose. More rapid loss of motility of ejaculated sperm was noted on the second versus the first day of dosing, but total sperm numbers also decreased from 330×10^6

TABLE 25-9. Comparison of RS-68287 and RS-51801 Concentrations in Semen and Plasma

	SEMEN CONCENTRATION (μg/ml)		PLASMA CONCENTRATION (μg/ml)		SEMEN-TO-PLASMA RATIO	
SAMPLE TIME (hr)	RS-68287	RS-51801	RS-68287	RS-51801	RS-68287	RS-51801
4	9.7	2.2	18.5	3.9	0.52	0.56
24	0.5	1.0	1.7	5.4	0.29	0.18

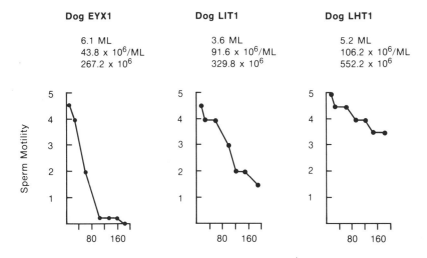

Dog EYX1

6.1 ML
43.8 x 10^6/ML
267.2 x 10^6

Dog LIT1

3.6 ML
91.6 x 10^6/ML
329.8 x 10^6

Dog LHT1

5.2 ML
106.2 x 10^6/ML
552.2 x 10^6

Minutes After Ejaculation

FIG. 25-7. Effect of total sperm numbers and sperm concentration on motility over time of ejaculated sperm obtained 4 hours after single oral administration of 60 mg/kg of RS-29984 to male beagle dogs. Motility was scored on an increasing scale of 0 through 4 on aliquots of the ejaculate kept at 37°C in a closed humid system.

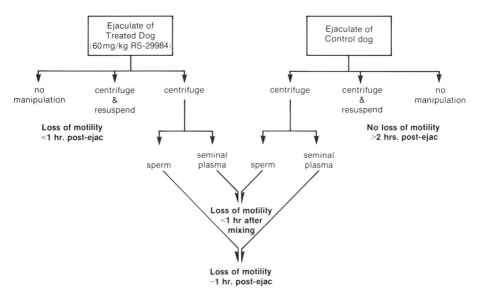

FIG. 25-8. Schematic of manipulations and results of separation and recombination experiment using ejaculates from a dog treated with RS-29984 and an untreated dog. Sperm motility was inhibited in all samples containing either sperm or seminal plasma from the treated dog.

the first day to 260×10^6 the second day. This effect could not be replicated by further studies with this or other related compounds.

FERTILITY TRIALS

In preliminary fertility trials, two dogs each were dosed with 30 mg/kg or 90 mg/kg of RS-90847. Four hours after dosing, the dogs were either ejaculated manually (one from each dose) and the ejaculate used to inseminate an estrous bitch artificially, or alternatively (remaining dogs) mated each with an estrous bitch. All bitches conceived and carried to term.

The result for the direct breeding may be in part explained by the findings in a subsequent study in which split ejaculates were collected from dosed dogs (Tables 25-10 and 25-11). It became clear that the early sperm-rich fractions of the ejaculate either were not exposed to, or were less sensitive to, the effects of the compound. The artificial inseminations were performed with combined ejaculates, however, which should have corresponded with previous in vitro evaluations. This suggests either that sperm reached the site of fertilization prior to being immobilized, or, alternatively, that the ultimate motility of these sperm is in some way different after insemination than when incubated in a test tube.

It should be noted that the dog differs from many other species in that 1) ovulation takes place before sexual receptivity and mating, so that the egg awaits the sperm, and 2) there is no seminal coagulation in the dog. In species in which ovulation is not so precisely timed to mating and in which entrapment of sperm in a coagulum takes place, such fertility trials may well have a different outcome.

CONCLUSIONS

An exciting lead to post-testicular male contraception has been identified that would differ from all previous agents in the extreme rapidity of onset of action (Fig. 25-9). Spermicidally active compounds have been found that are already present in the seminal plasma 1 to 4 hours after oral administration.

There are, however, a number of potential problems that need to be addressed. The degree of mixing of seminal plasma with the sperm that is required for efficacy, the fractional concentration of compound, and the time to immobilization of sperm after ejaculation, all appear to impede the efficacy of these agents in the dog. It should be noted, however, that the dog ejaculate, in contrast to that of humans, does not coagulate, and the bitch breeds only after ovulation, so that the ovum is always waiting for the arrival of sperm. In humans we would expect that the entrapment of sperm in contact with seminal plasma for some time in the coagulum, the believed requirement for time to elapse for capacitation, and the less stringent relationship between times of intercourse and ovulation, might all favor agents such as these. Rapid transport of sperm within the female tract has been noted for a variety of species including humans, but it is suggested that, on morphologic considerations, these are not the fertilizing sperm.[39,50]

TABLE 25-10. Effect of 30 mg/kg RS-90847 Administered Orally to Dogs on Sperm Motility in Split Ejaculate Fractions

| DOG | FRACTION (ml) IN ORDER OF COLLECTION | MINUTES AFTER START OF EJACULATION | POSTEJACULATION MOTILITY | | SPERM CONCENTRATION (×10⁶/ml) |
			MOTILITY/ FORWARD PROGRESSION (%)	MOTILITY/ FORWARD PROGRESSION (%) (at 2 hr)	
LIT1	0.2	20	90/83	NS*	1.7
	0.4	24	97/84	92/89	422.0
	0.3	27	92/98	97/86	708.0
	0.25	30	92/54	12/0	71.0
	0.3	35	93/63	85/0	11.2
	0.4	40	97/26	82/0	12.3
	0.5	49	97/0	0/0	18.7
	2.2	53	97/9	0/0	5.6
LI90	0.6	—	—	—	No sperm
	0.4	24	93/99	30/0	102.0
	0.7	30	100/93	93/7	26.6
	0.7	33	100/95	93/66	837.0
	1.1	34	95/72	97/0	114.8
	5.6	38	92/34	0/0	20.5
	Equal part mix†	43	95/93	23/0	126.3
JL11	0.5	18	97/86	83/90	33.5
	0.6	22	97/81	97/81	217.0
	0.7	25	100/88	93/0	38.0
	0.8	28	98/77	23/0	27.6
	7.0	32	98/31	8/0	1.3
	Equal part mix†	37	97/79	22/0	27.5

* NS, not sufficient sample
† One half of each fraction, combined

TABLE 25-11. Effect of 90 mg/kg RS-90847 Administered Orally to Dogs on Sperm Motility in Split Ejaculate Fractions

DOG	FRACTION (ml) IN ORDER OF COLLECTION	MINUTES AFTER START OF EJACULATION	POSTEJACULATION MOTILITY		SPERM CONCENTRATION ($\times 10^6$/ml)
			MOTILITY/ FORWARD PROGRESSION (%)	MOTILITY/ FORWARD PROGRESSION (%) (at 2 hr)	
LI90	0.6	—	—	—	No sperm
	0.5	—	—	—	No sperm
	0.6	20	65/0	0/0	1.2
	0.6	24	25/0	0/0	9.5
	0.6	28	88/89	42/0	443.0
	0.7	31	25/0	10/0	94.0
	5.2	34	10/0	0/0	16.0
	Equal part mix†	36	35/0	25/0	48.0
LIT1	0.8	23	85/92	0/0	0.9
	0.5	29	93/93	90/93	396.8
	0.7	35	87/48	0/0	447.0
	0.7	43	60/0	0/0	15.9
	2.2	48	62/0	0/0	9.4
	Equal part mix†	53	65/3	0/0	101.2

† One half of each fraction, combined

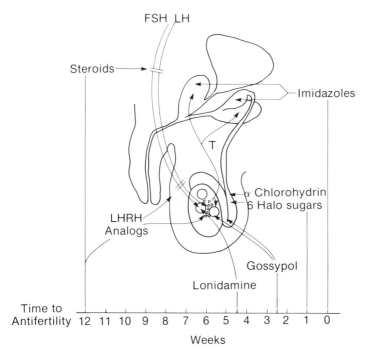

FIG. 25-9. Schematic representation of site(s) of action and latency from time of first dose to expression of antifertility with some representative male contraceptive agents.

The interaction of frequency of ejaculation (or of abstinence) on the secretion rate of the accessory organs has not been explored fully. Such an interaction might play a major role in eventual efficacy. Finally, the requirement that these agents be well absorbed, poorly metabolized, and delivered into the seminal plasma, raises the possibility of reabsorption in the female after intercourse, so that safety and tolerance would need to be satisfied in both male and female. The answers to these questions can probably be gained only in the primate, and we may still require more potent or better distributed compounds for final efficacy. The eventual prize of an on-demand, rapid-onset, fully reversible male contraceptive, however, would appear worth the effort.

REFERENCES

1. CHANG MC, GU ZP, SAKSENA SK: Effects of gossypol on the fertility of male rats, hamsters and rabbits. Contraception 21:461–469, 1980
2. COPPOLA JA: Extragonadal male antifertility agent. Life Sci 8:43–48, 1969
3. COULSTON F, BEYLER AL, DROBECK HP: The biologic actions of a new series of bis (dichloroacetyl) diamines. Toxic Appl Pharmacol 2:715–731, 1960
4. DANESHMEND TK, WARNOCK DW, TURNER A, ROBERTS CJC: Pharmacokinetics of ketoconazole in normal subjects. J Antimicrob Chemother 8:299–304, 1981
5. ELIASSON R, DORNBUSCH K: Levels of trimethoprin and sulphamethoxazole in human seminal plasma. Andrologia 9:195–202, 1977

6. ELIASSON R, DORNBUSCH K: Secretion of metronidazole into the human semen. Int J Androl 3:236–242, 1980
7. ELIASSON R, MALMBORG A-S: Concentrations of doxocycline in human seminal plasma. Scand J Infect Dis (Suppl) 9:32–36, 1976
8. ELIASSON R, MALMBORG AS, DORNBUSCH K, KVIST U: Excretion of erythromycin into human semen: Methodological, experimental and clinical aspects. In SIEGENTHALER W, LUTHY R (eds): Current Chemotherapy, Vol 1, pp 648–649. Washington, Publications American Society of Microbiology, 1978
9. ELLINWOOD WE, RESKO JA: Sex differences in biologically active and immunoreactive gonadotropins in the fetal circulation of rhesus monkeys. Endocrinology 107:902–907, 1980
10. ERICSSON RJ: A post-testicular antifertility drug. J Reprod Fertil 18:156, 1969
11. ERICSSON RJ: α-Chlorohydrin (Epibloc®): A toxicant–sterilant as an alternative in rodent control. In MARSH RE (ed): Proc 10th Vertebrate Pest Conference, pp 6–9. Davis, CA, University of California, 1982
12. ERICSSON RJ, BAKER VF: Male antifertility compounds: Biological properties of U-5897 and U-15,646. J Reprod Fertil 21:267–273, 1970
13. ERICSSON RJ, CONNOR ND: Lesions of the rat epididymis and subsequent sterility produced by U-5897 (3-chloro-1,2-propanediol), (abstr 49). Davis, California, Proc 2nd Ann Meeting of Soc Study Reprod, 1969
14. FARNSWORTH NR, WALLER DP: Current status of plant products reported to inhibit sperm. In ZATUCHNI GI (ed): Research Frontiers in Fertility Regulation Vol 2, No 1, pp 1–16. Chicago, PARFR, 1982
15. FAUNDES A, BRACHE V, LEON P, SCHMIDT F, ALVAREZ-SANCHEZ F: Sperm suppression with monthly injections of medroxyprogesterone acetate combined with testosterone enanthate at a high dose (500 mg). Int J Androl 4:235–245, 1981
16. FORD WCL: The effect of 6-deoxy-6-fluoroglucose on the fertility of male rats and mice. Contraception 25:535–545, 1982
17. FORD CL, WAITES GMH: Chlorinated sugars: A biochemical approach to the control of male fertility. Int J Androl (Suppl) 2:541–564, 1978
18. GOODPASTURE JC, BERGSTRÖM K, VICKERY BH: Comparison of the spermicidal efficacy of two nonoxynol-containing preparations with that of a new agent, using a novel "no-mix" assay. Contracep Deliv Syst 3:167, 1982
19. HADLEY MA, LIN YC, DYM M: Effects of gossypol on the reproductive system of male rats. J Androl 2:190–199, 1981
20. HAHN DW, RUSTICUS C, PROBST A, HOMM R, JOHNSON AN: Antifertility and endocrine activities of gossypol in rodents. Contraception 24:97–105, 1981
21. HECKEL NJ, ROSSO WA, KESTEL L: Spermatogenic rebound phenomenon after administration of testosterone propionate. J Clin Endocrinol 11:235–245, 1951
22. HEIBERG JK, SVEJGAARD E: Toxic hepatitis during ketoconazole treatment. Br Med J 283:825–826, 1981
23. HEITFELD F, MCRAE GI, VICKERY BH: Antifertility effect of 6-chloro-6-deoxy-glucose in the male rat. Contraception 19:543–555, 1979
24. HELLER CG, LAIDLAW WM, HARVEY HT, NELSON WO: Effects of progestational compounds on the reproductive processes of the human male. Ann NY Acad Sci 71:649–665, 1958
25. HELLER CG, MOORE DJ, PAULSEN CA, NELSON WO, LAIDLAW WM: Effects of progesterone and synthetic progestins on the reproductive physiology of normal men. Fed Proc 18:1057–1065, 1959
26. HELLER CG, FLAGEOLLE BY, MATSON LJ: Histopathology of the human testis as affected by *bis* (dichloroacetyl) diamines. Exp Mol Pathol (Suppl) 2:107–114, 1963
27. HOMONNAI ZT, SHILON M, PAZ GF: Phenoxybenzamine: An effective male contraceptive pill. Contraception 29:479–491, 1984
28. JACKSON H, FOX BW, CRAIG AW: The effect of alkylating agents on male rat fertility. Br J Pharmacol 14:149–157, 1959
29. JONES AR, FORD SA: The action of (S)-α-chlorohydrin and 6-chloro-6-deoxyglucose on the metabolism of guinea pig spermatozoa. Contraception 30:261–269, 1984
30. KING TO, BERLINER VR, BLYE RP: Pharmacology of 2,4-dinitropyrroles: A new class of antispermatogenic compounds. Biochem Pharmacol 12:69, 1963
31. KIRTON KT, ERICSSON RJ, RAY JA, FORBES AD: Male antifertility compounds: Efficacy of U-5897 in primates (Macaca mulatta). J Reprod Fertil 21:275–278, 1970
32. LIN ZQ, LIU GZ, HEI LS, ZHANG RA, YU CZ: Clinical trial of gossypol as a male antifertility

agent. In FEN CC, GRIFFIN D (eds): Recent Advances in Fertility Regulation, pp 160–163. Geneva, Atar SA, 1981
33. LOHIYA NK, SHARMA OP: Reversible inhibition of spermatogenesis by danazol with combination of testosterone enanthate in rabbit. Andrologia 16:72–75, 1984
34. MACLEOD J, TIETZE C: Control of reproductive capacity. Ann Rev Med 15:299–314, 1964
35. MAKSYMIUK AW, LEVINE HB, BODEY GP: The pharmacology of ketoconazole, a new orally administered antifungal (abstr 104). Twentieth Interscience Conference on Antimicrobial Agents and Chemotherapy, New Orleans, Sept. 22–24, 1980
36. MALMBORG AS, DORNBUSCH K, ELIASSON R, LINDHOLMER C: Concentrations of various antibacterials in human seminal plasma. In DANIELSSON D, JUHLIN L, MARDH P-A (eds): Genital Infections and Their Complications, pp 307–312. Stockholm, Almqvist & Wiksel, 1975
37. NELSON WO, BUNGE RG: The effect of therapeutic dosages of nitrofurantoin (furadantin) upon spermatogenesis in man. J Urol 77:275–281, 1957
38. NIELSEN OS, FRIMODT-MOLLER N, MAIGAARD S, MADSEN PO: Nitroimidazoles in the canine prostate, vagina and urethra. The Prostate 2:71–78, 1981
39. OVERSTREET JW, COOPER GW: Sperm transport in the reproductive tract of the female rabbit. 1. The rapid transport phase of transport. Biol Reprod 19:101–114, 1978
40. OVERSTREET JW, KATZ DF, BRAZIL C, VICKERY BH: Assessment of a new spermicidal agent against human seminal sperm in vitro. Contracep Deliv Syst 3:144, 1982
41. PAGET GE, WALPOLE AL, RICHARDSON DN: Nonsteroidal inhibitors of pituitary gonadotrophic function. Nature (Lond) 192:1191–1192, 1961
42. PATANELLI DJ (ed) Proceedings: Hormonal Control of Male Fertility U.S. Dept. of Health Education and Welfare, DHEW Publication No. (NIH) 78-1097, 1977
43. PAZ GF, SHILON M, HOMONNAI ZT: The possible use of phenoxybenzamine as a male contraceptive drug: Studies on male rats. Contraception 29:189–195, 1984
44. PONT A, WILLIAMS PL, AZHAR S, REITZ RE, BOCHRA C, SMITH ER, STEVENS DA: Ketoconazole blocks testosterone synthesis. Arch Int Med 142:2137–2140, 1982
45. PONT A, WILLIAMS PL, LOOSE DS, FELDMAN D, REITZ RE, BOCHRA C, STEVENS DA: Ketoconazole blocks adrenal steroid synthesis. Ann Int Med 97:370–372, 1982
46. PRASAD MRN, SINGH SP, RAJALAKSHMI M: Fertility control in male rats by continuous release of microquantities of cyproterone acetate from subcutaneous silastic capsules. Contraception 2:165–178, 1970
47. PRIOR JT, FERGUSON JH: Cytotoxic effects of nitrofuran on the rat testis. Cancer 3:1062–1072, 1950
48. ROY S, CHATTERJEE S, PRASAD MRN, PODDAR AK, PANDEY DC: Effects of cyproterone acetate on reproductive functions in normal human males. Contraception 14:403–420, 1976
49. SCHENCK B, NEUMANN F: Some comments on the use of antiandrogens for male contraception. Int J Androl (Suppl) 2:155–161, 1978
50. SETTLAGE DSF, MOTOSHIMA M, TREDWAY DR: Sperm transport from the external cervical os to the Fallopian tubes in women: a time and quantitation study. Fertil Steril 24:655–661, 1973
51. SHILON M, PAZ GF, HOMONNAI ZT: The use of phenoxybenzamine treatment in premature ejaculation. Fertil Steril 42:659–661, 1984
52. SMOJLIK E, CHANG MC: Antifertility activities of U-5897 (3-chloro-1,2-propanediol) on male rats, (abstr 50). Proc of 2nd Ann Meeting Soc Study Reprod, Davis, California, 1969
53. STEINBERGER E, BOCCABELLA A, NELSON WD: Cytotoxic effects of 5-chloro-2-acetyl thiophen (Ba 11044, CIBA) on the testis of the rat. Anat Rec 125:312–313, 1956
54. SWANSON BN, GORDON WP, LYNN RK, GERBER N: Seminal excretion, vaginal absorption, distribution and whole blood kinetics of D-methadone in the rabbit. J Pharmacol Exp Therap 206:507–514, 1978
55. TRACHTENBURG J, HALPERN N, PONT A: Ketoconazole: A novel and rapid treatment for advanced prostatic cancer. J Urol 130:152–153, 1983
56. VICKERY BH, ERICKSON GI, BENNETT JP: Mechanisms of action of low doses of α-chlorohydrin in the rat. J Reprod Fertil 38:1–10, 1974
57. VICKERY BH, GOODPASTURE JC, BERGSTRÖM K, WALKER KAM, OVERSTREET J, KATZ DF: Assessment of a new vaginal contraceptive agent against ejaculated dog and human spermatozoa in vitro. Fertil Steril 40:231–236, 1983
58. VICKERY BH, GOODPASTURE JC, LIN L-Y: Delivery of a new vaginal contraceptive. In

ZATUCHNI GI, GOLDSMITH A, SHELTON JD, SCIARRA JJ (eds): Long-Acting Contraceptive Delivery Systems, pp 228–240. Philadelphia, Harper & Row, 1984

59. VICKERY BH, BURNS J, ZANEVELD LJD, GOODPASTURE JC, CHAPLIN M: Studies towards a same day, orally administered, male contraceptive, (abstr). J Androl 6:P–37, 1985

60. WALLER DP, ZANEVELD LJD, FONG HHS: In vitro spermicidal activity of gossypol. Contraception 22:183–187, 1980

61. WALPOLE AL: Nonsteroidal agents inhibiting pituitary gonadotropic function. In AUSTIN CR, PERRY JS (eds): Agents Affecting Fertility. Biological Council Symposium on Drug Action, pp 159–179. London, J & A Churchill, 1965

62. WARREN LA, MCRAE G, VICKERY BH: Antifertility efficacy of twice daily administration of 6-chloro-6-deoxy-D-glucose in the male rat. Contraception 20:275–289, 1979

63. ZANEVELD LJD, BURNS JW, GOODPASTURE JC, VICKERY BH: Evaluation of the in vivo efficacy of a new vaginal contraceptive agent in stumptailed macaques. Fertil Steril 41:455–459, 1984

26

Discussion: Experimental Approaches for Male Contraception

MODERATORS: C. ALVIN PAULSEN

JEFFREY M. SPIELER

DOES THE HORMONAL MILIEU OF FEMALE ANIMALS CHANGE WHEN THEY ARE EXPOSED TO MALES?

Male animals developed elevated testosterone levels when exposed to females. One could imagine that GnRH might be released in females when exposed to males, and this could play a role in reflex ovulation in some animals. In reflex ovulators, enormous hormonal changes are known to result from the mechanical stimulation of mating. If any changes occur in animals that are not reflex ovulators, however, the changes are probably subtle and have not been investigated.

DOES TESTOSTERONE AFFECT LIBIDO BUT NOT POTENCY?

Studies at Stanford showed that hypogonadal men did not think about sex, but when they were stimulated appropriately, their responses were essentially normal, suggesting that the libidinal component of sexual behavior was androgen dependent. In studies of mating and nonmating behavior in the rat, using the GnRH antagonist-treated male rat as the model and then looking at the effect of administering graded concentrations of testosterone enanthate, investigators found an excellent dose-dependent correlation between the dose of testosterone, the serum levels, and androgen-dependent behavior.

Two anorchidic men who received biweekly injections of testosterone prior to undergoing testicle transplantation complained that immediately after their injections they desired sex three times a day. Their desire waned during the last few days of the 2-week interval, and then they had no interest in sex at

Panelists: R. John Aitken, Andrzej Bartke, Do Won Hahn, Danny H. Lewis, Patrizio Scorza Barcellona, Brian H. Vickery, Donald P. Waller, John P. Wiebe, L. J. D. Zaneveld; *Discussants:* Nancy J. Alexander, C. Wayne Bardin, Shalender Bhasin, William J. Bremner, Eric Chantler, Jean Cohen, Rune Eliasson, Erwin Goldberg, Kamran S. Moghissi, Eberhard Nieschlag, Rochelle Shain, Sherman J. Silber, Irving M. Spitz, Emil Steinberger, Kenneth S. K. Tung, Willem van Os, Gerald I. Zatuchni

all. They also experienced increased aggressiveness. Following the testicle transplant, with even physiologic levels of testosterone, their behavior pattern in terms of sex and aggressiveness evened out.

IS IT FEASIBLE TO USE SALIVARY TESTOSTERONE TO ESTABLISH A RELATIONSHIP BETWEEN TESTOSTERONE AND SEXUAL ACTIVITY?

Possibly. A group of investigators in reproductive medicine and psychology recently conducted a study in which volunteers were shown various films, some boring and some erotic, following which the volunteers' saliva was tested. With the erotic films, testosterone in the saliva increased.

DO VARIOUS STRAINS OF MICE DIFFER IN THEIR RESPONSE TO TESTOSTERONE?

Several years ago, investigators found that inbred mice differ from other mice in their sexual behavior. Under genetic control, this was mapped to genes within the major histocompatibility complex and could explain differences in responses to testosterone supplementation.

In Bartke's investigation, reported in this volume, the investigators did not look at the behavior response of testosterone administration, but the investigators have evidence to show that in a strain of mice with chronic low androgen levels, responsiveness of the seminal vesicles to testosterone is enhanced. This seems to explain the simultaneous existence of adequate accessory sex gland function and fertility. Furthermore, in the same strain there was an interesting behavioral characteristic in that these animals, which are genetically hypoandrogenic, also had an extremely long recovery time after mating, which seemed to provide a biologic compensation mechanism for the low sperm production.

In studies at the Population Council of the action of a variety of androgen-dependent genes in different strains of mice, every gene responded differently to a different dose of testosterone; there seemed to be gene-selective dependence of androgen action. Also, each gene was modified selectively by different modifier genes in different strains. Understanding individual variations in sexual behavior is difficult. Looking at individual structural genes within different strains of mice is so complex that it will take years to unravel the differences among single genes.

MIGHT DAILY RELEASE OF SMALL AMOUNTS OF GOSSYPOL FROM A LONG-ACTING DELIVERY SYSTEM BE PREFERABLE TO ORAL ADMINISTRATION IN TERMS OF TOXICITY?

Investigators currently are trying to develop a method to deliver gossypol to the testis. Microgram rather than milligram quantities may be sufficient to mediate the gossypol effects on the testis. Thus, only nanograms of gossypol would get into the systemic circulation and toxicity effects might be eliminated. If this could be accomplished, gossypol might have a good future.

COULD AN ANALOGUE OF GOSSYPOL BE FOUND THAT WOULD DISSOCIATE THE TOXICOLOGY FROM THE ANTIFERTILITY EFFECT?

If gossypol can be shown to exert a specific effect on the testis, then the search for analogues might be worthwhile, but to begin changing the structure of gossypol by adding side chains without knowing how gossypol acts is probably a waste of time. One should begin to develop analogues once the site and the mechanism of action have been identified.

DOES SULFASALAZINE INTERFERE WITH SPERM PRODUCTION?

Clinical data on the effect of sulfasalazine have come from men who were under treatment for ulcerative colitis, so there is some doubt whether the sulfasalazine or the underlying disease was interfering with sperm production.

About 10 years ago there was a flurry of interest in the idea that perhaps colchicine was an effective male contraceptive, based on similar kinds of data from colchicine-treated men. Investigators, accordingly, administered colchicine in commonly used therapeutic doses to normal men and showed that over a period of 6 months, it had no effect on sperm production or hormone levels. A similar study should be done with sulfasalazine.

DOES SULFASALAZINE INTERFERE WITH HORMONE PROFILES?

In addition to having no effect on serum testosterone, sulfasalazine appears not to cause significant changes in gonadotropins (LH and FSH).

IS A SIGNIFICANT FAILURE RATE LIKELY WHEN THE SHUG DEVICE HAS BEEN IN FOR A LONG TIME?

The Shug device appears to be a viable lead, but possibly there will be a significant failure rate in terms of reversibility when the device has been in place for a long time, because of epididymal damage. On the optimistic side, however, there may be some minor sperm leakage in this system, venting epididymal pressure, which does not occur in the normal closed-ended cautery vasectomy.

DO ACROSIN-INHIBITING COMPOUNDS CONSTITUTE AN IMPROVEMENT OVER THE PRESENTLY EXISTING SPERMICIDES?

Although some investigators believe that no compound will be able to inactivate all sperm before they get into the cervical mucus, contraception may be possible by preventing the rapid entry of spermatozoa into the cervical mucus, thereby giving the acrosin-inhibiting compound more chance to be effective. Investigators are now working to improve these compounds by making them of such a composition that they reach the spermatozoa more rapidly.

Surfactants have a slight disadvantage because they tend to stick to surfaces such as the semen coagulum and therefore do not move as rapidly as do low molecular weight inhibitors. Efficacy will depend on how many spermatozoa enter the cervical mucus. If 99.9% of the spermatozoa are inactivated, the preparation will be very effective; if only 75% of the spermatozoa are inactivated, the preparation may not be sufficiently effective. The delivery systems for these compounds can themselves have a contraceptive effect. Nonoxynol 9, when combined with a diaphragm, results in very few method failures; these new compounds, combined with an effective delivery system, should be even more effective.

WHAT IS THE MECHANISM OF ACTION OF THE ACROSIN INHIBITOR?

Proacrosin conversion to acrosin, at least in nonhuman species, seems to occur at least partially during the acrosome reaction; any further conversion occurs during the subsequent penetration of the zona. These inhibitors have been shown not only to inhibit human acrosin but also to prevent the conversion of proacrosin to acrosin. When human spermatozoa are incubated with inhibitors, and acrosin levels subsequently decrease, it is not clear if the proacrosin has been converted to acrosin and then the total amount of acrosin is inhibited, or whether proacrosin conversion to acrosin is itself inhibited. Presently, it appears that conversion of proacrosin to acrosin can be inhibited, but we do not know the mechanism. It may bind to the small amount of active acrosin involved in the conversion of proacrosin to acrosin, or bind the proacrosin directly, or it may inhibit some type of converting enzyme.

HOW DOES ORF-13904 INTERACT WITH MUCUS?

ORF-13904 is a polycation, and polycationic polymers have been shown to interact on a charge basis with a mucus glycoprotein. In the extreme interaction, precipitation may occur. One of the more important features one must look at in a compound of this nature is how easily it can diffuse into the mucus. The compound was mixed directly with the mucus in the present study. This type of interaction frequently has a negative effect on the movement of the compound into the mucus. When the compound was formulated in a water-base formulation, effectiveness was much improved over the oil-base.

HOW DO RESULTS OF OTHER STUDIES WITH INTRATESTICULAR INJECTIONS OF THP COMPARE WITH THE PRESENT STUDY?

Investigators using a protocol perhaps different from the one presented found that in testicular tissue from injected animals, everything was destroyed in the center of the injection site; even the Leydig cells were gone. Normal tissue was found only in the surrounding areas. The investigators also found permanent elevation of FSH but no change in testosterone levels. Saline alone, at the same osmolarity as the glycerol preparation, had the same effect.

Wiebe's group have done these studies in nearly 1000 rats, however, and on only a few occasions, in isolated areas within the testis, have the investigators seen such destruction. In their experience, the injected material simply pushed aside the tubules. Hormone determinations, performed many times in rats, revealed no changes in gonadotropins and testosterone.

Hormonal Approaches

27

Androgen-Progestogen Combinations

C. ALVIN PAULSEN

These past 15 years have seen concerted and systematic efforts to develop new chemical male contraceptive agents. Before these efforts were initiated, general guidelines were established as reasonable goals for such agents to be successful. When such agents are administered, the inhibition of sperm production would have to occur without any significant accompanying adverse reaction, and, when the chemical agent was discontinued, sperm production should return to previous levels and the subject should regain his previous state of fertility.

On the basis of available animal studies and clinical investigation data, one class of compounds appeared to be reasonable for study, namely, the synthetic progestational steroids. For some time it has been known that the 19-norprogestational compounds, such as norethindrone and norethynodrel, were potent when given orally in terms of suppressing gonadotropin secretion by the anterior pituitary. When they were administered to normal adult males, testicular function was effectively suppressed and sperm counts decreased sharply.[7] These preparations possessed two drawbacks, however; they also suppressed testosterone levels, and a decrease in libido and sexual potency was observed. Also, they exerted estrogenic effects when administered to men.[9,11] This was evidenced by the development of gynecomastia more frequently and much more severely than occurs with the administration of various forms of androgens. The decrease in testosterone levels could have been solved by simultaneously administering testosterone, but the latter could not.

This led to the consideration of using a less potent gonadotropin inhibitor, medroxyprogesterone acetate. This steroid does not possess estrogenic properties. For the clinical trials, both the oral form and the "depo" preparation, given intramuscularly, were compared for their efficacy in suppressing spermatogenesis. In addition, testosterone was added to the regimen both for its demonstrated synergistic action in inhibiting gonadotropin secretion and to ensure a reasonably steady level of testosterone so that libido and sexual potency would remain intact. These small, well-monitored clinical trials were conducted in several centers throughout the world, supported primarily by the World Health Organization, the Population Council, and the Ford Foundation.

Portions of this work were supported by grant P-50-HD 12629, WHO grant H9-445-20, Ford Foundation grant 730-0853, and a grant-in-aid from Upjohn Laboratories.

TESTOSTERONE AND ORAL MEDROXYPROGESTERONE ACETATE

One center studied the effects of methyltestosterone plus medroxyprogesterone acetate, both given orally. Bain reported that this combination induced oligospermia in only a few of his volunteers and none developed azoospermia.[1] The daily doses of methyltestosterone used were 5 mg, 10 mg, and 20 mg, whereas at the same time medroxyprogesterone acetate was administered in daily doses, ranging from 5 mg to 20 mg.

Even when the oral form of medroxyprogesterone acetate was used in conjunction with testosterone enanthate, 250 mg or 500 mg once monthly, the degree of oligospermia achieved was quite variable.

Several centers evaluated the effect of depomedroxyprogesterone acetate (DMPA) plus testosterone enanthate (TE) or cypionate (TC), both administered once monthly. The clinical trials supported by the Population Council have been reported previously.[3–5,12] These investigators used a variety of experimental regimens. With DMPA in monthly doses of 150 mg or higher plus TE, of 250 mg or 500 mg, oligospermia or azoospermia was induced in the majority of volunteers.

Three additional centers used a common protocol in terms of pre-drug, drug exposure, and recovery time periods with slightly different dose levels of DMPA plus TE or TC.[8,10,13] The periods called for 3-months pre-drug, 6-months drug exposure, and at least 3-months recovery periods. Seminal fluid samples (SFS) were collected at 2-week intervals throughout the study; physical examinations were performed monthly. At the same time, blood was drawn for toxicology studies and luteinizing hormone (LH), follicle-stimulating hormone (FSH), and testosterone determinations. For these studies, oligospermia was defined as three consecutive SFS showing sperm concentrations of $\leqslant 5$ M/ml. Azoospermia was defined as three consecutive SFS revealing no sperm, and recovery was achieved when three SFS showed sperm concentrations within the pre-drug exposure range for that man.

Dr. Lee reported that over 80% of his volunteers achieved either oligospermia or azoospermia with DMPA in monthly doses of 200 mg or 400 mg, plus TC in monthly doses of 200 or 400 mg.[8] Dr. Cheviakoff and colleagues, in a study supported by the WHO, observed similar results.[13] In our own study we found that a combination of 200 mg DMPA, plus 250 mg TC once monthly, produced azoospermia in 56% of men within 6 to 15 weeks (Fig. 27-1). Each of the remaining men achieved oligospermia within 20 weeks. Full recovery occurred in each man between 14 and 60 weeks. Only one man required 60 weeks to recover. All the remaining men showed recovery by 39 weeks (Fig. 27-2). These recovery data are in agreement with those of Brenner and co-workers.[3] No decrease in libido and sexual potency was noted by our volunteers during the drug exposure period. No laboratory changes occurred to indicate liver or other toxicity; but we did note a transient drop in mean HDL levels of 15% in each of the three dose groups of men. This transient drop occurred after drug exposure had been discontinued at this time, serum testosterone levels were still below the normal male range in 38% to 80% of the men, depending on the dose of DMPA (*e.g.,* 50 mg–200 mg DMPA 1×/mo). We have no clear explanation for this transient drop, which began 1 month after drug exposure was stopped and lasted approximately 3

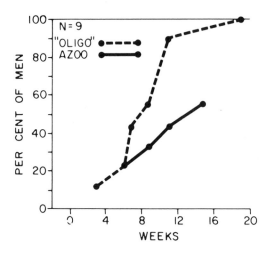

FIG. 27-1. Time to oligospermia and azoospermia when depomedroxyprogesterone acetate (200 mg/mo) in addition to testosterone cypionate (250 mg/mo) were given. (From Paulsen CA, Bremner WJ, Leonard JM: Male contraception: Clinical trials. In Mishell DR Jr (ed): Advances in Fertility Research, p. 157. New York, Raven Press, 1982)

months.[6] Additional nonestrogenic synthetic progestational agents could be studied beyond the few trials that already have been conducted, but these preparations do not appear to show any greater promise than do TE or TC plus DMPA.

Clearly, the issue of the transient drop in high-density lipoprotein (HDL) levels needs verification. Beyond that, the fundamental issue remaining is the presence of oligospermia in some of the volunteers and what it means in terms of an actual method failure rate. Barfield and associates have called attention to the possibility of unplanned pregnancies occurring in the presence of sperm counts below 1M/ml.[2] If the entire clinical experience with various steroidal agents, LHRH agonists, or the animal data of any other known compound is

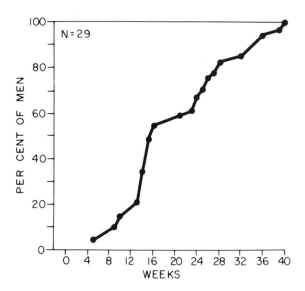

FIG. 27-2. Time to recovery when depo-medroxyprogesterone acetate and testosterone cypionate (250 mg/mo) were stopped. (From Advances in Fertility Research. New York, Raven Press, 1982)

considered, it seems evident that it is not possible to induce azoospermia in 100% of cases in a safe and reversible manner. This observation suggests that there is a need to determine the actual method failure rate associated with induction of oligospermia in a carefully designed, well-monitored, multicentered clinical trial. There would have to be a safeguard for stopping the trial; that is, if the failure rate appears to exceed that of condom use, the trial should be discontinued.

REFERENCES

1. BAIN J, ROCHLIS V, ROBERT E, KHAIT Z: The combined use of oral medroxyprogesterone acetate and methyltestosterone in a male contraceptive trial programme. Contraception 21:365, 1980
2. BARFIELD A, MELO J, COUTINHO E, ALVAREZ-SANCHES F, FAUNDES A, BRACHE V, LEON P, FRICK J, BARTSCH G, WEISKE WH, BRENNER P, MISHELL D JR, BERNSTEIN G, ORTIZ A: Pregnancies associated with sperm concentrations below 10 million/ml in clinical studies of a potential male contraceptive method, monthly depot medroxyprogesterone acetate and testosterone esters. Contraception 20:121, 1979
3. BRENNER PF, MISHELL DR JR, BERNSTEIN GS, ORTIZ A: Study of medroxyprogesterone acetate and testosterone enanthate as a male contraceptive. Contraception 15:679, 1977
4. FRICK J, BARTSCH G, WEISKE WH: The effect of monthly depo-medroxyprogesterone acetate and testosterone on human spermatogenesis. I. Uniform dosage level. Contraception 15:649, 1977
5. FRICK J, BARTSCH G, WEISKE WH: The effect of monthly depot medroxyprogesterone acetate and testosterone on human spermatogenesis. II. High initial dose. Contraception 15:669, 1977
6. FRIEDL KE, PLYMATE SR, PAULSEN CA: Transient reduction in serum HDL-cholesterol following medroxyprogesterone acetate and testosterone cypionate administration to healthy men. Contraception 31:409, 1985
7. HELLER CG, MOORE DJ, PAULSEN CA, NELSON WO, LAIDLAW WM: Effects of progesterone and synthetic progestins on the reproductive physiology of normal men. Fed Proc 18:1057, 1959
8. LEE HY, KIM SI, KWON EH: Clinical trial on reversible male contraceptive with long-acting sex hormones. Seoul J Med 20:1, 1979
9. PAULSEN CA: Progestin metabolism: Special reference to estrogenic pathways. Metabolism 14:313, 1965
10. PAULSEN CA, BREMNER WJ, LEONARD JM: Male contraception: Clinical trials. In MISHELL DR JR (ed): Advances in Fertility Research, p 157. New York, Raven Press, 1982
11. PAULSEN CA, LEACH RB, LANMAN J, GOLDSTON H, MADDOCK WO, HELLER CG: The inherent estrogenicity of norethindrone and norethynodrel: Comparison with other synthetic progestins and progesterone. J Clin Endocrinol 22:1033, 1962
12. SCHEARER SB, ALVAREZ-SANCHEZ F, ANSELMO J, BRENNER P, COUTINHO E, LATHAM-FAUNDES A, FRICK J, HEINILD B, JOHANSSON EDB: Hormonal contraception for men. Int J Androl 1 (Suppl 2): 680, 1978
13. Special Programme of Research, Development and Research Training in Human Reproduction. World Health Organization, Seventh Annual Report, Geneva, p 92, 1978

28

Testosterone–Estradiol Contraception in the Male Rhesus Monkey

LARRY L. EWING

Androgens have been tested extensively as male contraceptive agents in laboratory animals and in humans.[8,13] The major difficulty encountered by investigators in development of an androgenic male contraceptive has been inconsistent inhibition of spermatogenesis.[8,13] This problem led investigators to study androgen–progestogen,[5,14] androgen–danazol,[23,26] and androgen–estrogen[3,10] combinations. To date, androgen–progestogen and androgen–danazol combinations have failed to uniformly produce azoospermia.

Briggs and Briggs have shown that oral administration of methyltestosterone and ethynyl estradiol to five adult men caused azoospermia.[3] This azoospermia was accompanied by infertility. Return to pretreatment semen content of spermatozoa was attained within 35 weeks.[3] No sustained deleterious effects were observed.[3]

Some time ago we completed an extensive series of investigations testing the effect of testosterone–estradiol Silastic subdermal implants on spermatogenesis, sexual behavior, and fertility in male rats.[2,7,10,11,21] We discovered that there is a synergistic inhibition of spermatogenesis in rats (U.S. Patent #4,210,644) simultaneously administered testosterone and estradiol by means of subdermal Silastic implants.[10]

Contraceptive doses of testosterone–estradiol inhibit luteinizing hormone (LH) release, testicular testosterone production, spermatogenesis,[7,10] and subsequently, fertility.[11] Most importantly, the sterility in rats is reversible[11] and is achieved without alteration of either sexual or aggressive behavior and accessory sex organ weight.[11]

EFFECT OF TESTOSTERONE–ESTRADIOL SILASTIC IMPLANTS ON TESTIS FUNCTION OF MALE RHESUS MONKEYS (*MACACA MULATTA*)

Twenty monkeys were divided into two groups of ten to match body weight, seminal volume, and sperm output in control (n = 10) and the testosterone–estradiol-treated group (n = 10). Control monkeys received subdermal Silastic implants filled with cholesterol. The treated monkeys received

This review was supported in part by the National Institute of Child Health and Human Development through Research Grant #07204 and Population Center Grant #06268.

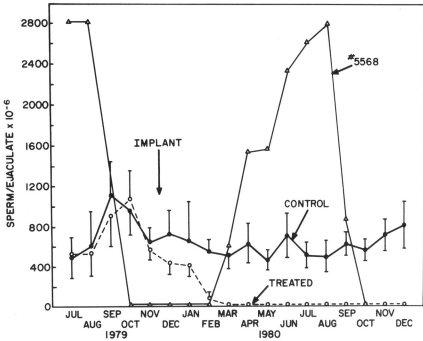

FIG. 28-1. Spermatozoa per ejaculate in control and testosterone–estradiol treated monkeys. With the exception of monkey #5568, each point represents the mean of data derived for semen collected twice per month by electroejaculation from ten control and nine treated monkeys. The vertical bars represent the standard error of the mean. (Ewing LL, Cochran RC, Adams RJ *et al.:* Testis function in Rhesus monkeys treated with a contraceptive steroid formulation. Contraception 27:347–362, 1983)

testosterone and estradiol Silastic implants designed to deliver 100 μg testosterone and 0.5 μg estradiol per kg body weight per day. Semen and blood samples were collected periodically for 18 months. The testosterone and estradiol Silastic capsules were implanted subdermally 5 months after initiation of the experiment. The monkeys were sacrificed 13 months after subdermal placement of the testosterone–estradiol Silastic implants (18 mo after initiation of blood and semen collection) by an overdose of sodium pentobarbital. Refer to Ewing and colleagues[9] for a complete description of materials and methods.

SPERM PRODUCTION

Seven hundred and twenty attempts were made to collect semen by means of electroejaculation from the twenty monkeys during the course of the experiment. Control monkeys provided measurable ejaculates 83% of the time; steroid-treated monkeys, 90% of the time. The results in Figure 28-1 show the number of spermatozoa per ejaculate of control and testosterone–estradiol treated monkeys. The sperm count of control monkeys varied from 500×10^6

to 1100×10^6. With the exception of monkey #5568, the sperm production of treated monkeys decreased dramatically after implantation of the steroid-filled capsules. Monkey #5568 was obviously aberrant, becoming azoospermic 6 weeks prior to the initiation of steroid treatment. Unexpectedly, the sperm production of this monkey increased to 2800×10^6 spermatozoa per ejaculate during the course of the steroid treatment, then declined rapidly, and the monkey remained azoospermic thereafter.

The percentage and rate of sperm motility were measured using a scale of 0% to 100% for percentage and 0 to 4 for rate of motility. The average percent and rate of sperm motility in control monkeys was 62% and 2.8, respectively. Ejaculates from steroid-treated monkeys contained too few poorly motile spermatozoa to assess the percentage and rate of motility accurately, however, the low numbers of sperm present in the ejacula of steroid-treated monkeys showed little progressive motility.

PERIPHERAL BLOOD HORMONE CONCENTRATIONS

Male rhesus monkeys exhibit a dramatic diurnal variation in serum concentration of LH and testosterone.[20,25] The serum concentration of FSH, LH, testosterone, and estradiol in control and steroid-treated monkeys therefore was measured in serum collected between 0900 and 1100 hours (morning, with lights on) and between 2100 and 2400 hours (evening, with lights off). The results also were expressed as the mean of the light and dark period (morning + evening).

The results in Figure 28-2 show that there was no difference in serum FSH concentration between control and treated monkeys at any time of the day. In contrast, serum LH concentrations were lower in steroid-treated monkeys than in the controls during the dark period (2100–2400 hrs, evening, with lights off), when serum LH is elevated in control monkeys. Identical results were obtained when LH was measured by means of a bioassay procedure.[9] Thus, the testosterone–estradiol treatment significantly inhibited LH but not FSH production.

Figure 28-3 shows the serum concentrations of testosterone (left panels) and estradiol (right panels) in control and steroid-treated monkeys during the morning, evening, and the average of both. Although the serum testosterone concentration in steroid-treated monkeys was elevated compared to control monkeys during the morning, there was no significant difference between treatments during the evening or the average of morning and evening values (left panels, Fig. 28-3). In contrast, the serum concentration of estradiol was significantly ($p < 0.05$) higher in treated than control monkeys regardless of the time of day (upper, middle, and lower right panels, Fig. 28-3). These observations raise the question of whether the treatment effects on serum testosterone and estradiol concentrations actually reflect biologically important elevations in steroid production rate.

TESTOSTERONE AND ESTRADIOL BLOOD PRODUCTION RATE

The concentration of testosterone and estradiol in peripheral blood is the net result of production from steroid-secreting organs and peripheral conversion of steroidogenic precursors versus metabolism and excretion. The 24-hour

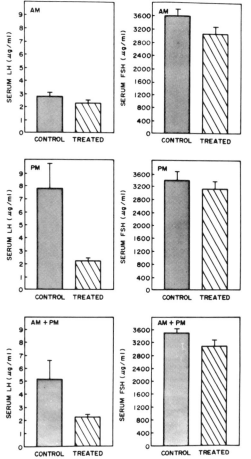

FIG. 28-2. Upper, middle, and lower left panels show serum LH concentrations during morning (lights on), evening (lights off) and the average of both. Upper, middle, and lower right panels show serum FSH concentrations during morning (lights on), evening (lights off) and the average of both. Each bar represents the mean. The morning and evening panels represent the mean of 10 monkeys from which blood was collected on two separate dates in the fall of 1980. The T represents the standard error of the mean. Stippled bars equal control; cross-hatched bars, testosterone–estradiol treated monkeys. (Ewing LL, Cochran RC, Adams RJ *et al.:* Testis function in Rhesus monkeys treated with a contraceptive steroid formulation. Contraception 27:347–362, 1983)

blood production rate (P_B) of testosterone and estradiol is derived by multiplying the metabolic clearance rate (MCR) of each steroid by its concentration in peripheral blood.

Testosterone and estradiol MCRs were determined for control (n = 10) and treated (n = 10) monkeys, which were divided further into groups in which MCR was determined during the period from 0900 to 1100 hours (n = 5) or from 2100 to 2400 hours (n = 5). There was no significant effect of treatment or time of day on the MCR of either steroid. The MCR for each steroid in each monkey was multiplied by the serum steroid concentration measured during MCR determination to calculate 24-hour P_B. There was no effect of time of day on P_B of either steroid and therefore results are expressed as mean P_B of testosterone or estradiol during the morning plus evening in Figure 28-4. There was no significant effect of treatment on the 24-hour P_B of either testosterone or estradiol (Fig. 28-4).

Taken together, these results show that the testosterone–estradiol contraceptive formulation inhibits LH release, and subsequently spermatogenesis, in

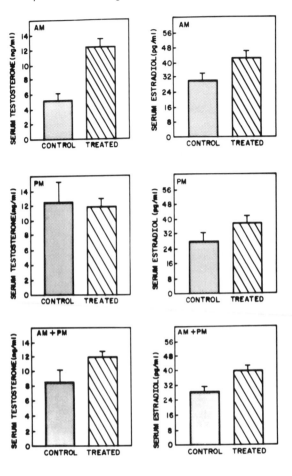

FIG. 28-3. Upper, middle, and lower left panels show serum testosterone concentrations during morning (lights on), evening (lights off), and the average of both. Upper, middle, and lower right panels show serum estradiol concentrations during morning (lights on), evening (lights off), and the average of both. Each bar represents the mean. The morning and evening panels represent the mean of 10 monkeys from which blood was collected on two separate dates in the fall of 1980. The T represents the standard error of the mean. Stippled bars equal control; cross-hatched bars, testosterone-estradiol treated monkeys. (Ewing LL, Cochran RC, Adams RJ *et al.:* Testis function in Rhesus monkeys treated with a contraceptive steroid formulation. Contraception 27:347–362, 1983)

adult rhesus monkeys. The amount of exogenous testosterone (100 μg/kg/ day) and estradiol (0.5 μg/kg/day) needed to inhibit testis function approximates the amount of testosterone and estradiol produced endogenously in rhesus males because the 24 hour P_B of testosterone and estradiol are not significantly different in steroid-treated monkeys compared to controls.

These latter results raise two important questions about the mechanisms by which the testosterone and estradiol combination induce severe oligospermia–azoospermia. First, why are testosterone and estradiol 24-hour P_B *not* increased significantly in testosterone–estradiol-treated monkeys compared to controls? The answer is that endogenous testicular contributions of testosterone and estradiol are depressed dramatically by the testosterone–estradiol Silastic implant treatment. This was shown when testes from control and testosterone–estradiol-treated monkeys were perfused in vitro at the termination of the experiment with concentrations of LH, which stimulated steroidogenic response of the testis maximally. Testes from control and steroid-treated monkeys secreted, respectively, 23 ± 4 (n = 9) and 1.3 ± 0.3 μg testosterone/testis/hr. Testes from control and steroid-treated monkeys secreted 15.6 ± 1.9 (n = 9) and 3.5 ± 0.6 (n = 9) ngE/testis/hr, respectively.

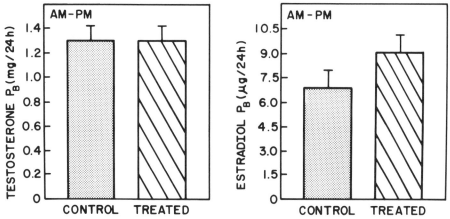

FIG. 28-4. Left panel shows testosterone blood production rate (P_B) and right panel shows estradiol blood production rate (P_B). Each bar represents the mean of five monkeys from which blood was collected from 0900 to 1100 hours, plus 5 monkeys from which blood was collected from 2100 to 2400 hours. The T represents the standard error of the mean. Stippled bars equal control; cross-hatched bars, testosterone–estradiol treated monkeys. (Ewing LL, Cochran RC, Adams RJ *et al.:* Testis function in Rhesus monkeys treated with a contraceptive steroid formulation. Contraception 27:347–362, 1983)

These results suggest that the testicular capacity to produce testosterone and estradiol are inhibited 94% and 78%, respectively. This, combined with the small dose of estradiol required to synergize with testosterone, results in a 24-hour P_B rate of testosterone and estradiol in treated monkeys that is not significantly different than controls. Spermatogenesis fails in the treated monkeys because testosterone emanating from the Silastic capsule is insufficient to maintain the high intratesticular testosterone concentration required for meiosis.

Second, how do what appear to be normal 24-hour P_B rates of testosterone and estradiol suppress circulating LH concentrations so dramatically? At this juncture, the answer to this question is not evident. We can only suggest that this effect is due to a combination of the synergistic interaction between testosterone and estradiol,[10] and that the sustained release of steroids from the Silastic implants exerts a more effective negative feedback on the hypothalamohypophyseal complex than endogenously produced steroids.

SOMATIC AND ACCESSORY SEX ORGAN TISSUE RESPONSES OF MALE RHESUS MONKEYS TO TESTOSTERONE–ESTRADIOL SILASTIC IMPLANTS

We examined the longitudinal effects of testosterone–estradiol Silastic implants on several aspects of somatic and accessory sex organ function in the control and the steroid-treated monkeys described above during a 13-month period. Nineteen of these twenty monkeys were autopsied 13 months after the

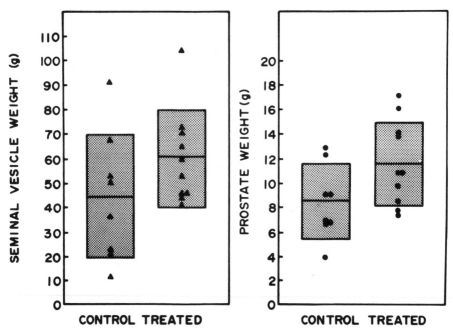

FIG. 28-5. Weight of seminal vesicles and prostate glands from control and treated monkeys. Each point represents organ weight from an individual animal autopsied at the termination of the experiment. The horizontal lines in the middle of each cross-hatched rectangle represents the mean. The hatched area represents one standard deviation about the mean. (Ewing LL, Huber AC, Strandberg JD *et al.:* Somatic tissue responses of male Rhesus monkeys treated with a contraceptive steroid formulation. Contraception 27:363–381, 1983)

subdermal placement of the testosterone–estradiol Silastic implants. Refer to Ewing and colleagues for complete description of methods.[12]

GROSS PATHOLOGY

Control and treated monkeys were identical in weight and both were free of major lesions in the musculoskeletal, circulatory, gastrointestinal, endocrine, and central nervous systems. Particularly noteworthy was the lack of steroid effects on the liver, because hepatic adenomas have been associated with the administration of contraceptive steroids to the human female[27,28] and to rats.[29]

Testes of steroid-treated monkeys were significantly smaller than controls (7.2 g ± 0.9 g versus 22.6 g ± 2.9 g, respectively). These results are reminiscent of those reported for human males treated with androgens.[18,24] To date, this reduction in testicular size has not been perceived to be a problem in males electing treatments that inhibit spermatogenesis.[24]

The results in Figure 28-5 show that seminal vesicles and prostate glands of testosterone–estradiol treated monkeys were slightly, but not significantly heavier than controls. The results in Figure 28-6 show that ejaculate volume

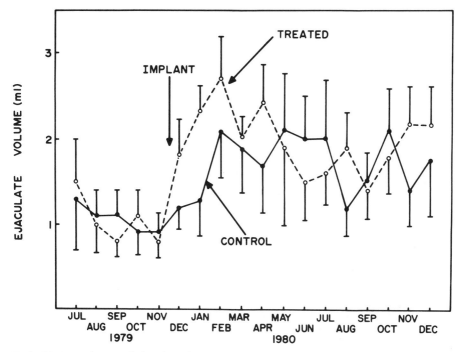

FIG. 28-6. Volume of ejaculate from control and treated monkeys. Each point represents the mean of two semen collections per month from 10 monkeys. The vertical lines represent the standard deviation about the mean. (Ewing LL, Huber AC, Strandberg JD *et al.*: Somatic tissue responses of male Rhesus monkeys treated with a contraceptive steroid formulation. Contraception 27:363–381, 1983)

was significantly ($p < 0.05$) higher in steroid-treated than in control monkeys. The higher mean value (2.3 ± 0.1 ml) for the treated monkeys was within the range of seminal volumes observed for controls, however. Seminal plasma fructose concentrations also were significantly ($p < 0.05$) higher in treated than in control monkeys (15.3 ± 2.0 versus 9.2 ± 2.3 mg/ml; $\bar{x} \pm$ SEM), respectively.

HISTOPATHOLOGY

Somatic Tissues

No histopathologic lesions were observed in the musculoskeletal, circulatory, gastrointestinal, endocrine, and central nervous systems of control and treated monkeys.

Reproductive Tissues

Testes of monkeys receiving the testosterone–estradiol treatment were atrophied, and spermatogenesis was arrested at either the primary or secondary spermatocyte stage. Mature spermatids were observed only occasionally. Epi-

TABLE 28-1. Hematology: Red Blood Cells

CRITERIA	CONTROL		TREATED	
Red blood cells $\times$ 10^3/mm^3	5,812	$\pm$ 138*	6,413	$\pm$ 552
Hematocrit (%)	43	$\pm$ 0.3	43	$\pm$ 0.3
Hemoglobin (g/dl)	14	$\pm$ 0.1	14	$\pm$ 0.1
MCV (μm^3)	76	$\pm$ 0.6	74	$\pm$ 0.6
MCH (pg)	26	$\pm$ 0.3	25	$\pm$ 0.3
MCHC (%)	30	$\pm$ 0.2	30	$\pm$ 0.2
Reticulocytes (%)	0.5 $\pm$	0.2	0.9 $\pm$	0.2

* Mean $\pm$ SEM of 13 blood samples collected from the femoral vein of 10 control and 10 treated monkeys between 0900 and 1100 hours at approximately monthly intervals from November 1979 to December 1980. (Ewing LL, Huber AC, Strandberg JD, Adams RJ, Cochran RC, Desjardins C: Somatic tissue responses of male rhesus monkeys treated with a contraceptive steroid formulation. Contraception 27:363–381, 1983)

didymal tubules of steroid-treated monkeys contained some immature and abnormal spermatozoa.

Seminal vesicles of control and treated monkeys were similar in histologic appearance. The caudal lobe of the prostate of steroid-treated monkeys was characterized by an increased epithelial height and a decreased luminal core of alveoli. The prostatic epithelium did not appear to be "piled up," however, and did not appear to contain a higher proportion of papillary infoldings, which are characteristic of glandular hyperplasia in accessory sex structures.

Apparently, the accessory sex organs of testosterone–estradiol treated monkeys are mildly stimulated, however, these changes are small, and the values for the steroid-treated monkeys are well within the range of values described for control monkeys.

There was no demonstrable effect of the testosterone–estradiol treatment on mammary tissue.

HEMATOLOGY

The results in Tables 28-1 and 28-2 show that the number of red blood cells, hematocrit, hemoglobin, corpuscular volume, corpuscular hemoglobin concentration, reticulocytes, lymphocytes, monophils, and eosinophils were unaffected by treatment of monkeys with testosterone–estradiol Silastic implants.

BLOOD CLOTTING

The values for clotting time, prothrombin time, and partial thromboplastin time were identical for control and steroid-treated monkeys (Table 28-3) and were within the range of values considered normal for male rhesus monkeys.[15,19]

TABLE 28-2. Hematology: White Blood Cells

CRITERIA	CONTROL	TREATED
White blood cells per mm^3	7053 ± 173*	6954 ± 173
Total neutrophils (%)	55 ± 0.8	56 ± 0.8
Lymphocytes (%)	37 ± 0.7	37 ± 0.7
Monophils (%)	3.8 ± 0.16	3.8 ± 0.16
Eosinophils (%)	4.2 ± 0.27	3.4 ± 0.27

* Mean ± SEM of 13 blood samples collected from the femoral vein of 10 control and 10 treated monkeys between 0900 and 1100 hours at approximately monthly intervals from November 1979 to December 1980. (Ewing LL, Huber AC, Strandberg JD, Adams RJ, Cochran RC, Desjardins C: Somatic tissue responses of male rhesus monkeys treated with a contraceptive steroid formulation. Contraception 27:363–381, 1983)

BLOOD CHEMISTRY

Elements

The results in Table 28-4 show that serum calcium, phosphorus, sodium, potassium, chloride, iron, and magnesium concentrations were similar in both control and treated monkeys, and within the range considered normal for healthy male rhesus monkeys.[1,4,16]

Proteins and Enzymes

The results in Table 28-5 show that total protein albumin, albumin/globulin, SGPT, SGOT, γ-glutamyl transpeptidase, and LDH were similar in both control and treated monkeys. In contrast, the alkaline phosphatase level (Table 28-5) was significantly ($p < 0.05$) lower in the blood of treated compared to control monkeys. However, the values for treated monkeys were within the normal range reported by the Animal Reference Laboratory (Division of Medical Technology, Tetersboro, NJ).

TABLE 28-3. Blood Clotting

CRITERIA	CONTROL	TREATED
Blood clotting (sec)	243 ± 7*	239 ± 8
Prothrombin time (sec)	14 ± 0.1	14 ± 0.1
Partial thromboplastin time (sec)	58 ± 0.5	58 ± 0.5

* Mean ± SEM of 13 blood samples collected from the femoral vein of 10 control and 10 treated monkeys between 0900 and 1100 hours at approximately monthly intervals from November 1979 to December 1980. (Ewing LL, Huber AC, Strandberg JD, Adams RJ, Cochran RC, Desjardins C: Somatic tissue responses of male rhesus monkeys treated with a contraceptive steroid formulation. Contraception 27:363–381, 1983)

TABLE 28-4. Blood Chemistry: Elements

CRITERIA	CONTROL	TREATED
Calcium (mg/dl)	9.7 ± 0.05*	9.8 ± 0.05
Phosphorus (mg/dl)	3.7 ± 0.06	3.6 ± 0.06
Sodium (mMol/l)	145 ± 0.7	146 ± 0.7
Potassium (mMol/l)	3.8 ± 0.03	3.8 ± 0.03
Chloride (mMol/l)	107 ± 0.5	107 ± 0.5
Iron (μg/dl)	143 ± 2.7	146 ± 2.7
Magnesium (meq/l)	1.57 ± 0.01	1.61 ± 0.01

* Mean ± SEM of 13 blood samples collected from the femoral vein of 10 control and 10 treated monkeys between 0900 and 1100 hours at approximately monthly intervals from November 1979 to December 1980. (Ewing LL, Huber AC, Strandberg JD, Adams RJ, Cochran RC, Desjardins C: Somatic tissue responses of male rhesus monkeys treated with a contraceptive steroid formulation. Contraception 27:363–381, 1983)

Organics

The results in Table 28-6 show that triglyceride, uric acid, total bilirubin, direct bilirubin, BUN, creatinine, and BUN/creatinine levels were similar in both control and treated monkeys and were within the range reported for normal male rhesus monkeys.[1,4,16] In contrast, the results in Table 28-6 show that the blood cholesterol level was higher and blood glucose concentrations were lower in steroid-treated compared to control monkeys.

The marginal changes in alkaline phosphatase, cholesterol, and glucose probably are not clinically important, for several reasons. First, we did not observe these changes in another group of monkeys treated identically with

TABLE 28-5. Blood Chemistry: Proteins

CRITERIA	CONTROL	TREATED
Total protein (g/dl)	7.0 ± 0.05*	7.0 ± 0.05
Albumin (g/dl)	4.1 ± 0.04	4.1 ± 0.04
Albumin/globulin	1.5 ± 0.02	1.5 ± 0.02
SGPT (IU/L)	50.3 ± 1.5	56.5 ± 1.5
SGOT (IU/L)	48.8 ± 1.7	48.1 ± 1.7
Alkaline phosphatase (IU/L)	60.5 ± 1.6	50.9 ± 1.6†
r-Glutamyl transpeptidase (IU/liter)	28.9 ± 0.4	29.1 ± 0.4
LDH (IU/liter)	506 ± 16	490 ± 15

* Mean ± SEM of 13 blood samples collected from the femoral vein of 10 control and 10 treated monkeys between 0900 and 1100 hours at approximately monthly intervals from November 1979 to December 1980. (Ewing LL, Huber AC, Strandberg JD, Adams RJ, Cochran RC, Desjardins C: Somatic tissue responses of male rhesus monkeys treated with a contraceptive steroid formulation. Contraception 27:363–381, 1983)

† p < 0.05

TABLE 28-6. Blood Chemistry: Organics

CRITERIA	CONTROL	TREATED
Cholesterol (mg/dl)	135 ± 1.9*	151 ± 1.9†
Triglycerides (mg/dl)	92 ± 3	82 ± 3
Uric acid (mg/dl)	0.24 ± 0.01	0.23 ± 0.01
Total bilirubin (mg/dl)	0.23 ± 0.02	0.21 ± 0.02
Direct bilirubin (mg/dl)	0.08 ± 0.002	0.07 ± 0.002
Glucose (mg/dl)	81.7 ± 1.4†	68.4 ± 1.4†
BUN	23.3 ± 0.4	21.6 ± 0.04
Creatinine (mg/dl)	1.6 ± 0.02	1.6 ± 0.02
BUN/creatinine	15.3 ± 0.3	14.0 ± 0.3

* Mean ± SEM of 13 blood samples collected from the femoral vein of 10 control and 10 treated monkeys between 0900 and 1100 hours at approximately monthly intervals from November 1979 to December 1980. (Ewing LL, Huber AC, Strandberg JD, Adams RJ, Cochran RC, Desjardins C: Somatic tissue responses of male rhesus monkeys treated with a contraceptive steroid formulation. Contraception 27:363–381, 1983)

† p < 0.05

testosterone–estradiol Silastic implants.[17] Second, the increase in alkaline phosphatase occurred in the control rather than in the steroid-treated monkeys. Third, none of the changes was statistically significant when analyzed in terms of a mixed linear model analysis of variance, which removed the effect of time as a source of variance. Instead, this type of analysis showed a significant effect of time, which suggested significant variance in serum alkaline phosphatase, cholesterol, and glucose concentrations during the 13-month experiment. We suggest that these slight changes in blood serum alkaline phosphatase, cholesterol, and glucose concentrations are due to random variation in blood sampling, batch-to-batch variation in food sources, and analytical procedures, rather than to meaningful pathophysiologic changes.[6]

In summary, these results demonstrate that the testosterone–estradiol formulation inhibits spermatogenesis without significantly perturbing somatic tissues, the ionic, chemical, and formed elements of blood, or secondary sex structures, including the mammary gland.

CONTRACEPTIVE EFFICACY OF TESTOSTERONE–ESTRADIOL IMPLANTS IN MALE RHESUS MONKEYS

Given the above positive results, the question of the contraceptive efficacy of testosterone–estradiol Silastic implants in rhesus monkeys was addressed. Ten rhesus monkeys were selected from a group of fertile males. Five were assigned randomly to control and five to a treated group, which received 100 μgT and 0.5 μgE per kg body weight per day.

Lobl and colleagues provide a complete description of this study.[17] Briefly, the experiment was divided into three parts: pretreatment, treatment, and post-treatment, which lasted for 6, 40, and 30 weeks, respectively. Breeding trials were carried out, and blood and semen samples were collected at various

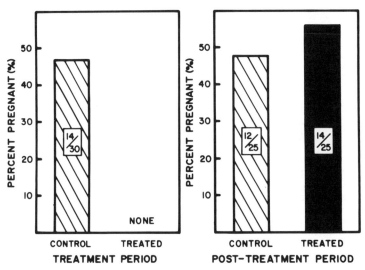

FIG. 28-7. The left panel shows the percent pregnant for control (*cross-hatched*) and treated (*black*) monkeys during the treatment phase of the study. The right panel shows the percent pregnant for control (*cross-hatched*) and treated (*black*) monkeys during the post-treatment phase of the study. The insert in each bar shows the number of pregnancies attained per the number of successful matings. (Lobl TJ, Kirton KT, Forbes AD *et al.*: Contraceptive efficacy of testosterone–estradiol implants in male Rhesus monkeys. Contraception 27:383–389, 1983)

times during the course of the study.[17] Two breeding trials were completed: one during the treatment and another during the post-treatment phase of the study.

Males were mated with fertile females until each had completed six (during treatment phase) and five (during post-treatment phase) successful matings, as evidenced by the presence of a seminal plug in the cage. The bred females were maintained until pregnancy was diagnosed by manual palpation.

FERTILITY

Figure 28-7 shows the results of breeding trials completed during the treatment period (left panel) and post-treatment period (right panel). Results in the left panel of Figure 28-7 shows that while 47% of control matings were fertile, none of the 30 matings by the contracepted monkeys were fertile. The results in the right panel of Figure 28-7 show that the fertility of the treated males was restored to control levels during the post-treatment period after removal of the testosterone–estradiol Silastic implants. Sexual behavior in the treated monkeys probably was unaffected by the steroid treatment because seminal plugs were observed in the cages of control and treated monkeys with the same frequency. The complete and reversible infertility in rhesus monkeys caused by the testosterone–estradiol treatment was identical to that observed in rats[11] and humans[3] treated with androgen–estrogen formulations. No other male contraceptive formulation has been reported to be as efficacious.

TABLE 28-7. The Effect of Testosterone-Estradiol Treatment on Semen Volume, Spermatozoa Numbers, Motility, and Morphology During the Treatment Phase of the Study

CRITERIA	CONTROL	TREATED
Semen volume (ml)	1.8 ± 0.2*	2.0 ± 0.4
Spermatozoa/ejaculate × 10⁶	1046 ± 102	74 ± 28†
Motility rate (0–4)	2.4 ± 0.3	0.2 ± 0.1†
Motile spermatozoa (%)	82 ± 3	18 ± 6†
Normal morphology (%)	75 ± 4	11 ± 4†

 * Mean ± SEM of 10 semen samples collected from 5 control and 5 treated monkeys 16 weeks and 40 weeks after implantation of the contraceptive steroids.

 † p < 0.01 (Lobl TJ, Kirton KT, Forbes AD, Ewing LL, Kemp PL, Desjardins C: Contraceptive efficacy of testosterone–estradiol implants in male rhesus monkeys. Contraception 27:383–389, 1983)

SEMEN CHARACTERISTICS

The results in Table 28-7 show that semen volume was identical in control and treated monkeys but that sperm per ejaculate, motility rate, percent motile spermatozoa, and percent normal morphology were significantly (p < 0.01) lower in treated than in control monkeys. Spermatozoa per ejaculate declined below 1×10^6 in only one of five treated monkeys. Therefore, azoospermia is not essential to render rhesus monkeys infertile. Presumably, infertility results because the few remaining sperm in the ejaculate are abnormal in form and/ or weakly motile.

This raises the issue of whether abnormal spermatozoa in an oligospermic contracepting male can result in an increased incidence of congenital abnormalities, should pregnancy occur. Several points are worth considering. The results of the present study show clearly that the weakly motile and/or abnormally shaped spermatozoa were incapable of creating a palpable embryonic–placental mass in test females.[17] Therefore, if fertilization occurred, the abnormal embryos were resorbed. This latter possibility probably was not the case because we found no evidence of prolonged menstrual cycles in females mated with treated rhesus males.[17]

Finally, there is little reason to expect that weakly motile and/or abnormally shaped sperm in men treated with an antispermatogenic contraceptive formulation will cause an increased incidence of congenital abnormalities because the ejaculates of normal men contain a high percentage of abnormal forms of spermatozoa.[22] In fact, a human semen sample is considered normal by some authors even if it contains 40% abnormal forms.[22]

CONCLUSION

Treatment of male rhesus monkeys with 100 µg testosterone plus 0.5 µg estradiol per kg body weight per day by means of subdermal Silastic implants inhibits endogenous LH production, testosterone production, and subsequently spermatogenesis. This is accomplished with doses of steroid that do not significantly increase the 24-hour blood production rate of testosterone and estradiol in treated monkeys above that of control monkeys.

In contrast to the dramatic inhibition of spermatogenesis and decrease in testis size, there are no clinically important side-effects of the testosterone–estradiol formulation on the gross pathology or histopathology of somatic and accessory sex organs, and no clinically important changes in red blood cell number and function, white blood cell number, blood clotting characteristics, and blood chemistry.

Importantly, the testosterone–estradiol contraceptive formulation causes a complete and reversible infertility in mature monkeys that is accompanied by dramatic changes in sperm number per ejaculate and motility of spermatozoa. The complete and reversible infertility caused by the testosterone–estradiol contraceptive formulation coupled with the lack of secondary complications provides justification for further evaluation of this contraceptive technique in human males.

Experiments should next be completed on the long-term effects of the testosterone–estradiol contraceptive formulation on canine somatic tissues and prostatic structure and function because the aged dog, like man, has a significant incidence of benign prostatic hyperplasia. In addition, high-dose toxicology studies, including assessment of somatic tissues, breast, and accessory sex organ structure and function, must be completed in nonhuman primates. Finally, a practical method of delivering testosterone and estradiol to human males must be developed.

REFERENCES

1. ANDERSON DR: Normal values for clinical blood chemistry tests of the *Macaca mulatta* monkey. Am J Vet Res 27:1484–1489, 1966
2. BERNDTSON WE, DESJARDINS C, EWING LL: Inhibition and maintenance of spermatogenesis in rats with polydimethylsiloxane capsules containing various androgens. J Endocrinol 62:125–135, 1975
3. BRIGGS MH, BRIGGS M: Oral contraceptive for men. Nature 252:585–586, 1974
4. CAISEY JD, KING DJ: Clinical chemical values for some common laboratory animals. Clin Chem 26:1877–1879, 1980
5. COUTINHO EM, MELO JF: Successful inhibition of spermatogenesis in man without loss of libido: a potential new approach to male contraception. Contraception 8:207–17, 1973
6. DESJARDINS C: Potential sources of variation affecting studies on pituitary-gonad function. In ALEXANDER N (ed): Animal Models for Research on Contraception and Fertility, pp 13–32. Hagerstown, MD, Harper & Row, 1979
7. DYKMAN DD, COCHRAN R, WISE PM, BARRACLOUGH CA, DUBIN NH, EWING LL: Temporal effects of testosterone–estradiol polydimethylsiloxane subdermal implants on pituitary, Leydig cell, and germinal epithelium function and daily serum testosterone rhythm in male rats. Biol Reprod 25:235–243, 1981
8. EWING LL, ADAMS RJ, COCHRAN RC: The effects of chemicals on spermatogenesis and epididymal maturation of spermatozoa: Experimental principles. In ALEXANDER NJ (ed): Animal Models for Research on Contraception and Fertility, pp 326–343. Hagerstown, Harper & Row, 1979
9. EWING LL, COCHRAN RC, ADAMS RJ, DARNEY KJ JR, BERRY SJ, BORDY MJ, DESJARDINS C: Testis function in rhesus monkeys treated with a contraceptive steroid formulation. Contraception 27:347–362, 1983
10. EWING LL, DESJARDINS C, IRBY DC, ROBAIRE B: Synergistic interaction of testosterone and estradiol on the inhibition of spermatogenesis in rats. Nature 269:409–411, 1977
11. EWING LL, GORSKI RA, SBORDONE RJ, TYLER JV, DESJARDINS C, ROBAIRE B: Testosterone-estradiol–filled polydimethylsiloxane subdermal implants: Effect on fertility and masculine sexual behavior and aggressive behavior. Biol Reprod 21:765–772, 1979

12. EWING LL, HUBER AC, STRANDBERG JD, ADAMS RJ, COCHRAN RC, DESJARDINS C: Somatic tissue responses of male rhesus monkeys treated with a contraceptive steroid formulation. Contraception 27:363–381, 1983
13. EWING LL, ROBAIRE B: Endogenous antispermatogenic agents: Prospects for male contraception. Ann Rev Pharmacol Toxicol 18:167–187, 1978
14. FRICK J: Control of spermatogenesis in men by combined administration of progestin and androgen. Contraception 8:191–206, 1973
15. HUSER H-J: Atlas of Comparative Primate Hematology, pp 1–154. New York, Academic Press, 1970
16. LEWIS JH: Comparative hematology: Rhesus monkeys *Macaca mulatta.* Comp Biochem Physiol 56A:379–383, 1977
17. LOBL TJ, KIRTON KT, FORBES AD, EWING LL, KEMP PL, DESJARDINS C: Contraceptive efficacy of testosterone-estradiol implants in male Rhesus monkeys. Contraception 27:383–389, 1983
18. MAUSS J, BORSCH G, BORMACHER K, RICHTER E, LEYENDECKER G, NOCKE W: Seminal fluid analyses, serum FSH, LH, and testosterone in seven males before, during, and after 250 mg testosterone oenanthate weekly over 21 weeks. In PATANELLI DJ (ed): Proceedings of Hormonal Control of Male Fertility, pp 93–121. Washington, DC, DHEW Pub. No. (NIH) 78–1097, 1977
19. MCCLURE HM: Hematologic, blood chemistry, and cerebrospinal fluid data for Rhesus monkey. In The Rhesus Monkey, Vol. II, Management, Reproduction and Pathology, pp 409–429. New York, Academic Press, 1975
20. PLANT TM: Time course of concentration of circulating gonadotropin prolactin, testosterone, and cortisol in adult male rhesus monkeys *Macaca mulatta* throughout the 24h light–dark cycle. Biol Reprod 25:244–252, 1981
21. ROBAIRE B, EWING LL, IRBY DC, DESJARDINS C: Interactions of testosterone and estradiol-17β on the reproductive tract of the male rat. Biol Reprod 21:455–463, 1979
22. SHERINS RJ, HOWARDS SS: Male infertility. In HARRISON JH, GITTES RF, PERLMUTTER AD, STAMEY TA, WALSH PC (eds): Campbell's Urology, Vol. 1, pp 715–776. Philadelphia, WB Saunders, 1978
23. SKOGLUND RD, PAULSEN CA: Danazol–testosterone combination: A potentially effective means for reversible male contraception. A preliminary report. Contraception 7:357–365, 1973
24. SWERDLOFF RS, PALACIOS A, MCCLURE RD, CAMPFIELD LA, BROSMAN SA: Clinical evaluation of testosterone enanthate in the reversible suppression of spermatogenesis in the human male: Efficacy, mechanism of action and adverse effects. In PATANELLI DJ (ed): Proceedings of Hormonal Control of Male Fertility, pp 41–69. Washington, DC, DHEW Pub. No. (NIH) 78-1097, 1977
25. STEINER RA, PETERSON AP, YU JYL, CONNER H, GILBERT M, TERPENNING B, BREMNER WJ: Ultradian luteinizing hormone and testosterone rhythms in the adult male monkey, *Macaca fascicularis.* Endocrinol 107:1489–1542, 1980
26. ULSTEIN M, NETTO N, LEONARD J, PAULSEN CA: Changes in sperm morphology in normal men treated with Danazol and testosterone. Contraception 12:437–444, 1975
27. VANA J, MURPHY G: Primary malignant liver tumors: Association with oral contraceptives. NY State J Med 79:321–325, 1979
28. VESSEY MP, KAY CR, BALDWIN JA, CLARKE JA, MACLEOD IB: Oral contraceptives and benign liver tumours. Br Med J 6068:1064–1065, 1977
29. YAGER JD JR, YAGER R: Oral contraceptive steroids as promotors of hepatocarcinogenesis in female Sprague–Dawley rats. Cancer Res 40:3680–3685, 1980

29

19-Nortestosterone for Male Fertility Regulation

ULRICH A. KNUTH

HERMANN BEHRE

LUTZ BELKIEN

HINRICH BENTS

EBERHARD NIESCHLAG

It has long been known that administration of gonadal steroids may impair spermatogenesis.[10,11,15] Testosterone alone or androgens in combination with gestagens have been tested for their potential as agents for male fertility regulation (for review see Patanelli and colleagues[17]). To date, no treatment schedule nor any combination of hormones has been able to induce azoospermia in 100% of participating volunteers. Even in men responding with complete disruption of spermatogenesis, testosterone esters have to be given at least every 10 to 12 days to maintain azoospermia because of the relatively short half-life of available preparations.[23]

THE NEED FOR LONG-ACTING ANDROGEN PREPARATIONS WITHOUT INITIAL SERUM PEAK FORMATION AFTER INJECTION

Data from nonhuman primates suggest that testosterone alone may be sufficient to maintain or reinitiate spermatogenesis even in the absence of detectable gonadotropin values.[3,16] One could speculate that peak values of serum testosterone, reached after injection with available testosterone esters, may be high enough to maintain spermatogenesis to a certain extent. Intratesticular testosterone levels under substitution therapy are likely to be much lower than physiologic concentrations. Binding to the androgen receptor is not a linear function of testosterone concentrations, however. Because binding follows a sigmoid curve or logarithmic function, even low concentrations of testosterone may cause sizable receptor occupancy during peaks of serum testosterone concentrations with consequent maintenance of spermatogenesis. To avoid this, a slow-release formulation of an androgen devoid of high-peak concentrations after injection would be required for male fertility control.

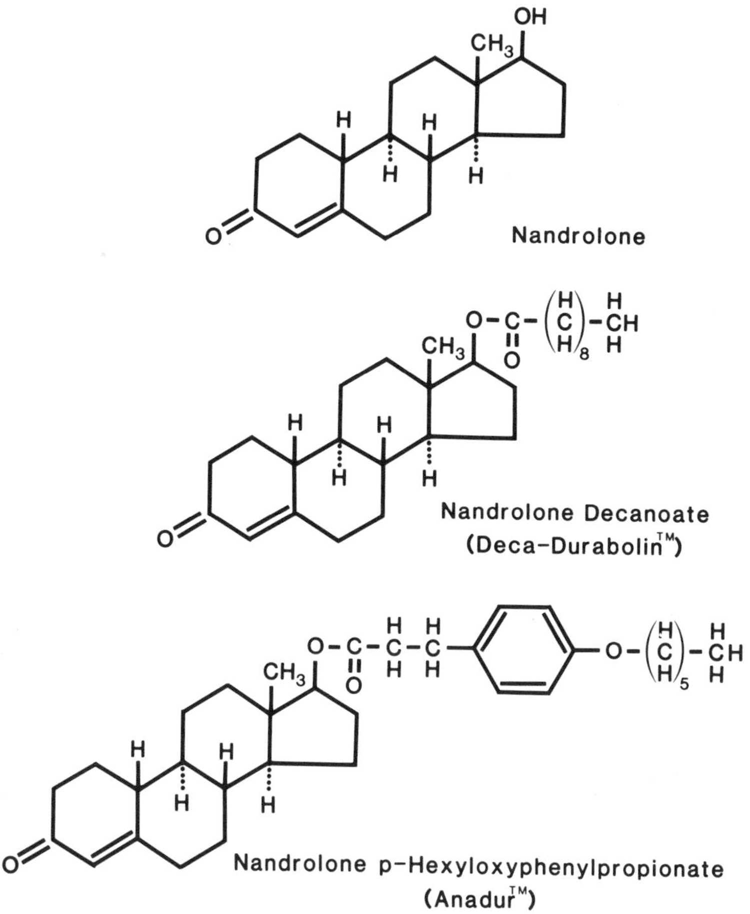

FIG. 29-1. 19-Nortestosterone and its esters.

THE SEARCH FOR AN APPROPRIATE ANDROGEN

Since commercially available testosterone preparations do not provide this characteristic, we looked for other androgenic substances already available on the market.[20,22] In the course of this search, our attention was called to nandrolone (19-nortestosterone, 19NT) and its esters (Fig. 29-1). Since their synthesis and initial testing, they have been used widely as anabolic substances and proved to be without toxic side-effects during many years of clinical use.[6]

PHARMACOKINETIC STUDIES

To characterize commercially available nandrolone esters most suitable for the intended purpose, pharmacokinetic studies with nandrolone hexyloxy-phenylpropionate (Anadur; 19NT-HPP) and nandrolone decanoate (Deca-

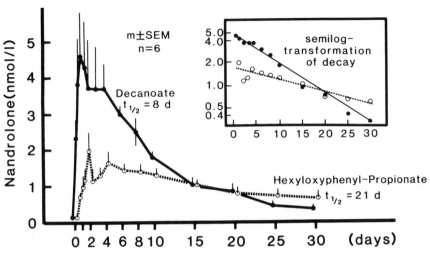

FIG. 29-2. Nandrolone serum levels after IM administration of 50 mg nandrolone decanoate or nandrolone hexyloxyphenylpropionate in a group of six volunteers. (Redrawn after Belkien L, Schürmeyer T, Hano R *et al.*: Pharmacokinetics of 19-nortestosterone esters in normal men. J Steroid Biochem 22:623–629, 1985)

Durabolin; 19NT-D) were conducted using HPLC separation in combination with a specific radioimmunoassay for detection of 19NT in serum.[1] Both preparations led to rapidly increasing levels of 19NT in the peripheral blood after intramuscular injection. Peak levels were reached within 8 hours of 19NT-D administration, whereas 19NT-HPP injections caused a considerably slower release from the injection site; 24 hours were required to reach maximal serum concentrations of nandrolone (Fig. 29-2). Magnitude of peak serum levels showed an inverse relation with a pronounced peak following 19NT-D injection and a more blunted increase after the 19NT-HPP treatment. In five out of the six volunteers tested in a crossover design, the elimination of 19NT was slower after administration of 19NT-HPP compared to 19NT-D. The mean half-life (±SD) of 19NT-HPP was 21 ± 12 days versus 8 ± 5 days for the decanoate. Based on these data for half-life and peak formation, 19NT-HPP was chosen as the androgen ester suitable for further use in clinical trials for a male antifertility agent.

ANDROGENIC PROPERTIES OF NANDROLONE

Although considered to be mainly an anabolic steroid, the parent compound, nandrolone (19NT), exerts a strong inhibitory effect on gonadotropin secretion. Compared to testosterone, nandrolone binds to the androgen receptor with 54% higher affinity and possesses some gestagenic activity.[5,19,24,25] Like testosterone, 19NT is metabolized by 5-alpha-reductase to the reduced compound, dihydronandrolone (DHNT). In contrast to dihydrotestosterone (DHT), binding affinity of DHNT to the androgen receptor is considerably lower (Fig. 29-3). Binding data imply stronger androgenic activity in all target

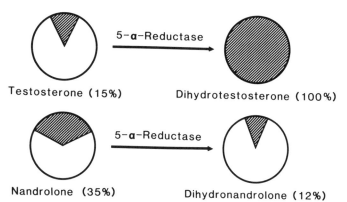

FIG. 29-3. Relative binding of testosterone, nandrolone, and their metabolites to the androgen receptor. (Redrawn after Toth M, Zakar T: Relative binding affinities of testosterone, 19-nortestosterone and their 5-alpha-reduced derivatives to the androgen receptor and to other androgen binding proteins: A suggested role of 5-alpha-reductive steroid metabolism in the dissociation of "myotropic" and "androgenic" activities of 19-nortestosterone. J Steroid Biochem 17:653–660, 1982 and from Toth M, Zakar T: Different binding of testosterone, 19-nortestosterone and their 5-alpha-reduced derivatives to the androgen receptor of the rat seminal vesicle: A step toward the understanding of the anabolic action of nortestosterone. Endokrinologie 80:163–172, 1982)

tissue without 5-alpha-reductase activity and very low androgenic activity in organs with DHT dependence.

PREVIOUS STUDIES WITH ANABOLIC STEROIDS

In view of the favorable pharmacokinetic background, it is surprising that 19NT has not been tested previously for its potential as a male antifertility agent. To our knowledge, no clinical studies have been performed by other groups. Anabolic steroids alkylated in position 17 have been studied for their effects on gonadotropin and testosterone production, but detailed studies on spermatogenesis are virtually nonexistent.[2,4,13,18] A case report has appeared, and a significant reduction in sperm density after 1 and 2 months of daily treatment with methandienone was reported by Holma.[13] In this study three out of fifteen men became azoospermic,[12,14] however treatment time was too short to allow a comprehensive analysis.

CLINICAL TRIALS

PILOT STUDY

To test the potential of 19NT-HPP as a male antifertility agent in more detail, we conducted a pilot study in a small number (n = 5) of volunteers.[21] All of them engaged in heavy physical exercise to improve muscle mass and they expected additional improvement of strength by the anabolic action of the substance to be used.

Participants received 100 mg/week IM injections of 19NT-HPP for 3 weeks, followed by 200 mg/week for the subsequent 10 weeks. Follow-up continued until sperm density again reached more than 20 mil/ml.

During treatment, despite testosterone levels in the range of orchidecto-mized men, none of the volunteers reported a loss of libido or potency. Azoospermia was first observed in one subject after 7 weeks of treatment (Fig. 29-4). By week 13, all participants were azoospermic. Azoospermia persisted for 4 to 14 weeks after treatment. Seminal measurements returned to normal 8 weeks after treatment in one subject, 14 weeks in another, and 20 weeks in two. In the fifth volunteer normalization of seminal parameters took more than 24 weeks, when sperm density was still below 1 mil/ml. During week 30, however, all parameters returned to normal.

During treatment, body weight increased from 87.5 ± 0.9 kg to 94.0 ± 1.9 kg, whereas testicular size was reduced by 50%, lagging behind the fall in sperm count. Since all participants were involved in heavy weight lifting dur-ing the study period, it is difficult to decide whether the increase in weight was caused by the anabolic steroid alone or was attributable to an increase in muscle mass consequent to extreme training.

The absence of impaired libido and impotence in spite of severely reduced testosterone values proved the androgenic potency of 19NT-HPP. Since no other side-effects became apparent, a certain potential of 19NT as a male antifertility agent seemed to be established.

LONG-TERM STUDY

Because of the promising results of the pilot study, the antifertility potential of 19NT-HPP was investigated in greater detail in a larger group of normal volunteers. To exclude bias by extreme exercise and related habits of body-builders, only men with average physical activity, who were not interested in increasing their strength, were recruited for a second study.

Twelve volunteers received 200 mg/wk of 19NT-HPP IM for 7 weeks to allow gradual accumulation of effective 19NT serum levels in a minimum of time. After this initial phase, injection intervals varied between 1 and 3 weeks in an effort to maintain effects on serum gonadotropin values and spermato-genesis at a lower dose of nandrolone administration. Total treatment lasted 25 weeks, succeeded by follow-up examinations for 17 additional weeks. The regimen was supplemented by a final test at week 52. Possible changes in general well-being and sexuality were monitored by standardized tests and specially designed protocols.[7]

Differences in injection intervals during the second half of the treatment phase did not influence any of the parameters measured, except 19NT serum levels themselves. This demonstrates the advantageous influence of the long half-life of the ester used.

As in the pilot study, 19NT treatment generally suppressed serum gonado-tropins below detection limits. This was followed by testosterone levels well in the castrate range. Complete suppression persisted up to week 28.

The subsequent inhibition of spermatogenesis caused azoospermia in two volunteers as early as 9 weeks after the first injection of 19NT-HPP, with an

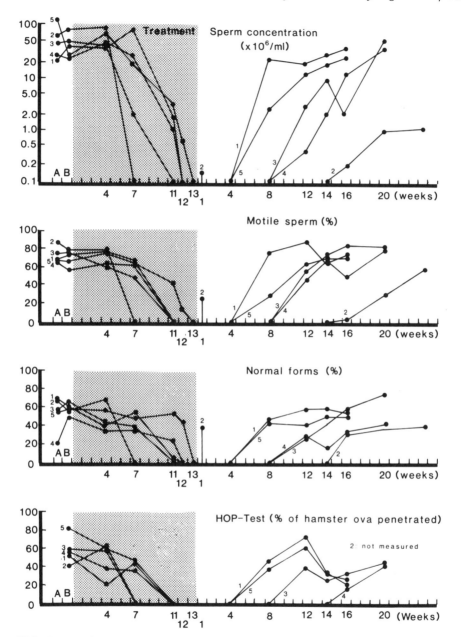

FIG. 29-4. The effect of 19-nortestosterone administration on sperm parameters in five volunteers. Treatment phase of 13 weeks is indicated by shaded area. A and B represent pretreatment control values. (Redrawn after Schürmeyer TH, Knuth UA, Belkien L *et al.:* Reversible azoospermia induced by the anabolic steroid 19-nortestosterone. Lancet i:417–420, 1984)

increasing number of men throughout the following treatment period. Twenty-one days after the last injection, 27 weeks after the start of treatment and theoretically the point at which a maximal impact of treatment could be expected, six volunteers presented with azoospermia; two additional volunteers showed only single sperm in the sediment of the ejaculate, and two had sperm counts below 5 mil/ml. Only two out of twelve men treated with 19NT-HPP revealed sperm counts in the normal range above 20 mil/ml with unimpaired motility, representing a failure rate of 17%. One of them, however, had been azoospermic after 9 and 12 weeks of treatment, with a recovery of sperm counts thereafter.

Normalization in the other participants with sperm concentrations above 20 mil/ml occurred as early as 15 weeks after the last injection and was complete in eleven of the twelve men after 28 weeks of follow-up. The volunteer with sperm counts below 5 mil/ml at week 52 presented with normal values 8 weeks later.

In contrast to the study in body-builders, no significant weight increase occurred. In spite of low testosterone concentrations, no effect on libido or potency became apparent when weekly protocols on several parameters of sexual activity, desire, and functions were evaluated. Complaints about impaired somatic functions or reduction of general well-being were not reported by any of the volunteers.

Administration of 19NT-HPP did not affect liver enzymes, creatinine, uric acid, serum electrolytes or serum lipids; however, hemoglobin, erythrocytes, hematocrit, and mean corpuscular volume (MCV) were significantly elevated following 13 weeks of treatment when compared to pretreatment values. They did not exceed the range considered normal by our laboratory standards, however.

EVALUATION

Both studies presented here provide evidence that 19NT may be used to suppress spermatogenesis in men while its androgenic property is strong enough to maintain libido and potency.

The ideal result of complete azoospermia in all participants at the end of the treatment phase during the small pilot study (with body-builders undergoing extreme physical exercise) could not be achieved in a larger number of men.[21] Nevertheless, the rate of 83% of azoospermia or severe oligospermia with sperm concentrations below 5 mil/ml observed at the end of treatment compares favorably to results achieved with testosterone esters at more frequent injections (for review see Patanelli and colleagues[17]). Because of its long half-life, 19NT-HPP offers a considerable advantage over available testosterone esters, since azoospermia can be maintained in a large number of men with longer intervals between single injections.

Besides the long half-life of the 19NT-ester used and its slow release without pronounced peak levels after injection, the effectiveness of 19NT as a potential male antifertility agent (compared to testosterone) seems to depend greatly on the unique binding characteristics of the parent substance and its reduced metabolite to the androgen receptor already discussed above. We have yet not tried to find the minimal effective dose, but it is to be expected that the psychosexual effect on libido and potency as well as the inhibitory effect on gonadotropin secretion is still maintained at lower concentrations of 19NT. This effect is probable because mediating central brain areas are devoid of 5-alpha-reductase activity and the higher endogenous androgenic activity of nandrolone compared to nonreduced testosterone is of influence.

A potential antifertility agent used by a healthy person has to be beyond the possibility of any adverse effect on general health and well-being, especially when taken for extended periods. In contrast to 17-alkylated steroids, no changes in liver function have been reported with 19NT. Our studies to date also demonstrate the lack of liver toxicity since transaminases were unchanged throughout the entire periods under investigation.

Considering the suppressive action of testosterone on HDL and stimulating effects on LDL (for review see Goldberg and associates[8]) with the consequence of an increased risk of cardiovascular problems, it is of special interest to note that 19NT at doses used did not alter serum triglycerides, cholesterol, or LDL and HDL concentrations.[9]

In summary, one can conclude that 19NT-HPP seems to offer advantages over available testosterone esters as a male antifertility agent. Ongoing and future studies using different dose regimens or the combination with other substances will reveal whether 19NT-HPP will maintain its position in the front line of potential methods for male fertility regulation.

REFERENCES

1. BELKIEN L, SCHÜRMEYER T, HANO R, GUNNARSSON PO, NIESCHLAG E: Pharmacokinetics of 19-nortestosterone esters in normal men. J Steroid Biochem 22:623–629, 1985
2. BIJLSMA JWJ, DUURSMA SA, BOSCH R, HUBER O: Lack of influence of the anabolic steroid nandrolonedecanoate on bone metabolism. Acta Endocrinol (Copenhagen) 101:140–143, 1982
3. BINT AKHTAR F, MARSHALL GR, WICKINGS EJ, NIESCHLAG E: Reversible induction of azoospermia in rhesus monkeys by constant agonist infusion of a gonadotropin-releasing hormone agonist using osmotic minipumps. J Clin Endocrinol Metab 56:534–540, 1983
4. CLERICO A, FERDEGHINI M, PALOMBO C, LEONCINI R, DEL CHICCA MG, SARDANO G, MARIANI G: Effect of anabolic treatment on serum levels of gonadotropins, testosterone, prolactin, thyroid hormones and myoglobin of male athletes under physical training. J Nucl Med Allied Sci 25:279–288, 1981
5. DELETTRÉ J, MORNON JP, LEPICARD G, OJASOO T, RAYNAUD JP: Steroid flexibility and receptor specificity. J Steroid Biochem 13:45–59, 1980
6. DICZFALUSY E, FERNÖ O, FEX H, HÖGBERG B: Long-acting p-alkoxyhydrocinnamic acid esters of steroid hormones. Acta Chem Scand 17:2536–2547, 1963
7. FAHRENBERG J: Die Freiburger Beschwerdeliste FBL. Z Klin Psychiatrie 4:79–100, 1975
8. GOLDBERG RB, RABIN D, ALEXANDER AN, DOELLE GC, GETZ GS: Suppression of plasma testosterone leads to an increase in total and high-density lipoprotein cholesterol and apoproteins A-I and B. J Clin Endocrinol Metab 60:203–207, 1985
9. HAMILTON JB, MESTLER GE: Mortality and survival: Comparison of eunuchs with intact men and women in a mentally retarded population. J Gerontol 24:395–411, 1969
10. HECKEL NJ: Production of oligospermia in a man by the use of testosterone propionate. Proc Soc Exp Biol Med 40:658–659, 1939
11. HELLER CG, NELSON WO, HILL IB, HENDERSON E, MADDOCK WO, JUNGCK EC, PAULSEN CA, MORTIMER GE: Improvement in spermatogenesis following depression of the human testis with testosterone. Fertil Steril 1:415–422, 1950
12. HOLMA PK: Effects of an anabolic steroid (metandienone) on spermatogenesis. Contraception 15:151–162, 1977

13. HOLMA P, ADLERCREUTZ H: Effect of an anabolic steroid (metandienon) on plasma LH, FSH, and testosterone and on the response to intravenous administration of LRH. Acta Endocrinol (Copenhagen) 83:856–864, 1976
14. KILSHAW BH, HARKNESS RA, HOBSON BM, SMITH AWM: The effects of large doses of the anabolic steroid methandrostenolone on an athlete. Clin Endocrinol 4:537–541, 1975
15. LUDWIG DJ: The effect of androgen on spermatogenesis. Endocrinology 46:453–481, 1950
16. MARSHALL GR, WICKINGS EJ, LÜDECKE DK, NIESCHLAG E: Stimulation of spermatogenesis in stalk-sectioned Rhesus monkeys by testosterone alone. J Clin Endocrinol Metab 57:152–159, 1983
17. PATANELLI DJ (ed): Hormonal control of male fertility, Pub. No. 78-1097. Washington, DC, U.S. Dept of Health, Education and Welfare, National Institute of Health, 1978
18. REMES K, VUOPIO P, JÄRVINEN M, HÄRKÖNEN M, ADLERCREUTZ H: Effects of short-term treatment with an anabolic steroid (methandienone) and dihydroepiandrosterone sulphate on plasma hormones, red cell volume and 2,3-diphosphoglycerate in athletes. Scand J Clin Lab Invest 37:577–586, 1977
19. SAARTOK T, DAHLBERG E, GUSTAFSSON JA: Relative binding affinity of anabolic-androgenic steroids: Comparison of the binding to the androgen receptors in skeletal muscle and in prostate, as well as to sex hormone-binding globulin. Endocrinology 114:2100–2106, 1984
20. SCHÜRMEYER TH, NIESCHLAG E: Comparative pharmacokinetics of testosterone enanthate and testosterone cyclohexanecarboxylate as assessed by serum and salivary testosterone levels in normal men. Int J Androl 7:181–187, 1984
21. SCHÜRMEYER TH, KNUTH UA, BELKIEN L, NIESCHLAG E: Reversible azoospermia induced by the anabolic steroid 19-nortestosterone. Lancet i:417–420, 1984
22. SCHULTE-BEERBÜHL M, NIESCHLAG E: Comparison of testosterone, dihydrotestosterone, luteinizing hormone, and follicle-stimulating hormone in serum after injection of testosterone enanthate or testosterone cypionate. Fertil Steril 33:201–203, 1980
23. STEINBERGER E, SMITH KD: Effect of chronic administration of testosterone enanthate on sperm production and plasma testosterone, follicle-stimulating hormone, and luteinizing hormone levels: A preliminary evaluation of a possible male contraceptive. Fertil Steril 28:1320–1328, 1977
24. TOTH M, ZAKAR T: Relative binding affinities of testosterone, 19-nortestosterone and their 5-alpha-reduced derivatives to the androgen receptor and to other androgen binding proteins: A suggested role of 5-alpha-reductive steroid metabolism in the dissociation of "myotropic" and "androgenic" activities of 19-nortestosterone. J Steroid Biochem 17:653–660, 1982
25. TOTH M, ZAKAR T: Different binding of testosterone, 19-nortestosterone and their 5-alpha-reduced derivatives to the androgen receptor of the rat seminal vesicle: A step toward the understanding of the anabolic action of nortestosterone. Endokrinologie 80:163–172, 1982

30

Dissociating Antifertility Effects of a GnRH Antagonist from Its Adverse Effects on Mating Behavior: The Critical Importance of Testosterone Dose

SHALENDER BHASIN

THOMAS J. FIELDER

RONALD S. SWERDLOFF

RATIONALE FOR COMBINED TREATMENT WITH GnRH ANALOGUES AND TESTOSTERONE

Observations that hypophysectomized men and those deficient in LH and FSH are azoospermic have led to attempts to suppress gonadotropins by pharmacologic means as a method for reversible male contraception. Initially, long-acting esters of testosterone were tested, but these agents failed to induce azoospermia predictably in normal men.[19,20] More recently, agonist and antagonist analogues of gonadotropin-releasing hormone (GnRH) have been explored as approaches toward inhibition of gonadotropin secretion.[2,3,5,8,10,16] Such agents, however, result in concomitant decrease in serum testosterone. For example, chronic treatment with GnRH agonist not only leads to reversible oligospermia, but also results in concomitant decrease in serum testosterone, which is attended by an unacceptable decrease in libido and potency.[10] Thus, contraceptive agents that act by suppressing gonadotropins require concomitant androgen replacement to prevent agonist induced changes in libido and potency.

The antagonist analogue for these studies was generously provided by Marvin J. Karten of the Contraceptive Development Branch of the National Institutes of Health. The agonist analogue, nafarelin, used in the GnRH agonist-related studies, was kindly provided by Syntex Research, Palo Alto, CA. The histologic examinations of the testes were performed by Dr. Luciano Zamboni, Professor and Chairman, Department of Pathology, Harbor–UCLA Medical Center, Torrance, CA.

STUDIES WITH GnRH AGONIST AND ANDROGEN IN MAN

Studies with GnRH agonists by our group and several others have demonstrated that the actions of GnRH agonist are biphasic, with an initial stimulatory and a subsequent down regulatory phase.[5,10] Long-term treatment with single daily injections of 200 μg of D(Nal$_2$)[6] GnRH (Syntex Research, Palo Alto, CA) combined with bimonthly injections of testosterone enanthate led to a mean 85% decline in sperm count and to a nadir of 17.4 ± 6.3 mil/ml.[5] One subject did not show significant suppression of sperm count as assessed by regression analysis, however. Thus, this combined regimen of intermittent agonist injection and bimonthly injections of testosterone did not induce azoospermia. These results are similar to those of Doelle and colleagues, who also noted only partial suppression of spermatogenesis with a combined regimen that employed a subsuppressive dose of testosterone.[8]

In more recent studies, in which we administered a higher dose of GnRH agonist (400 μg) by constant subcutaneous infusion combined with bimonthly injections of 200 mg of testosterone enanthate, more consistent suppression of spermatogenesis was achieved but only one out of five subjects, who have completed these studies so far, achieved azoospermia. These data are similar to those reported by Schurmeyer and associates, which also failed to demonstrate predictable azoospermia in men with constant infusion of a relatively smaller dose of buserelin combined with oral testosterone undecanoate.[16] It remains to be seen whether a still higher dose of the GnRH agonist will result in greater suppression of spermatogenesis.

DOES TESTOSTERONE ATTENUATE THE ANTIFERTILITY EFFECTS OF GnRH ANALOGUES?

Whereas the studies in the rat suggested that the addition of androgens to an LHRH agonist regimen treatment would potentiate inhibitory effects of LHRH agonist,[8,9] Akhtar and co-workers reported attenuation of the antifertility effects of an LHRH agonist in the male rhesus monkey by testosterone supplementation.[1] Three adult rhesus monkeys were treated with the LHRH agonist, buserelin, using osmotic minipumps implanted subcutaneously. Testosterone was administered subcutaneously by means of Silastic capsules. All the animals were oligospermic within 8 to 15 weeks of treatment. Azoospermia was, however, not achieved even after 22 weeks of treatment, although in a previous study by the same authors, in which LHRH agonist had been administered alone, azoospermia was achieved after 8 to 10 weeks. These investigators concluded from their data that, in this primate species, testosterone supplementation attenuates the suppressive effects of LHRH agonist infusion on spermatogenesis. This finding highlighted the need to exercise caution in selecting a testosterone substitution regimen when developing a method for male infertility control based on GnRH agonists or antagonists.

POTENTIAL ADVANTAGES OF GnRH ANTAGONISTS OVER ITS AGONIST

Whereas agonist analogues of GnRH have proven to be highly effective in clinical situations in which complete suppression of gonadal function is not required and partial suppression is enough to achieve the therapeutic end point (*e.g.*, in precocious puberty, endometriosis, etc.), trials of these analogues for contraception have been unsuccessful in humans because complete suppression of spermatogenesis is not achieved. This appears at least in part due to the fact that although there is progressive down regulation of gonadotropins with continued agonist treatment, the stimulatory effects persist at a lower magnitude. Thus, a state of "medical hypophysectomy" (as assessed by radioimmunoassay or bioassay of serum LH) is never achieved. GnRH antagonists, as outlined below, can achieve complete suppression of LH and gonadal function and are thus likely to be effective in inducing desired suppression of spermatogenesis.

The effects of the agonist analogues are biphasic, with an initial stimulatory and a subsequent downregulatory phase. The stimulatory phase leads to considerable delay in the onset of the desired inhibitory effects.

Antagonist analogues, being devoid of stimulatory effects, lead to prompt inhibition of gonadal function.

There has been concern about the changes in testicular histology, such as calcification of some experimental animals, induced by GnRH agonist. The histologic picture after antagonist treatment is similar to that seen after hypophysectomy.

DOSE RESPONSE STUDIES WITH A GnRH ANTAGONIST IN THE MALE RAT

To assess the effective dose of the antagonist (Ac-D2 Nal^1, 4 ClD-Phe^2, D Trp^3, D Arg^6, D Ala^{10}) GnRH–HoAc (GnRH–Ant), we administered a single dose of 1 μg, 10 μg, 50 μg, 100 μg, and 250 μg of this antagonist to sexually mature male Wistar rats. The maximal suppression of serum testosterone and LH was only about 50% and was seen at doses of 100 μg and 250 μg per rat. A similar degree of suppression (50%) of serum LH, testosterone and accessory organ weights was seen when the animals were treated for 5 days. When the same antagonist (250 μg/rat or 1 mg/kg) was given by simple daily injections for 60 days, however, serum LH concentrations were undetectable. Serum testosterone concentrations were in the castrate range (25 ng/dl) and the testis and accessory organ weights were similar to those seen after hypophysectomy. All the rats were azoospermic, and testicular histology showed complete arrest of spermatogenesis uniformly in all the tubules.

These studies demonstrated 1) that the inhibitory effects of this antagonist are cumulative, and 2) that a dose of 1 mg/kg, when chronically administered, effectively induces medical hypophysectomy and azoospermia in the male rat.

These data also indicated that the single-dose studies may be misleading with regard to the potency estimates desired for long term contraceptive studies.

DISSOCIATING ANTIFERTILITY EFFECTS OF A GnRH ANTAGONIST FROM ITS ADVERSE EFFECTS ON MATING BEHAVIOR

THE IMPORTANCE OF TESTOSTERONE DOSE

Chronic treatment with the antagonist analogues of GnRH alone inhibits spermatogenesis in the rat, but the concomitant decline in serum testosterone leads to loss of mating. Akhtar and colleagues recently reported that replacement with supernormal doses of testosterone attenuates antifertility effects of GnRH agonist by supporting spermatogenesis.[1] We wondered if antifertility effects of GnRH–Ant could be dissociated from its effects on mating behavior by combining it with a small dose of androgen. We hypothesized that testosterone levels required to maintain mating would be much lower than those required to support spermatogenesis. To test this hypothesis, we treated six groups of male Wistar rats for 70 days as follows:

Group 1 Controls
Group 2 GnRH–Ant
Group 3 GnRH–Ant + 0.05 mg testosterone enanthate (TE)
Group 4 GnRH–Ant + 0.15 mg TE
Group 5 GnRH–Ant + 0.5 mg TE
Group 6 GnRH–Ant + 1.5 mg TE.[4]

Dose of 250 μg/day GnRH–Ant was shown in preliminary experiments to maximally suppress serum testosterone. Mating behavior was studied twice prior to treatment and at two, four, and eleven weeks during treatment. At the end of the experiment, the animals were mated with two cycling female rats for 5 days.

Serum LH concentrations were undetectable in all groups except controls (Fig. 30-1). Testes and prostate weights were similar to those seen after hypophysectomy in the GnRH–Ant-treated animals. Addition of graded concentrations of TE to GnRH–A led to a dose-dependent increase in prostate and seminal vesicle weights with an ED_{50} of 145 mg for both the accessory organs. Serum FSH concentrations were markedly reduced in the animals treated with GnRH–Ant alone; however, addition of progressively higher doses of TE to the GnRH–Ant led to progressive increase in serum FSH concentrations (Table 30-1). The reasons for this paradoxical increase in serum FSH with increasing dose of TE are not entirely clear.

GnRH–Ant treatment alone led to azoospermia in five out of six rats and markedly impaired mating behavior in all rats (Table 30-1). Addition of increasing dose of TE to GnRH–Ant led to a dose-dependent increase in sperm count; however, all animals in groups 3 and 4 receiving 0.05 mg and 0.15 mg TE were infertile and retained mating behavior. Animals treated with higher

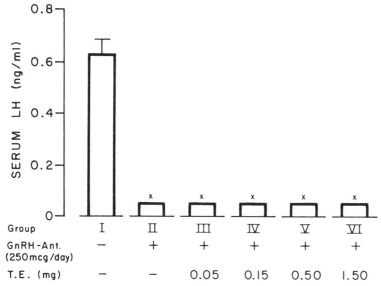

FIG. 30-1. Effect of GnRH antagonist and testosterone on serum LH in the male rat. Data are mean ± SEM (n = 6 in each group).

doses of the TE retained spermatogenesis as well as mating behavior (Table 30-1).

Testicular histology confirmed the observations from intratesticular sperm counts. Testes from animals in Groups 1, 3, and 4 showed complete arrest of spermatogenesis at the spermatogonial stage, whereas those from Groups 5 and 6 showed normal spermatogenesis.

These data are similar to those of Rivier and co-workers and demonstrate that the antifertility effects of the GnRH–Ant can be dissociated from its

TABLE 30-1. Effects of GnRH Antagonist and Testosterone in the Male Rat

GROUPS*	1	2	3	4	5	6
Serum LH (ng/ml)	0.63 ± 0.06	X	X	X	X	X
Serum FSH (ng/ml)	7.5 ± 0.6	1.6 ± 0.1	1.7 ± 0.1	2.5 ± 0.1	2.8 ± 0.2	3.5 ± 0.2
Intratesticular sperm count million/testis	161 ± 22.1	0 in 5 1.5 in 1	0 in 6/6	0 in 1 2.9 ± 1.7	92 ± 16.3	148 ± 14.3
Number of pups/rats	13.5 ± 0.5	0	0	0	10.1 ± 2.2	14.4 ± 0.5
Mating	Maint.	Impaired	Maint.	Maint.	Maint.	Maint.

X, Below limit of detection

* The animals were grouped as follows: 1, controls; 2, GnRH–Ant alone; 3, GnRH–Ant + T.E. 0.05 mg; 4, GnRH–Ant + T.E. 0.15 mg; 5, GnRH–Ant + T.E. 0.50 mg; 6, GnRH–Ant + T.E. 1.5 mg. Data are mean ± SEM.

N = 6 in each group.

adverse effects on mating behavior by combining it with an appropriate dose of testosterone.[14] These data also point out the critical importance of the testosterone dose to the success of the male contraceptive approaches directed at suppressing pituitary gonadotropin secretion. Superphysiologic doses of testosterone can attenuate the antifertility effects of the antagonist by supporting spermatogenesis while subphysiologic doses may have adverse effects on the bone and protein metabolism.

These data suggest feasible application of combined GnRH–Ant and androgen treatment for male contraception.

LIMITATIONS OF THE CURRENT METHODS OF ANDROGEN REPLACEMENT

The three methods of androgen replacement in current use are the long-acting injectable testosterone esters, oral testosterone, and testosterone implants.[7,15,18,19,20] These preparations also cause several side-effects, including pain at the site of injection, breast tenderness, weight gain, and skin oiliness. Studies of Akhtar and colleagues have raised considerable concern that supraphysiologic levels of testosterone achieved with this preparation may adversely influence the antifertility effects of GnRH analogues.[1] Marked variability in absorption of testosterone undecanoate results in marked variability in serum testosterone concentrations between different subjects and in the same subject on different occasions.[7,12,17] Cantrill and associates, in a controlled comparison of the three methods of testosterone replacement, reported overall unsatisfactory clinical responses in hypogonadal patients.[7] The dose of oral testosterone undecanoate currently being recommended is equivalent to 100 mg of testosterone, which represents a large steroid load to the liver, the long-term effects of which have not been studied. Finally, oral testosterone undecanoate is by far the most expensive method and is not available in the United States for general use.

The use of subcutaneous implantation of fused pellets of testosterone was popular in the 1940s,[6] but has decreased in recent years for reasons not altogether clear. The main problems were the rather painful subcutaneous administration by a trocar and spontaneous extrusion of pellets. In a recent study, Cantrill and others reported that testosterone implants in hypogonadal men produced a gradual rise in serum testosterone followed by a slow decline, even though the testosterone levels remained within the normal range for 4 to 5 months. Thus, even though clinical responses were satisfactory, steady nonfluctuating square wave pattern of serum testosterone was not achieved.

It is evident from these results that the current methods of testosterone substitution are far from satisfactory.[17]

CONCLUSION

The metabolic effects of testosterone in humans remain poorly understood, so that the long-term consequences of underreplacement or overreplacement on protein, bone, mineral, and lipid metabolism and sexual behavior remain unknown. It is, however, evident from the emerging data that the mode and dose of androgen replacement remains critical to the success of contraceptive approaches directed toward inhibiting pituitary gonadotropin secretion.

REFERENCES

1. AKHTAR FB, MARSHALL GR, NIESCHLAG E: Testosterone supplementation attenuates the antifertility effects of an LHRH agonist in male rhesus monkeys. Int J Androl 6:461, 1983
2. AKHTAR FB, MARSHALL GR, WICKINGS EJ *et al.:* Reversible induction of azoospermia in rhesus monkeys by constant infusion of a GnRH agonist using osmotic minipumps. J Clin Endocrinol Metab 56:534, 1983
3. BERGQUIST C, NILLIUS SJ, BEIGHT R *et al.:* Inhibitory effects on gonadotropin secretion and gonadal function in men during chronic treatment with a potent LHRH analog. Acta Endocrinol 91:601–608, 1979
4. BHASIN S, FIELDER T, ZAMBONI L *et al.:* Dissociating antifertility effects of a GnRH antagonist from its adverse effects on mating behavior: The importance of testosterone dose. (submitted for publication)
5. BHASIN S, HEBER D, HANDELSMAN DJ *et al.:* Hormonal effects of a GnRH agonist in the human male. III: Effects of long term combined treatment with GnRH agonist and testosterone. J Clin Endocrinol Metab (in press)
6. BISKIND GR, ESCAMILLA RF, LISSER H: Implantation of testosterone compounds in cases of male eunuchoidism. Acta Endocrinol 1:38, 1941
7. CANTRILL JA, DAVIS P, LARGE DM: Which testosterone replacement therapy? Clin Endocrinol 21:97, 1984
8. DOELLE GC, ALEXANDER AN, EVANS RM *et al.:* Combined treatment with a LHRH agonist and testosterone in man: Reversible oligospermia without impotence. J Androl 4:298–302, 1983
9. HEBER D, SWERDLOFF RS: Gonadotropin releasing hormone analogue and testosterone synergistically inhibit spermatogenesis. Endocrinology 108:2019, 1981
10. LINDE R, DOELLE GC, ALEXANDER N *et al.:* Reversible inhibition of testicular steroidogenesis and spermatogenesis by a potent GnRH agonist in normal men. N Engl J Med 305:663, 1981
11. NIESCHLAG E: Current status of testosterone substitution therapy. Int J Androl 5:225, 1982
12. NIESCHLAG E, MAUSS J, COERT A *et al.:* Plasma androgen levels in men after oral administration of testosterone or testosterone undecanoate. Acta Endocrinol (Copenhagen) 79:366, 1975
13. NIESCHLAG E, CUPPERS HJ, WIEGELMANN W *et al.:* Bioavailability and LH suppressing effects of different testosterone preparations in normal and hypogonadal men. Horm Res 7:138, 1976
14. RIVIER C, RIVIER J, VALE W: Effect of a potent GnRH antagonist and testosterone propionate on mating behavior in the male rat. Endocrinology 110:1998, 1981
15. SCHULTE-BEERBUHL M, NIESCHLAG E: Comparison of testosterone, DHT, LH and FSH in serum after injection of testosterone enanthate or testosterone cypionate. Fertil Steril 33:201, 1980
16. SCHURMEYER TH, KNUTH UA, FREISCHMEN CW *et al.:* Suppression of pituitary and testicular function in normal men by constant GnRH agonist infusion. J Clin Endocrinol Metab 59:19, 1984
17. SKAKKEBACK NE, BANCROFT J, DAVIDSON DW *et al.:* Androgen replacement with oral testosterone undecanoate in hypogonadal men: A double-blind controlled study. Clin Endocrinol 14:49, 1981
18. SOKOL RZ, PALACIOS A, CAMPFIELD LA *et al.:* Comparison of the kinetics of injectable testosterone in eugonadal and hypogonadal men. Fertil Steril 37:425, 1982
19. SWERDLOFF RS, CAMPFIELD LA, PALACIOS A *et al.:* Suppression of human spermatogenesis by depot androgen: potential for male contraception. J Steroid Biochem 11:663, 1979
20. SWERDLOFF RS, PALACIOS A, MCCLURE RD *et al.:* Male contraception: Clinical assessment of chronic administration of testosterone enanthate. Int J Androl (Suppl) 2:731, 1978

31

Overview of Controlled Release Systems for Male Contraception

DANNY H. LEWIS

THOMAS R. TICE

LEE R. BECK

Recent developments in biotechnology have afforded clinical investigators an opportunity for major advances in human fertility regulation. These new products are usually chemical replicas of the natural products, and although highly potent and specific regarding their biologic functions, most are difficult to administer clinically because they are orally inactive and have extremely short biologic half-lives when given as parenteral dosage formulations. Consequently, before widespread benefit of these new products is realized, a parallel development of new drug delivery systems to improve bioavailability will be required.

Several comprehensive review papers and proceedings of symposia on the topic of long-acting contraceptive systems are available.[2-4,6,21] Delivery systems under current development include subcutaneous polymeric implants, vaginal rings, medicated intrauterine devices, injectable depot formulations, and injectable polymeric formulations. Each of these delivery systems, with the exception of the injectable depot formulations, utilizes a polymeric membrane to separate the drug from the body fluids and control the rate of hormone release.

The ultimate aim in the regulation of fertility in the male is the development of suitable methods that reversibly interfere with fertilizing capacity without compromising libido and potency. At the present time, however, no acceptable pharmacologic method is available for the safe and reversible control of male fertility. The current status of research on hormonal contraception in the male has been summarized in Chapters 17 and 27.

Recently, luteinizing hormone-releasing hormone (LHRH), a hypothalamic neurohormone, and its analogues have received considerable attention as potential new nonsteroidal contraceptives.[1,5,7,11,15,20] LHRH and its analogues exhibit poor bioactivity when administered orally. Parenteral administration is therefore essential. Consequently, these novel compounds are ideally suited for controlled-release dosage forms.

The authors would like to acknowledge Mr. Richard M. Gilley, Dr. Robert J. Flores, Mr. Thomas E. Stonecypher, Mr. R. Gerard Carter, Mr. Thomas Forman, and Mr. Daniel Sherman for their assistance in developing the microcapsule formulations.

CRITERIA FOR CONTROLLED RELEASE MALE CONTRACEPTIVES

Because of the extensive investigations of long-acting contraceptives for the female and recent advances in male contraception, it is now possible to establish criteria for an ideal formulation for human males. These criteria should include the following. The method

Should be highly effective

Should exhibit maximum bioavailability and minimal dosage (optimal pharmacokinetics)

Should not compromise libido and potency

Should allow for flexibility in drug selection

Should not require action by the user at the time of coitus

Should not require frequent action by the user (maximum, $1\times$/mo)

Should not cause pain or discomfort at the time of administration or during the treatment period

Should be free from metabolic effects (serum lipid levels, carbohydrate mechanism, etc)

Should be inexpensive

Should not require highly trained medical personnel to administer

Should be reversible

Should allow immediate return to fertility after discontinuation

The composite of these design specifications can be used as a theoretical standard for the critical evaluation of potential long-acting male contraceptives. It is not likely that an ideal system meeting all of these criteria will be readily achieved; however, some systems currently under development for female application and potentially useful in male contraception are described here.

CONTROLLED-RELEASE SYSTEMS FOR STEROIDS

No single class of drugs or human health problem has received more study in regard to controlled drug delivery than steroidal contraceptives. This unparalleled attention is primarily due to the relatively high priority placed on these new systems by various government funding agencies. Some of the more significant advances in controlled-release technology were direct results of programs sponsored during the 1970s by the U.S. Agency for International Development, through PARFR, U.S. National Institutes of Health, the World Health Organization, and the Population Council. Most of the research and development projects involved a lipophilic steroid such as norethindrone, progesterone, levonorgestrel, or testosterone as the active agent. The various polymeric delivery systems currently under study as female contraceptives have been recently reviewed.[3,21] Some of these novel controlled release systems have potential utility in the area of male contraception.

SUBCUTANEOUS SYSTEMS

The subdermal implant is the oldest form of controlled delivery system for hormones. Three types of implants have been developed: steroid pellets; nonbiodegradable implants made of silicone in the form of pellets and rods; and biodegradable implants made from polyesters such as polycaprolactone, polylactic and polyglycolic acids, and polyorthoesters. One of the currently available formulations of steroid pellets is Oretron (Schering AG), 75-mg pellets of testosterone used for treatment of testosterone deficiency syndrome. Steroid pellets have not been widely accepted because of variable release rates.

Implants made of polycaprolactone, a biodegradable polyester, and filled with levonorgestrel, have been tested in animals. Early clinical trials are under way. The drug is released by diffusion, after which the polymer biodegrades. The system is designed to deliver contraceptive doses of levonorgestrel for 6 to 12 months.[14]

Contraceptive implants have the advantages of requiring minimal patient compliance, providing continuous low-dose therapy at predictable levels for up to several years following a single treatment, and easy reversibility. Their disadvantages include requirement for skilled personnel to perform insertion and removal, typical steroid-induced side-effects, and pain associated with treatment and reversal. Additionally, systems that are capable of very long-term efficacy pose the potential problem of decreased physician contact. The implants based on biodegradable polymers are potentially suitable for delivery of agents employed in male contraception.

MEDICATED FIBERS

Fibrous delivery systems for the delivery of various contraceptive steroids have recently been developed.[8] Nonbiodegradable fibers loaded with steroids, which are released at constant rates in vivo for extended periods, have been developed and are undergoing animal testing. Biodegradable polymers are now being studied and appear to offer promise in drug delivery.[8] These systems have potential uses in reversible vas occlusion approaches in the male.

Fibrous polymers offer unique advantages in controlled drug delivery. The fibers allow a wider selection of geometric configurations and a high surface area for release. The fibers are highly uniform and can be produced at low cost compared with other controlled release systems. These products are at an early stage of development and have not yet been tested clinically.

INJECTABLE DELIVERY SYSTEMS

Small particulate systems have been widely studied for delivery of contraceptive steroids. Advantages of such systems include conventional administration as a parenteral formulation and greater surface area allowing for higher release rates. Because of dose-response capabilities and multiple delivery routes, small particulate systems offer one of the most versatile approaches to the development of long-acting systems for contraceptive formulations. A disadvantage of using the injectable particle is its obviously nonreversibility.

Microspheres and microcapsules have been the most widely used forms of small particles for the administration of steroids. *Microcapsules* are spherical particles that contain the drug as a solid suspension or liquid in the core (reservoir devices). *Microspheres* are solid spherical particles that contain the drug in either solution or crystalline form dispersed throughout the polymer. Release of the drug from both types is by diffusion, leaching, erosion, or a combination of these mechanisms.

Injectable microsphere and microcapsule systems have been developed for the controlled release of steroid hormones.[2-4,12] A microsphere system for the steroid norethindrone has been tested extensively in primates and recently has been evaluated in phase I clinical trials.[3] Other steroids recently microencapsulated in biodegradable polymers and evaluated as injectable long-acting female contraceptives include norgestimate, progesterone,[12] and levonorgestrel.[13] Formulation parameters that affect pharmacokinetics with the microsphere system can be summarized as follows:

Polymer composition and molecular weight
Microsphere drug content (loading)
Size distribution of the microspheres
Quality of the microspheres
Sterilization parameters
Quantity of microspheres injected

Testosterone and testosterone derivatives have been microencapsulated in biodegradable lactide/glycolide copolymers as injectable hormone formulations.[12] A proprietary solvent–evaporation microencapsulation process (Stolle Research and Development Corporation) was utilized to produce testosterone microspheres containing approximately 50% by weight of the steroid.[12] These novel testosterone delivery systems have been used successfully in the control of the wild horse population of the western United States. Stallions were injected with a testosterone microsphere formulation designed to inhibit sperm production over a 6-month period.[17]

In lieu of using a synthetic derivative of testosterone for a human male contraceptive, our approach has been to use natural testosterone and to incorporate it into a long-acting, injectable delivery system. The delivery system developed consists of biocompatible, biodegradable microcapsules, with testosterone encapsulated in a poly(DL–lactide–coglycolide) excipient. The microcapsules can be referred to as either monolithic microcapsules or microspheres. The microcapsule product obtained is a free-flowing powder of spherical particles no larger than 125 μ in diameter. After being suspended in an aqueous injection vehicle, the microcapsules can be administered intramuscularly with a conventional hypodermic needle.

Because natural testosterone is not a very potent compound, it is estimated that as much as 2 mg to 6 mg of testosterone will have to be delivered per day to achieve a contraceptive effect in the human male. Of course, this dose may be reduced dramatically, as often seen before, by using a controlled-release microcapsule formulation. Another aspect to take into consideration is that the microcapsule formulation would be more acceptable to the patient if it delivered testosterone for a period of 3 months following a single injection.

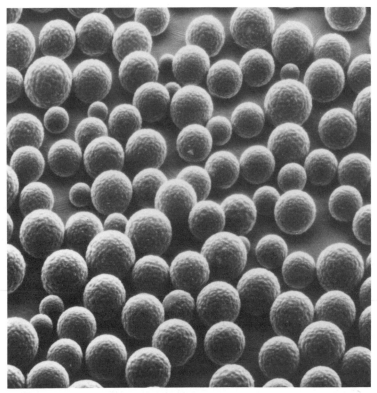

FIG. 31-1. Photomicrograph taken by scanning electron microscopy of 42%-loaded testosterone microcapsules. The bar represents 100 μ.

Therefore, considering the potency of testosterone and the need for a 3-month delivery system, the challenge has been to fabricate highly loaded testosterone microcapsules having as constant as possible release characteristics to minimize the quantity of microcapsules one would have to administer to a patient.

Microcapsules with loadings ranging from 38 wt % to 67 wt % testosterone were prepared. The 67%-loaded microcapsules released their drug too quickly in vitro because the surface of the microcapsules was of poor quality. More specifically, the surface of the 67%-loaded microcapsules was very porous. By titrating down to lower loadings, we found with the process conditions we had employed that the best quality microcapsules could be prepared at a loading of about 42 wt % (Fig. 31-1).

To optimize the release characteristics of 42%-loaded testosterone microcapsules, we assessed the in vitro release kinetics of testosterone microcapsules isolated as two size fractions, 45 μ to 90 μ and 90 μ to 125 μ. The in vitro release method we used to determine these kinetics is described elsewhere.[2] Briefly, the method involves shaking microcapsules at 37°C in a receiving fluid containing 27.5 wt % aqueous ethanol. The amount of testosterone released into the receiving fluid is then quantified spectrophotometrically.

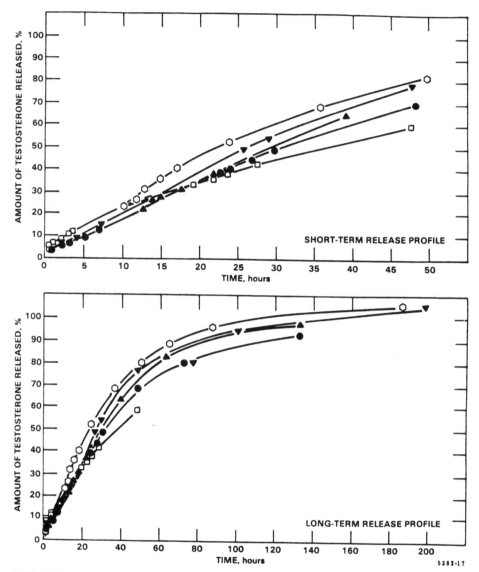

FIG. 31-2. Results of a study to determine the reproducibility of the in vitro release method for testosterone microcapsules. The receiving fluid was 27.5 wt % aqueous ethanol maintained at 37°C.

The in vitro release kinetics are accelerated because ethanol is used in the receiving fluid. Figure 31-2 indicates the reproducibility of the in vitro release method. This reproducibility study was achieved by testing a single batch of testosterone microcapsules several times.

As shown in Figure 31-3, smaller microcapsules release testosterone at a faster rate. This result follows theory, in which smaller microcapsules release faster because they have a higher surface area per unit mass than do larger

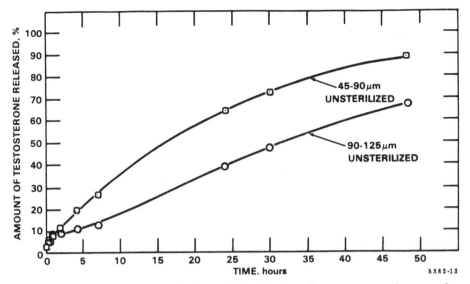

FIG. 31-3. Comparison of the in vitro release kinetics of testosterone microcapsules from two different size fractions (45 μ–90 μ and 90 μ–125 μ).

microcapsules. In addition, it can be seen that the rate of release of testosterone from the microcapsules; that is, the slope of the tangent to the release curve decreases with time. This type of release curve is indicative of monolithic microcapsules. Because the microcapsules are highly loaded and their internal structure is approaching that of reservoir microcapsules, however, their release curves are almost linear, indicating near zero-order release kinetics.

Another parameter that was manipulated to optimize the release kinetics of the microcapsules was the dose of gamma radiation used to sterilize the microcapsules. With other steroid microcapsules prepared with poly(DL-lactide-coglycolide) excipients, we have observed that gamma radiation increases the rate of release of the steroid from the microcapsules.[3] This effect also was seen with testosterone microcapsules (Fig. 31-4). We have shown, and described elsewhere (Chap. 32), by varying the dose of gamma radiation, one can predictably alter the release kinetics of testosterone microcapsules.

In summary, by combining the effect of microcapsule size and the sterilizing dose of gamma radiation, a wide range or family of in vitro release curves can be obtained with 42%-loaded testosterone microcapsules (see Chap. 32).

CONTROLLED RELEASE SYSTEMS FOR LHRH AND LHRH ANALOGUES

The remarkable advance of biotechnology has made available a new family of potent hormones as potential contraceptive agents. Because of their physical and chemical properties, these recent materials (LHRH, GnRH) have pre-

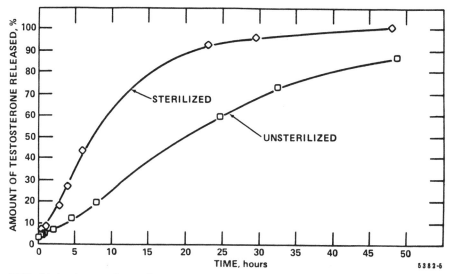

FIG. 31-4. Comparison of the in vitro release kinetics of sterilized and unsterilized testosterone microcapsules. The sterilization dose was 2.8 Mrad of gamma radiation.

sented a new challenge to the designers of controlled-release formulations. Little has been reported until recently on the delivery of polypeptides by controlled-release formulations.[9,11,16] The water-soluble polypeptides require considerably different formulation techniques and design considerations when compared to the steroidal formulations. LHRH delivery systems generally have been limited to injectable microsphere formulations.

LHRH MICROSPHERES

Since 1980, rather intense effort has been devoted by several groups to the development of LHRH microspheres based on poly(lactide-coglycolide) as the biodegradable excipient.[10,18,19] Continuous administration of these LHRH agonists from such microspheres appears to offer promise in female and male contraception, treatment of endometriosis, and metastatic carcinoma.

The most promising formulations comprise a 50:50 (lactide:glycolide) co-polymer and 1% to 10% by weight of active hormone. The microspheres are generally 10 μ to 100 μ in diameter and are prepared by conventional phase-separation microencapsulation techniques. This specific type of formulation has been shown to afford efficacious levels of drug for 30 to 50 days following a single intramuscular injection in animals. The microspheres are administered as a suspension in an aqueous vehicle such as saline or saline containing various surfactants and thickening agents. A typical LHRH microsphere formulation is shown in Figure 31-5.

The LHRH material is released from the polymeric matrix through combination mechanisms of leaching and bioerosion of the polymer. It is generally believed that very little true diffusion of the polypeptide occurs in the polymers. The copolymer composition has been selected to allow rapid biodegra-

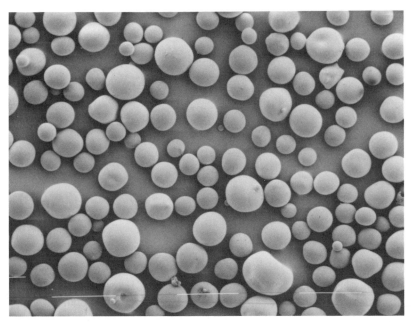

FIG. 31-5. Photomicrograph taken by scanning electron microscopy of 10%-loaded LHRH microspheres designed to release over a 30-day period.

dation to occur following treatment. The 50:50 (lactide:glycolide) copolymer undergoes complete biodegradation in 4 to 8 weeks, depending on molecular weight parameters.

Although most studies to date have been aimed toward formulations with a 30-day duration of activity, longer durations are possible with the versatile microsphere approach. Polymeric excipients with longer biodegradation profiles are readily available and are suitable for delivery of the LHRH materials. Problems yet to be overcome completely with the LHRH microspheres include optimization of the microencapsulation procedure to allow better drug entrapment efficiency and reproducibility, improvement in the synthesis procedures for the copolymer excipients, and a better understanding of the release mechanism so that in vivo performance will be more reproducible and predictable. Solutions to these problems appear to be well within reach, and it is obvious that this technology offers tremendous potential.

CONCLUSION

Several controlled-release technologies applicable to female contraception have now been demonstrated. Some of these approaches may be suitable for use in long-acting contraceptives for the human male. Injectable biodegradable microsphere formulations of testosterone and LHRH agonists appear to offer immediate promise in this area. These small particulate systems seem to offer the greatest potential as long-acting male contraceptives because they have greater flexibility with regard to the mechanism of release and dose selection. These systems are well-suited for combination therapy such as testosterone–LHRH treatment in the male or progestin–estrogen therapy in the female.

REFERENCES

1. ASCH RH, ROJAS FJ, BARTKE A, SCHALLEY AV, TICE TR, KLEMCKE HG, SILER-KHODR TM, BRAY RW, HOGAN MP: Prolonged suppression of plasma LH levels in male rats after a single injection of an LHRH agonist in DL-lactide:Glycolide microcapsule. J Androl: 1985
2. BECK LR, COWSAR DR, POPE VZ: Long-acting steroidal contraceptive systems. In ZATUCHNI GI (ed): Research Frontiers in Fertility Regulation, pp 1–16. Chicago, Program for Applied Research on Fertility Regulation, Vol 1, No 1, 1980
3. BECK LR, POPE VZ: Controlled-release delivery systems for hormones. Drugs 27:528, 1984
4. BECK LR, TICE TR: Poly(lactic acid) and poly(lactic acid-co-glycolic acid) contraceptive delivery systems. In MISHELL DR JR (ed): Long-Acting Steroid Contraception. New York, Raven Press, 1983
5. BELCHETZ PE, PLANT TM, NAKAI Y, KEOGH EJ, KNOBIL E: Hypophysical responses to continuous and intermittent delivery of hypothalamic gonadotropin-releasing hormone. Science 202:631–633, 1978
6. BENAGIANO G, GABELNICK HL: Biodegradable systems for the sustained release of fertility regulating agents. J Steroid Biochem 11:449, 1979
7. BERGQUIST C, NILLIUS SJ, WIDE L: Long-term intranasal luteinizing hormone-releasing hormone agonist treatment for contraception in women. Fertil Steril 38:190–193, 1982
8. DUNN RL, LEWIS DH: Fibrous polymers for the delivery of contraceptive steroids to the female reproductive tract. In LEWIS DH (ed): Controlled Release of Pesticides and Pharmaceuticals, pp 125–146. New York, Plenum Press, 1981
9. KENT JS, SANDERS LM, MCRAE GI, VICKERY BH, TICE TR, LEWIS DH: Feasibility studies on the controlled release of an LHRH analogue from subcutaneously injected polymeric microspheres: Early in vivo studies. Contracep Deliv Syst 3:58, 1982
10. KENT JS, SANDERS LM, TICE TR, LEWIS DH: Microencapsulation of the peptide nafarelin acetate for controlled release. In ZATUCHNI GI, GOLDSMITH A, SHELTON JD, SCIARRA JJ (eds): Long-Acting Contraceptive Delivery Systems, pp 169–179. Philadelphia, Harper & Row, 1983
11. KENT JS, VICKERY BH, MCRAE GI: The use of cholesterol matrix pellet implants for early studies on the prolonged release in animals of agonist analogues of luteinizing hormone-releasing hormone. Seventh International Symposium on Controlled Release of Bioactive Materials, Controlled Release Society, Fort Lauderdale, FL, 1980
12. LEWIS DH, TICE TR: Polymeric considerations in the design of microencapsulated contraceptive steroids. In ZATUCHNI GI, GOLDSMITH A, SHELTON JD, SCIARRA JJ (eds): Long-Acting Contraceptive Delivery Systems, pp 77–95. Philadelphia, Harper & Row, 1983
13. NUWAYSER ES, WILLIAMS DL, KERRIGAN JH, NUCEFORA WA, ARMSTRONG JC: Microencapsulation of contraceptive steroids. In ZATUCHNI GI, GOLDSMITH A, SHELTON JD, SCIARRA JJ (eds): Long-Acting Contraceptive Delivery Systems, pp 64–76. Philadelphia, Harper & Row, 1983
14. PITT CG, SCHINDLER A: Capronor: A biodegradable delivery system for levonorgestrel. In ZATUCHNI GI, GOLDSMITH A, SHELTON JD, SCIARRA JJ (eds): Long-Acting Contraceptive Delivery Systems, pp 48–63. Philadelphia, Harper & Row, 1983
15. REDDING TW, SCHALLEY AV, TICE TR, MEYERS WE: Long-acting delivery systems for peptides: Inhibition of rat prostate tumors by controlled release of (D-Trp[6])-LHRH from injectable microcapsules. Proc Nat Acad Sci 81:5845–5848, 1984
16. SANDERS LM, KENT JS, MCRAE GI, VICKERY BH, TICE TR, LEWIS DH: Feasibility studies on the controlled release of an LHRH analogue from subcutaneously injected polymeric microspheres: Formulation characteristics. Contr Deliv Syst 3:60, 1982

17. TICE TR: Personal communication, 1984
18. TICE TR, MEYERS WE, SCHALLEY AV, REDDING TW: Inhibition of rat prostate tumors by controlled release of (D-Trp^6)-LHRH from injectable microspheres. Eleventh International Symposium on Controlled Release of Bioactive Materials, Controlled Release Society, Fort Lauderdale, FL, 1984
19. VICKERY BH, MCRAE GI, SANDERS LM, KENT JJ, NESTOR JJ JR: In vivo assessment of long-acting formulations of luteinizing hormone-releasing hormone analogs. In ZATUCHNI GI, GOLDSMITH A, SHELTON JD, SCIARRA JJ (eds): Long-Acting Contraceptive Delivery Systems, pp 180–189. Philadelphia, Harper & Row, 1983
20. VICKERY BH, MCRAE GI: Antagonism by an LHRH agonist of the steroidogenic effects of exogenous human chorionic gonadotrophin in the female primate. Life Sci 27:1409–1413, 1980
21. ZATUCHNI GI, GOLDSMITH A, SHELTON JD, SCIARRA JJ (eds): Long-Acting Contraceptive Delivery Systems. Hagerstown, Harper & Row, 1983

32

Preliminary Results on the Effects of Testosterone Microcapsules

RICARDO H. ASCH

TERI O. HEITMAN

RICHARD M. GILLEY

THOMAS R. TICE

Controlled-release formulations can provide programmed durations of drug action ranging from days to months from a single injection, and parenteral administration of controlled-release drugs may soon become more popular than the oral route. Controlled-release microcapsules offer several profound advantages over conventionally administered medications. First, patient compliance with the dose regimen is ensured because dosing is automatic. Second, the plague of the first-pass effect inherent in the oral route can be forgotten. Third, the ability of maintaining the minimal effective level of drug in the blood allows minimization of the amount of drug used, and, because adverse side-effects usually are dose related, many of the toxicologic problems of drugs can be obviated by parenteral microcapsules.

Controlled-release microcapsule products designed for parenteral administration are powders consisting of spherical particles, preferably less than 125 μm in diameter. Microcapsules of this size can be administered easily to the patient by suspending them in a suitable vehicle followed by injection with a conventional syringe using an 18- or 20-gauge needle.

Polymers chosen as excipients for parenterally administered microcapsules must meet several requirements, including suitable mechanical properties and biodegradation kinetics, tissue compatibility, drug compatibility, drug permeability, and ease of processing. One class of polymers that is currently popular for this purpose is the polyesters poly(lactic acid) and poly(glycolic acid)—also referred to as polylactide and polyglycolide—and copolymers of lactide and glycolide, that is, poly(lactide-co-glycolide). These polymers biodegrade by undergoing random, nonenzymatic, hydrolytic scissioning of their ester linkages to form lactic acid and glycolic acid, normal metabolic compounds. Because these materials have proven to be biocompatible and have extensive

Support (PARFR-361) for this project was provided by the Program for Applied Research on Fertility Regulation, Northwestern University, under a Cooperative Agreement with the United States Agency for International Development (AID) (DPE-0546-A-00-1003-00). The views expressed by the authors do not necessarily reflect the views of AID.

toxicologic documentation (*e.g.*, from their use as resorbable sutures), their approval by the FDA for use as microcapsule excipients should be less costly and more straightforward than the use of new polymers for excipients.[3]

This chapter describes the in vivo testing of a testosterone microcapsule delivery system developed to serve as a long-acting male contraceptive. The delivery system consisted of testosterone encapsulated in a matrix of poly(DL-lactide-co-glycolide) (DL-PLG). The system was designed to deliver testosterone for a duration of 3 months. Being a 3-month system, an 86:14 (mol/mol) DL-PLG was selected as the excipient. This particular DL-PLG was chosen based on excipients used previously in other injectable, steroid-releasing microcapsule systems. In microcapsule form, an 86:14 DL-PLG will biodegrade completely within 6 months.[3] This is a reasonable resorption rate for a 3-month delivery system because polymer buildup will not become a problem. More specifically, polymer from the first dose will be completely resorbed by the time the patient receives the third dose. With respect to the mechanism of drug release, it is believed that the release of testosterone from the microcapsules is initially due to drug diffusion through the rate-controlling DL-PLG matrix (during months 1 and 2), followed by release due to drug diffusion and biodegradation of the DL-PLG excipient (during the third month).

The three factors that control the release characteristics of testosterone microcapsules, namely, 1) core loading, 2) size, and 3) the sterilizing dose of gamma radiation, were optimized to produce four formulations of testosterone microcapsules. These four formulations have distinctly different in vitro release kinetics. The purpose of the pharmacokinetics studies described below was to assess the effects of these different microcapsule formulations on steroid and protein hormone blood levels and on blood chemistries in castrated male rhesus monkeys.

MATERIALS AND METHODS

TESTOSTERONE MICROCAPSULES PREPARATION

Testosterone microcapsules were prepared by a patented microencapsulation process.[11] Briefly, testosterone (Sigma) and 86:14 DL-PLG were dissolved in methylene chloride maintained at about 38°C. This solution was then emulsified in an aqueous solution consisting of deionized water and 7 wt % polyvinyl alcohol (Vinol 205C, Air Products and Chemicals). After a stable oil-in-water emulsion formed, the contents of the resin kettle was stirred under reduced pressure to evaporate a portion of the methylene chloride. Then the microcapsules were poured into a large volume of water to extract the remaining methylene chloride. The microcapsules were then separated into various size fractions using stainless steel sieves and dried at room temperature for 72 hours.

The drug content of the microcapsules (core loading) was determined by dissolving a known amount of microcapsules in a known volume of methylene chloride. After the microcapsules had dissolved, the amount of testosterone in the sample was quantified spectrophotometrically at 240 nm, and the core loading was calculated in terms of weight percent testosterone.[6]

TABLE 32-1. Characteristic of 42%-Loaded Testosterone* Microcapsule Formulations Tested in Vivo

FORMULATION	MICROCAPSULE DIAMETER (μm)	GAMMA RADIATION (Mrad)
A	45–90	2.8
B	45–90	0.5
C	90–125	2.0
D	90–125	0.5

* Total testosterone content was constant in all formulations at 55 mg.

The in vitro rate of release of testosterone from the microcapsule formulations was determined by adding a weighed sample of microcapsules to a receiving fluid consisting of 27.5 wt % aqueous ethanol. The receiving fluid was maintained at 37°C and shaken slowly to keep the microcapsules suspended. Periodically, aliquots were removed from the receiving fluid and quantified for testosterone spectrophotometrically at 247 nm. A more detailed description to the in vitro release method is described elsewhere.[3]

Four testosterone microcapsule formulations (containing about 42 wt % testosterone) were tested. These formulations differed in size (either 45 μm to 90 μm to 125 μm) and in the dose of sterilizing gamma radiation they received (0.5 Mrad–2.8 Mrad, Table 32-1). The total content of testosterone in each microcapsule formulation remained constant at 55 mg.

ANIMAL EXPERIMENTAL DESIGN

Twelve adult male rhesus monkeys of proven fertility were placed under quarantine for 45 days at the Laboratory Animal Facilities of the University of Texas Health Science Center at San Antonio. After the quarantine period, baseline levels of various hormones testosterone (T), dihydrotestosterone (DHT), follicle-stimulating hormone (FSH), and luteinizing hormone (LH) were established. Animals were then castrated bilaterally with simultaneous removal of the epididymis under ketamine HCl sedation (7–10 mg/kg). After castration, blood samples were collected daily for 1 week to determine acute changes in hormone values. For 3 weeks thereafter postcastration hormone levels were determined periodically. Thirty days after castration, animals were divided into three groups of four animals each. Different formulations of testosterone microcapsules were administered to each group as follows:

Group 1 = Microcapsule diameter 45 μm to 90 μm and gamma radiation 0.5 Mrad (formulation B)

Group 2 = Microcapsule diameter 90 μm to 125 μm and gamma radiation 0.5 Mrad (formulation D)

Group 3 = microcapsule diameter 90 μM to 125 μM and gamma radiation 2.0 Mrad (formulation C)

Blood samples were drawn every day for 10 days, then every other day for 1 month, and then every third day for 2 subsequent months.

Serum concentrations of FSH, LH, T, and DHT were determined by RIA techniques described elsewhere.[1,2,4] Assay sensitivity for FSH and LH were

750 ng/ml and 165 ng/ml, respectively, and the interassay and intra-assay coefficients of variation (%) were 9 and 2.8, 12 and 5.3, respectively. Assay sensitivity for T and DHT were 11 pg/ml and 24.5 pg/ml, respectively. Interassay and intra-assay coefficients of variations (%) were 15 and 4.7, and 12.4 and 10.2 respectively, for T and DHT.

Blood chemistry profiles (SMAC 24) were determined using: ultracentrifugation and phosphotungstate precipitation for lipoproteins–cholesterol,[5,7] enzymatic, colorimetric and/or flame photometric analysis for 24 test chemical profile,[12] and quantitative, colorimetric determination for acid phosphatase.[10]

Special attention was placed to record any changes in body weight, as well as upper arm, thigh, neck, chest, and abdomen diameters throughout the study.

RESULTS

After we had determined that the maximum core loading was 42 wt % drug for the process conditions employed, we prepared microcapsule doses for testing in vivo. These microcapsule doses were prepared to establish baseline in vivo data that could be used to optimize the microcapsule formulation. More specifically, 42% loaded testosterone microcapsules (45 μm–90 μm and 90 μm–125 μm in diameter) were prepared and sterilized with gamma radiation.

After sterilization, the microcapsules were thoroughly characterized. Photomicrographs taken by scanning electron microscopy (SEM) show that these microcapsules consist of relatively spherical particles with slightly irregular surfaces; however, the polymer coating of the microcapsules appears continuous. Figure 32-1 shows the in vitro release profiles for formulations A and B (45 μm–90 μm). As expected, the rate of testosterone release from these microcapsules increased as the dose of gamma radiation increased. Figure 32-2 shows the in vitro release profiles for formulations C and D (90 μm–125 μm). Again, the testosterone release rate varied directly with the dose of gamma radiation that the microcapsules received. Because the microcapsules in formulations C and D were larger than those in formulations A and B, they did demonstrate slower release rates at equivalent radiation doses, however.

Within 1 month of castration, blood levels of T, DHT, FSH, and LH changed drastically, serum T and DHT levels fell 90% to 98% and 80% to 92% respectively from baseline (Figs. 32-3, 32-4, 32-5, 32-6). During the same period, FSH and LH levels rose 700% to 1145% and 180% to 340%, respectively. One month after the microcapsule injections, T and DHT levels rose to T—group 1, 40% to 60%; group 2, 24% to 30%; and group 3, 60% above precastration baseline levels. DHT—group 1, 0% to 12%; group 2, 112% to 132%; and group 3, 112% to 195% above precastration baseline values. One month after LH drug administration, LH levels in group 1 remained at 200% above baseline, whereas in groups 2 and 3 LH dropped to 72% to 92% and 64% to 68% above baseline levels, respectively. At that time FSH levels in group 1 were 580%; group 2, 450%; and group 3, 500% to 600% above baseline values. Two months after the microcapsules injection, T and DHT

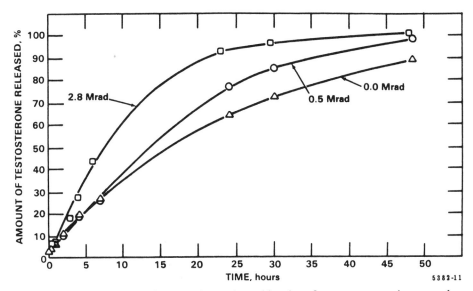

FIG. 32-1. Comparison of the in vitro release kinetics of testosterone microcapsules that had received 2.8 Mrad (formulation A); 0.5 Mrad (formulation B); and 0.0 Mrad of gamma radiation. Microcapsules are 45 μm to 90 μm in diameter, and the receiving fluid was 27.5 wt % aqueous ethanol.

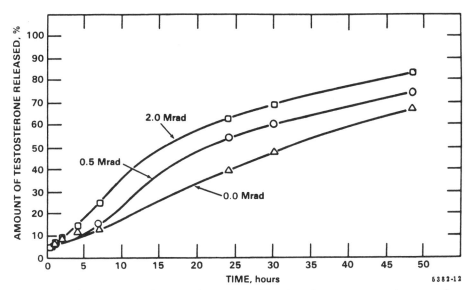

FIG. 32-2. Comparison of the in vitro release kinetics of testosterone microcapsules that had received 2.0 Mrad (formulation C); 0.5 Mrad (formulation D); and 0.0 Mrad of gamma radiation. Microcapsules are 90 μm to 125 μm in diameter, and the receiving fluid was 27.5 wt % aqueous ethanol.

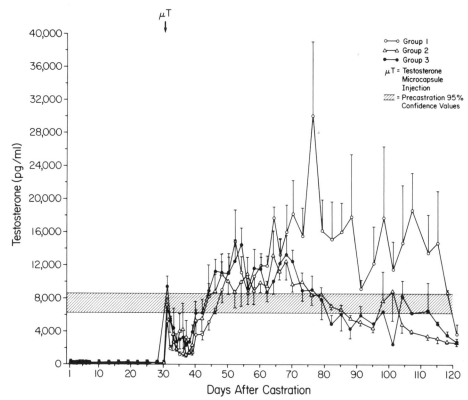

FIG. 32-3. Serum testosterone concentrations in animals from groups 1 to 3, following castration (day 0) and injection of testosterone microcapsule formulation (μT).

levels in group 1 were 120% to 150% and 16% to 168% above baseline levels respectively. T levels in group 2 and group 3 were both 0% to 50% below baseline, whereas DHT levels were 0% to 88% above baseline in group 2 and from 30% below to 80% above precastration levels in group 3. FSH levels remained high: group 1, 500% to 600%; group 2, 520% to 570%; and group 3, 460% to 500% above baseline. By 2 months postinjection, LH levels in all groups dropped: group 1, 108% to 124%; group 2, 40% to 90%; and group 3, 35% to 70% above baseline. By three months after the injection, T levels in group 1 were 18% to 150% above; group 2, 30% to 60% below; and group 3, 12% to 60% below baseline levels. DHT values in group 1 ranged from 30% below to 44% above; group 2, 35% below to 56% above, and group 3, 15% to 58% below baseline precastration levels. FSH levels in all groups remained high at 500% to 600% above baseline precastration levels. After 3 months, LH levels in group 1 were 120% to 190%; group 2, 90% to 160%; and group 3, 40% to 80% above baseline.

The results of blood chemistries are shown in Figures 32-7, 32-8, and 32-9. The normal values for our colony ($\bar{X} \pm$ SEM) are shown in Table 32-2.

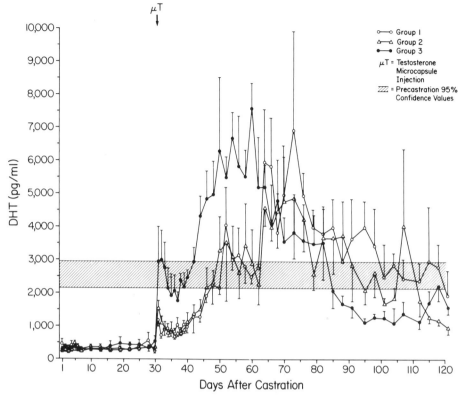

FIG. 32-4. Serum DHT concentrations in animals from groups 1 to 3, following castration (day 0) and injection of testosterone microcapsule formulations (μT).

These results are comparable to those reported previously in the literature for rhesus monkeys.[8]

No major changes were observed in any of the parameters tested (cholesterol, triglycerides, HDL, LDL, VLDL, SMAC 22) after castration, or following the different microcapsule formulation injections. Even though some determinations showed increase in triglyceride, inorganic phosphorus, and alkaline phosphate levels 1 month after microcapsule injections, the levels remained within the normal ranges for rhesus monkeys. No significant changes in body weight or muscle diameters were observed throughout the study.

DISCUSSION

The results of the preliminary pharmacokinetics study demonstrated the need to optimize the testosterone microcapsule formulation so they would release the drug at a more constant release rate. To achieve this goal, it would be necessary to slow down the initial release of testosterone from the microcap-

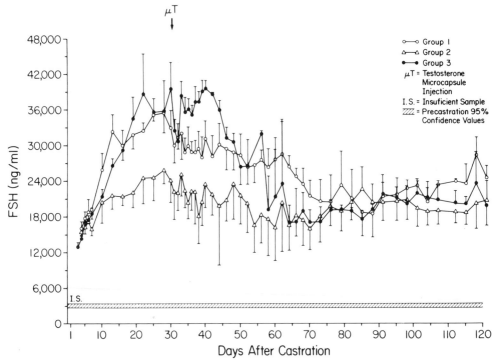

FIG. 32-5. Serum FHS concentrations in animals from groups 1 to 3, following castration (day 0) and injection of testosterone microcapsule formulations (μT).

sules, that is, the release occurring during the first 50 days in vivo. There are several mechanisms that can be employed to reduce the rate of release of drug from microcapsules that are releasing drugs primarily by diffusion. These formulation modifications include reducing the core loading of the microcapsules, increasing the diameter of the microcapsules, and reducing the dose of gamma radiation used in the sterilization process.

Because of the high dose of testosterone needed to maintain efficacious serum levels, we did not examine lower core loadings as a means of reducing the in vivo release rate of the testosterone microcapsules. Instead, we investigated the effect of slightly larger microcapsules and lower doses of gamma radiation. With diffusion-controlled systems, the release of drug is dependent on the surface area of the microcapsules, which in turn is related to the size of the microcapsules. That is, the release of drug is slower from larger microcapsules because they have a smaller surface area per unit mass. The rate of release of testosterone can therefore be reduced by increasing the average microcapsule diameter.

The rate of release of drug from microcapsules also can be reduced by decreasing the dose of gamma radiation that the microcapsules receive during the sterilization process. It is well documented that gamma radiation will

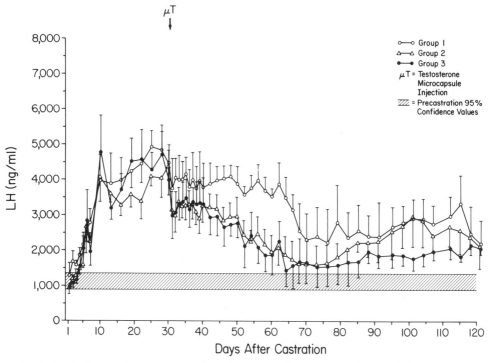

FIG. 32-6. Serum LH concentrations in animals from groups 1 to 3, following castration (day 0) and injections of testosterone microcapsule formulations (μT).

break polymer chains, particularly the chains of polyesters. This results in a decrease in the polymer molecular weight. Experience has shown that gamma radiation increases the rate of release of steroids from microcapsules with DL-PLG excipients. The rate of release of testosterone microcapsules can be reduced, therefore, by lowering the gamma radiation dose, that is, by reducing the break down of the DL-PLG excipient during sterilization.

Using the above-mentioned modifications, we prepared three new microcapsule formulations for testing in vivo, formulations B, C, and D. Although the release profiles for each formulation differed, they all released testosterone at a lower rate than formulation A, which was tested in the first pharmacokinetics study. Each of the new formulations had core loadings similar to formulation A (about 42 wt % testosterone). Although formulation B contained microcapsules of the same size as formulation A (45 μm–90 μm), it differed in that the dose of gamma radiation it received was lower, 0.5 Mrad instead of 2.8 Mrad. Formulations C and D differed from formulation A with respect to both microcapsule diameter and sterilization dose. Formulations C and D contained larger microcapsules (90 μm–125 μm) than did formulation A. Formulation C was sterilized with 2.0 Mrad of gamma radiation, whereas formulation D received 0.5 Mrad, both lower doses than that received by formulation A.

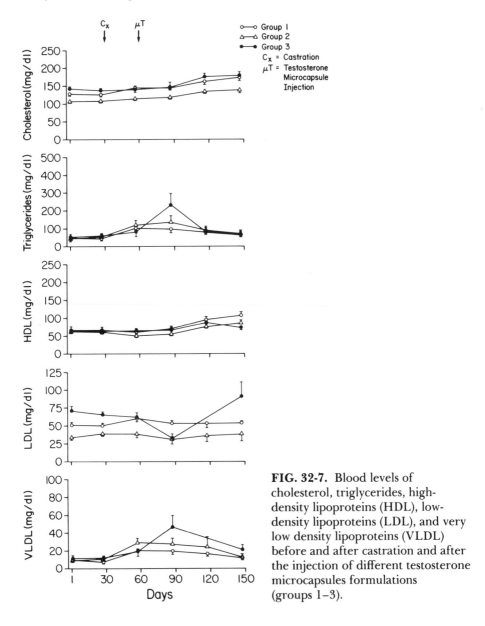

FIG. 32-7. Blood levels of cholesterol, triglycerides, high-density lipoproteins (HDL), low-density lipoproteins (LDL), and very low density lipoproteins (VLDL) before and after castration and after the injection of different testosterone microcapsules formulations (groups 1–3).

The results of the present studies revealed that a single injection of testosterone microcapsules produced serum T and DHT concentrations similar to those observed before castration for up to 3 months. Differential results were observed in the effect of testosterone microcapsules on gonadotropin levels. Although LH levels return to almost precastration values in most animals through the study, FSH levels failed to show significant decreases over the

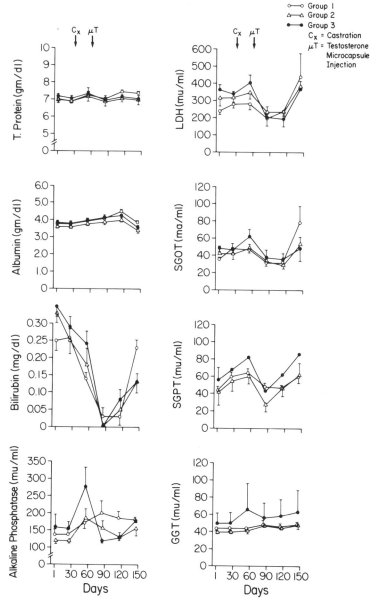

FIG. 32-8. Blood levels of total protein (T-protein), albumin, bilirubin, alkaline phosphatase, lactic dehydrogenase (LDH), aspartate transaminase (SGOT), alanine transaminase (SGPT), and gamma glutamine transferase (GGT), before and after castration and following the injection of different testosterone microcapsule formulations (μt T) (groups 1–3).

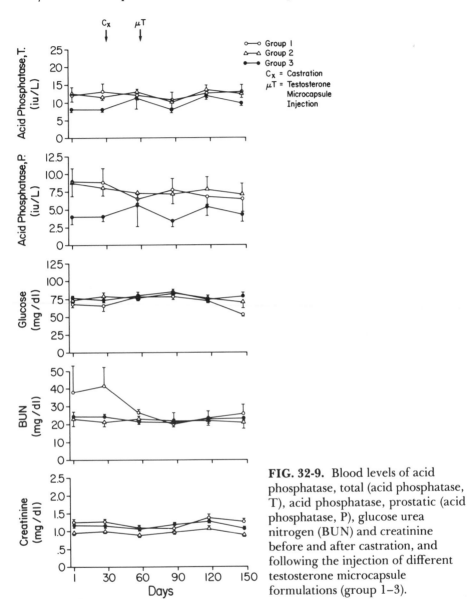

FIG. 32-9. Blood levels of acid phosphatase, total (acid phosphatase, T), acid phosphatase, prostatic (acid phosphatase, P), glucose urea nitrogen (BUN) and creatinine before and after castration, and following the injection of different testosterone microcapsule formulations (group 1–3).

entire periods of follow up after the microcapsule injection. These results differ from those of Plant and co-workers,[9] who postulated that testosterone inhibited both FSH and LH to a same degree in male rhesus monkeys, casting doubt on the hypothesis of the presence of a testicular "inhibin" that controls FSH secretion specifically.

From the present pharmacokinetic studies it appears that the microcapsule formulations C and D (groups 3 and 2, respectively), provided the more

TABLE 32-2. Normal Ranges of Blood Chemistries in the Rhesus Monkey Colony

	$\bar{X} \pm$ SEM	RANGE
Cholesterol (mg/deciliter)	144.11 ± 3.53	99–221
Triglycerides (mg/deciliter)	92.34 ± 7.81	25–341
HDL (mg/deciliter)	65.38 ± 1.4	43–95
LDL (mg/deciliter)	60.78 ± 2.81	25–138
VLDL (mg/deciliter)	18.42 ± 1.56	5–68
Sodium (meq/liter)	143.81 ± 0.47	130–151
Potassium (meq/liter)	3.79 ± 0.04	3.3–4.6
Chloride (meq/liter)	106.19 ± 0.33	99–111
CO_2 (meq/liter)	25.46 ± 0.4	18–30
Anion gaps	15.95 ± 0.38	8.6–24.8
Osmolality (mosm/kg)	299.93 ± 1.13	2.71–322
Total protein (g/deciliter)	7.08 ± 0.06	6.1–8.4
Albumin (g/deciliter)	3.77 ± 0.06	2.7–5.0
T. Bilirubin (mg/deciliter)	0.18 ± 0.02	0.0–0.4
Alkaline phosphatase (mu/ml)	251.16 ± 23.96	72–1050
LDH (mu/ml)	299.13 ± 13.71	101–561
SGOT (mu/ml)	46.8 ± 1.86	17–78
SGPT (mu/ml)	58.64 ± 5.12	10–178
GGT (mu/ml)	56.72 ± 2.78	29–116
Acid phosphatase, T (IU/liter)	10.35 ± 0.48	4.5–28.3
Acid phosphatase, P (IU/liter)	5.55 ± 0.43	1.5–23.3
Glucose (mg/deciliter)	68.09 ± 2.09	28–101
BUN (mg/deciliter)	23.61 ± 1.66	15–86
Creatinine (mg/deciliter)	1.0 ± 0.03	0.5–1.4
Calcium (mg/deciliter)	9.15 ± 0.067	8.3–10.5
Inorganic phosphorus (mg/deciliter)	3.91 ± 0.14	2.2–7.2
Calcium (mg/deciliter)	4.02 ± 0.04	3.5–4.7

* University of Texas Health Sciences Center at San Antonio

physiologic levels of circulating T and DHT. Further studies are necessary to determine the maximum length of steroid release from newer formulations.

The absence of any side-effects or major changes in lipid profile, blood chemistries, and serum acid phosphatase level also suggest that the microcapsule formulations used in this study do not induce a nonphysiologic hyperandrogenic or hypoandrogenic state.

The results of these preliminary studies warrant further research in the area of testosterone microcapsule formulations because the availability of such long-lasting biodegradable systems may open new approaches of androgen administration, with possible uses both as a male contraceptive and in the treatment of hypogonadal men.

REFERENCES

1. ASCH RH, BALMACEDA JP, BORGHI MR, NIESVISKY R, COY DH, SCHALLY AV: Suppression of the positive feedback of estradiol benzoate on gonadotropin secretion by an inhibitory analogue of LHRH in oophorectomized rhesus monkeys. Evidence for a necessary synergism between LH-RH and estrogens. J Clin Endocrinol Metab 57:367–372, 1983

2. ASCH RH, SILER-KHODR TM, PAUERSTEIN CJ: Steroid and peptide hormonal concentrations in human seminal plasma. Int J Fertil 29:15–22, 1984

3. BECK LR, TICE TR: Poly(lactic acid) and poly(lactic acid-co-glycolic acid) contraceptive delivery systems. In MISHELL DR (ed): Advances in Human Fertility and Reproductive Endocrinology, Vol 2, pp 175–199. New York, Raven Press, 1983

4. BURGOS-BRICENO LA, SCHALLY AV, BARTKE A, ASCH RH: Inhibition of serum luteinizing hormone and testosterone with an inhibitory analog of luteinizing hormone-releasing hormone in adult male rhesus monkeys. J Clin Endocrinol Metab 59:601–607, 1984

5. BURSTEIN M, SCHOLNICK HR, MORFIN R: Rapid method for the isolation of lipoproteins from human serum by precipitation with polyanions. J Lipid Res 11:583–595, 1970

6. COWSAR DR, TICE TR, GILLEY RM, ENGLISH JP: Poly(lactide-co-glycolide) microcapsules for controlled release of steroids. In Methods in Enzymology 112:101–116, 1985

7. FRIEDEWALD WT, LEVY RI, FREDRICKSON DS: Estimation of the concentration of low-density lipoprotein cholesterol in plasma, without use of the preparative ultracentrifuge. Clin Chem 18:499–502, 1972

8. MITRUKA BM, RAWNSLEY HM: Clinical biochemistry. In Clinical Biochemical and Hematological Reference Values in Normal Experimental Animals, pp 154–157. New York, Masson Publishers, 1977

9. PLANT TM, HESS DL, HOTCHKISS J, KNOBIL E: Testosterone and the control of gonadotropin secretion in the male Rhesus monkey, *macaca mulatta*. Endocrinol 103:535–541, 1977

10. SHAW LM, BRUMMUND W, DORIO RJ: An evaluation of a kinetic acid phosphatase method. Am J Clin Pathol 68:57–62, 1977

11. TICE TR, LEWIS DH: Microcapsulation process. U.S. Patent No. 4,389,330. (Issued June 1983)

12. WARD PCJ: Chemical profiles of disease. Human Pathology 4:47–65, 1973

33

Preclinical Studies with LHRH Antagonists

ERIC C. PETRIE

ALVIN M. MATSUMOTO

JOHN J. NESTOR, JR.

BRIAN H. VICKERY

KENNETH M. GROSS

MOLLY B. SOUTHWORTH

WILLIAM J. BREMNER

The elucidation of the structure of LHRH stimulated attempts to develop clinically useful antagonistic analogues.[4] Initial attempts were only minimally successful, however, and early antagonists were of low potency. More recently, much progress has been made in increasing the potency of LHRH antagonists, with net increases of many thousandfold being achieved.[2,5,6,7] We have assessed the potency and duration of action of several of these antagonists in rats and have initiated studies of the suppressive effects of one compound in monkeys.

MATERIALS AND METHODS

ANIMALS

Adult male Sprague-Dawley rats (Tyler Laboratories) were individually housed under a 12:12 hr, light–dark cycle, with free access to food and water. They were castrated under ether-induced anesthesia a minimum of 3 weeks before use in the assay except in study B, when they were studied 1 to 2 days after castration. Animals were approximately 90 days old at the time of testing.

We appreciate the technical assistance of Patricia Gosciewski, Patricia Payne, and Vasumathi Sundarraj, and the help of Elaine Rost and Maxine Pollock in manuscript preparation.

This work was supported by NIH Grant P-50-HD-12629, the Veterans Administration, Syntex Research, and March of Dimes Grant No. 8-83-59.

TABLE 33-1. Structure of LHRH Antagonists

NUMBER	STRUCTURES
1	[N-Ac-Pro^1,D-pF-Phe^2,D-Nal(2)^{3,6}]-LHRH
2	[N-Ac-D-Nal(2)^1,D-pF-Phe^2,D-Trp^3,D-hArg(Me$_2$)^6]-LHRH
3	[N-Ac-D-Nal(2)^1,D-pF-Phe^2,D-Trp^3,D-hArg(Et$_2$)^6]-LHRH
4	[N-Ac-D-Nal(2)^1,D-pCl-Phe^2,D-Trp^3,D-hArg(Et$_2$)^6,D-Ala^{10}]-LHRH

LHRH ANTAGONISTS

The structures of the LHRH antagonists are shown in Table 33-1. The compounds were administered as solutions in either corn oil or a 1:1 mixture of propylene glycol and normal saline (PGSA).

BLOOD SAMPLING

Samples in studies A and B were drawn from unanesthetized, unrestrained animals by means of a Silastic jugular catheter that had been placed with the animals under ether anesthesia 1 to 2 days prior to the experiment. In studies C and D, the samples were obtained by jugular venipuncture performed with the animals under light ether anesthesia.

EXPERIMENTAL DESIGN

Study A

For an initial assessment of the time course and dose–response effects of antagonist 1, castrated male rats (n = 5–6 per group) were injected subcutaneously with 25, 100, or 500 μg/kg of analogue or with PGSA vehicle alone. At 0, 1, 2, 4, 8, 24, 48, and 72 hours postinjection, 1.5-ml blood samples were drawn for measurement of LH and FSH content. To maintain blood volume and to ensure maintained patency of the catheter, 1.5 ml of heparinized saline (50 units/ml) were infused after each sample was withdrawn.

Study B

To characterize more fully the rapidity of response to low doses and to monitor for changes in the pulsatile pattern of LH release,[8] antagonist 1 was administered intravenously and blood sampled frequently. During a baseline sampling period of 3 hours, 50-μl blood samples were obtained from the jugular catheter at 6-minute intervals. The animals (n = 4–5 per group) then received an IV injection of analogue (10 μg/kg) or PGSA vehicle alone given as a bolus. Blood sampling was continued for another 3 hours, and the LH concentration was measured in each sample.

Study C

The rats (n = 5–6 per group) were injected intramuscularly with vehicle or with 50 μg/kg of antagonists 2 or 3 in corn oil. Blood samples (1 ml) were obtained at 0, 2, 24, and 48 hours postinjection.

Study D

Castrate male rats (n = 5 per group) were injected intramuscularly with corn oil or 25 or 50 μg/kg of antagonist 4. Blood sampling times were as in study C.

HORMONE ASSAYS

Blood samples from studies A, C, and D were allowed to clot at 4°C, centrifuged, and the serum stored at −20°C. In study B, duplicate blood samples (25 μl) were deposited directly into tubes containing 225 μl of assay buffer and stored at −20°C. LH and FSH levels in these samples were determined subsequently by radioimmunoassay.

The LH assay utilized NIAMDD reagents including reference standard RP-2, S-5 antibody and ^{125}I-labeled LH (I-5) as tracer. For assays of the diluted whole blood samples from study B, aliquots of 50% washed red cells in assay buffer were added to the tubes of the standard curve. Intra-assay and interassay coefficients of variation (CV) were 7% and 9% for serum assays, and 10% and 12% for whole-blood assays. Minimum detectable level was 0.15 ng/ml.

The FSH assay used NIAMDD reference standard RP-1, antibody S-10 and ^{125}I-labeled FSH (I-5) as tracer. Intra-assay and interassay CVs were 8% and 10% respectively.

DATA ANALYSIS

Data from Studies A, C, and D were evaluated using analyses of variance. Post hoc comparisons were made with the Newman-Keuls procedure. LH pulse data (study B) were analyzed by a modified version of the computer program of Santen and Bardin followed by paired t-tests of pulse parameters.

RESULTS

STUDY A

LH levels were maximally suppressed within 2 hours of 100 μg/kg or 500 μg/kg of antagonist 1 injection (Fig. 33-1). This suppression persisted for 8 hours at the lower dose and for 24 hours with the higher dose. LH suppression was less marked, slower in onset, and less persistent at the 25 μg/kg dose level.

Changes in FSH levels were less pronounced and much delayed. FSH levels in antagonist-treated animals did not differ from those of controls at 1, 2, 4, or 8 hours postinjection. At 24 hours postinjection, only the 500-μg/kg dose group had lower FSH levels than did the controls (means ± SEM were 65.4 ± 45 versus 1380.0 ± 164 ng/ml respectively). By 48 hours postinjection, no differences from control animals were detected.

STUDY B

Intravenous injection of 10 μg/kg of antagonist 1 caused a decline in blood LH levels within minutes, and the levels continued to fall for approximately 1 hour after infusion ceased (Fig. 33-2). To eliminate the effect of this rapidly

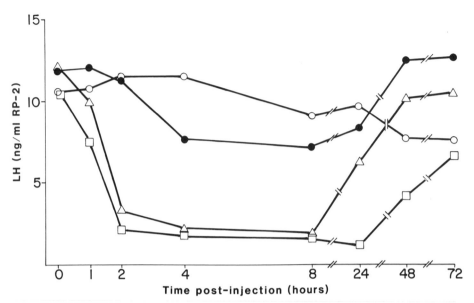

FIG. 33-1. Mean serum LH levels in study A. Castrated male rats received an SC injection of 50% propylene glycol vehicle (○ — ○, n = 5) or antagonist 1 at doses of 25 μg/kg (● — ●, n = 6), 100 μg/kg (△ — △, n = 5), or 500 μg/kg (□ — □, n = 6).

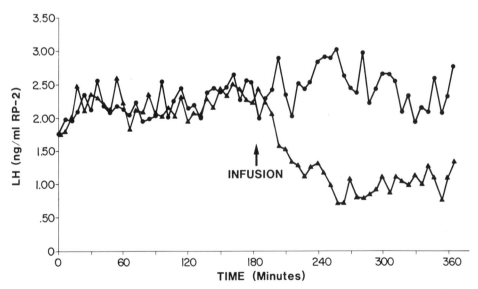

FIG. 33-2. Study B. Mean serum LH levels in castrated male rats before and after IV infusion of 10 μg/kg antagonist 1 in 50% propylene glycol vehicle (▲ — ▲, n = 5), or vehicle alone (● — ●, n = 4). Blood samples were drawn by means of a jugular catheter at 6-minute intervals.

TABLE 33-2. LH Pulse Parameters in Study B: Mean ± SEM

TREATMENT	PREINFUSION			POSTINFUSION		
	*MEAN LH**	*PULSES/ HR*	*AMPLITUDE**	*MEAN LH**	*PULSES/ HR*	*AMPLITUDE**
10 μg/kg Antagonist 1	2.21 ± 0.22	2.70 ± 0.41	0.84 ± 0.09	1.00 ± 0.10	2.00 ± 0.27	0.62† ± 0.10
50% Propylene Glycol vehicle	2.23 ± 0.15	2.37 ± 0.31	0.77 ± 0.10	2.49 ± 0.25	1.87 ± 0.24	1.01 ± 0.09

* ng/ml of RP-2 standard.

† P < 0.05 vs. vehicle and preinfusion.

changing baseline on the computer analysis of LH pulse characteristics, data from the first postinfusion hour were excluded from analysis.

As shown in Table 33-2, mean LH levels in the antagonist-treated group declined following infusion (p < 0.05) as did LH pulse amplitude (p < 0.05). The number of pulses per hour was not affected significantly. There were no significant changes in mean LH levels, pulse amplitude or pulse frequency in the animals receiving vehicle alone.

STUDY C

Antagonists 2 and 3 caused a marked decline in circulating levels of LH by 2 hours postinjection (Fig. 33-3). LH levels in the groups receiving 50 μg/kg of antagonists 2 and 3 remained suppressed at 24 hours postinjection. Levels of LH had returned to control in both groups by 48 hours postinjection.

FSH levels changed less rapidly. At 24 hours postinjection, FSH levels were significantly suppressed in both groups receiving analogues (mean ± SEM of 786.2 ± 82.6 ng/ml). Control values at 24 hours postinjection were 1813 ± 86.7 ng/ml.

STUDY D

Both the 25 μg/kg and 50 μg/kg doses of antagonist 4 produced a significant (p < 0.05) decline in LH levels by 2 hours postinjection (Fig. 33-4). LH suppression persisted for a full 24 hours in both dose groups; FSH levels changed less rapidly in the antagonist-treated animals and were significantly (p < 0.05) suppressed only at 24 hours postinjection. At that time FSH levels (mean ± SEM) were 786.2 ± 119.2 ng/ml in the 50 μg/kg dosage group, 893.0 ± 209.2 ng/ml in the 25 μg/kg group and 1728.4 ± 67.2 ng/ml in the vehicle control group.

DISCUSSION

All analogues tested caused a rapid decrease in circulating levels of LH and a more gradual suppression of FSH levels. The initial decrease in LH occurred

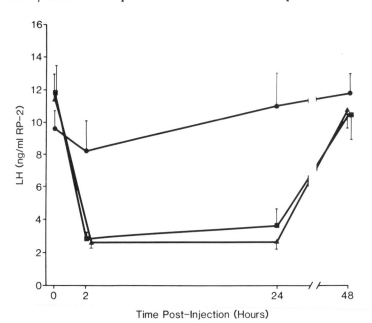

FIG. 33-3. Mean serum LH levels in study C. Castrated male rats were injected IM with corn oil (● — ●, n = 6) or a 50 μg/kg dose of antagonist 2 (■ — ■, n = 5), or antagonist 3 (▲ — ▲, n = 5), in the same vehicle.

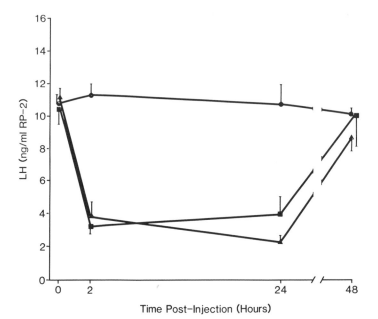

FIG. 33-4. Serum LH levels in study D. Castrated male rats were injected IM with corn oil (● — ●, n = 6) or with antagonist 4 in the same vehicle at a dose of 25 μg/kg (■ — ■, n = 6) or 50 μg/kg (▲ — ▲, n = 6).

within minutes of the administration of the antagonists. This presumably reflects the high affinity of the agents for pituitary LHRH receptors. Interestingly, low dosages of antagonist 1 (study B) led to decreases in the pulse amplitude of LH secretory episodes but no change in pulse frequency, implying that the analogue induced partial pituitary desensitization to endogenous episodic LHRH production.

In contrast to the rapid changes in serum LH caused by the antagonists, FSH levels declined slowly. Significant reductions in FSH levels were not evident until 24 hours after analogue administration. The delayed response to antagonist treatment is consistent with other studies, showing that FSH levels may persist for up to 24 hours following neutralization of releasing factor stimulation.[3] It may reflect differences between the circulatory half lives of the two gonadotropins as well as the persistence of FSH secretion for up to 24 hours following LHRH removal.

These studies have demonstrated that antagonist 4 is a very potent compound, with duration of action exceeding 24 hours in the dosages used here. Because of this evidence of effectiveness and the fact that we noted no apparent side-effects in the rats, we went on to study this compound in the adult male monkey (*M. fascicularis*).

In the first monkey study,[1] a single injection of 5 µg/kg or more of antagonist 4 into castrated animals markedly reduced plasma LH and FSH levels by 4 hours (the first time measurements were obtained). Nadir levels (40% of preinjection control values) of both gonadotropins were reached 24 hours after administration of 250 or 500 µg/kg, and these hormones remained significantly suppressed for over 48 hours following the highest dose.

In the second monkey study,[1] using intact animals, a single injection of 50 µg/kg or more of antagonist 4 markedly reduced plasma LH and T levels within 6 hours. Doses of 250 or 500 µg/kg maintained LH and T levels at <30% of control levels for over 24 hours. In a third study, using intact adult animals, 250 µg/kg daily for 3 weeks resulted in near-castrate levels of T throughout the course of antagonist administration. Daily injection of 100 µg/kg, on the other hand, were ineffective in suppressing T levels. In a fourth study, which is ongoing, we are assessing the effects on hormone levels and sperm production of dosages of 250 and 750 µg/kg as daily injections with or without the addition of testosterone replacement therapy. Obviously, the key question is whether sperm production can be eliminated while plasma testosterone levels are held within the normal range by a combination of antagonist and testosterone administration.

CONCLUSION

For clinical utility, LHRH antagonists need to exert both profound suppressive effects on gonadotropin secretion and a duration of action of many hours. The rat assay used here has monitored both parameters, and several of the analogues appear to meet the criteria. Compound 4, the most potent of the series, shows promise from the monkey studies for gonadosuppression by once-daily administration. This compound is currently undergoing clinical evaluation in man.

REFERENCES

1. ADAMS LA, BREMNER WJ, NESTOR J, VICKERY B, STEINER RA: Primate studies with a new, potent gonadotropin-releasing hormone (GnRH) antagonist. J Clin Endocrinol Metab 62:58–63, 1986
2. COY DH, HORVATH A, NEKOLA MV, COY EJ, ERCHEGYI J, SCHALLY AV: Peptide antagonists of LHRH: Large increases in antiovulatory activities produced by basic D-amino acids in the six position. Endocrinology 110:1445, 1982
3. LINCOLN GA, FRASER H: Blockade of episodic secretion of luteinizing hormone in the ram by the administration of antibodies to luteinizing hormone releasing hormone. Biol Reprod 21:1239, 1979
4. MATSUO H, BABA Y, NAIR RMG, ARIMURA A, SCHALLY AV: Structure of the porcine LH- and FSH-releasing hormone. Part I. Proposed amino acid sequence. Biochem Biophys Res Commun 43:1334, 1971
5. MCRAE GI, VICKERY BH, NESTOR JJ, BREMNER WJ, BADGER TM: Biological activity of a highly potent LHRH antagonist. In VICKERY BH, NESTOR JJ, HAFEZ ESE (eds): LHRH and Its Analogs: Contraceptive and Therapeutic Applications, pp 137–151. Lancaster, England, MTP Press, 1983
6. NESTOR JJ, TAHILRAMANI R, HO TL, MCRAE GI, VICKERY BH, BREMNER WJ: New luteinizing hormone-releasing factor antagonists. In HRUBY VJ, RICH DH (eds): Peptides: Structure and Function, pp 861–864. Pierce Chemical Company, Rockford, IL, 1983
7. RIVIER J, RIVIER C, PERRIN M, PORTER J, VALE W: LHRH analogs as antiovulatory agents. In VICKERY BH, NESTOR JJ, HAFEZ ESE (eds): LHRH and Its Analogs: Contraceptive and Therapeutic Applications, pp 11–22. Lancaster, England, MTP Press, 1983
8. STEINER RA, BREMNER WJ, CLIFTON DK: Regulation of luteinizing hormone pulse frequency and amplitude by testosterone in the adult male rat. Endocrinology 111:2055, 1982

34

Preclinical and Clinical Trials with LHRH Agonists and Antagonists

EBERHARD NIESCHLAG

ERIK MICHEL

GERHARD F. WEINBAUER

Because spermatogenesis is under hormonal control, the possibility of interfering with spermatogenesis by means of endocrinologic mechanisms appears to be a reasonable approach to male fertility regulation. Although the endocrine suppression of ovulation in women has proven to be an extremely efficient and also practicable method, the endocrine approach to male fertility regulation is associated with special problems. The production of sperm and male hormones in the testes is so closely connected that it is difficult to suppress sperm production selectively without simultaneously suppressing androgens that are responsible for erythropoesis, protein anabolism, bone metabolism, secondary sex and behavioral characteristics as well as libido and potency (see Chap. 37). Therefore, unless it is possible to interfere selectively with spermatogenesis without affecting Leydig cell function, or unless the substance used has androgenic properties itself (see Chap. 29) these methods will require androgen substitution.

One of the promising endocrine approaches to male fertility regulation is the use of LHRH analogues in combination with androgen substitution. These analogues are either more active than the native decapeptide; that is, they function as LHRH agonists or superagonists, or, they block the function of LHRH; that is, they are antagonistic in nature. Whereas the LHRH agonists given in high doses desensitize the pituitary, the LHRH antagonists block the pituitary LHRH receptors. In the end, the effect of both substances is identical, namely, suppression of pituitary gonadotropin secretion. These effects are not only interesting in the context of male fertility regulation, but also are being applied in the treatment of androgen-dependent tumors. In fact, after extensive testing, LHRH agonists became available for clinical use in the treatment of prostatic carcinoma. Parallel to their development for the treatment of prostatic carcinoma, LHRH agonists have been tested in clinical trials for male fertility regulation (trials summarized in Table 34-1). LHRH antagonists with sufficiently high specific activity only recently have been synthesized and have not been tested in humans beyond phase I studies.

TABLE 34-1. Clinical Trials With LHRH Agonists for Male Fertility Regulation

	SUBJECTS (number)	AGONIST	DAILY DOSE (μg/day)	ROUTE OF ADMINISTRATION	WEEKS	ANDROGEN	EFFECT ON SPERM COUNTS
Bergquist et al 1979	4	Buserelin	5	SC injection	17	None	None
Linde et al 1981	8	D-Trp⁶-Pro⁹-NEth	50	SC injection	6–10	None	Azoosp. in 1/8
Doelle et al 1983	6	DTO	50	SC injection	20	TE 100 mg biweekly	$12 \pm 4^*$
Rabin et al 1984	8	DTO	100–500	SC injection	20	TE 100 mg biweekly	5.5^*
Bhasin et al 1983	7	Nafarelin	200	SC injection	16	TE 100 mg biweekly	$17 \pm 6^*$
Schürmeyer et al 1984	7	Buserelin	118	SC infusion	12	TU daily	$18 \pm 5^*$
	4	DTO	230	SC infusion	12	TU daily	$10 \pm 3^*$
Michel et al 1985	7	DTO	440	SC infusion	12	TU daily	$44 \pm 14^*$

* Lowest mean values (mil/ml)

TE, Testosterone enanthate

TU, Testosterone undecanoate

LHRH-AGONIST TRIALS IN NONHUMAN PRIMATES

Before testing the potential of LHRH agonists in clinical trials, we investigated their effectiveness in suppressing spermatogenesis and possible side-effects of the LHRH agonist buserelin in rhesus monkeys (Akhtar and associates).[4] We were able to show that chronic infusion implemented by subcutaneously implanted osmotic minipumps was the most effective form of application and led to azoospermia while intermittent injections, of even high doses, were ineffective.[1,2,16] We also found that the required testosterone substitution attenuates the antigonadal effect of the GnRH agonist[3] and that therefore testosterone substitution should not be applied simultaneously with the LHRH agonist, but only when a testosterone decrease is noted.

CLINICAL TRIALS WITH LHRH AGONISTS

The lack of side-effects plus achievement of azoospermia in the primate studies gave us reason to conduct our first clinical trial with an LHRH-agonist infusion.[13] Because constant release of the LHRH agonist appeared mandatory, but the subcutaneous implantation of osmotic minipumps or the use of mechanical pumps was precluded, the osmotic pumps were worn extracorporeally in a small reservoir, and their content was delivered subcutaneously by means of a small infusion set. For 12 weeks, eleven volunteers participating in the trial received 180 μg/day (n = 7) or 230 μg/day (n = 4) of buserelin from osmotic minipumps changed weekly or biweekly (Table 34-1).

After an initial rise, serum LH, FSH, and testosterone levels decreased below the normal range. After 4 weeks of treatment, the LH response to acute LHRH stimulation was abolished in the high-dose group and severely impaired in the low-dose group (Fig. 34-1). Androgen substitution using the orally effective testosterone undecanoate was initiated when androgen levels fell below 10 nmol/liter or when the volunteers complained of signs of androgen deficiency. Initiation of testosterone substitution ranged from the third to the ninth week of treatment. Although sperm counts were suppressed in both groups, this effect occurred sooner and to a higher degree in the high-dose group. Azoospermia, however, as a prerequisite for fertility regulation in men, was not observed in any volunteer. All subjects tolerated this type of treatment well and no side-effects were encountered.

Although the ultimate goal for male fertility regulation, namely azoospermia, could not be achieved, the results were encouraging. Because a dose dependence of the sperm suppression could be noted in the foregoing studies, a further study employing an even higher dose of buserelin, that is, 440 μg/day, was initiated. Testosterone was substituted with the orally effective testosterone undecanoate and 80 mg, administered from the fifth week, was increased to 120 mg/day from the eighth week of treatment. Although LHRH stimulation tests performed at the end of treatment showed pituitary desensitization and significant suppression of serum testosterone levels, the subjects' emotional well-being remained unchanged. With this regimen only a moderate decrease in sperm counts was observed, however, and severe oligozoospermia was not achieved.[10]

LHRH tests in normal volunteers before, during
and after constant LHRH agonist infusion

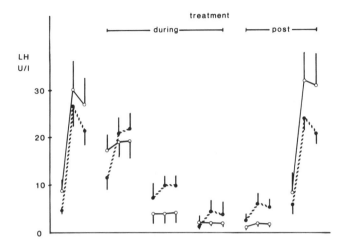

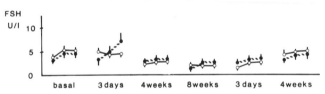

FIG. 34-1. Serum LH and FSH responses (mean ± SD) 25 minutes and 45 minutes after 25 µg LHRH bolus injection in volunteers receiving constant LHRH agonist (buserelin) infusion. Seven men receiving on average 118 ± 24 µg/day (*broken line*); four men receiving on average 230 ± 27 µg/day (*solid line*). (From Schürmeyer T, Knuth UA, et al.: Suppression of pituitary and testicular function in normal men by constant gonadotropin-releasing hormone agonist infusion. J Clin Endocrinol Metab 59:19, 1984)

Although there is reason to assume that not only in nonhuman (as discussed before) but also in human primates,[14] sustained release of the LHRH agonist is more effective than single injections, our studies with constant infusion of buserelin did not lead to the expected and required results. The possibility remains that androgen replacement is counterproductive and may sustain spermatogenesis. The importance of testosterone administration in this type of clinical trials is highlighted further by Linde and colleagues[9] and Doelle and co-workers.[8] In the first study, LHRH agonists were injected without testosterone substitution, whereas in the second study testosterone enanthate was administered simultaneously with the LHRH agonist. When no testosterone was given, the suppression of sperm counts was more pronounced and occurred sooner than when testosterone was given simultaneously. In our trial the mode of testosterone application may have been particularly suited to

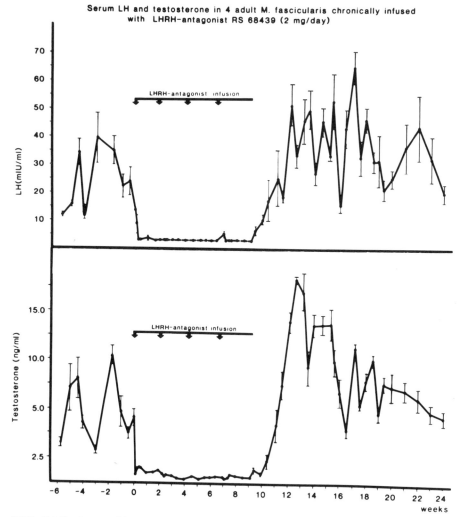

FIG. 34-2. Serum bio-LH and testosterone in four adult *M. fascicularis* monkeys chronically infused with the LHRH antagonist RS 68439 (2 mg/day). (From Weinbauer GF, Surmann FJ et al.: Reversible inhibition of testicular function by a gonadotropin hormone-releasing hormone antagonist in monkeys (*Macaca fascicularis*). Fertil Steril 42:906, 1984)

maintain spermatogenesis. The administration of two or three testosterone undecanoate capsules per day produced two or three distinct serum testosterone peaks that may have been sufficient to counteract the sperm suppression achieved by the down-regulatory effects of the LHRH agonist. Thus, in future studies even more care has to be exerted in the administration of testosterone and, ideally, a constant-release preparation resulting in physiologic concentrations in circulation would be required.

LHRH ANTAGONISTS

The treatment with LHRH agonists has the disadvantage that pituitary and testes are stimulated at the beginning of treatment before suppression is achieved. It therefore appears more reasonable to use LHRH antagonists that directly block pituitary LHRH receptors and do not achieve their effects by means of desensitization.

Thus far, LHRH antagonists have only been assessed for male fertility regulation on a long-term basis in preclinical monkey studies. The antagonist N-Ac-D-Nal (2)[1], D-pCl-Phe[2], D-Trp[3], D-hArg(Et2)[6]-D-Ala[10] LHRH (RS-68439, Syntex Research) was administered by constant infusion from osmotic minipumps at a dose of 2 mg/day for 9 weeks to four cynomolgus monkeys.[15] An immediate and precipitous decline of LH and testosterone levels was found, which persisted uniformly during the entire treatment period (Fig. 34-2). Testicular volumes underwent a drastic decrease, and at the nadir, 25% of the basal levels were measured. Three of the four monkeys were azoospermic after 7 to 9 weeks of treatment, and the fourth produced only 4×10^6 sperm/ejaculate as compared to $>50 \times 10^6$ sperm/ejaculate in the pretreatment phase. Histology revealed disruption of spermatogenesis, decreases in tubular diameter, thickening of the tubular wall, and atrophy of Leydig cells. The endocrine parameters normalized within 2 weeks of cessation of treatment. Normal seminal parameters were found 14 to 16 weeks post-treatment. Despite severe histologic alterations, all effects were fully reversible. Similar results were achieved in another group of cynomolgus monkeys treated with another potent LHRH antagonist (Org 30276, Organon Scientific Development Group).[5]

Thus, LHRH antagonists appear to have an even better potential for male fertility regulation than do the agonists. Before clinical trials can be initiated, however, toxicology of the compounds has to be fully assessed. From animal studies it appears that the problems with testosterone substitution may be similar for both LHRH antagonists and agonists,[12] and this point will require careful consideration in the pending clinical trials.

REFERENCES

1. AKHTAR FB, WICKINGS EJ, ZAIDI P, NIESCHLAG E: Pituitary and testicular functions in sexually mature rhesus monkeys under high-dose LHRH-agonist treatment. Acta Endocrinol 101:113, 1982
2. AKHTAR FB, MARSHALL GR, WICKINGS EJ, NIESCHLAG E: Reversible induction of azoospermia in rhesus monkeys by constant infusion of a GnRH agonist using osmotic minipumps. J Clin Endocrinol Metab 57:534, 1983
3. AKHTAR FB, MARSHALL GR, NIESCHLAG E: Testosterone supplementation attenuates the antifertility effects of an LHRH agonist in male monkeys. Int J Androl 6:461, 1983
4. AKHTAR FB, WICKINGS EJ, NIESCHLAG E: Male fertility control with an LHRH-agonist: Primate studies. In VICKERY BH, NESTOR JJ JR, HAFEZ ESE (eds): LHRH and its Analogs: Contraceptive and Therapeutic Applications, p 77. Lancaster, England, MTP Press, 1984
5. AKHTAR FB, WEINBAUER GW, NIESCHLAG E: Acute and chronic effects of a gonadotropin-releasing hormone antagonist on pituitary and testicular function in monkeys. J Endocrinol 104:345, 1985
6. BERGQUIST C, NILLIUS SJ, BERGH T, SKARIN G, WIDE L: Inhibitory effects on gonadotropin secretion and gonadal function in men during chronic treatment with a potent stimulatory luteinizing hormone-releasing hormone analogue. Acta Endocrinol 91:601, 1979

7. BHASIN S, HEBER D, STEINER B, PETERSON M, JANG M, ATIENZA V, SWERDLOFF RS: Combined treatment with a GnRH agonist and testosterone in man: An approach toward reversible oligospermia without impotence (abstr). Fertil Steril 40:418, 1983
8. DOELLE GC, ALEXANDER AN, EVANS RM, LINDE R, RIVIER J, VALE W, RABIN D: Combined treatment with an LHRH agonist and testosterone in man: Reversible oligospermia without impotence. J Androl 4:298, 1983
9. LINDE R, DOELLE GC, ALEXANDER N, KIRCHNER F, VALE W, RIVIER J, RABIN D: Reversible inhibition of testicular steroidogenesis and spermatogenesis by a potent gonadotropin-releasing hormone agonist in normal men. N Engl J Med 305:663, 1981
10. MICHEL E, BENTS H, AKHTAR FB, HÖNIGL W, SANDOW J, NIESCHLAG E: Failure of high-dose sustained release GnRH agonist plus testosterone to suppress male fertility, p. 37, (abstr). J Androl (Suppl) 6: 1985
11. RABIN D, EVANS RM, ALEXANDER AN, DOELLE GC, RIVIER J, VALE W, LIDDLE GW: Heterogeneity of sperm density profiles following 20-week therapy with high-dose LHRH analog plus testosterone. J Androl 5:176, 1984
12. REA MR, MARSHALL GR, WEINBAUER GF, NIESCHLAG E: Testosterone maintains pituitary and serum FSH and spermatogenesis in GnRH antagonist-suppressed rats. J Endocrinol 1986 (in press)
13. SCHÜRMEYER T, KNUTH UA, FREISCHEM CW, SANDOW J, AKHTAR FB, NIESCHLAG E: Suppression of pituitary and testicular function in normal men by constant gonadotropin-releasing hormone agonist infusion. J Clin Endocrinol Metab 59:19, 1984
14. SWERDLOFF RS, BHASIN S: Suppression of gonadal function by constant infusion of GnRH agonist in the human male (abstract). J Steroid Biochem 20 No. 6 B:1347, 1984
15. WEINBAUER GF, SURMANN FJ, AKHTAR FB, SHAH GV, NIESCHLAG E: Reversible inhibition of testicular function by a gonadotropin hormone-releasing hormone antagonist in monkeys (*Macaca fascicularis*). Fertil Steril 42:906, 1984
16. WICKINGS EJ, ZAIDI P, NIESCHLAG E: Effects of chronic, high-dose LHRH-agonist treatment on pituitary and testicular functions in rhesus monkeys. J Androl 2:72, 1982

35

Discussion: Hormonal Approaches

MODERATORS: ANDRZEJ BARTKE

EBERHARD NIESCHLAG

ARE HIGH DOSES OF TESTOSTERONE AND NORTESTOSTERONE DERIVATIVES SAFE FOR MEN?

There is more concern about using estrogens in men. In clinical experience, pseudohermaphrodite patients and transvestites who are genetically male but want to change their gender and so are treated with estrogens are very sensitive to estrogens (*e.g.*, in terms of blood clotting and thrombosis). There may be a much higher risk of blood clotting from estrogen than from androgens. We do not know the long-term effects in those men treated with testosterone.

In a study based on 17 men given androgenic hormones, it is only slightly reassuring to find no change in total high-density lipoprotein (HDL) cholesterol levels and low-density lipoprotein (LDL) cholesterol levels.

The lack of HDL suppression with the 19-nor compound is interesting because the data do not show a correlation with HDL suppression in humans and androgenic activity. For example, testosterone is a much more potent androgen than levonorgestrel on a weight basis, but they are almost equally potent in suppressing HDL at clinically effective doses.

In addition, although there is a good epidemiologic correlation with HDL levels and atherosclerosis as it occurs in the normal population, the effect of drugs that change HDL levels and their ability to influence atherosclerosis is not clearly established. In a 4-year study just completed on monkeys, in which investigators compared normal males, normal females, females treated with levonorgestrel and estradiol, and males treated with levonorgestrel and ethinyl estradiol, the levonorgestrel-treated animals had the lowest HDL levels and the atherosclerotic index was greater in males than in levonorgestrel plus estradiol-treated females. Thus, in two levonorgestrel-treated groups that had very low HDL levels, one group was protected from atherosclerosis and the other was not.

Panelists: Ricardo Asch, William J. Bremner, Larry L. Ewing, Ulrich A. Knuth, Eberhard Nieschlag, C. Alvin Paulsen; *Discussants:* C. Wayne Bardin, Philippe Bouchard, Shalender Bhasin, Paul Franchimont, Alfredo Goldsmith, Walter L. Hermann, Erkki Hirvonen, Danny H. Lewis, Diana Petitti, Carlos A. Schaffenberg, Brian Vickery, Gerald I. Zatuchni

The investigators could not predict from HDL levels what the coronary artery index would be between groups, but they could make this prediction within groups. Several groups studying lipids reported that women could tolerate much lower HDL levels than men and not develop atherosclerosis, indicating that between males and females there is something other than HDL level correlating to atherosclerosis. When a steroid is found not to change HDL, it should be studied.

ARE THERE STUDIES IN MONKEYS TO ASSESS WHETHER STEROID ADMINISTRATION WILL PRODUCE AZOOSPERMIA?

It would be impossible to do the matrix study in monkeys that was done in rats, so investigators spent nearly two years trying different doses of testosterone and estradiol in the same group of monkeys, putting them on treatment and leaving them on for several months; it was not possible to do enough different doses to show really clearly whether there was a synergistic effect in the monkey.

IN MALE FERTILITY CONTROL STUDIES, WHY DO SOME MEN NOT ACHIEVE AZOOSPERMIA?

Investigators should find an answer to this question before going ahead. One study compared the responders and nonresponders by doing 20-minute blood sampling just before the next injection and then measuring luteinizing hormone (LH) and follicle-stimulating hormone (FSH) and testosterone levels; over a 4-hour period of time the investigators did not find pulses of LH, but they did not have the resources to monitor the gonadotropins continuously throughout the month in which the men received their medication. From other data that have resulted from trying to suppress sperm production in men with testosterone alone, given in 200 mg doses three times a week, and measuring gonadotropins, the lack of response does not appear to reside in the gonadotropin.

HAS AN ATTEMPT BEEN MADE TO EXPLAIN WHY TWO MEN BECAME AZOOSPERMIC AND THEN REACHED NORMAL SPERM LEVELS AFTER TREATMENT WITH 19-NORTESTOSTERONE?

There was no change or deviation from the normal range of sperm counts or hormone levels; however, the two men who went through a period of azoospermia and then returned to normal showed an escape of their suppressive activity of LH levels. In all the other men the LH levels were below detection, but suddenly in those two men the LH levels returned to a range of 1.5 to just above detection limit. Possibly if their LH levels could be suppressed by another substance, their spermatogenesis also could be suppressed. The investigators are thinking now of combining the 19-nortestosterone with some additional agent, perhaps LHRH.

Another group of investigators saw similar effects with danazol plus testosterone; when maximum suppressability was reached, they gave danazol the first week of each month plus testosterone once a month, and saw escaping or fluctuation and lack of suppressability.

WITH LEVONORGESTREL, WERE A CORRELATION AND A CHANGE IN INDEX FOUND WITH ESTRADIOL AND PROGESTIN?

In monthly lipid studies, the investigators drew a good correlation between either total cholesterol or HDL cholesterol and the amount of atherosclerosis in a given group of animals. This was the case with all the fractions measured, regardless of how the data were related, whether they were correlated to total cholesterol, LDL cholesterol, HDL, or some ratio in which the cholesterol was normalized with the HDL cholesterol. This also has been done with humans. Usually the ratio is that of total cholesterol divided by the HDL cholesterol, and there is a good correlation within a group of men or women between those values. This held in the monkeys, as long as females and males within a group, were not compared; however, a given HDL cholesterol in a male was much different from the same HDL cholesterol in a female.

On the issue of LDL–HDL concentrations, one group of investigators has looked at total cholesterol LDL and HDL concentrations during the course of GnRH agonist studies in the human and were surprised at the absence of any significant changes. It appears, however, that there are several difficulties: one is the stability of the samples; HDL concentrations tend to change in stored samples so they need to be measured immediately or within a few days at best. The subfractions of HDL and the LDL and HDL-associated apoprotein concentrations also may show divergent changes, so that overall concentration of HDL may not change, yet HDL_3 may in fact decrease significantly. That fraction is best correlated with risk for cardiovascular disease.

ARE PROSTATIC PROBLEMS LIKELY TO RESULT FROM THE USE OF ANDROGENS?

About 1976 a consultant team supported by the World Health Organization (WHO) on the potential of increasing prostatic disease sharply with the use of androgens, looked at whether a marker could provide a monitor for detecting early prostatic disease. None was found. Moreover, there appeared to be no way to separate or identify those persons that might be more susceptible to prostatic changes. It also is apparent that distribution of testosterone throughout the body is poorly understood. Despite studies on seminal fluid testosterone, we really do not know what the concentration of testosterone is within the prostate, seminal vesicles, and other parts of the tissue when we administer testosterone.

Although there is a clear relationship between testosterone levels and the volume of the prostate, there is a part of the prostate both in dogs and in men that is more responsive to estrogens. Paradoxically, although levels of testosterone slowly decrease in men with age, at the same time the prostate begins to enlarge. When this happens, aromatase activity increases. The production of estradiol and possibly the benign prostatic hypertrophy seems related more to this distorted ratio than to testosterone alone. Some studies are needed on aromatase inhibitors.

SHOULD THE GnRH ANALOGUES BE USED AT ALL IN HUMANS?

In both the male and female, a contraceptive effect is achieved by performing a selective pharmacologic hypophysectomy for gonadotrophs, a deficiency that then has to be corrected. Contraception in women is sometimes achieved by producing a pharmacologic oophorectomy, which subsequently must be corrected; if it is performed halfway, then one must worry about unopposed estrogen. In males, one of the immediate problems has been that the men soon became impotent, so that even collecting semen specimens was impossible. Testosterone was then added, paradoxically, taking it away and then adding it again.

On the other hand, if one says it is ridiculous to substitute testosterone, the concept of oral contraceptives for the female is also ridiculous, because you take progestins, "knock out" the pituitary and the ovary, and then substitute estrogens. Why then should it not work for the male to "knock out" the pituitary and substitute testosterone?

There is no problem in the concept of replacing testosterone. That is how we treat medically hypophysectomized men. If we had a delivery system such as microcapsules that could deliver both the GnRH antagonist or the agonist and also could deliver testosterone, there is no conceptual problem in that kind of drug system, were it effective. To date, no agent except the antagonist has been able to induce medical hypophysectomy, and for the first time we have seen that it predictably does induce azoospermia in animals.

The tricky question is one of antagonist toxicity. Some of the newer-generation antagonists that biochemists are working with have a much higher therapeutic index of safety. The rat is also a peculiar organism with regard to histamine release, and therefore investigators testing antagonists in the female have seen some local reactions but no systemic toxicity that could be attributed to histamine release. The GnRH analogues are a very promising group of drugs.

The issue of toxicity still needs study, and some of the new analogues look promising in that regard. Some studies with the Syntex antagonist have illuminated this problem when very high doses were given; the effect was transient over a few minutes. Investigators have not seen the localized swelling in the primate studies that has been seen in some rat studies.

The remaining major question is whether one can produce either azoospermia or low enough sperm counts to induce infertility. That is the main question in male contraceptive development. The delivery systems and a lot of the other problems will be straightened out if such a system can be shown to be effective.

IS DIRECT ACTION OF AGONIST OR ANTAGONIST POSSIBLE AT THE GONAD LEVEL?

In the rat there are receptors for GnRH; also in primates some receptors exist, but with less affinity than the high-affinity receptor observed in the rat gonad.

Investigators have not found any evidence of any direct effect of either GnRH agonists or antagonists at the gonad level. Some investigators have infused into the ovarian artery of rhesus monkey doses of DTrp[6] LHRH without changes in progesterone production or progesterone concentration in the ovarian vein that drains that particular ovary. They have looked at binding status and at alanine and cyclase effects and have been unable to see any effect in either human or nonhuman gonads.

Several investigators have studied this effect in species other than the rat, also with very negative results. A few studies suggest that it could be a local, direct effect, but in humans, receptor activity has not been demonstrated.

WHEN EVALUATING CONSTANT RELEASE SYSTEMS, CAN SERUM CONCENTRATIONS BE USED AS ENDPOINTS?

Investigators noted in previous studies in rats and castrated rats with testosterone implants that when 20-mm implants were given to castrated male rats, the prostate weight returned to normal. When the serum testosterone was measured in rats that had 20-mm testosterone implants, however, the serum testosterone concentrations were one third of normal.

They have seen the same thing with GnRH antagonists; when a single daily injection of GnRH agonist is given and measurements are integrated with the 24-hour concentrations, they are totally different from when the same daily dose is given by constant infusion.

In vivo release rates must be related to whatever effect is being studied, either protein metabolism, libido or potency, or mineral metabolism; trying to find the dose that results in normal testosterone levels in the rhesus monkey may be the wrong endpoint.

WOULD THE FDA APPROVE USE OF TESTOSTERONE MICROCAPSULES IN A PHASE I CLINICAL TRIAL?

Using testosterone in polymer microcapsules has been discussed with various investigators, and the possibility of approving such trials is very good. Many things must be considered: the volume to be injected, the duration of effect, whether individuals can tolerate the injection locally, whether azoospermia or marked oligospermia will last over a period of 2 or maybe 3 months, then what happens when the drug is used for 6 months or longer. An IND to test these things will be welcome when the methodology is at hand.

Immunologic Approaches

36

Immunopathologic Consideration of Antifertility Vaccine

KENNETH S. K. TUNG

An immunologic approach to contraception, in the form of an antifertility vaccine, has received serious consideration in recent years.[5,14,72] Reproductive hormones and antigens of the male and female gametes have been the most prominent antigen candidates. Female experimental animals, including subhuman primates, have been rendered infertile by immunization with these antigenic preparations. Whereas the question of feasibility of contraceptive vaccine development will be handled by the other contributors to this volume, this chapter considers the *potential* hazards of immunization with antigens of the gametes. Because immunization in female subjects is the primary focus of antifertility vaccine development,[5] the discussion confines itself to the female. Sperm antigens may be cross reactive with endogenous antigens of the immunized subject, and zonae pellucidae antigens normally are present in the ovaries; thus autoimmune response and autoimmune disease will constitute the major considerations. These potential problems are discussed in the light of our understanding of immunologic diseases. Specifically, this chapter considers the immunopathologic events that may follow 1) immunization with sperm antigens, and 2) immunization with zonae pellucidae antigens. The potential complications of immunization of reproductive hormones have been discussed elsewhere.[61,73]

POTENTIAL COMPLICATIONS OF IMMUNE RESPONSE TO SPERM ANTIGENS

Experimental autoimmune orchitis (EAO) is the best-studied example of immunopathologic sequelae of immune response to sperm.[62] Although EAO is not a consideration in the females immunized with sperm antigens, findings of EAO research are relevant to potential complications of immune response to sperm in general. Immune reactants to sperm in the female may lead to immunologic diseases by reacting with 1) self or fetal tissue antigens that happen to cross react with sperm antigens, 2) ovarian (zonae pellucidae) antigens by means of anti-idiotype antibodies to the zona receptors of sperm, and

The author thanks Cherrie Brown for sharing her unpublished data and for helpful discussion, and Danna Richards for preparation of the manuscript. The study was supported by NIH grant HD-12247 and HD-14504.

TABLE 36-1. Correlation Between Autoantibody Responses to Sperm Surface Antigens and Autoimmune Orchitis Susceptibility in Inbred Mice and Guinea Pigs

ANIMAL	STRAIN	MHC HAPLOTYPE	ANTISPERM AUTOANTIBODY RESPONSE*	SUSCEPTIBILITY TO EXPERIMENTAL AUTOIMMUNE ORCHITIS
Mouse	BALB/cBY	d	High	Susceptible
	A/J	k/d	High	Susceptible
	DBA/2	d	High	Resistant
	DBA/1	q	High	Resistant
	B10.BR	k	Low	Resistant
	CBA	k	Low	Resistant
	B10.D2	d	Low	Susceptible
	C57BL/6	b	Low	Susceptible
Guinea pig	XIII		High	Susceptible
	Poly-L-Lysine responder		Low	Susceptible

* Based on a solid phase radioimmunobinding assay. Sera are from orchiectomized mice immunized against autologous sperm/testis in CFA, or vasectomized guinea pigs.

3) sperm antigens in the genital tract. As the third mechanism might be equivalent to the intended operative mechanism of the contraceptive vaccine, complication from hypersensitivity (or allergic) reactions could arise if the immune response in a susceptible subject provokes a preferentially strong IgE or T cell-mediated (such as delayed hypersensitivity) immune response.

STUDIES ON EXPERIMENTAL AUTOIMMUNE ORCHITIS: SPERM ANTIGEN USAGE IN ANTIFERTILITY VACCINE

Defining the EAO Responder Phenotype

Recent studies clearly indicate that susceptibility to EAO, an immunopathologic consequence of immunization with sperm antigen, can be influenced by genetic and environmental factors. Studies based on well-defined inbred congeneic mice have shown that H-2 genes, including H-2D^d and the H-2s haplotype, control orchitis susceptibility, whereas non–H-2 genes (of the DBA/2 mice) may code for disease resistance.[57] Apart from genetic influence (which will be expanded on in Chap. 40), evidence for significant environmental influence has emerged in a recent study on a substrain of BALB/c mice. Whereas these mice obtained directly from the Jackson Laboratory were high responders, mice from the 1-year-old colony of the same substrain in the National Institutes of Health, which were established with breeder pairs from the Jackson Laboratory, were nonresponders.[56]

In studies on mice and guinea pigs, antisperm antibody response and development of EAO were found to be discordant (Table 36-1).[25,66] This is not surprising because antisperm autoantibody response is but one of many factors that influence the induction of EAO.[62] It is probable that the antifertility effect of sperm immunization in the female also is affected by complex immunologic and nonimmunologic factors. Thus, studies that attempt to define the responder phenotype to the sperm antifertility vaccine should evaluate not only the factors that influence the immune response but also factors that influence the biologic consequence of the immune response.

Therefore, the phenotype of a responder to antifertility vaccine may be complex enough that nonresponders to sperm vaccine antigen can exist potentially in a heterogeneous population, and that the responder phenotype can be influenced by genetic and environmental factors. Whether careful selection of adjuvants and carrier antigens will succeed in driving such population to uniform responders can be answered only by future experimentation.

The Nature of Immune Response to Sperm–Testis Antigens

The immune response of guinea pig to sperm–testis antigens clearly have included anaphylactic antibody, complement-activating antibodies, and lymphokine-secreting T cell components.[62] By varying adjuvants or antigen preparation for immunization, it is possible preferentially to elicit anaphylactic or complement-activating antibody responses.[60,67] Furthermore, local sperm antigen–antibody complexes associated with tissue injury have been detected in the testes of vasectomized rabbits,[8] rabbits and mice with EAO,[28,68] and the infertile dark mink.[64] These findings indicate the potential of sperm–testis antigens in eliciting immune responses that can lead to various hypersensitivity (allergic) reactions.

IMMUNOPATHOLOGY RESULTING FROM IMMUNE RESPONSE TO ANTIGENS THAT CROSS REACT WITH SPERM ANTIGENS

Antigens or Antigenic Determinants Common to Testis or Sperm and the Central Nervous System

That antigens common to the testes and the brain may exist was documented serologically over 30 years ago.[30–32] The testis and the central nervous system (CNS) have common glycolipid antigens, including galactocerebrosidelike molecules.[58] Rabbits immunized with galactocerebroside in complete Freund's adjuvant have been found to develop autoimmune neuritis.[55] Moreover, Lewis rats immunized with testicular antigens developed focal pathology in the brain indistinguishable from that of experimental autoimmune encephalomyelitis.[42] In some of the immunized rats, granulomatous inflammation in the hypothalamus has been found.[43] These histopathologic changes were not observed when rats were immunized with other tissue antigens; however, the existing experimental findings indicative of biologic significance of cross-reactive antigens between the CNS and sperm are either preliminary in nature, or they have not yet been confirmed by other laboratories. Nevertheless, there are sufficient data to warrant the concern that immune response to testicular antigens may lead to immunologic diseases of the CNS. A systematic analysis of the nature of the putative cross-reactive antigens should now be implemented.

TABLE 36-2. Immunization of Female Animals with Spermatozoa or Sperm Antigens: Reduction of Fertility Resulting from Embryo Loss

ANIMAL	IMMUNIZATION	RESULTS	REFERENCE
Rabbit	Rabbit semen or testis in CFA	Embryos transferred to immunized rabbits do not survive.	38
Rabbit	Rabbit sperm in CFA	Embryos transferred to immunized rabbits do not survive.	29
Rabbit	Rabbit sperm antigens not extractable with lithium di-iodosalicylate in CFA	Embryos transferred to immunized rabbits do not survive.	41
Mouse	Allogeneic sperm	Reduction of number of litter without effect on fertilization or number of implantation sites.	65
Heifer	Bull semen or testis in CFA	Embryo loss frequent	39
Heifer	Bull semen in CFA at different times after insemination	Early embryo loss; delayed return to estrus	37
Guinea pig	Testis in CFA	Reduction in embryo survival	27
Guinea pig	Sperm or sperm antigens, P, in CFA	Increased stillborns	13

CFA = Complete Freund's adjuvant

Antigen Shared Between Sperm and Embryo

Infertility in the female animals immunized with sperm have resulted from reduced fertilization rate, or increased embryo loss, or both.[63] The effect of sperm immunity on embryo survival appears well established (Table 36-2).[13,27,29,37,38,39,41,65] Mice immunized with sperm developed infertility associated with normal ovulation, unaltered fertilization rate, and normal implantation frequency. In addition, embryos did not survive well when transferred to pseudopregnant recipients that were immunized with sperm. That these experimental findings may have clinical relevance is shown by the finding that women with antisperm antibodies had higher prevalence of spontaneous abortion.[24,36,40]

The existence of cross-reactive antigens between sperm and embryo also is supported by the finding that active immunization of female mice with teratocarcinoma (OTT6050 and F9), in vitro models of the embryo, could lead to a reduction of fertility and fertilization in vitro.[20,70] In these animals, both prefertilization and postfertilization, preimplantation state may have been interrupted.[19]

Several studies have identified cross-reactive antigens that exist between sperm and syngeneic embryo tissues.[19] Immunochemical analysis of OTT6050 cell surface antigens revealed the presence of low molecular weight antigens, presumably glycolipids in nature, which also are found on the surface of epididymal sperm.[69] Moreover, monoclonal antibodies to teratocarcinoma, Nulli-SCCl, recognized a Forssman glycolipid antigen, which is also present on testicular cells and sperm.[51]

Antigen of Sperm and Oncofetal Antigen

Several years ago, the possibility was suggested that immunization with sperm could lead to immune response against antigens shared between sperm and oncofetal antigens (*e.g.*, F9), and this in turn may lead to enhancement of tumor bearing the oncofetal antigenic markers.[61] This idea since has been supported by the important observation that vasectomized mice were associated with a significantly high prevalence of neoplasia.[6] Although a causal relation between postvasectomy antisperm immune response and carcinogenesis is not established, the study is worthy of future exploration.

MAY ANTIBODY TO CERTAIN SPERM MOLECULES ELICIT ANTI-IDIOTYPE ANTIBODIES THAT REACT WITH ANTIGENS OF ZONAE PELLUCIDAE?

This theoretical consideration (see Fig. 36-1) has been stimulated by the finding that an increasing number of human diseases are mediated by antireceptor antibodies,[54] by the discovery that anti-idiotype to antibody against a biologically active ligand can react with the physiologic receptor for the ligand,[48] and by the recent elucidation of a glycoprotein (ZP3) of mouse zonae pellucidae as sperm receptors.[9] For this proposed mechanism to be operative, however, the immunizing sperm antigen would have to include the sperm receptor(s) for the zonae pellucidae. Although there are studies that provided indirect evidence for the lack of immunogenicity of sperm receptor on zonae pellucidae,[1,2] this finding may not apply to the immune response against the antisperm receptor idiotope. The possible immunopathologic consequence of immune response to the zona pellucida will be considered later.

HYPERSENSITIVITY REACTIONS TO SPERM ANTIGENS IN THE FEMALE GENITAL TRACT

Introduction of antigens to a susceptible host previously sensitized to the antigen could lead to undesirable hypersensitivity (or allergic) reactions, including: 1) IgE-mediated anaphylactic type reaction; 2) T cell-mediated delayed type hypersensitivity reaction, and 3) immune complex-mediated inflammation and tissue injury. In subjects immunized with sperm antifertility vaccine, these reactions could occur locally in the genital tract following unprotected sexual intercourse. That this could happen is illustrated by the occurrence of hypersensitivity reactions to seminal plasma antigen.[7,18] It is therefore important to review briefly the pertinent predisposing factors to hypersensitivity reactions.

There have been important recent advances in our understanding of the control of IgE immune responses.[26,50] IgE antibody response clearly is regulated at two levels. The first is the regulation of antigen-specific IgE antibody response, which is under the control of Ir genes mapped within the major histocompatibility complex. A second mechanism is the isotype-specific control of the total serum IgE level. Many factors have been shown to influence

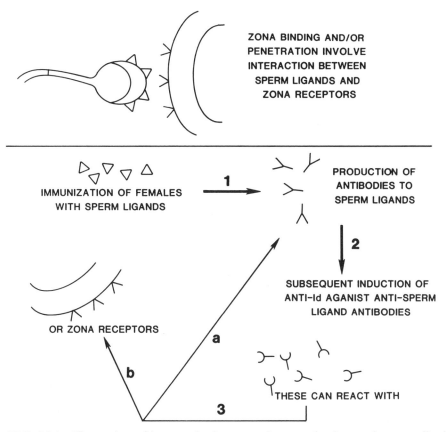

FIG. 36-1. Illustration of immunologic events that may lead to antizona antibody response in female subjects immunized with sperm molecules. The top figure illustrates sperm ligands that normally react with receptors on zonae pellucidae. As illustrated below that, females immunized with sperm ligands will produce antibody to the ligand (*1*). The antibody in turn can elicit anti-idiotype antibody (*2*), which can react with the antisperm ligand antibody (*3b*). In some instances, the anti-Id antibody can also react with the receptors on the zona (*3b*).

the isotype-specific IgE response, including antigen dose, adjuvant selection, existence of parasitic diseases, low-dose irradiation, and treatment with cyclophosphamide.[22] Moreover, total serum IgE levels often are elevated in patients with different types of immunodeficiencies.[12]

Factors that influence isotype-specific IgE response have been shown to increase the propensity of a subject to make a high IgE antibody response. Thus, rats injected with a protein antigen followed by *Schistosoma mansonii* or *Nipponstrongylus brasiliensis* infection produce a predominant IgE antibody response to the protein antigen.[10,46] The duration of the immune response varied depending on the parasite. Parasitic infection in humans is also associated with high serum levels of IgE.[23] It is known that atopic patients have elevated serum IgE levels, and hypersensitivity reaction to seminal antigens is more prevalent in atopic subjects.[7] It is therefore conceivable that a high prevalence of IgE anaphylactic response to sperm will be found in sperm-vaccinated subjects in geographical areas where parasitic infections are endemic or epidemic. Furthermore, one should also take into consideration in the selection of adjuvant that alum preferentially elicits a high IgE antibody response.[21]

Induction of local immune complex reaction requires the presence of antibody of IgG or IgM class, capable of complement activation. Both of these antibody classes are known to increase in mucosal secretions of patients with selective IgA deficiency,[44] which has been estimated to occur in 1 of 1000 subjects.[4] Finally, mucosal T cell response can be detected and may lead to cell-mediated hypersensitivity.[26,59]

Two additional factors that might influence the likelihood of local hypersensitivity reaction to sperm antigens should be considered. Because immunosuppressive properties normally may circumvent the development of immunologic reaction against antigenic components of semen,[35,45,52] hypersensitivity reactions may develop only when the immunosuppressive property of the sexual partner's semen is defective. Second, if immunization by means of the mucosal route becomes the method of choice, one could expect considerable variations in response between individuals. Some may develop both mucosal and systemic responses, others may develop mucosal response but systemic tolerance to the antigen, whereas in still others, immunologic tolerance in both mucosal and systemic responses may ensue.[53] Because of the expectant individual variation in the response to mucosal antigenic stimulation, it may be difficult to carry out meaningful experiments that will predict the probability of hypersensitivity reactions as possible sequelae of sperm immunization.

POTENTIAL COMPLICATIONS OF IMMUNE RESPONSE TO ANTIGENS OF THE ZONAE PELLUCIDAE

Immunization of female animals with heterologous zonae pellucidae or soluble or purified antigens can lead to temporary or prolonged infertility.[49] This has been documented in rabbits,[33] dogs,[33] and subhuman primates.[15,47] following immunization with porcine zona, as well as in rats immunized with heterologous rodent zona.[3,69] The resultant infertility correlated well with the level of circulating antizona antibodies. Presumed antizona antibody (as IgG) can be detected in the zona in vivo. Furthermore, antizona antibodies effectively blocked fertilization in vitro, and sufficient antibody titer was elicited with relatively harmless adjuvant, including alum. These extremely promising results have been dampened somewhat by the recent discovery that animals immunized with zona antigen may also develop irreversible ovarian disease with the loss of ova. At the moment, the pathogenesis of the ovarian disease is poorly understood, and it is unclear whether the ovarian disease and fertilization prevention by antizona antibody are dissociable events. It is therefore pertinent that we briefly review these findings.

In 1981, Wood and co-workers observed that rabbits immunized with intact and heat-solubilized porcine zona antigens failed to ovulate in response to hCG.[71] The ovaries were small and contained very few or no visible mature follicles. Histologically, a reduction of tertiary follicles was noted 6 weeks after immunization.

In 1982, Mahi-Brown and colleagues documented abnormal estrus cycle in dogs immunized with porcine zonae pellucidae.[34] The abnormal reproductive response subsequently was characterized to include 1) prolonged estrogen secretion associated with absence of progesterone rise in estrus and metestrus (Fig. 36-2), 2) absence of preovulatory or postovulatory cycles at proestrus or estrus, 3) presence of multiple follicular cysts in the ovaries, and 4) loss of oocytes from follicles.[11] Thus, bitches immunized with zona not only failed to ovulate, they also developed severe ovarian diseases compatible with permanent sterility. Histologic and immunohistochemical studies demonstrated no inflammatory changes in the ovaries of the immunized bitches or the rabbits, although in vivo binding of presumed antizona antibody was observed.

Ovarian disease since has been found in subhuman primates as a result of zona immunization. Gulyas and associates found that zona-immunized cynomologus monkeys failed to ovulate and had depressed levels of estradiol and progesterone.[15] The ovaries of some monkeys showed massive loss of follicles, particularly the large antral follicles. Sacco immunized squirrel monkeys with porcine zona antigen that had been purified by gel filtration, ion exchange chromatography, and lectin affinity chromatography, and found significant reduction in oocyte number during ovulation.[47] In addition, the ovaries were reduced in size.

Two pathogenetic mechanisms for the ovarian disease are being considered. It is possible that the immunizing zona antigens are contaminated by antigens other than zona antigens, and immune response to the contaminants is responsible for the ovarian disease. If this were the only mechanism, ovarian disease theoretically could be circumvented by applying truly purified or synthetic zona antigens as immunogens. Alternatively, ovarian disease is the result of immune response to zona antigens, and the occurrence of ovarian disease parallels the magnitude of the antizona antibody response. In this case, unless ovarian disease and fertilization prevention are mediated by immune response to different antigens or antigenic epitopes in the zonae pellucidae, this mechanism may well negate the application of zonae pellucidae antigen in antifertility vaccine.

SUMMARY AND CONCLUSIONS

This chapter has discussed the potential immunopathologic complications of immunization of the females with antigens of the spermatozoa and the zonae pellucidae. Immune responses to sperm antigens may elicit immune responses against antigens shared between sperm and the CNS, between sperm and the embryo, and between sperm and oncofetal antigens. The biologic consequences of these cross-reactive immune responses may, respectively, be autoimmune diseases of the nervous system, embryotoxic effect, and increased

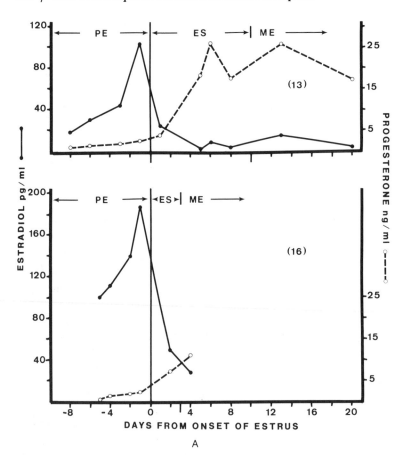

FIG. 36-2. (*A*) Estradiol 17B and progesterone patterns in control bitches (#13 and #16) that were immunized and unbred. Day 0 is the day of onset of estrus. *PE,* proestrus; *ES,* estrus; *ME,* metestrus. (*B*) Estradiol and progesterone patterns in bitches #4 and #9 immunized with crude porcine zona pellucida and developing high antizona antibody titers. For bitch 4, day 0 is the day of onset of estrus. Bitch 9 did not enter estrus, so that the abscissa indicates days of proestrus. Note absence of progesterone rise in both immunized bitches. (From Mahi-Brown CA, Yanagimachi R, Hoffman JC, Huang TTF Jr: Fertility control in the bitch by active immunization with porcine zonae pellucidae: Use of different adjuvants and patterns of estradiol and testosterone levels in estrous cycles. Biol Reprod 32:761, 1985)

occurrence of neoplasia. It is postulated that antibody to sperm ligand (for the zona receptor) may elicit anti-idiotype antibodies that cross react with the zona receptor.

Although immunization with zonae pellucidae has been shown to reduce the fertility rate of female animals unequivocally, the recent demonstration of irreversible ovarian disease in the immunized animals has raised serious ques-

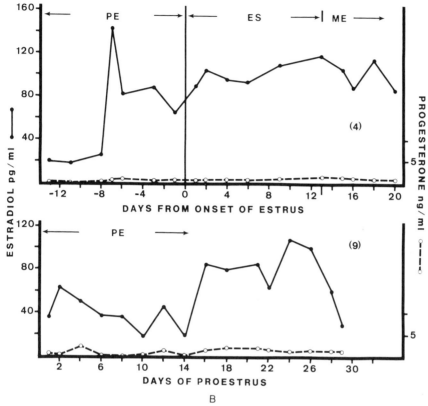

FIG. 36-2. (*Continued*)

tions on the feasibility of this approach. The chapter further discussed the possibility of hypersensitivity reactions against sperm antigens occurring locally in the female genital tract, and some of the factors that could potentiate these reactions. Finally, based on recent findings on the complex nature of factors that control the induction of autoimmune orchitis, it is suggested that the characteristics that differentiate responders from nonresponders to antifertility vaccine also may be difficult to define.

It should be emphasized that much of the experimental evidence on which the theoretical discussions were based is far from being fully established. Because of their relevance to an understanding of the possible complications of antifertility vaccine, however, these studies should now be subjected to critical experimentation, and they should be included in the consideration and evaluation of antifertility vaccine safety. Finally, the lack of experimental data does not permit an estimation of the likelihood of the complications outlined. Because of this, the important question of whether the risk of antifertility vaccination is worth the benefit of an alternate form of contraception cannot yet be answered.

REFERENCES

1. AHUJA KK, TZARTOS SJ: Investigation of sperm receptors in the hamster zona pellucida by using univalent (Fab) antibodies to hamster ovary. J Reprod Fertil 61:257, 1981
2. AITKEN RJ, HOLME E, RICHARDSON DW, HULME M: Properties of intact and univalent (Fab) antibodies raised against isolated, solubilized mouse zonae pellucidae. J Reprod Fertil 66:327, 1982
3. AITKEN RJ, RICHARDSON DW: Immunization of rats with cumulus free mouse ova: Induction of infertility and antibody titers. J Exp Zool 216:149, 1981
4. AMMANN AJ, HONG R: Selective IgA deficiency and autoimmunity. Clin Exp Immunol 7:833, 1971
5. ANDERSON DJ, ALEXANDER NJ: A new look at antifertility vaccines. Fertil Steril 40:557, 1983
6. ANDERSON DJ, ALEXANDER NJ, FULGHAM DL, PALOTAY JL: Spontaneous tumors in long-term vasectomized mice: Increased incidence in association with antisperm immunity. Am J Pathol 111:129, 1983
7. BERNSTEIN IL, ENGLANDER BE, CALLAGHER JS, NATHAN P, MARCUS ZH: Localized and systemic hypersensitivity reactions to human seminal fluid. Ann Intern Med 94:459, 1981
8. BIGAZZI PE, KOSUDA LL, HSU KC, ANDRES GA: Immune complex orchitis in vasectomized rabbits. J Exp Med 143:382, 1976
9. BLEIL JE, WASSARMAN PM: Mammalian sperm-egg interaction: Identification of a glycoprotein in mouse egg zonae pellucidae possessing receptor activity for sperm. Cell 20:873, 1980
10. BLOCH KJ, OHMAN JL JR, WALTIN J, CYGAN RW: Potentiated reagin response: Initiation with minute doses of antigen and alum followed by infection with nippostrongylus brasiliensis. J Immunol 110:197, 1973
11. BROWN CA: Personal communication, 1985
12. BUCKLEY RH, BECKER WG: Abnormalities in the regulation of human IgE synthesis. Immunol Rev 41:288, 1978
13. D'ALMEIDA N, VOISIN GA: Resistance of female guinea pig fertility to efficient iso-immunization with spermatozoa autoantigens. J Reprod Immunol 1:237, 1979
14. DICZFALUSY E (ed): Karolinksa Symposia on Research Methods in Reproductive Endocrinology. Stockholm, Karolinska Institute, 1974
15. GULYAS BJ, GWATKIN RDL, YUAN LC: Active immunization of cynomolgus monkeys (*Macaca fascicularis*) with porcine zonae pellucidae. Gamete Res 4:299, 1983
16. GWATKIN RBL, WILLIAMS DT: Immunization of female rabbits with heat-solubilized bovine zonae: Production of antizona antibody and inhibition of fertility. Gamete Res 1:19, 1978
17. GWATKIN RB, WILLIAMS DT, CARLO DJ: Immunization of mice with heat solubilized hamster zonae: Production of antizona antibody and inhibition of fertility. Fertil Steril 28:871, 1977
18. HALPERN BN, KY T, ROBERT B: Clinical and immunological study of an exceptional case of reaginic type sensitization to human seminal fluid. Immunol 12:247, 1967
19. HAMILTON MS: Maternal immune responses to oncofetal antigens. J Reprod Immunol 5:249, 1983
20. HAMILTON MS, MAY RD, BEER AE, VITETTA ES: The influence of immunization of female mice with F9 teratocarcinoma cells on their reproductive performance. Transplant Proc 11:1069, 1979
21. ISHIZAKA K: Cellular events in the IgE response. Adv Immunol 23:1, 1976
22. ISHIZAKA K: Regulation of IgE synthesis. Ann Rev Immunol 2:159, 1984
23. JOHANSSON SGO, MELLBIN T, VAHLQUIST B: Immunoglobulin levels in Ethiopian pre-school children with special reference to high concentrations of immunoglobulin (E IgND). Lancet i:1118, 1968
24. JONES WR: Immunological aspects of infertility. In SCOTT JS, JONES WR (eds): Immunology of Reproduction, p 375. New York, Academic Press, 1976
25. KASAI K, TEUSCHER C, TUNG KSK: Unpublished data, 1985
26. KATZ DH: Recent studies on the regulation of IgE antibody synthesis in experimental animals and man. Immunology 41:1, 1980
27. KIDDY CA, ROLLINS RM: Infertility in female guinea pigs injected with testis. Biol Reprod 8:545, 1973

28. KOHNO S, MUNOZ JJ, WILLIAMS TM, TEUSCHER C, BERNARD CCA, TUNG KSK: Immunopathology of murine experimental allergic orchitis. J Immunol 130:2675, 1983
29. KUMMERFELD HL, FOOTE RH: Infertility and embryonic mortality in female rabbits immunized with different sperm preparations. Biol Reprod 14:300, 1976
30. LEWIS JH: Antigenic relationship of alcohol-soluble fractions of brain and testicle. J Immunol 27:437, 1934
31. LEWIS JH: The antigenic relationship of alcohol-soluble substances of corpus luteum to those of testis and brain. Am J Pathol 17:725, 1941
32. LEWIS JH: The immunologic specificity of brain tissue. J Immunol 24:193, 1933
33. MAHI-BROWN CA, HUANG TTF JR, YANAGIMACHI R: Infertility in bitches induced by active immunization with porcine zonae pellucidae. J Exp Zool 222:89, 1982
34. MAHI-BROWN CA, YANAGIMACHI R, HOFFMAN JC, HUANG TTF JR: Fertility control in the bitch by active immunization with porcine zonae pellucidae: Use of different adjuvants and patterns of estradiol and testosterone levels in estrous cycles. Biol Reprod 32:761, 1985
35. MARCUS ZH, FREISHSEM JH, HOUK JL, HERMAN JH, HESS EV: In vitro study in reproductive immunology. 1. Suppression of CMI response by human spermatozoa and fractions isolated from human seminal plasma. Clin Immunol Immunopathol 9(3):318, 1978
36. MATHUR S, BAKER ER, WILLIAMSON HO, DERRICK FC, TEAQUE KJ, FUDENBERG HH: Clinical significance of sperm antibodies in infertility. Fertil Steril 36:486, 1981
37. MENGE AC: Early embryo mortality in heifers isoimmunized with semen and conceptus. J Reprod Fertil 18:67, 1969
38. MENGE AC: Fertilization, embryo and fetal survival rates in rabbits isoimmunized with semen, testis and conceptus. Proc Soc Exp Biol Med 127:1271, 1968
39. MENGE AC: Induced infertility in cattle by iso-immunization with semen and testis. J Reprod Fertil 13:445, 1967
40. MENGE AC, MEDLEY NE, MANGIONE CM, DIETRICH JW: The incidence and influence of antisperm antibodies in infertile human couples on sperm-cervical mucus interactions and subsequent fertility. Fertil Steril 38:439, 1982
41. MENGE AC, PEEGEL H, RIOLO ML: Sperm fractions responsible for immunologic induction of pre- and post-fertilization infertility in rabbits. Biol Reprod 20:931, 1979
42. PATTERSON PY: Experimental allergic encephalomyelitis and autoimmune disease. Adv Immunol 5:131, 1966
43. PATTERSON PY, HARWIN SM: In vivo cross/reactivity of the central nervous system (CNS), testis and ovary tissues causes two types of CNS lesions in rats sensitized to these tissues. In SPECTOR NH (ed): Proceedings of the First International Neuroimmunomodulation Workshop (in press)
44. POLMER SH, WALDMAN TA, BALESTRA ST, JOST MC, TERRY WD: Immunoglobulin E in immunologic deficiency diseases. I. Relation of IgE and IgA to respiratory tract disease in isolated IgE deficiency, IgA deficiency and ataxia telangiectasia. J Clin Invest 51:326, 1972
45. PRAKASH C, LANG RW: Studies on immune infertility: A hypothesis on the etiology of immune infertility based on the biological role of seminal plasma immune response inhibitor. Mt Sinai J Med 47:491, 1980
46. ROUSSEAUX-PREVOST R, BAZIN H, CAPRON A: IgE in experimental schistosomiasis. 1. Serum levels after infection by schistosoma mansoni in various strains of rats. Immunology 33:501, 1977
47. SACCO AG, SUBRAMANIAN MG, YUREWICZ EC, DEMAYO FJ, DUKELOW WR: Hetero-immunization of squirrel monkeys (*Saimiri sciureus*) with a purified zona antigen (Tpcza) immune response in biologic activity antiserum. Fertil Steril 39:350, 1983
48. SECHTER Y, MARON R, ELIAS D, COHEN IR: Autoantibodies to insulin receptor spontaneously develop as anti-idiotypes in mice immunized with insulin. Science 216:542, 1982
49. SHIVERS CA, SIEG PM: Antigens of oocytes and their environments. In DHINDSA DS, SCHUMACHER GFB (eds): Immunological Aspects of Infertility and Fertility Regulation, p 173. New York, Elsevier/North Holland, 1980
50. SPIEGELBERG HL: Lymphocytes bearing Fc receptors for IgE. Immunol Rev 56:199, 1981
51. STERN PL, WILLSON KR, LENNOX E, GAFFRE G, MILSTEIN C, SECHER D: Antibodies as probes for differentiation in tumor associated antigens: A Frossman specificity on teratocarcinoma stem cells. Cell 14:775, 1978
52. STITES DT, ERICKSON RT: Suppressive effect of seminal plasma on lymphocyte activation. Nature 253:727, 1975

53. STROBER W, RICHMAN LK, ELSON CO: The regulation of gastrointestinal immune responses. Immunology Today 2:156, 1981
54. Symposium: Immunopathology of Receptors. Fed Proc 38:2606, 1979
55. TAKAHIKO S, SAIDA K, DORFMAN SH, SILBERBERG DH, SUMNER AJ, MANNING MC, LISAK RP, BROWN MJ: Experimental allergic neuritis induced by sensitization with galactocerebroside. Science 204:1103, 1979
56. TEUSCHER C, POTTER M, TUNG KSK: Unpublished data, 1985
57. TEUSCHER C, SMITH SM, GOLDBERG EH, SHEARER GM, TUNG KSK: Experimental autoimmune orchitis in mice: Genetic control of susceptibility and resistance to induction of orchitis. Immunogenetics 22:323, 1985
58. TEUSCHER C, WILD C, TUNG KSK: Personal data, 1981
59. TOMASI TB: The secretory immune system. In STITES DP, STOBO JD, FUDENBERG HH, WELLS JV (eds): Basic and Clinical Immunology, 5th ed, p 187. Los Altos, CA, Lange Medical, 1984
60. TOULLET F, VOISON GA, NEMINOVSKY M: Histochemical localization of three guinea pig spermatozal autoantigens. Immunology 24:635, 1973
61. TUNG KSK: Antifertility vaccines: Considerations of their potential immunopathologic complications. Int J Fertil 21:197, 1976
62. TUNG KSK: Autoimmunity of the testis. In DHINDSA DF, SCHUMACHER GFB (eds): Immunologic Aspects of Infertility and Fertility Regulation, p 33. New York, Elsevier/North-Holland, 1980
63. TUNG KSK: Models of autoimmunity to spermatozoa and testis. In WEGMANN TG, GILL TJ, III (eds): Immunology of Reproduction, p 387. Oxford, Oxford University Press, 1983
64. TUNG KSK, ELLIS L, TEUSCHER C, MENG A, BLAUSTEIN JC, KOHNO S, HOWELL R: The black mink (*mustela vison*): A natural model of immunologic male infertility. J Exp Med 154:1016, 1981
65. TUNG KSK, GOLDBERG EH, GOLDBERG E: Immunobiological consequence of immunization of female mice with homologous spermatozoa: Induction of infertility. J Reprod Immunol 1:145, 1979
66. TUNG KSK, TEUSCHER C, GOLDBERG EH, WILD C: Genetic control of antisperm autoantibody response in vasectomized guinea pigs. J Immunol 127:835, 1981
67. TUNG KSK, UNANUE ER, DIXON FJ: Immunological events associated with immunization by sperm in incomplete Freund's adjuvant. Int Arch Allerg Appl Immunol 41:565, 1971
68. TUNG KSK, WOODROFFE AJ: Immunopathology of experimental allergic orchitis in the rabbit. J Immunol 120:320, 1978
69. WEBB CG: Characterization of antisera against teratocarcinoma OTT 6050: Molecular species recognized on embryoid bodies, preimplantation embryos and sperm. Develop Biol 76:203, 1980
70. WEBB CG: Decreased fertility in mice immunized with teratocarcinoma OTT 6050. Biol Reprod 22:695, 1980
71. WOOD DM, LIU C, DUNBAR BS: Effect of alloimmunization and heteroimmunization with zonae pellucidae on fertility in rabbits. Biol Reprod 25:439, 1981
72. World Health Organization Symposium Varna, 1975: Development of vaccines for fertility regulation. Copenhagen, Scriptor, 1976
73. WHO Task Force on Immunological Methods for Fertility Regulation: Evaluating the safety and efficacy of parental antigen vaccines for fertility regulation. Clin Exp Immunol 33:360, 1978

37

Reasons for Abandoning Immunization Against FSH As an Approach to Male Fertility Regulation

EBERHARD NIESCHLAG

Between 1977 and 1983 our group performed preclinical studies exploring the possibility of suppressing spermatogenesis and achieving male fertility regulation by immunization against FSH. The rationale underlying immunization against FSH as an approach to male fertility regulation should be reviewed before the reasons for abandoning it are discussed.

RATIONAL BASIS FOR IMMUNIZATION WITH FSH

The classical concept of the pituitary–testicular feedback control mechanism attributes the regulation of Leydig cell function to LH and the control of spermatogenesis to FSH.[8] Both compartments are believed to be well-separated entities. If this concept holds true, the selective suppression or neutralization of FSH activity should lead to a suppression of spermatogenesis, and consequently to azoospermia. Because Leydig cell function would remain intact, the selective inhibition of FSH would then provide an ideal method for male fertility regulation.

In the 1970s, evidence accumulated that inhibin, postulated by McCullagh in 1932 as an FSH suppressing hormone of testicular origin,[16] may be a reality and that this hormone might eventually become available for clinical testing as an FSH and spermatogenesis-suppressing modality.

In contrast to the classical concept of feedback control described so far, studies in the rat provided evidence that although FSH is indeed required for the initiation of spermatogenesis,[10] it might be dispensable for the maintenance of spermatogenesis in this species.[7] It was found that testosterone alone could maintain spermatogenesis in rats.[6,24] If these findings also were to hold

The studies reported in this review were initially supported by the Special Program in Human Reproduction of the World Health Organization and in later phases by funds from the Deutsche Forschungsgemeinschaft and the Max Planck Society. The secretarial help provided by Ina Oberschachtsiek in preparing this manuscript is gratefully acknowledged.

true in the human, selective inhibition of FSH would not lead to suppression of spermatogenesis.

In men, however, the situation remained rather controversial. On the one hand, clinical evidence was presented to support the requirement of FSH in the spermatogenic process,[9,25] whereas on the other, there were reports that testosterone alone can maintain spermatogenesis in men once initiated by FSH.[22] Because the experiments required to illuminate the role of FSH in human spermatogenesis are restricted by ethical considerations, it was necessary to turn to suitable nonhuman primate models. Therefore, studies in monkeys with well-characterized reproductive functions[21] were initiated to elucidate the role of FSH in spermatogenesis.

The logical first choice for experimental approach would have been to hypophysectomize monkeys, replace FSH and/or LH, and evaluate the effects on the testis. Such studies, however, are impossible because monkey gonadotropins are not available in quantities sufficient for such studies. Furthermore, human gonadotropins or those from other species are highly antigenic in monkeys, thus precluding their use for the pending experiments. In earlier studies aimed at clarifying the role of steroids in pituitary–gonadal feedback control, immunization against hormones had provided a rather powerful tool.[19,20] Therefore, neutralization of FSH bioactivity by antibodies seemed a valid approach in defining the role of FSH in control of spermatogenesis.

PASSIVE IMMUNIZATION AGAINST FSH

In the first experiment, adult rhesus monkeys in season were immunized passively against ovine FSH.[26] A drastic fall in testicular volume and in sperm counts (although not to azoospermia) was observed, although serum testosterone concentrations and ejaculatory behavior were not influenced. Testicular histology showed a decrease in tubular diameter and in the height of the seminiferous epithelium, but no influence on Leydig cells.

Although azoospermia was not reached, the study showed that immunization against FSH resulted in a clear suppression of spermatogenesis without affecting Leydig cell function. Thus, the role of FSH in maintaining spermatogenesis in primates was established. This experiment had not only contributed to the clarification of the role of FSH in spermatogenesis, but also showed that immunization against FSH might provide an approach to male fertility regulation. This approach was tested in the study described below.

ACTIVE IMMUNIZATION AGAINST FSH

Because passive immunization requiring frequent injections of antiserum was impractical, active immunization was chosen for the second study. The trial was conducted as a long-term study extending over $4\frac{1}{2}$ years to answer the question whether long-term active immunization would result in suppression of spermatogenesis sufficient to warrant fertility regulation. The study also addressed the question of potential side-effects arising from the possible formation of immune complexes due to immunization against a normal body constituent.

Four adult male rhesus monkeys were immunized with highly purified ovine FSH in complete Freund's adjuvant using the multiple-site intradermal technique for primary immunization, followed by intramuscular booster injections. The animals developed high antibody titers capable of neutralizing rhesus FSH but without cross reactivity to rhesus LH.

Soon after primary immunization, the testicular volumes decreased from high in-season values to volumes in the range of hypophysectomized animals. Values were lowest 6 months after immunization and slowly increased over the remaining period so that volumes of approximately half the normal size were reached in the final year.

Serum testosterone remained in the normal range, indicating that the endocrine testicular function was unaffected. As a sign of normal androgenicity, the animals maintained normal ejaculatory behavior. Sperm counts during the first 2 years of immunization were severely reduced, and azoospermia was observed occasionally. Thereafter, sperm counts remained in approximately the lower normal range and were even higher in a few instances. Sperm motility and morphology remained generally normal. Mating studies were not performed, but when tested in the third year of immunization, the sperm were able to penetrate zona pellucida-free hamster eggs, indicating their functional integrity.

Spermatogenesis, as evidenced by testicular biopsies performed 1 year after immunization, was severely impaired. The tubular diameter was reduced to almost half the control values. Some tubules contained Sertoli cells and spermatogonia only. Testicular histology after $4\frac{1}{2}$ years, at the end of the study, showed that spermatogenesis had been reestablished, but the cell number (in particular the number of spermatids per cross-section) was reduced. The tubular diameter also had slightly increased compared to the biopsies from the first year but was still below normal. All cell types were present, but the epithelium appeared quantitatively reduced.

Immune complexes could not be detected in circulation; nor could precipitated immune complexes be found by immunofluorescence techniques in tissues removed from kidney, heart, aorta, lung, brain, liver, spleen, pancreas, eye, muscle, testis, prostate, and vas deferens.

To summarize, although active immunization with FSH produced a severe reduction in spermatogenesis, azoospermia was not achieved consistently. The degree of oligospermia and the high variability in the sperm counts did not indicate that the animals were infertile over the entire period. Meanwhile, another group had immunized *Macaca fascicularis* monkeys with ovine FSH or the ovine FSH β-subunit.[11] The authors observed a reduction of sperm counts but not azoospermia. Although that study lasted for only 5 to 8 months, it corroborated our results. A third group of investigators immunized bonnet monkeys passively with FSH up to 8 months.[17,18] The authors also found a reduction in sperm count and no azoospermia, but they reported a loss of fertility in the immunized animals. The loss of fertility in the presence of is difficult to explain, and the question remains whether the number of animals was great enough to draw firm conclusions from the mating studies. Nevertheless, all three studies agreed in that a reduction in spermatogenesis and in sperm counts, but not azoospermia, was seen under FSH immunization. Azoospermia, however, appears to be a prerequisite for effective fertility regulation in men.[4]

EMERGING THEORIES FOR THE REGULATION OF TESTICULAR FUNCTION

The results of the long-term study that had absorbed much effort and hope were disappointing and—at first sight—puzzling. The possibility that the antibodies had lost their neutralizing capacity would have provided an explanation but could be excluded almost with certainty. Investigations of the relative importance of FSH and LH/testosterone for spermatogenesis in primates from our laboratory and others helped to explain why the FSH immunization failed to lead to azoospermia.

Observations in hypopituitary patients by Baranetsky and Carlson made it likely that testosterone alone may maintain spermatogenesis in humans.[3] Experiments in hypophysectomized monkeys provided further evidence that testosterone alone may maintain spermatogenesis, albeit only in a qualitative fashion.[14] When intact mature male rhesus monkeys were treated with high doses of LHRH agonists, testicular atrophy and azoospermia occurred after several weeks of treatment.[1] When testosterone was administered in physiologic doses along with the LHRH agonist, the testes atrophied at a slower rate, and azoospermia was not reached in comparable treatment phases.[2] This again demonstrates that testosterone, even in physiologic concentrations, exerts a maintaining influence on spermatogenesis.

Furthermore, testosterone alone could initiate spermatogenesis in immature monkeys[13] and could reinitiate spermatogenesis in monkeys with atrophied testes due to severance of the pituitary stalk.[12] It also was shown that in men with gonadotropin secretion suppressed by testosterone enanthate administration, spermatogenesis could be reinitiated with either hCG or hLH alone.[5,15]

In all these experimental situations, however, testosterone alone could initiate, maintain, and reinitiate spermatogenesis only to a qualitatively but not to a quantitatively normal degree. Another factor appears necessary for quantitatively normal spermatogenesis, and this factor is most likely FSH. Only the combined action of FSH and testosterone appears to guarantee fully normal spermatogenesis in primates.

WHY FSH IMMUNIZATION FAILS TO PRODUCE AZOOSPERMIA

Extrapolation of the foregoing experiments to the situation in the FSH-immunized monkey leads to the conclusion that blocking of FSH bioactivity suppresses spermatogenesis, but the unaltered intratesticular testosterone is "counterproductive" and maintains spermatogenesis to a certain level. As a result, sperm counts are reduced but are not low enough for male fertility regulation. An effective endocrine method for male fertility regulation must therefore suppress not only FSH, but also LH and testosterone. Because fertility regulation in the human cannot be achieved at the expense of virility, such a method will require testosterone substitution to maintain extratesticular androgen actions.

Although immunization with FSH in monkeys led to new insights in the control of testicular function, it did not result in a feasible approach to male fertility regulation. At the onset of studies, possible immunologic side-effects could not be predicted or excluded with certainty. Although the observations are restricted to a small number of animals, the studies show that immunologic side-effects may not preclude immunization against FSH a priori (or another body constituent) as a method for male fertility regulation. Other ancillary problems arising from the immunologic approach, such as the clinical use of adjuvants, the genetically determined interindividual variability of the immune response, the unpredictability of the duration of antibody production, and the difficulties in its termination, remained unaddressed. These problems were not responsible for abandoning our experiments. New insights into the endocrine control of testicular function emerging during the course of our studies led to the conclusion that the selective elimination of FSH bioactivity was conceptually inadequate as an approach to male fertility regulation.

REFERENCES

1. AKHTAR FB, MARSHALL GR, WICKINGS EJ, NIESCHLAG E: Reversible induction of azoospermia in rhesus monkeys by constant infusion of a GnRH agonist using osmotic minipumps. J Clin Endocrinol Metab 56:534–540, 1983
2. AKHTAR FB, MARSHALL GR, NIESCHLAG E: Testosterone supplementation attenuates the antifertility effects of an LHRH agonist in male monkeys. Int J Androl 6:461–468, 1983
3. BARANETSKY NG, CARLSON HE: Persistence of spermatogenesis in hypogonadotropic hypogonadism treated with testosterone. Fertil Steril 34:477–482, 1980
4. BARFIELD A, MELO J, COUTINHO E, ALVAREZ-SANCHEZ F, FAUNDES A, BRACHE V, LEON P, FRICK J, BARTSCH G, WEISKE WH, BERNER P, MISHELL D JR, BERNSTEIN G, ORTIZ A: Pregnancies associated with sperm concentrations below 10 million/ml in clinical studies of a potential male contraceptive method, monthly depot medroxyprogesterone acetate and testosterone esters. Contraception 20:121–127, 1979
5. BREMNER WJ, MATSUMOTO AM, SUSSMAN AM, PAULSEN CA: Follicle-stimulating hormone and human spermatogenesis. J Clin Invest 68:1044–1052, 1981
6. CUNNINGHAM GR, HUCKINS C: Persistence of complete spermatogenesis in the presence of low intratesticular concentrations of testosterone. Endocrinology 105:177–186, 1979
7. DYM M, RAJ HGM, LIN YC, CHEMES HE, KOTITE NJ, NAYFEH SN, FRENCH FS: Is FSH required for maintenance of spermatogenesis in adult rats? J Reprod Fertil (Suppl) 26:175–181, 1979
8. GREEP RO, FEROLD HL, HISAW FL: Effect of two hypophyseal gonadotropic hormones in the reproductive system of the rat. Anat Rec 65:261, 1936
9. JOHNSEN SG: A study of human testicular function by the use of human menopausal gonadotropin and of human chorionic gonadotropin in male hypogonadotrophic eunuchoidism and infantilism. Acta Endocrinol 53:489, 1966
10. RAJ HGM, DYM M: The effects of selective withdrawal of FSH or LH on spermatogenesis in the immature rat. Biol Reprod 14:489–494, 1976
11. RAJ HGM, MURTY GSRC, SAIRAM MR, TALBERT LM: Control of spermatogenesis in primates: Effects of active immunization against FSH in the monkey. Int J Androl (Suppl) 5:27–33, 1982
12. MARSHALL GR, WICKINGS EJ, LÜDECKE DK, NIESCHLAG E: Stimulation of spermatogenesis in stalk-sectioned rhesus monkeys by testosterone alone. J Clin Endocrinol Metab 57:152–159, 1983
13. MARSHALL GR, WICKINGS EJ, NIESCHLAG E: Testosterone can initiate spermatogenesis in an immature nonhuman primate, *Macaca fascicularis*. Endocrinology 114:2228–2233, 1984

14. MARSHALL GR, JOCKENHÖVEL F, LÜDECKE DK, NIESCHLAG E: Maintenance of spermatogenesis in hypophysectomized monkeys with testosterone (T). In 7th International Congress of Endocrinology, Abstracts, p. 1074. Excerpta Medica, International Congress Series 652. Amsterdam, Elsevier Science Publishers, 1984

15. MATSUMOTO AM, PAULSEN CA, BREMNER WJ: Stimulation of sperm production in gonadotropin-suppressed normal men by administration of follicle-stimulating hormone. J Clin Invest 72:1005–1015, 1983

16. MCCULLAGH DR: Dual endocrine activity of testes. Science 76:19–20, 1932

17. MOUDGAL NR: A need for FSH in maintaining fertility of adult male subhuman primates. Arch Androl 7:117–125, 1981

18. MURTY GSRC, RANI CSS, MOUDGAL NR, PRASAD MRN: Effect of passive immunization with specific antiserum to FSH on the spermatogenic process and fertility of adult male bonnet monkeys (*Macaca radiata*). J Reprod Fertil (Suppl) 26:147–163, 1979

19. NIESCHLAG E (ed): Immunization With Hormones in Reproduction Research. Amsterdam and New York, North–Holland/American Elsevier, 1975

20. NIESCHLAG E, WICKINGS EJ: Biological effects of antibodies to gonadal steroids. In Vitamins and Hormones, Vol 36. London, Academic Press, 1978

21. NIESCHLAG E, WICKINGS EJ: Does the rhesus monkey provide a suitable model for human testicular functions? In SERIO M, MARTINI L (eds): Animal Models in Human Reproduction. New York, Raven Press, 1980

22. SHERINS RJ: Clinical aspects of treatment of male infertility with gonadotrophins: Testicular response of some men given hCG with and without Pergonal. In MANCINI RE, MARTINI L (eds): Male Fertility and Sterility, Vol 5, pp 545–556. New York, Raven Press, 1974

23. SRINATH BR, WICKINGS EJ, WITTING C, NIESCHLAG E: Active immunization with follicle-stimulating hormone for fertility control: A 4½-year study in male rhesus monkeys. Fertil Steril 40:110–117, 1983

24. STEINBERGER E: Hormonal control of mammalian spermatogenesis. Physiol Rev 51:1, 1971

25. TROEN P, YANAIHARA T, NANKIN HR, TOMINAGA T, LEVER H: Assessment of gonadotrophin therapy in infertile males. In ROSENBERG E, PAULSEN CA (eds): The Human Testis, pp 591–602. New York, Plenum Press, 1970

26. WICKINGS EJ, USADEL KH, DATHE G, NIESCHLAG E: The role of follicle-stimulating hormone in testicular function of the mature rhesus monkey. Acta Endocrinol 95:117, 1980

38

Partial Purification of Inhibin from Ovine Rete Testis Fluid

JEAN RIVIER

RICHARD McCLINTOCK

JOAN VAUGHAN

GAYLE YAMAMOTO

HARRY ANDERSON

JOACHIM SPIESS

WYLIE VALE

JOSEF VOGLMAYR

C. YAN CHENG

C. WAYNE BARDIN

The existence of water-soluble substances of gonadal origin that can suppress FSH secretion selectively has been suspected for more than 50 years.[4] The quest to chemically characterize these molecules (referred to as inhibin in the male and folliculostatin in the female) has not succeeded to date.[1,2,3] The primary structures of a 31-peptide and 94-peptide with inhibin like activities recently were reported by Ramasharma and colleagues[6] and Seidah and associates.[13] More recently, Robertson and others reported the isolation of folliculostatin from bovine follicular fluid; this entity was purified over 3000-fold and had an apparent molecular weight (MW) of 56,000.[12] Under reducing conditions it could be dissociated into two subunits of MW 14,000 and 44,000. We reported on a 27,000-fold folliculostatin preparation purified from porcine follicular fluid (PFF), the apparent molecular weight of which

The collection and fractionation of ram rete testis fluid was supported by USAID Grant pha-G-116 and Cooperative Agreement No. DPE-3005-A-00-3003-00. Synthetic efforts were supported by Contract NOI-HD-2-2824 with the Contraceptive Development Branch, Center for Population Research, NIH. Research conducted in part by the Clayton Foundation for Research, California Division (W. Vale and J. Spiess are Clayton Foundation Investigators).

The authors wish to thank A. Corrigan, D. Dalton, R. Azad, D. Karr, and W. Woo for expert technical help. We also thank B. Hensley and R. Schachne for preparation of the manuscript. We are grateful to the Endocrine Society sections for the FSH RIA kits.

Boc-His(Tos)-Asn(Xan)-Lys(2ClZ)-Gln(Xan)-Glu(Bzl)-Gly-
Arg(Tos)-Asp(Bzl)-His(Tos)-Asp(Bzl)-Lys(2ClZ)-Ser(OBzl)-
Lys(2ClZ)-Gly-His(Tos)-Phe-His(Tos)-Arg(Tos)-Val-Val-Ile-
His(Tos)-His(Tos)-Lys(2ClZ)-Gly-Gly-Lys(2ClZ)-Ala-His(Tos)-
Arg(Tos)-Gly-CM resin.

FIG. 38-1. Synthetic protected inhibin 31-OH. Tos is the abbreviation for the Tosyl group used for the side chain protection of arginine and histidine. OBzl is the abbreviation for benzyl ether of the side chain hydroxyl group of serine. Bzl is the abbreviation for the side chain benzyl ester protection for aspartic and glutamic acids; 2ClZ is the abbreviation for the 2-chlorocarbobenzoxy group used to protect the side chain of lysine. Xan is the abbreviation for the xanthyl group used in glutamine and asparagine protection. This peptide was deprotected as described in the text.

was significantly lower.[11] Independently of this latter isolation project, we have also investigated methods for the large-scale purification of inhibin from ram rete testis fluid (RTF). This preliminary report describes an approximate 3000- to 5000-fold purification that led to a preparation that we estimate to be in the range of 10% to 30% pure. In addition, we report that under the conditions tested, synthetic inhibin 31-OH does not have the biologic properties expected for inhibin or folliculostatin.

SYNTHESIS AND ASSAY OF INHIBIN 31-OH

Synthetic inhibin 31-OH was synthesized *de novo* using the solid phase approach of Merrifield on a classic chloromethyl resin.[5] N-Boc protection was used for each of the amino acids throughout the synthesis. The protected peptide resin is shown in Figure 38-1.

Cleavage and complete deprotection of the peptide from the resin was performed by stirring the peptide-resin, 10 g at 0°C, with 120 ml hydrofluoric acid. Anisole (25 ml) was added to the peptide resin prior to treatment with hydrofluoric acid as a scavenger for carbonium-ion species generated during this treatment. After removal of the hydrofluoric acid under vacuum, the peptide was treated with ether, filtered, and taken in dilute acetic acid and lyophilized.

Purification of the desired product from the crude mix was accomplished through HPLC procedures on a Waters Prep LC500A instrument.[9] Conditions were: Vydac C18 silica (15 μm–20 μm) packed into cartridges (5 × 30 cm). Gradient was 50% A (A = 0.1% HFBA), 50% B (B = 60% CH_3CN/40% and H_2O/0.1% HFBA) to 25% A, 75% B in 60 min (flow rate 125 ml/min). It was found that neither TEAP nor TFA buffer with acetonitrile allowed the hydrophilic peptide to be retained long enough on the column to achieve the desired purification. The purified fractions were pooled and lyophilized to yield the HFBA salt of inhibin 31-OH. Amino acid analysis and sequence analysis* confirmed that the peptide was at least 85% pure. Analytical HPLC in different systems failed to uncover UV-absorbing (210 nm) impurities.

---

* Courtesy of Dr. W. Gray, University of Utah, Salt Lake City, UT.

TABLE 38-1. In vivo Assay of Synthetic Inhibin 31-OH

GROUP	NUMBER OF RATS	SERUM FHS ng/ml
1. Intact + saline × 3	6	11 ± 2.2
2. Castrate + saline × 3	5	30 ± 6.3
3. Castrate + inhibin 5 μg × 3	4	26 ± 1.4
4. Castrate + inhibin 10 μg × 3	5	28 ± 4.3

Sprague-Dawley rats (34 days old) in groups 2, 3, and 4 were orchiectomized and injected immediately with saline, 5 μg inhibin 31-OH or 10 μg inhibin 31-OH respectively. Inhibin 31-OH was dissolved in saline. The animals received the same treatment at 8 and 24 hours. Blood was obtained at 30 hours and serum was assayed for FSH by radioimmunoassay.

The synthetic inhibin 31-OH was tested for biologic activity in acutely castrated male rats; the results of this study are shown in Table 38-1. The peptide did not prevent the rise of FSH in these animals at the highest dose tested. Using similar doses of the native peptide, Ramasharma and colleagues reported an 80% suppression of FSH.[6]

PURIFICATION OF INHIBIN FROM RAM RETE TESTIS FLUID

Cannulae were inserted into the rete testes of adult rams under halothane anesthesia. Rete testis fluid was collected, pooled, and stored at $-20°C$. Protein content was approximately 500 μg/ml RTF.

Inhibin was assayed in vitro based on its ability to lower basal FSH secretion by cultured rat anterior pituitary cells. This assay is a modified version of the cell culture method developed in 1972[14] and further refined.[15] Parallel dose response curves (3–5 points) gave relative potency estimates versus an internal standard of crude RTF. Based on this assay, RTF maximally suppresses basal FSH release at around 10 μl RTF per milliliter of culture medium.

Reverse-phase, high-pressure liquid chromatography (RP-HPLC) is described.[7,8,9] (Exact conditions are reported in Table 38-2.) In view of the low protein content of RTF (~250 mg/500 ml), as determined by amino acid analysis, it was thought that both the precipitation and the gel permeation steps, which we have used for the partial purification of folliculostatin from follicular fluid,[10] could be bypassed and that this material could be applied directly to RP-HPLC. Pilot experiments were implemented, and we were able to demonstrate good recovery under specific conditions, such as those shown in Table 38-2.

Whereas step 1 (Table 38-2) was preparative, the subsequent steps were carried out on an analytical column that, for natural products, had been found to be considerably more resolutive than the prepacked, semipreparative cartridges, and more often, for that matter, than the prepacked semipreparative columns, at least under the conditions tested. In all cases, we chose the triethylammonium phosphate buffer at pH 6.5. Under these conditions and using CH_3CN as the organic modifier, we were able to achieve considerable resolution, as illustrated in Fig. 38-2, as well as good recovery of biologic activity.

(Text continues on p. 406)

TABLE 38-2. Partial Purification of Inhibin from 525 ml of Ram Testicular Fluid

HPLC STEP*	FLOW RATE (ml/min)	SOLVENT COMPOSITION†		LOAD		GRADIENT	RV§ (ml)	TEMPERATURE (°C)
		A	B	Ml-eq‡	VOLUME (ml)			
1	75	0.1% TEAP pH 6.5	80% CH_3CN 20% A	525.0	525	25%–80% B in 40 min	1350–1600	25
2	0.8	0.1% TEAP pH 6.5	80% CH_3CN 20% A	52.5	30	30%–70% B in 45 min	23.2–24.8	60
3	0.8	0.1% TEAP pH 6.5	80% CH_3CN 20% A	16.8	3	30%–70% B in 45 min	23.2–24.4	60

* Silicas were from Vydac. Step 1 used a 5 × 30 cm cartridge filled with 15 μm–20 μm C_4.[10] Steps 2, 3 used 0.46 × 25 cm columns filled with 5 μm C_4.

† TEAP buffer was 0.1% H_3PO_4 titrated to pH with redistilled triethylamine. Except for Step 1, the active fractions (partially concentrated in Savant rotary evaporator and diluted with an equal volume of H_2O) were loaded 1.0 ml at a time into a 2-ml injector loop.

‡ For accounting purposes and to gain an appreciation of recovery at each step of the purification, 1 ml RTF is equal to 1 ml equivalent (1 ml-eq) as the purification progresses. Ml-eq is the unit use in dose response curves.

§ Retention volume (RV) of the active zone was measured in ml from the start of the gradient (not including loading volume). Fractions were stored at 3°C–5°C. Aliquots for assays (0.1%–1% of total fraction volume, never less than 4 μl) were measured with micropipettes and plastic tips and were transferred into polypropylene tubes containing bovine serum albumin (10 μl; 10 mg/ml) and dried in a Savant rotary evaporator. Losses prior to assays and inconsistent results could be minimized in this manner. When 52.5 ml-eq RTF were loaded (step 2), ten identical runs were performed to process the total 525 ml-eq available. Manual column fractionation was based on OD patterns.

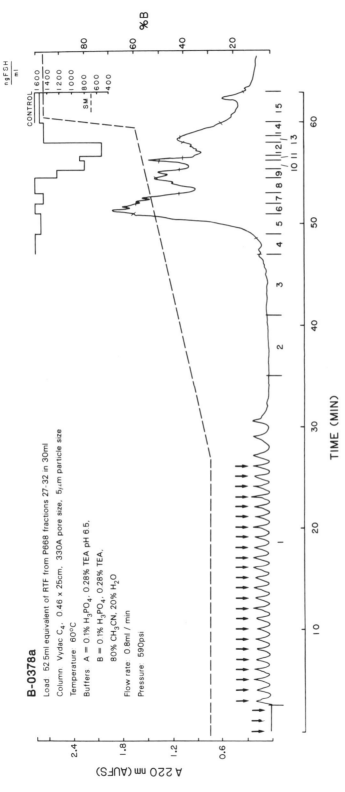

FIG. 38-2. Chromatogram of step 2 (see Table 38-2) in the fractionation of inhibin activity in ram rete testis fluid. Inhibin activity is shown by the suppression of basal FSH secretion by rat anterior pituitary cells. Starting material (*SM*); active fractions 10 to 12 are significantly different from the controls.

405

Indeed, throughout these steps we observed maximal inhibition of basal FSH release at doses of 10 μl eq/ml of tissue culture medium. As shown in Figure 38-2, repetitive loading of a twofold diluted fraction from the previous run (*i.e.,* step 1) in 1-ml increments, as indicated by multiple arrows on the chromatogram, is a very effective way of concentrating fractions. Because the separation may be repeated, equivalent fractions can be collected in the same tubes. We have been able to reproduce this separation at weekly intervals on multiple occasions.

Step 3 (Table 38-2) was run to investigate whether a lower load (16.8 ml-eq) of a highly purified material would behave identically to a higher load, because it is known that one of the earlier pitfalls of RP-HPLC was that small amounts of protein could be lost only to reappear as "ghost peaks" in subsequent fractionations. Under the selected conditions, no loss of biologic potency occurred, and most activity was found in a fraction that encompassed approximately $\frac{1}{3}$ of total OD. Amino acid analysis after acid hydrolysis of the starting material used in this last step showed that we had applied approximately 3 μg protein/10 ml-eq. With the active fraction being maximally active at 10 μl-eq, and in view of the fact that this fraction corresponded to an estimated $\frac{1}{3}$ of total peptide weight, we can suggest that this fraction maximally inhibited FSH secretion as about 1 ng protein/ml culture fluid. If we assume a molecular weight of 20,000 daltons (or slightly higher) as suggested by several laboratories, we can propose that inhibin will be maximally active at 50 fM concentrations.

Based on in vitro bioassay showing similar biologic responses with 10 μl-eq/ml of starting material and the final product, we have achieved a 3000- to 5000-fold increase in specific activity of inhibin over that in RTF. Loss of inhibin activity due to absorption by test tubes or chemical alteration, as well as to the very small quantities available, prevented us from further characterizing this fraction. Larger batches, allowing for better quantitation, will have to be run to obtain enough material for sequence analysis. It is our estimate at the present time that we may need another 3- to 10-fold purification in order to obtain a pure protein. Whether this will be feasible and whether at the very end a practical desalting step will allow us to submit the sample to structural analysis must await the availability of significantly larger amounts of starting material.

REFERENCES

1. CHANNING CP, GORDON WL, LIU V-K, WARD DN: Minireview: Physiology and biochemistry of ovarian inhibin. Biol Medicine 178:339–361, 1985
2. DEJONG FH: Inhibin—fact or artifact. Mol Cell Endocrinol 13:1–10, 1979
3. DUBAS M, BURGER HG, HEARN MTW, MORGAN FJ: Isolation of inhibin from ovine follicular fluid using reversed-phase liquid chromatography. Mol Cell Endocrinol 31:187–198, 1983
4. MCCULLAGH DD: Dual endocrine activity of the testis. Science 76:19–20, 1932
5. MERRIFIELD RB: Solid-phase peptide synthesis. I. The synthesis of a tetrapeptide. J Am Chem Soc 85:2149, 1963
6. RAMASHARMA K, SAIRAM MR, SEIDAH NH, CHRÉTIEN M, MANJUNATH P, SCHILLER PW, YAMASHIRO D, LI CH: Isolation, structure, and synthesis of a human seminal plasma peptide with inhibin-like activity. Science 223:1199–1202, 1984
7. RIVIER J: Use of trialkylammonium phosphate (TAAP) buffers in reverse-phase HPLC for high resolution and high recovery of peptides and proteins. J Liquid Chromatogr 1:343–367, 1978

8. RIVIER J, RIVIER C, SPIESS J, VALE W: High-performance liquid chromatographic purification of peptide hormones: Ovine hypothalamic amunine (corticotropin-releasing factor). Anal Biochem 127:258–266, 1983

9. RIVIER J, MCCLINTOCK R, GALYEAN R, ANDERSON H: Reversed phase HPLC: Preparative purification of synthetic peptides. J Chromatogr 288:303–328, 1984

10. RIVIER J, MCCLINTOCK R, VAUGHAN J, RIVIER C, SPIESS J, VALE W: Partial purification of a high molecular weight fraction of folliculostatin to be used as a possible reference preparation. Biol Reprod (in press)

11. RIVIER J, MCCLINTOCK R, SPIESS J, VAUGHAN J, DALTON D, CORRIGAN A, AZAD R, VALE W: Isolation from porcine follicular fluid of a protein exhibiting potent inhibin-like biological activity. Proc 7th Intl Cong Endocrinol 655:1141–1144, 1985

12. ROBERTSON DM, FOULDS LM, LEVERSHA L, MORAN FJ, HEARN MTW, BURGER HG, WETTENHALL REH, KRETSEN DMV DE: Isolation of inhibin from bovine follicular fluid. Biochem Biophys Res Commun 126:220–226, 1985

13. SEIDAH NG, ARBATTI NJ, ROCHEMONT J, SHETH AR, CHRÉTIEN M: Complete amino acid sequence of human seminal plasma-inhibin. FEBS 175:349–355, 1984

14. VALE W, GRANT G, AMOSS M, BLACKWELL R, GUILLEMIN R: Culture of enzymatically dispersed anterior pituitary cells: Functional validation of a method. Endocrinology 91:562–572, 1972

15. VALE W, VAUGHAN J, SMITH M, YAMAMOTO G, RIVIER J, RIVIER C: Effects of synthetic ovine CRF, glucocorticoids, catecholamines, neurohypophysial peptides and other substances on cultured corticotropic cells. Endocrinology 113:1121–1131, 1983

39

Inhibin and Gonadal Parahormones: Possible Contraceptive Agents

PAUL FRANCHIMONT

Cell-to-cell communications are assessed by various mechanisms: hormones are released from an endocrine gland into the bloodstream and reach the target organ, where they bind to a specific receptor. Neuromediators are involved in synaptic transmission; neurohormones are mediators produced by neurons and released in the circulation most often in a portal system.

Autocrine regulation is related to the mediators that influence the cell from which they have been secreted, leading to an intracellular feedback regulation.

Paracrine communication is a mechanism by which a substance is secreted by a cell and moves through interstitial spaces to act on a neighboring target cell. These paracrine communications are mediated by substances of various natures (polypeptides, glycoproteins, steroids) and often act by inhibitory mechanisms.

Paracrine control is a generalized biologic process that already has been well investigated for the gonadal functions. Several identified factors may be involved in the paracrine control of the gonads: steroids (androgens, estrogens) and polypeptides such as oxytocin, pro-opiomelanocortin, gonadotropin-releasing hormone (GnRH), and GnRH-like peptides. Other polypeptide parahormones have been identified in the gonads but not yet characterized biochemically. Thus, several biologic effects have been identified in follicular fluid and in rete testis fluid.[17,19] They are not related to steroids or to known proteins or peptides. Among these reported biologic effects are the inhibition of progesterone secretion,[26] of oocyte maturation,[1] of follicle-stimulating hormone (FSH) and luteinizing hormone (LH) receptor binding,[28] and of aromatase.[9] Some of the substances involved in these inhibitory effects are in the process of being purified, and all of them are possible factors of prime importance in the physiology and pathophysiology of reproduction. Inhibin is a real hormone, regulating FSH secretion by pituitary gland; it may also act locally in the gonads.[16]

INHIBITION OF OOCYTE MATURATION

The presence of an oocyte maturation inhibitor (OMI) in follicular fluid was first suggested by Chang.[1] OMI appears to be a peptide of 1000 to 2000 molecular weight (MW).[45] The best preparations have been purified about

---

The study described in this chapter was supported by grant No. 3.4501.80 of FRSM.

TABLE 39-1. Effect of a Fraction of Rete Testis Fluid on Germinal Vesicle Breakdown of a Rat Oocyte in Culture and Progesterone Production by Bovine Granulosa Cell in Culture

CONCENTRATION OF RTF_{2-4} $\mu g/ml^{-1}$	GERMINAL VESICLE BREAKDOWN (%)	IN VITRO PROGESTERONE PRODUCTION BY GRANULOSA CELLS ng/ml^{-1}
Control	85 (75)	98.7 ± 22
15 μg	68 (51)	82.4 ± 14
25 μg	62 (53)	66.3 ± 12*
30 μg	52 (51)	59.9 ± 6*
50 μg	46 (135)	47.7 ± 12*
50 μg heated (90°–15′)	79 (39)	47.7 ± 12*

( ) Number of oocytes
* P < 0.005

15,000-fold. Besides the presence of OMI in follicular fluid, evidence has been presented to demonstrate that granulosa cells are a source of OMI.[45] Using such cultured cells, some investigators have looked at the effects of adding various hormones to the culture medium on the regulation of OMI secretion. It appears that FSH stimulates the formation of OMI-like activity, whereas testosterone or androstenedione prevents its formation. Furthermore, prolactin may act on the granulosa cell to enhance its secretion. Estradiol or LH has no effect.[3]

Besides inhibiting oocyte maturation, the biologically active fractions have been shown to reduce progesterone secretion by cultured granulosa cells and to inhibit cumulus cell outgrowth in culture.[26] The inhibitory action on progesterone secretion per se is not responsible for OMI inhibition of oocyte maturation because incubation of cumulus-enclosed oocytes with aminoglutethimide inhibits progesterone secretion by the cumuli but does not alter oocyte maturation.[26] The mechanism is not known whereby OMI acts on the cumulus cells to retain the oocyte in the immature (dictyate) stage until normal maturation and ovulation occur. It needs the presence of cumulus oophorus cells. Even if one assumes that OMI is indeed responsible for maintaining the oocytes in the arrested state of meiosis, however, it remains to be determined what selectively releases a given follicle from its influence.

Recently, our group has proposed evidence for the presence of OMI-like activity in fractions purified from ram rete testis fluid.[19] Like the female OMI, this factor inhibits oocyte maturation in vitro, and progesterone secretion by cultured granulosa cells (Table 39-1). The relationship with the meiosis-preventing substance (MPS) that has been identified in epididymides and testes of fetal human males, which prevents male germ cells enclosed in seminiferous cords during fetal and infantile life from entering meiosis,[22] has not yet been investigated.

Although the establishment of the exact physiologic role of OMI requires complete purification of the active molecule, one can hypothesize that factor(s) with biologic properties similar to those of female OMI might play an important role in regulating mitosis and meiosis of spermatogonia and spermatocytes.

OMI has potentially contraceptive action by keeping oocytes immature and therefore incapable of being fertilized, and by inhibiting meiosis of primary spermatocytes. A major advantage of such substances is the reversibility of their actions. Inhibitory effect on germinal vesicle breakdown disappears when OMI is discarded from the culture medium for 4 hours.[2]

FSH-RECEPTOR BINDING INHIBITOR (FSH-RBI)

Fractions with FSH-RBI activity have been found in aqueous extracts of testis,[34] follicular fluid,[7] and serum.[35] FSH-RBI activity appears to be associated with a small molecular weight peptide (about 700 daltons) that lacks carbohydrate residues.[36] Recently, Reichert identified a peptide of 11 amino acids possessing FSH-RBI activity. The addition of biologically active fractions to Sertoli cells or granulosa cells causes a reduction of FSH binding to these cells. In granulosa cells, this inhibition is accompanied by a decrease in FSH stimulation of progesterone secretion and a reduction in the number of binding sites for LH.[28] The concentration of FSH-RBI is higher in follicular fluid pooled from small follicles than in follicular fluid pooled from large follicles of either pregnant or luteal phase cows. Furthermore, the concentration of FSH-RBI is positively correlated with relative degree of follicular atresia, based on the concentration of androgens and the ratio of androgens to estrogens in follicular fluid.[41] At present, the mechanism of action of FSH-RBI remains unknown. Whether it competes with FSH for its receptors or it interacts directly with FSH and as a consequence inhibits FSH binding remains to be determined. The physiologic role of FSH-RBI still is being discussed. It is well known that FSH stimulates aromatase activity and estrogen production by granulosa cells. Estrogens and FSH allow follicular growth. Furthermore, FSH induces the expression of LH receptor on the cellular membrane of granulosa cells. FSH-RBI would thus be capable of inhibiting estrogen production in granulosa cells with accumulation of androgens and defect of follicular growth process. The lack of FSH stimulation and estrogen production thus would lead to atresia. In males, FSH-RBI could depress Sertoli cell functions that are involved in maturation of germ cells. FSH-RBI could be considered a candidate for contraceptive purposes.

AROMATASE INHIBITOR

Recently, a heat- and trypsin-labile protein(s) has been identified in venous effluent from the ovaries containing the dominant follicle, but not from anovulatory ovaries,[9] and in porcine and human follicular fluid.[11] This factor suppresses follicular response to gonadotropins, HMG-mediated increases in rat ovarian weight, and serum estradiol concentrations. Furthermore, spent media from human granulosa cell culture inhibits rat ovarian weight gain and estradiol production in response to gonadotropin stimulation.[12] Moreover, in vitro, this protein fraction inhibits the conversion of pregnenolone to progesterone and the aromatase activity in porcine granulosa cells. Addition of FSH or removal of aromatase inhibitor allows the recovery of progesterone secretion, whereas FSH does not overcome the inhibitory effect of the fraction, and aromatase activity does not return to normal following the removal of these regulatory follicular proteins. Finally, they inhibit FSH induction of granulosa cell LH receptors.

The molecular weight of the substance ranges between 12,500 and 16,000 dalton with isoelectric points of 4.5 and 6.1. It does not bind to concanavalin A. When injected into a regularly menstruating monkey twice daily (3 mg each injection) for the first 14.5 days of the menstrual cycle, purified porcine follicular fluid protein(s) disrupts folliculogenesis, resulting in either anovulatory cycles (2 cases on 5 monkeys) or in long follicular phases followed by luteal phase insufficiencies (3 cases on 5). All the cases are characterized by low follicular and luteal phase serum estradiol concentrations and subnormal luteal progesterone production. Serum gonadotropin concentrations are not affected by the follicular fluid protein(s). These data demonstrate in the non-human primates that porcine follicular fluid contains a protein(s) that acts at the ovarian level to inhibit gonadotropin action.[13] As a result of assays in human follicular fluid, a positive correlation has been found between estradiol concentration and the aromatase inhibitor, and a negative correlation between progesterone levels and aromatase inhibitor. These correlations imply that as the follicle continues its preovulatory maturation, aromatase inhibitor may increase. Once luteinization begins, however, there may be an overall diminution of aromatase inhibitor activity.[10]

It is tempting to speculate that this peptide may mediate dominance of the preovulatory follicle by an active process, such that after the selection of the dominant follicle, the gonadotropin responsivity of other follicles on the same and contralateral ovaries is suppressed. Furthermore, it is well known that estrogens stimulate granulosa cell proliferation and enhance granulosa cell FSH and LH binding.[37] They act as a central regulator of follicular maturation. This inhibition of estrogen formation by such a protein(s) would suppress continued follicle maturation to ovulatory status in favor of atresia. These properties then could be used as the basis of a contraceptive agent.

INHIBIN

Since 1972, numerous investigations have been directed toward demonstrating the existence of inhibin, a gonadal peptide that specifically or preferentially decreases the secretion of FSH.

Inhibin has been detected in and partially purified from human seminal fluid; bovine seminal fluid; ram rete testis fluid (RTF); extracts of spermatozoa; testicular extracts; ovarian extracts; bovine, porcine, and human follicular fluid; as well as the culture medium of Sertoli cells and granulosa cells.[17]

Several investigators have attempted to purify this hormone; however, few believe that a completely pure preparation can be achieved. Its chemical structure and physicochemical properties are still highly controversial. The physiologic role of this hormone, its action on the pituitary, the hypothalamus, and the gonads, and its synergism with the sex steroids make it a possible agent capable of modifying the fertility of animals and human beings.

INTERRELATIONSHIPS BETWEEN FSH, INHIBIN, AND SPERMATOGENESIS IN MALE ANIMALS

Spermatogenesis is the process that leads to the development and maturation of the germ cells. It involves the participation of two cell types, the germ cell proper, the differentiation of which results in the formation of spermatozoa, and the Sertoli cell. The role of the Sertoli cells appears to be of great importance, although incompletely elucidated, through metabolic steps such as testosterone aromatization to 17 β-estradiol,[14] production of androgen-binding protein (ABP) under the influence of FSH[20] and testosterone,[42] and inhibin secretion, which is involved directly and through FSH in the control of spermatogenesis.[16]

The hormonal control of this testicular function still remains open to considerable discussion, but it appears that FSH is involved in the initiation and maintenance of spermatogenesis. During puberty, FSH increases testicular weight and the diameter of the seminiferous tubules.[21,38] It also is involved in the multiplication and differentiation of types A_0 and A_1 spermatogonia following hypophysectomy in rats or lambs, a process in which testosterone is also required.[27] Treatment of 25-day-old immature male rats for 15 days with specific anti-FSH serum leads to the arrest of spermatogenesis, without any adverse effects on accessory organs and their functions.[39] Thus, germ cells, particularly type A spermatogonia, pachytene spermatocytes, and spermatids are markedly reduced. Furthermore, according to Chemes and colleagues administration of anti-FSH serum to immature rats from the day of birth reduces preleptotene spermatocytes and step 7 to 8 spermatids, suggesting a requirement for FSH in some of the steps leading to the differentiation of type A spermatogonia into preleptotene spermatocytes, and for normal early spermiogenesis.[4] These data indicate that FSH is essential to the maintenance of different cells in the seminiferous epithelium during the completion of the first wave of spermatogenesis.

In hypophysectomized adult rats, the absence of gonadotropins suppresses the proliferation and/or the differentiation of the various generations of differentiated spermatogonia, resulting in a significant reduction in the total yield of type B spermatogonia.[5] In contrast, maturation of pachytene spermatocytes, meiotic division, and spermatogenesis are testosterone dependent. FSH maintains the reserve of spermatogonia as well as restoring their divisions, whereas meiosis and spermiogenesis are all maintained effectively by LH and testosterone.[27]

These effects of FSH on the early stages of spermatogenesis confirm the previous studies of Means.[30] Means showed that FSH increases the mitotic rate and reduces degeneration in spermatogonia. Furthermore, Orth and Christensen using autoradiography, have shown that FSH-binding sites are found over the surface of spermatogonia in concentrations similar to those of Sertoli cells in the basal compartment of the seminiferous tubules.[33]

The work of Murty and associates similarly shows that FSH is required for the maintenance of spermatogenesis in the adult.[31] Thus, chronic withdrawal of FSH in subhuman primates affects the fertility of the adult male. The administration of antisera directed specifically against FSH reduces the fertility rate to zero and the number of spermatozoa to 44% of that found in control animals, whereas the number of living spermatozoa is no greater than 7.4%. The results of Nieschlag and co-workers confirm that FSH is required to maintain spermatogenesis in male monkeys. Thus, active and passive immunization of monkeys against FSH selectively inhibits spermatogenesis, which reduces sperm counts, periods of azoospermia, and tubuli depleted of germinal epithelium, some with Sertoli cells only. Testicular volumes and tubular diameters are reduced. In contrast, Leydig cells appear histologically normal, and serum testosterone and bioassayable LH levels never fall below control values.[32,46] It thus seems logical to conclude that spermatogenesis is controlled by FSH as well as by other hormones. FSH acts particularly on spermatogonial multiplication.

The mechanism and site of action of FSH are still obscure, however. This hormone appears to act directly on germ cells but also through the Sertoli cells, which possess FSH receptors. It is known that the latter cells secrete androgen-binding protein (ABP) under the influence of FSH and testosterone. This transport protein binds androgens that, originating in the Leydig cell, are secreted in the seminiferous tubules, and also facilitates the transfer of androgen to the specific receptors of germ cells.

A hormone that can lower the secretion of FSH without altering that of LH at certain dosage levels could be used to block FSH-dependent steps in gametogenesis. In humans, and in the rat, initiation of spermatogenesis during puberty is brought about by increases in FSH levels.[15,40,44] It is conceivable that treatment with inhibin during puberty would impair initiation of the spermatogenesis without disturbing the androgen-dependent processes of pubertal maturation, which are modulated by normal LH secretion.

Few experiments have been undertaken to study the effects of inhibin on spermatogenesis. De Jong gave bovine follicular fluid, devoid of steroids, for 12 days to 21-day-old male rats and were able to show a delay in pubertal development of the testes compared with control animals, as well as reduction of testicular weight, retardation of spermatogenesis, and decrease in the number of pachytene spermatocytes. These effects were produced even though the levels of FSH were reduced only during the first 4 days of treatment and the levels of LH were significantly increased.

We have given different inhibin preparations and extracts of human seminal fluid and RTF inhibin in doses totaling 160 μg/100 g body weight, administered as four injections intraperitoneally over 36 hours to rats of different ages.[18] We measured the incorporation of tritiated thymidine injected 3 hours before sacrifice into testicular DNA and the labeling of germinal cells by autohistoradiography. The inhibin preparations markedly reduced the incorporation of tritiated thymidine into testicular DNA and the uptake by intermediate and type B spermatogonia compared with the same preparation previously degraded by trypsin and heated to 60°C for 1 hour. This effect was apparent in a 42- to 49-day-old rat in which spermatogenesis commences and progresses at the same time as a significant incorporation of thymidine into testicular DNA is observed. In contrast, in adult rats, no effect was observed on the incorporation of (^{3}H) thymidine, which is ten times less than that seen in pubertal rats.[18] Inhibin preparations specifically act on testicular DNA synthesis because they induce no modification of thymidine incorporation into hepatic DNA.

Inhibin thus appears to inhibit the synthesis of DNA implicated in the mitoses of germinal cells (particularly, spermatogonia type B) and intermediate in pubertal animals. These cells, as they divide, signal the beginning of spermatogenesis. This effect doubtless is mediated by the reduction of the secretion of FSH. It is known, in fact, that after FSH withdrawal by injection of specific anti-FSH serum, there is also an inhibition of (^{3}H) thymidine incorporation into DNA.[31] A direct effect of inhibin on the multiplication of germinal cells disclosed by the incorporation of tritiated thymidine in the testicular DNA has been observed in vitro with preparations of inhibin, however. The action of these inhibin preparations, as much in vivo as in vitro, resembles that of testicular chalones.[6] These substances extracted from testes exert an inhibitory effect on germ cells, particularly on the multiplication of spermatogonia type A.

In adults, inhibin may have no detectable effect because the frequency of mitoses is insufficient for an effect to be observed, or because cell multiplication ceases to be dependent on FSH and, secondarily, on inhibin. Steinberger showed that in adult rats, spermatogenesis can be maintained by testosterone alone.[43]

In the adult male, the reduction of FSH levels by inhibin could directly or indirectly (in lowering ABP secretion by Sertoli cells) alter the process of spermatogenesis by an action at different levels. It is known that an optimal concentration of testosterone is required for the process of meiosis (primary spermatocytes to secondary spermatocytes); for spermatocyte maturation, ABP may be important in the maintenance of such concentrations in the seminiferous tubular compartment of the testis. FSH also appears to be necessary for the transformation of spermatids to spermatozoa.[29]

CONCLUSIONS: RELATIONSHIPS AMONG FSH, INHIBIN, AND FOLLICULAR MATURATION IN ANIMALS

Inhibin is produced by granulosa cells. The production is increased with the maturation of the follicles, which may be appreciated by the aromatase activity.[24] In contrast, luteinization of granulosa cells leads to a decrease of inhibin production, as shown by an inverse relationship between inhibin and progesterone production by granulosa cells.[23]

In females, a reduction by the administration of inhibin of the FSH increment at the beginning of the follicular phase of the menstrual cycle and at ovulation could also interfere with fertility potential. These actions could prevent the maturation of the primordial follicle and interfere with the formation of the corpus luteum.

Channing and colleagues showed that the pattern of FSH secretion was modified during the estrous cycle of the rat by the injection of porcine follicular fluid previously treated with charcoal.[2] Thus, the elevation of blood FSH levels that appears between proestrus and estrus in response to the natural preovulation peak of LH or an artificial peak of LH (induced by the inhibition of the natural preovulation peak of LH by pentobarbital and replaced by exogenous LH) can be suppressed by the steroid-free fluid given intraperitoneally in two 0.5-ml doses. This inhibitory factor does not alter the LH levels or modify estradiol and progesterone secretion rates and does not affect rupture of the follicle. Under these experimental conditions, treatment by steroid-free porcine follicular fluid inhibited the second elevation of FSH, which may recruit follicles for the next cycle.

De Jong and co-workers obtained somewhat different results in long-term experiments with much smaller doses of follicular fluid.[8] These investigators injected adult female rats with charcoal-treated bovine follicular fluid daily over five estrous cycles. The dose was 0.25 ml/100 g body weight for the first 17 days, subsequently 1 ml/100 g. Under these conditions, the authors did not observe any changes in vaginal smears. Furthermore, the number of ova in the tubes from the second to the fifth estrous cycle was no different from controls treated with bovine plasma. FSH levels fell 8 hours after the first injection, there was then an increase in FSH and LH levels, as compared with control values. The blood levels are, nevertheless, difficult to interpret because they were not taken systematically during the five estrous cycles but at very wide intervals.

A most interesting experiment was performed by Channing and associates, who demonstrated that inhibin inhibits follicular maturation and can modify the midcycle FSH peak in monkeys.[2]

Porcine follicular fluid (PFF) from small and medium follicles was pooled, charcoal treated, and injected intraperitoneally in 4-ml doses every 8 hours between days 1 and 4 of the menstrual cycle of four rhesus monkeys. Treatment was followed by laparotomy on days 12 to 14 of the cycle, with recovery of the preovulatory follicle. Serum FSH levels were measured in daily blood samples for one control menstrual cycle prior to treatment and throughout one treatment cycle. The PFF caused a significant decrease in serum FSH levels within 24 to 36 hours of the start of the treatment in the 4 animals. FSH levels returned to preinjection control levels within 1 to 3 days of cessation of treatment. There was a decline of less than 5% in serum LH levels. The follicle present on days 12 to 14 of the treatment cycle was smaller than normal and contained few granulosa cells (0.1×10^6 cells) compared to control preovulatory follicles, which contained 2 to 50×10^6 cells, that is, fewer than 10% of the normal number of granulosa cells. The action of inhibin on follicular maturation is certainly mediated by FSH, but a direct effect of inhibin on the follicle is not excluded.

Two monkeys were given PFF for 4 days at midcycle. In one case in which the treatment was started 1 day prior to the expected midcycle surge of FSH, the midcycle FSH surge was delayed until after cessation of PFF treatment. In the other monkey, in which treatment was started 8 hours after the start of the FSH surge, the surge was shortened to about one third of normal.

Interestingly, active immunization with follicular fluid inhibin seems to be a potential means of increasing fecundity in sheep.[25] Thus, the ovulation rates of the ewes immunized with the inhibin preparation were significantly higher than those of the control ewes: 2.06 ± 0.16 (SEM) versus 1.31 ± 0.06 ovulations per ewe.

SUMMARY

Some functional protein and polypeptide substances have been identified in male and female gonads; these are capable of inhibiting progesterone production, aromatase activity, FSH-induced LH receptor formation, oocyte maturation, and FSH secretion. If these substances can be obtained in a pure form, they may have potential as contraceptive agents.

REFERENCES

1. CHANG G: The maturation of rabbit oocytes in culture and their maturation activation, fertilization and subsequent development in the fallopian tube. J Exp Zool 128:378–405, 1955
2. CHANNING CP, ANDERSON LD, HODGEN GD: Inhibitory effect of charcoal-treated porcine follicular fluid upon serum FSH levels and follicular development in the rhesus monkey. In CHANNING CP, MARSH J, SADLER W (eds): Ovarian Follicular and Corpus Luteum Function, pp 407–428. New York, Plenum Press, 1979
3. CHANNING CP, EVANS VW: Stimulatory effect of ovine prolactin upon cultured porcine granulosa cell secretion of inhibitory activity of oocyte maturation. Endocrinology 111:1746–1748, 1982
4. CHEMES HE, PODESTA E, RIVAROLA MA: Action of testosterone, dihydrotestosterone and 5-androstan-3 α, 17 β oestradiol on the spermatogenesis of immature rats. Biol Reprod 14:332–338, 1976
5. CHOWDHURY AK: Dependence of testicular germ cells on hormones: A quantitative study in hypophysectomized testosterone-treated rats. J Endocrinol 82:331–340, 1979
6. CLERMONT Y, MAUGER A: Existence of a spermatogonial chalone in the rat testis. Cell Tissue Kinet 7:165–172, 1974
7. DARGA NS, REICHRET LE: Some properties of the interaction of follicle-stimulating hormone with bovine granulosa cells and its inhibition by follicular fluid. Biol Reprod 19:235–241, 1978
8. DE JONG FH, WELSCHEN R, HERMANS WP, SMITH SD, VAN DER MOLEN HJ: Effects of testicular using "in vitro" and "in vivo" systems. Int J Androl (Suppl) 2:125–138, 1978
9. DI ZEREGA GS, GOEBELSMANN U, NAKAMURA R: Identification of proteins secreted by the preovulatory ovary which suppresses the follicle response to gonadotropins. J Clin Endocrinol Metabol 54:1091–1096, 1982
10. DI ZEREGA GS, CAMPEAU JD, NAKAMURA RN, UJITA EL, LOBA R, MARRS RP: Activity of a human follicular fluid protein(s) in spontaneous and induced ovarian cycle. J Clin Endocrinol 57:838–846, 1983
11. DI ZEREGA GS, MARRS RP, ROCHE CP, CAMPEAU JD, KLING OR: Identification of proteins in pooled human follicular fluid which suppress follicular response to gonadotropins. J Clin Endocrinol Metabol 56:35–41, 1983
12. DI ZEREGA GS, MARRS RP, CAMPEAU JD, KLING OR: Human granulosa cell secretion of protein(s) which suppress follicular response to gonadotropins. J Clin Endocrinol Metabol 56:147–155, 1983
13. DI ZEREGA GS, WILKS JW: Inhibition of the primate ovarian cycle by a porcine follicular fluid protein(s). Fertil Steril 41:635–638, 1984
14. DORRINGTON JH, FRITZ IB: Cellular localization of 5 α-reductase and 3 α-hydroxysteroid dehydrogenase in the seminiferous tubule in the rat testis. Endocrinology 96:879–889, 1975
15. FRANCHIMONT P, CHARI S, HAGELSTEIN MT, DURAISWAMI S: Existence of a follicle-stimulating hormone inhibiting factor "inhibin" in bull seminal plasma. Nature (Lond) 257:402–404, 1975
16. FRANCHIMONT P, VERSTRAELEN-PROYARD J, HAZEE-HAGELSTEIN MT, RENARD C, DEMOULIN A, BOURGUIGNON JP, HUSTIN J: Inhibin: From concept to reality. Vitam Horm 37:243–302, 1979
17. FRANCHIMONT P, CHANNING CP: Intragonadal Regulation of Reproduction. London, Academic Press, 1981
18. FRANCHIMONT P, CROZE F, DEMOULIN A, BOLOGNE R, HUSTIN J: Effect of inhibin on rat testicular desoxyribonucleic acid (DNA) synthesis in vivo and in vitro. Acta Endocrinol 98:312–320, 1981
19. FRANCHIMONT P, BOLOGNE R, HAZEE-HAGELSTEIN MT, LECOMTE-YERNA MJ, DEMOULIN A: OMI (oocyte maturation inhibitor) like material in ram rete testis fluid. In 7th Interna-

tional Congress of Endocrinology. Montebello, Canada, Satellite Symposium on Gonadal Proteins and Peptides and Their Biological Significance. June 27–30, 1984

20. FRENCH FS, RITZEN EM: Androgen-binding protein in efferent duct fluid of rat testis. J Reprod Fertil 32:479–483, 1973

21. GREEP RO, VAN DYKE HB, CHOW BF: Gonadotropins of the swine pituitary. I. Various biological effects of purified thylakentrin (FSH) and pure metakentrin (ICSH). Endocrinology 30:635–649, 1942

22. GRINSTED J, BYSKOV AG: Meiosis inducing and meiosis preventing substances in human male reproductive organs. Fertil Steril 35:199–204, 1981

23. HENDERSON KM, FRANCHIMONT P: Regulation of inhibin production by bovine ovarian cells in vitro. J Reprod Fertil 63:431–442, 1981

24. HENDERSON KM, FRANCHIMONT P: Inhibin production by bovine ovarian tissue *in vitro* and its regulation by androgens. J Reprod Fertil 67:291–298, 1983

25. HENDERSON KM, FRANCHIMONT P, LECOMTE-YERNA MJ, HUDSON N, BALL K: Increase in ovulation rate after active immunization of sheep with inhibin partially purified from bovine follicular fluid. J Endocrinol 102:305–309, 1984

26. HILLENSJO T, POMERANTZ SH, SCHWARTZ-KRIPNER A, ANDERSON LD, CHANNING CP: Inhibition of cumulus cell progesterone secretion by low molecular weight fractions or porcine follicular fluid which also inhibit oocyte maturation. Endocrinology 106:584–591, 1980

27. HOCHEREAU-DE REVIERS MT, COUROT M: Sertoli cells and development of seminiferous epithelium. Ann Biol Bioch Biophys 18:573–583, 1978

28. LEDWITZ-RIGBY F, RIGBY BW: Ovarian inhibitors and stimulators of granulosa cell maturation and luteinization. In FRANCHIMONT P, CHANNING CP (eds): Intragonadal Regulation of Reproduction, pp 7–131. New York, Academic Press, 1981

29. LOSROTH AJ: Hormonal control of spermatogenesis. In SPILMAN CH, LOBI TJ, KIRTON KT (eds): Regulatory Mechanisms of Male Reproductive Physiology, p 13. Amsterdam, Excerpta Medica/Elsevier, 1976

30. MEANS AR: Biochemical effects of follicle-stimulating hormone on the testis. Handbook Physiol, Sect 7, Endocrinology 5:203–218, 1975

31. MURTY GSRC, SHEELA-RANI CS, MOUGDAL NR, PRASAD MRN: Effect of passive immunization with specific antiserum to FSH on spermatogenic process and fertility of adult male bonnet monkey (*Macaca radiata*). J Reprod Fertil (Suppl) 26:16–23, 1979

32. NIESCHLAG E, WICKINGS EJ, USADEL KH, DATHE G: Impairment of spermatogenesis in adult rhesus monkeys by active immunization against FSH. Proceedings of the VI International Congress of Endocrinology, Melbourne, (abstr) 565, 1980

33. ORTH J, CHRISTENSEN AK: Autoradiographic localization of specifically bound ^{125}I-labelled follicle-stimulating hormone on spermatogonia of the rat testis. Endocrinology 103:1944–1951, 1978

34. REICHERT LE JR, ABOU-ISSA H: Studies on a low molecular weight testicular factor which inhibits binding of FSH to receptor. Biol Reprod 17:614–621, 1977

35. REICHERT LE JR, SANZO MA, DARGA NS: Studies on a low molecular weight follicle-stimulating hormone binding inhibitor from human sperm. J Clin Endocrinol Metab 49:866–872, 1979

36. REICHERT LE JR, SANZO MA, DIAS JA: Studies on purification and characterization of gonadotropin-binding inhibitors and stimulators from human sperm and seminal plasma. In FRANCHIMONT P, CHANNING CP (eds): Intragonadal Regulation of Reproduction, pp 61–80. New York, Academic Press, 1981

37. RICHARDS JS, IRELAND JJ, RAO MC, BERNATH GA, MIDGLEY AR, REICHERT LE: Ovarian follicular development in the rat: Hormone receptor regulation by estradiol, follicle-stimulating hormone and luteinizing hormone. Endocrinology 99:1562–1569, 1976

38. SIMPSON ME, LI CH, EVANS HM: Synergism between pituitary follicle-stimulating hormone (FSH) and human chorionic gonadotropin (hCG). Endocrinology 48:370–383, 1951

39. SIVASHANKARS S, PRASAD MRN, THAMPAN TNRV: Effects of a highly purified antiserum to FSH on testicular function in immature rats. Ind J Exp Biol 15:845–851, 1977

40. SIZONENKO CP, BURR I, KAPLAN SL, GRUMBACH HM: Hormonal changes in puberty. II. Correlation of serum luteinizing hormone with stages of puberty and bone age in normal girls. Pediatric Res 4:36–45, 1970

41. SLUSS PM, FLETCHER PW, REICHERT LE: Inhibition of ^{125}I human FSH binding to receptor by a low molecular weight fraction of bovine follicular fluid: Inhibitor concentration is

related to biochemical parameters of follicular development. Biol Reprod 29:1105–1113, 1983

42. STEINBERGER E, STEINBERGER A, SANBORN BM: Molecular mechanisms concerned with hormonal control of the seminiferous epithelium. In FABBRINI A, STEINBERGER E (eds): Recent Progress in Andrology, pp 143–178. New York, Academic Press, 1978

43. STEINBERGER E: Hormonal control of mammalian spermatogenesis. Physiol Rev 52:1–22, 1971

44. SWERDLOFF RS, WALSCH PS, JACOBS HS, ODELL WD: Serum LH and FSH during sexual maturation in the male rat: Effect of castration and cryptorchidism. Endocrinology 88:120–128, 1971

45. TSAFRIRI A, BAR-AMI S, DEKEL N: Follicular regulation of oocyte maturation. In FUJUU T, CHANNING CP (eds): Non Steroidal Regulators in Reproductive Biology and Medicine, pp 123–130. Oxford, Pergamon Press, 1982

46. WICKINGS EJ, USADEL KH, DATHE G, NIESCHLAG E: The role of follicle-stimulating hormone in testicular function of the mature rhesus monkey. Acta Endocrinol 95:117–128, 1980

40

Immunogenetic Considerations in the Development of Contraceptive Vaccines Based on Testicular or Sperm Antigens

DEBORAH J. ANDERSON

Immunogenetics, defined in a broad sense, is that specialty of immunology concerned with genetic factors affecting immune responses. Classically this field has centered on a subregion of the major histocompatibility complex (MHC) containing a set of genes called *immune response* (Ir) genes that directly influence the magnitude of immunologic response directed against a foreign antigen. It has been determined that the Ir genes encode cell surface molecules that play critical roles in antigen presentation and immunoregulation, and that the efficiency of these functions varies considerably between subjects within a population and also depends on the type of antigen administered. Surprisingly little is known about other genetic factors that affect the immune system. In this chapter, concepts of classical and nonclassical immunogenetics will be reviewed briefly to provide a background for an analysis of the types of immunologic problems that may be encountered when contraceptive vaccines are administered to genetically heterogeneous populations. Because this chapter deals with a unique antigen system, that of the male reproductive tract autoantigens, genetic factors affecting the immunologic status of the male reproductive tract will also be reviewed.

CLASSICAL IMMUNOGENETICS: MHC CONTROL OF HUMORAL IMMUNE RESPONSES

The immune system consists of a complex network of interacting cellular and soluble elements. Antibody production by lymphocytes of the B cell lineage is generally induced by macrophage-processed antigen and modulated by signals passed among different types of thymic (T)-dependent lymphocytes and other regulatory cells that determine antibody type and affinity, as well as onset, intensity, and duration of the response (Fig. 40-1). The main cell types

I am grateful to Arlene Haury, who assisted with the preparation of this manuscript, and to my technical and postdoctoral staff who contributed much of the data. These studies were supported by grant CA-32132 and AICA-21141 from the National Institutes of Health.

POSITIVE CONTROL OF THE HUMORAL IMMUNE RESPONSE

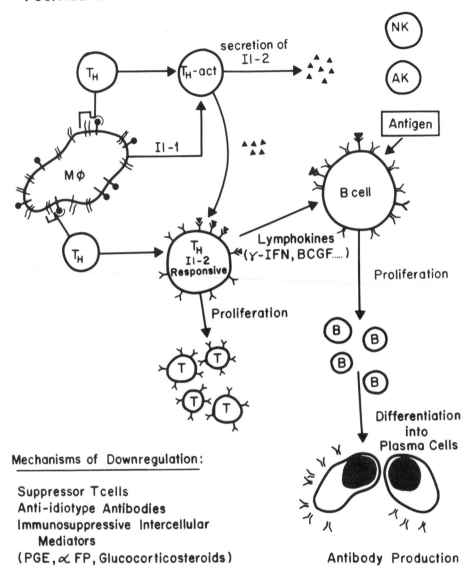

Mechanisms of Downregulation:

Suppressor T cells
Anti-idiotype Antibodies
Immunosuppressive Intercellular
   Mediators
(PGE, α FP, Glucocorticosteroids)

Antibody Production

$\langle\!\langle$ = MHC Class II antigens   ❖ = Foreign antigen   ▲ = Il-2

Y = Il-2 receptor   Y = Antibody (B cell antigen receptor)

FIG. 40-1. Schematic diagram of key cells involved in the generation and regulation of humoral immune responses.

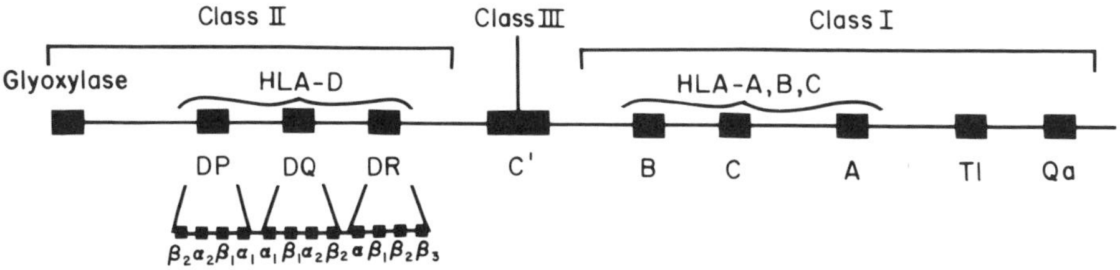

FIG. 40-2. Chromosomal map of the human major histocompatibility complex, which contains the immune response genes (HLA-D region). HLA-D region products are expressed by some immunologic effector cells and are thought to play a role in antigen presentation and immunoregulation.

involved in activation and regulation of B cell antibody production to T-dependent (most) antigens are macrophages (antigen-presenting cells), helper T cells (immunopotentiators), and suppressor T cell (immunoregulators). Few antigens activate B cells directly; these are called T-independent antigens and are usually polysaccharides with multiple repeating units.

The Ir genes that regulate immune responses to T-dependent antigens were first defined by analysis of immune responses of mice following administration of various synthetic polypeptide antigens. Some strains of mice produced high antibody titers whereas others made no response to a particular antigen; furthermore, strains developing high titers to one antigen could be low responders to other antigens. Back-cross studies of responder strains with nonresponder strains revealed that a single autosomal dominant genetic region, mapping between the H-2K and Ss loci of the MHC, controlled immunologic responsiveness in such well-defined experimental systems. Expression of Ir gene products, Ia antigens in mouse and HLA-D region (Fig. 40-2) antigens in humans, is limited to only a few cell types, many if not all of which have antigen presentation capabilities: macrophages, dendritic cells, B cells, activated T cells, thymic epithelium, and a few others. Activation of helper T cells, which play a crucial role in the generation of T-dependent antibody responses and cell-mediated immune responses, depends on presentation of antigen in association with Ir gene products on the antigen-presenting cell (APC) surface.[15,24] Immune regulation by Ir products therefore may be achieved through 1) quantitative differences in the amount of Ia or HLA-D antigen expressed by APC, 2) qualitative (*i.e.*, polymorphic or glycosylation) differences in Ir gene products, and 3) defective T-helper cell antigen receptors (which must recognize Ia or HLA-D products in combination with antigen). Each of these mechanisms is supported by experimental evidence.[14,18] That Ir genes can affect immune functions by contributing to the activation of suppressor T cells has also been described.[21,29] Antigen presentation mechanisms may also underlie this effect: ineffective antigen processing may result in increased levels of soluble (circulating) antigen that can directly stimulate suppressor but usually not helper T cells.[30] Ir gene influences on immunologic responses have been shown to affect resistance and/or susceptibility to pathologic agents and autoimmune disease, and clearly have implications for vaccine administration. With contraceptive vaccines, in which a 95% or greater efficacy rate is desirable, it would be useful to identify nonresponder individuals before or immediately after vaccination. Immunologists are now exploring ways to bypass Ir gene restriction mechanisms through several approaches (discussed below), and it is anticipated that these methods will decrease the number of nonresponder subjects in an immunized population.

OTHER INTRINSIC FACTORS THAT AFFECT SYSTEMIC IMMUNOLOGIC RESPONSES

Hundreds of genetic loci encode molecular structures used by the immune system, and any genetic condition leading to decreased or otherwise altered production of cells, cell surface structures, or soluble mediators involved in immune responses (see Fig. 40-1) could affect immunologic functions. Such defects are probably common; however, the complexity of the immune system provides a number of parallel regulatory mechanisms and alternate pathways that probably compensate for defects in specific immune functions. This suggests that the mechanisms underlying a given immune response are not necessarily identical in all subjects.

Other variables known to affect immune responsiveness are

1. Steroid hormones. Glucocorticosteroids and androgens can have potent immunosuppressive effects,[3,10] and levels of these steroids and their receptors vary within individuals of a population.[10,12]
2. The influence of the thymus on immune reactivity. Cell-mediated immunologic functions and T cell participation in humoral immunologic responses steadily decline with age; decreased activity is associated with thymic involution and a progressive decrease in thymic function. Animal studies suggest that the age-associated decline in T cell immune function is genetically programmed because it occurs at different rates in different inbred strains.[5]
3. Sex. Females usually produce better antibody responses than males. This is attributable to differences in steroid levels, and to X- and Y-chromosome–encoded factors that regulate immune responses.[10,20]

EVIDENCE FOR IMMUNOGENETIC VARIABILITY IN ANTISPERM OR TESTICULAR CELL IMMUNE RESPONSES

Sperm immunity studies in genetically defined inbred strains of experimental animals have revealed high and low responder strains,[6] providing evidence that sperm immune responses are under genetic control. Back-cross studies performed by Tung and colleagues in the high- and low-responder vasectomized guinea pig model indicate that the humoral immune response to a testicular antigen, TSDA, is controlled by a single dominant gene, although it

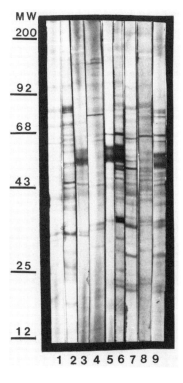

FIG. 40-3. Western blot profiles of sperm-immune mouse sera from 9 inbred strains (representative individuals): 1) C57B1/6, 2) C57L, 3) DBA-1, 4) DBA-2, 5) C3H, 6) Balb/c, 7) 129, 8) CBA, 9) A/J.

was unexpectedly found that the controlling element does not reside within the Ir region of the major histocompatibility complex.[35] This finding since has been confirmed by others using other model systems. Takami and others demonstrated non-MHC–associated genetic control of antisperm antibody responses in vasectomized rats.[32] Tarter and Alexander, studying sperm-immunized inbred mice, reported that immune responses to testicular and acrosomal sperm antigens are independent and controlled through more than a single non-MHC–associated genetic region.[33] Kille and associates reported strain differences in humoral immune responses of mice following challenge with homologous lactate dehydrogenase (LDH-C_4), a well-defined sperm antigen, and found no correlation between level of response and Ig allotype or H-2 type.[16] Recently Teuscher and co-workers reported that experimental autoimmune orchitis induced by *Bordetella pertussis* in mice is controlled by at least two genes: a disease-susceptibility gene mapping to the H-2 region, and a disease-resistance gene controlled by a non-MHC–associated region in orchitis-resistant strains.[34]

In a recent study of antisperm antibody specificities generated by immunization of mice from nine different inbred strains with syngeneic whole sperm we found enormous interstrain heterogeneity in sperm antigens generating humoral immune responses in subjects of different genetic backgrounds (Fig. 40-3).[19] Only one antigen of 38 KD-generated antibodies in all subjects tested

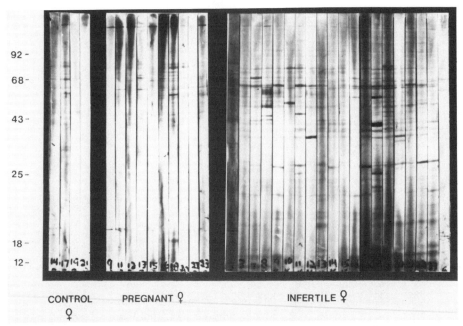

FIG. 40-4. Western blot profiles of sperm-antibody–positive infertility sera, pregnancy sera and control sera tested against sperm extracts (single donor). 25 KD and 50 KD bands react with several infertility sera and are nonreactive with pregnancy or control sera. For the most part, however, reactivity patterns are extremely heterogeneous, and specific antigens are detected by sera from only one or two individuals in the infertility panel.

in this study (detectable by Western blot). We have found similar highly heterogeneous results when analyzing human serum containing antisperm antibodies (Fig. 40-4). Other evidence that genetic factors affect antisperm humoral immune responses in men is provided by research on antisperm antibodies after vasectomy. Only 40% to 60% of vasectomized men develop detectable antisperm antibodies.[1] Because sperm continue to be produced after vasectomy, men that fail to develop antibodies may represent a nonresponder population. One group has reported an association between antisperm antibodies in vasectomized men and two HLA phenotypes: A-28 and B-22.[17] This finding provides evidence that antisperm antibody responses in men could be regulated by MHC-associated genes.

At least two studies have demonstrated that females develop higher titers of antisperm antibodies after immunization than do age-matched males of the same strain.[19,20] Western blot analysis also revealed that female mice responded to more sperm antigens than did male litter mates.[19] These observations could indicate that males are tolerant to certain sperm antigens, a hypothesis also supported by work from other laboratories.[11,31] Taguchi and associates reported that male mice of certain (not all) inbred strains develop spontaneous humoral and cellular autoimmune responses directed against sperm and testicular antigens following neonatal thymectomy.[31] Recently, these findings have been extended to reveal that Thy-1$^+$ (T cells) are principal effector cells of the orchitis reaction observed in thymectomized male mice, and these cells normally are suppressed in intact male mice by a Thy-1$^+$, Ly-2,3$^-$ suppressor cell population, which is reduced in number following neonatal thymectomy.[28] These data suggest that systemic suppressor cells actively inhibit antisperm responses in normal intact male mice of some genetic backgrounds.

ENVIRONMENTAL FACTORS THAT AFFECT IMMUNE RESPONSES

Environmental factors are numerous and include diet; previous exposure to the immunizing antigen (or cross-reactive antigens); health status with special regard to acute or chronic bacterial, viral, fungal, or parasitic infections; presence or generation of bacterial infection at the injection site; amount of antigen; route of immunization; and state of antigen (*i.e.*, degradation before immunization). Each of these factors interfaces with the immunogenetic framework of a subject and does not necessarily manifest the same effect in all subjects.

LOCAL FACTORS THAT AFFECT THE GENERATION AND ACTION OF IMMUNITY IN THE MALE REPRODUCTIVE TRACT

The male reproductive tract is an immunologically privileged site that sequesters developing germ cells and sperm behind Sertoli cell and epithelial cell barriers that impede the passage of immune cells and antibodies into the male reproductive tract. Extensive studies performed on the testis have shown that the Sertoli cell blood testis barrier is one of the most competent physical barriers in the body.[9,25] Less is known about the immunologic status of the epididymis, an area that should be further investigated. There are considerable species and perhaps even strain (individual) differences in the structure and competence of the immunologic barrier at this level; antibody passage into the intact epididymis has been reported for at least one species (the rabbit).[36] Most of the antibodies present in the human ejaculate are thought to enter the reproductive tract from the accessory glands at the time of ejaculation.[27] However, IgA has been detected in semen of infertility patients, which suggests that secretory antibodies can be produced locally in the human male reproductive tract.[7] Thus far no one has detected IgA-producing plasma cells in male reproductive tract tissues; however, Ritchie and colleagues have recently reported a large number of T cells of the T8 phenotype (a marker classically associated with suppressor or cytotoxic functions) lining the epididymal epithelium in men.[22] In the same report the human epididymal epithelium was demonstrated positive by immunoperoxidase assay for HLA-D region antigens, which raises the possibility that the human epididymis is an active immunologic site with antigen presentation capabilities (perhaps leading to the generation of suppressor cells). It is well established that several regions of the male reproductive tract contain potent soluble immunosuppressive factors that may function to suppress both humoral and cellular immunologic reactions directed against sperm or testicular germ cells located in the male reproductive tract.[2,13] All of these natural defense mechanisms are dependent on the expression of a number of genetic components, which are perhaps uniquely transcribed in the male reproductive tract. It is not yet known whether the levels or activity of the factors mediating these mechanisms vary between individuals within a population.

EFFECTIVE ADMINISTRATION OF TESTICULAR OR SPERM ANTIGEN VACCINES IN THE MALE

IR and other genetic restriction elements can be overcome or circumvented by a number of approaches.

1. Many adjuvants (agents that act nonspecifically to increase specific immune responses to an antigen) enhance the antigen presenting capabilities of macrophages or other antigen-presenting cells and can overcome genetic restrictions operating at that level. Other adjuvants such as lipopolysaccharide (LPS) are polyclonal B cell activators that bypass the need for helper T cells, and may be useful in boosting already existing immunologic responses.[4]

2. Anti-idiotype antibodies mimic antigen and can bind directly to receptors on helper T cells and B cells, and bypass the need for antigen processing and presentation by macrophages.[8,26]

3. Lymphokines could be administered to boost immune responses. For example, γ-interferon enhances Ia expression on APC, and II-2 partially bypasses the need for helper T cell activation in secondary immune responses.[14,23]

4. A multiple epitope (antigenic determinant) vaccine attached to a highly immunogenic carrier protein could be used to improve the chance of achieving an immune response in a population heterogeneous in Ir gene status.

REFERENCES

1. ALEXANDER NJ, ANDERSON DJ: Vasectomy: Consequences of autoimmunity to sperm antigens. Fertil Steril 32:253–260, 1979
2. ANDERSON DJ, TARTER TH: Immunosuppressive effects of mouse seminal plasma components in vivo and in vitro. J Immunol 128:535, 1982
3. ALLISON AC: Effects of glucocorticosteroids on lymphocytes and macrophages. Clin Exp Dermatol 4:135–138, 1979
4. ALLISON AC: Mode of action of immunological adjuvants. J Reticuloendothel Soc 26:619–630, 1979
5. ANDERSON DJ, WATSON ALM, YUNIS EJ: Environmental and genetic factors that influence immunity and longevity in mice. In: WOODHEAD AD, BLACKETT AD, HOLLAENDER A (eds): Molecular Biology of Aging, pp 231–240. New York, Plenum Press, 1985

6. BIGAZZI PE: Autoimmune responses to spermatozoa in vasectomized rats and mice of different inbred strains. In: ROSE NR, BIGAZZI PE, WARNER NL (eds): Genetic Control of Autoimmune Disease, p 445. New York: Elsevier/North Holland, 1978
7. BRONSON R, COOPER G, ROSENFELD D: Sperm antibodies and infertility (Letter). Fertil Steril 37:449–451, 1982
8. CUNNINGHAM AJ: Reliable vaccines using hybridoma products with defined idiotypes. In SERCARZ E, CUNNINGHAM AJ (eds): Strategies of Immune Regulation, p 497. New York, Academic Press, 1980
9. DYM M: The fine structure of the monkey (Macaca) Sertoli cell and its role in maintaining the blood–testis barrier. Anat Rec 175:639, 1973
10. GROSSMAN DJ: Interactions between the gonadal steroids and the immune system. Science 227:257, 1985
11. HERTENBACH U, MORGENSTERN F, BENNETT D: Induction of tolerance in vitro by autologous murine testicular cells. J Exp Med 151:1827, 1980
12. IVANYI P, GREGOROVA S, MICKOVA M, HAMPL R, STARKA L: Genetic association between a histocompatibility gene (H-2) and androgen metabolism in mice. Transplant Proc 5:189–191, 1973
13. JAMES K, HARGREAVE TB: Immunosuppression by seminal plasma and its possible clinical significance. Immunol Today 5:357–363, 1984
14. JANEWAY CA, BOTTOMLY K, BABICH J, CONRAD P, CONZEN S, JONES B, KAYE J, KATZ M, MCVAY L, MURPHY DB, TITE J: Quantitative variation in Ia antigen expression plays a central role in immune regulation. Immunology Today 5:99–105, 1984
15. KATZ DH, HAMAOKA T, BENACERRAF B: Cell interactions between histoincompatible T and B lymphocytes. II. Failure of physiologic cooperative interactions between T and B lymphocytes from allogeneic donor strains in humoral response to hapten–protein conjugates. J Exp Med 137:1405–1418, 1973
16. KILLE JW, WHEAT TE, MITCHELL G, GOLDBERG E: Strain differences in the immune response of mice to homologous sperm-specific lactate dehydrogenase (LDH-C$_4$). Exp Zool 204:259–266, 1978
17. LAW HY, BODMER WF, MATHEWS JD, SKEGG DC: The immune response to vasectomy and its relation to the HLA system. Tissue Antigens 14:115–139, 1979
18. LONGO DL, PAUL WE: Immune response genes and Ia antigens. The relationships between them and their role in lymphocyte interactions. In: PARHAM P, STROMINGER J (eds): Histocompatibility Antigens: Structure and Function, p 161–184. London, Chapman and Hall, 1982
19. MADRIGAL JA, ANDERSON DJ: Antisperm antibody titers and Western blot profiles in 9 inbred strains of mice following immunization with syngeneic sperm. J Reprod Immunol (in press)
20. MARSH JA, O'HERN P, GOLDBERG E: The role of an X-linked gene in the regulation of secondary humoral response kinetics to sperm specific LDH-C$_4$ antigen. J Immunol 126:100, 1981
21. PIERCE CW, KAPP JA: In SERCARZ EE, CUNNINGHAM AJ (eds): Strategies of immune regulation, p 315. New York, Academic Press, 1980
22. RITCHIE AWS, HARGREAVE TB, JAMES K, CHISHOLM GD: Intraepithelial lymphocytes in the normal epididymis: A mechanism for tolerance to sperm autoantigens? Br J Urol 56:79–83, 1984
23. ROBB RJ: Interleukin 2: The molecule and its function. Immunol Today 5:203–209, 1984
24. ROSENTHAL AS, SHEVACH EM: Function of macrophages in antigen recognition by guinea pig T lymphocytes. I. Requirement for histocompatible macrophages and lymphocytes. J Exp Med 138:1194–1212, 1973
25. ROSS MH: The Sertoli cell and the blood–testicular barrier: An electronmicroscopic study. Adv Androl 1:83, 1970
26. ROTH C, SOMME G, THEZE J: Induction of an anti-GAT response in genetically responder and nonresponder mouse strains by monoclonal anti-idiotypic antibodies. Table Ronde Roussel UCLAF 48:465, 1983
27. RUMKE P: The origin of immunoglobulins in semen. Clin Exp Immunol 17:287, 1974
28. SAKAGUCHI S, FUKUMA K, KURIBAYASHI K, MASUDA T: Organ-specific autoimmune diseases induced in mice by elimination of T cell subset 1. Evidence for the active participation

of T cell in natural self-tolerance; deficit of a T-cell subset as a possible cause of autoimmune disease. J Exp Med 161:72–87, 1985

29. SASAZUKI T, NISHIMURA Y, MUTO M, OHTA N: HLA-linked genes controlling immune response and disease susceptibility. Immunol Rev 70:51, 1983

30. STEINBERG AD: Autoimmunity In: SERCARZ EE, CUNNINGHAM AJ (eds): Strategies of Immune Regulation. New York, Academic Press, 1980

31. TAGUCHI O, NISHIZUKA Y: Experimental autoimmune orchitis after neonatal thymectomy in the mouse. Clin Exp Immunol 46:425, 1981

32. TAKAMI T, KUNZ HW, GILL TJ, BIGAZZI PE: Genetic control of autoantibody production to spermatozoa in vasectomized rats. Am J Reprod Immunol 2:5–7, 1982

33. TARTER TH, ALEXANDER NJ: Genetic control of humoral immunity to sperm acrosomal and cell surface antigens. J Reprod Immunol 6:213, 1984

34. TEUSCHER C, SMITH SM, GOLDBERG EH, SHEARER GM, TUNG KSK: Experimental autoimmune orchitis in mice: Genetic control of susceptibility and resistance to induction of orchitis. (in press)

35. TUNG KSK, TEUSCHER C, GOLDBERG EH, WILD G: Genetic control of antisperm autoantibody response in vasectomized guinea pigs. J Immunol 127:835, 1981

36. WEININGER RB, FISHER S, RIFKIN J, BEDFORD JM: Experimental studies on the passage of specific IgG to the lumen of the rabbit epididymis. J Reprod Fertil 66:251–258, 1982

41

Contraceptive Potential of Antisperm Antibodies

NANCY J. ALEXANDER

During spermatogenesis, a precise temporal proliferation of both somatic and germinal elements occurs. After the germinal cells (spermatogonia) leave the basal compartment, testicular germ cells begin to express unique gene products. Antigens not detected on spermatogonia are found on spermatocytes.[22,29] As early as the pachytene stage of meiosis in rats and mice, specific germ cell antigens can be identified.[4,6,31,36] For example, a glycolipid, sulfatoxygalactosylacylalkylglycerol, appears at the spermatocyte stage in rats.[25] Some antigens continue to be expressed, whereas others become undetectable by the elongated spermatid stage.[6] The mature spermatozoon is a highly differentiated cell with morphologically and functionally distinct contiguous antigenic membrane domains. Many of the antigens are integral parts of the sperm structure and persist during epididymal transit. As spermatozoa mature during epididymal transit, modifications occur. These include changes in electrophoretic characteristics and increases in the negative charge,[7] changes in lectin-binding patterns,[16] and alterations in the amount and type of surface glycoproteins.[8] These substances are important for sperm function. For example, antibodies developed against epididymal glycoproteins can block fertilization in rats.[11]

The spermatozoon is a unique and specialized cell sequestered from the male immunologic defense system during its production and maturation. At the time of ejaculation, the spermatozoon is exposed to additional antigens, that is, it is coated with seminal plasma. Antibodies to these coating antigens also can affect sperm function. For example, Shigeta and associates have developed a complement-dependent, sperm-immobilizing monoclonal antibody directed at a seminal plasma antigen similar to lactoferrin.[35]

ANTIBODIES TO SPERMATOZOA

Antisperm autoimmune and alloimmune responses can occur in both men and women. High titers of antisperm antibodies have been associated with infertility in both cases. About 3% to 8% of infertile men with otherwise normal

The work described in this chapter, Publication No. 1389 of the Oregon Regional Primate Research Center, was supported by National Institutes of Health grants RR-00163 and HD-14572.

semen profiles have antisperm antibodies.[13,15] Rümke observed an inverse correlation between antibody and fertility in men.[32] Fuchs and I have noted a similar association after vasovasostomy.[12] We found no pregnancies in couples in which the husband had an agglutinating antibody titer of 1:160 or higher. Likewise, Ayvaliotis and colleagues have demonstrated that the chance of conception is significantly greater for wives whose husbands have less than 50% of their sperm bound by immunoglobulins than for women whose husbands have higher amounts of their sperm bound by immunoglobulins.[3] Clearly, the nature and concentration of antibodies in seminal plasma can limit the fertilizing potential of sperm greatly. Such antibodies can block sperm function, as measured by a variety of in vitro tests. Most commonly, patients with putative immunologically mediated infertility have in their serum antibodies that, when exposed to spermatozoa, cause the sperm to become agglutinated, or, if complement is present, immobilized. Even sperm that are not so affected can be impaired. Penetration of cervical mucus is markedly reduced.[1] Sperm-bearing IgG are phagocytized and lysed to an enhanced degree by peritoneal macrophages.[20] In vitro penetration of eggs is impeded by the presence of antibodies to sperm.[1,9] Antibodies to spermatozoa also may react with early embryos, which express sperm antigens.

IMMUNOSUPPRESSIVE ASPECTS OF SEMINAL PLASMA

Seminal plasma contains a number of immunosuppressive factors that help minimize antisperm alloimmune responses after intercourse in females. Semen can affect natural killer cell activity,[14] macrophage function,[14] lymphocyte activation by mitogens,[2] complement-dependent antibody cytotoxicity,[37] and humoral immune responses to sperm and other antigens in vivo.[2] Different amounts of immunosuppressive substances can be found in seminal plasma of different men.[37] These substances may underlie immunologic infertility in their partners.

ANTIBODIES TO SPERM

Classic experimental animal systems, as well as autoantibodies and alloantibodies, can result in a variety of antisperm antibodies. Immunofluorescence studies have revealed antibodies that react with different parts of human sperm, that is, acrosomal, equatorial, postacrosomal, midpiece, tail, tip-of-tail, and nuclear (protamine) antigens. Standard clinical assessment of infertility involves sperm agglutination and immobilization tests.

Recent studies have indicated that an array of antibody specificities can be found in serum from infertile and vasectomized men. These antibodies are specific for antigens having molecular masses from 20 to over 150 Kd.

Monoclonal antibodies are highly specific immunoglobulins that recognize antigenic components of the cell surface. Such antibodies allow researchers to better understand the composition of the sperm plasma membrane and to deduce the roles of specific sperm antigens in germ cell differentiation, sperm maturation, sperm capacitation, and gamete interactions. My laboratory and others have been attempting to develop a series of cell lines that produce antibodies against sperm, whole sperm, or sperm membrane extracts. Although many monoclonal antibodies are exquisitely specific, some cross-react with antigens on spermatozoa of different species. O'Rand and Irons have developed monoclonal antibodies to rabbit sperm autoantigens RSA-1, RSA-2, and RSA-3 that cross-react with human ejaculated sperm.[27] The antigen is concentrated on the midpiece, and exposure of the monoclonal antibody to human sperm results in an inhibition of hamster egg penetration by sperm.

Glycoproteins are important in sperm–egg interactions. Both human and rabbit sperm appear to have similar low-molecular-weight families of membrane glycoproteins. Even after fertilization, the plasma membrane of the egg expresses glycoproteins RSA-1, RSA-2, and RSA-3.[28] The presence of sperm antigens on the surface of the fertilized egg indicates antisperm antibodies may affect fertility both before and after fertilization.

Some monoclonal antibodies immobilize motile sperm even though they are directed against seminal plasma antigens. For example, an antibody to a human seminal plasma antigen of 15 Kd can immobilize motile sperm in the presence of complement.[18,35] This antigen is from the seminal vesicles and is present on the postacrosomal and midpiece regions of sperm. Another example is a monoclonal antibody directed against an acrosome-stabilizing factor.[30] This factor is a 360-Kd glycoprotein that has been isolated from whole seminal plasma of rabbits. It is synthesized in the corpus epididymidis and is thought to maintain the intact acrosome during epididymal storage. Epididymal and seminal plasma-coating antigens are as relevant to the study of fertility as intrinsic sperm antigens.

By determining the location and the kinetics of expression, we may begin to understand the roles that various antigens play in fertilization. Lambert and Le have demonstrated sialylated glycoproteins of the sperm plasma membrane that can act as ligands for specific receptors on the egg surface.[19] Some monoclonal antibodies to either the sperm head or both the head and tail inhibit hamster egg penetration and in vitro fertilization by blocking sperm attachment to the zona pellucida and oolemma.[23] Our monoclonal antibody, MA-24, an IgG_{2a}, falls into this category. It is germ cell-specific and is bound to the postacrosomes, midpieces, and tails of both viable and methanol-fixed human sperm. It causes neither sperm agglutination nor sperm immobilization. The binding patterns are similar on noncapacitated, capacitated, and reduced (swollen sperm head) sperm treated with dithiotritol plus Triton-X. MA-24 reacts with a single 23-Kd protein band when a detergent-solubilized membrane preparation of human testis is used. It completely blocks binding and penetration of zona-free hamster ova, and it significantly inhibits in vitro fertilization of mouse eggs by murine sperm.[24]

CONTRACEPTIVE POTENTIAL

The concept that antibodies to sperm can cause immunologically mediated infertility is not a new one. As early as 1935, Baskin injected husband semen into wives in the hopes of causing infertility.[5] Sperm are highly immunogenic when administered in large amounts or with an appropriate adjuvant. As I have mentioned, antisperm antibodies from the serum of infertile men block sperm function in in vitro tests and may react with early embryos.[1,21] Koyama and co-workers demonstrated that antibody to spermatozoa in the presence of complement can impair the in vitro development of morulae to blastocysts in the rat.[17] It is not surprising that sperm antigens are being investigated for their contraceptive potential. With the advent of monoclonal antibody and genetic engineering technology, it may now be possible to produce specific antigens for immunization. My co-workers and I have demonstrated that monoclonal antibodies can block fertilization in vivo and in vitro.[24] Monoclonal antibodies are an important probe for determining which sperm-associated antigens are critical in fertilization.[33] Goldberg's group has been immunizing baboons with a synthesized decapeptide from the lactate dehydrogenase isoenzyme C (LDH-C$_4$) molecule. This peptide, when conjugated to diphtheria toxoid, provokes formation of antibody that reacts with native LDH-C$_4$. Mating studies have indicated a strong inhibition of fertility.

Although antisperm antibodies can occur in both men and women, development of high titers of antisperm antibodies with subsequent infertility seems more likely in females than males. The likelihood of autoimmune disease should be less when exposure to the antigen (sperm) is not constant. Aspermatogenic autoimmune orchitis will not be a concern. Furthermore, systemic antibody levels may be much less important than levels in the reproductive tract.

The cervix has its own secretory immunologic defense system. A local immune response has been induced in women intravaginally vaccinated with *Candida albicans*[38] and polio vaccine.[26] The cervix seems to be a site at which it is feasible to establish immunity. It is endowed with plasma cells that secrete IgA. Cytotoxic antisperm antibodies have been found in the cervical mucus of some infertile women.[10] Because an immune response can be activated in the gut, it may be possible to administer sperm antigens orally and thus achieve secretory antisperm antibody production in the cervix. With Shelton, Goldberg, and Wheat, I have been studying ways to activate the secretory immune system by stimulating the production of specific IgA-producing cells.[34] We administered primary and secondary immunization doses of LDH-C$_4$ and vaginal implants of antigen and concanavalin A. The secondary immunization was accomplished by way of bronchiole-associated lymphoid tissue (BALT) or gut-associated lymphoid tissue (GALT). Vaginal IgG and IgA levels rose, but oral levels were not elevated. Mating studies are currently being conducted.

Many steps must be taken before a vaccine can be realized. Although some good possibilities exist, we have yet to define fully which antigenic determinants are the most relevant. Through genetic engineering techniques, large quantities of antigen must be produced, and the best mode of administration must be considered. Perhaps a combination of several antigens will prove most efficacious as a contraceptive vaccine.

REFERENCES

1. ALEXANDER NJ: Antibodies to human spermatozoa impede sperm penetration of cervical mucus or hamster eggs. Fertil Steril 41:433–439, 1984
2. ANDERSON DJ, TARTER TH: Immunosuppressive effects of mouse seminal plasma components in vivo and in vitro. J Immunol 128:535–539, 1982

3. AYVALIOTIS B, BRONSON R, ROSENFELD D, COOPER G: Conception rates in couples where autoimmunity to sperm is detected. Fertil Steril 43:739–742, 1985
4. BALBONTIN J, BUSTOS-OBREGON E: Testicular specific soluble antigens and spermatogenic onset in the mouse. Arch Androl 9:159–166, 1982
5. BASKIN MJ: Temporary sterilization by injection of human spermatozoa: Preliminary report. Am J Obstet Gynecol 24:892–897, 1932
6. BECHTOL KB: Characterization of a cell-surface differentiation antigen of mouse spermatogenesis: Timing and localization of expression by immunohistochemistry using a monoclonal antibody. J Embryol Exp Morphol 81:93–104, 1984
7. BEDFORD JM: Changes in the electrophoretic properties of rabbit spermatozoa during passage through the epididymis. Nature 200:1178–1180, 1963
8. BOSTWICK EF, BENTLEY MD, HUNTER AG, HAMMER R: Identification of a surface glycoprotein on porcine spermatozoa and its alteration during epididymal maturation. Biol Reprod 23:161–169, 1980
9. BRONSON RA, COOPER GW, ROSENFELD DL: Complement-mediated effects of sperm head-directed human antibodies on the ability of human spermatozoa to penetrate zona-free hamster eggs. Fertil Steril 40:91–95, 1983
10. CHEN C, JONES WR: Application of a sperm microimmobilization test to cervical mucus in the investigation of immunologic infertility. Fertil Steril 35:542–545, 1981
11. CUASNICÚ PS, GONZÁLEZ-ECHEVERRÍA F, PIAZZA AD, CAMEO MS, BLAQUIER JA: Antibodies against epididymal glycoproteins block fertilizing ability in rat. J Reprod Fertil 72:467–471, 1984
12. FUCHS EF, ALEXANDER NJ: Immunologic considerations before and after vasovasostomy. Fertil Steril 40:497–499, 1983
13. HEKMAN A, RÜMKE P: Auto and isoimmunity against spermatozoa. In MIESCHER PA, MÜLLER-EBERHARD HJ (eds): Textbook of Immunopathology, pp 947–962. New York, Grune & Stratton, 1976
14. JAMES K, HARGREAVE TB: Immunosuppression by seminal plasma and its possible clinical significance. Immunology Today 5:357–363, 1984
15. JONES WR: Immunological factors in male and female infertility. In HEARN JP (ed): Immunological Aspects of Reproduction and Fertility, pp 105–142. Lancaster, MTP Press, 1980
16. KOEHLER JK: Lectins as probes of the spermatozoon surface. Arch Androl 6:197–217, 1981
17. KOYAMA K, HASEGAWA A, ISOJIMA S: Effect of antisperm antibody on the in vitro development of rat embryos. Gamete Res 10:143–152, 1984
18. KOYAMA K, TAKADA Y, TAKEMURA T, ISOJIMA S: Localization of human seminal plasma No. 7 antigen (Ferrisplan) in accessory glands of male genital tract and spermatozoa. J Reprod Immunol 5:135–143, 1983
19. LAMBERT H, LE AV: Possible involvement of a sialylated component of the sperm plasma membrane in sperm–zona interaction in the mouse. Gamete Res 10:153–163, 1984
20. LONDON SN, HANEY AF, WEINBERG JB: Macrophages and infertility: Enhancement of human macrophage-mediated sperm killing by antisperm antibodies. Fertil Steril 43:274–278, 1985
21. MENGE AC, FLEMING CH: Detection of sperm antigens on mouse ova and early embryos. Dev Biol 63:111–117, 1978
22. MILLETTE CF, BELLVÉ AR: Temporal expression of membrane antigens during mouse spermatogenesis. J Cell Biol 74:86–97, 1977
23. MOORE HDM, HARTMAN TD: Localization by monoclonal antibodies of various surface antigens of hamster spermatozoa and the effect of antibody on fertilization in vitro. J Reprod Fertil 70:175–183, 1984
24. NAZ RK, ALEXANDER NJ, ISAHAKIA M, HAMILTON MS: Monoclonal antibody to a human germ cell membrane glycoprotein that inhibits fertilization. Science 225:342–344, 1984
25. O'BRIEN DA, MILLETTE CF: Identification and immunochemical characterization of spermatogenic cell surface antigens that appear during early meiotic prophase. Dev Biol 101:307–317, 1984
26. OGRA PL, OGRA SS: Local antibody response to poliovaccine in the human female genital tract. J Immunol 110:1307–1311, 1973
27. O'RAND MG, IRONS GP: Monoclonal antibodies to rabbit sperm autoantigens. II. Inhibition of human sperm penetration of zona-free hamster eggs. Biol Reprod 30:731–736, 1984

28. O'RAND MG, IRONS GP, PORTER JP: Monoclonal antibodies to rabbit sperm autoantigens. I. Inhibition of in vitro fertilization and localization on the egg. Biol Reprod 30:721–729, 1984

29. O'RAND MG, ROMRELL LJ: Appearance of cell surface auto- and isoantigens during spermatogenesis in the rabbit. Dev Biol 55:347–358, 1977

30. REYNOLDS AB, OLIPHANT G: Production and characterization of monoclonal antibodies to the sperm acrosome-stabilizing factor (ASF): Utilization for purification and molecular analysis of ASF. Biol Reprod 30:775–786, 1984

31. ROMRELL LJ, O'RAND MG: Identification of surface autoantigens which appear during spermatogenesis. Gamete Res 5:35–48, 1982

32. RÜMKE P: The origin of immunoglobulins in semen. Clin Exp Immunol 17:287–297, 1974

33. SALING PM, RAINES LM, O'RAND MG: Monoclonal antibody against mouse sperm blocks a specific event in the fertilization process. J Exp Zool 227:481–486, 1983

34. SHELTON JA, GOLDBERG E, ALEXANDER NJ, WHEAT TE: Local secretory immunity to sperm-specific lactate dehydrogenase-C_4 in the reproductive tract of the female rhesus macaque (abstr). Biol Reprod (Suppl 1) 30:74, 1984

35. SHIGETA M, WATANABE T, MARUYAMA S, KOYAMA K, ISOJIMA S: Sperm-immobilizing monoclonal antibody to human seminal plasma antigens. Clin Exp Immunol 42:458–462, 1980

36. SÖDERSTRÖM K-O, ANDERSSON LC: Identification of the autoantigen-expressing cells in rat testis. Exp Mol Pathol 35:332–337, 1981

37. TARTER TH, ALEXANDER NJ: Complement-inhibiting activity of seminal plasma. Am J Reprod Immunol 6:28–32, 1984

38. WALDMAN RH, CRUZ JM, ROWE DS: Intravaginal immunization of humans with *Candida albicans*. J Immunol 109:662–664, 1972

42

Immunologic Properties of LDH-C$_4$ for Contraceptive Vaccine Development

ERWIN GOLDBERG

JOYCE A. SHELTON

Development of a contraceptive vaccine based on antigens specific for testes or spermatozoa would in all probability serve best for immunization of the female. Vaccination of the male has the potential for development of autoimmune disease. Nevertheless, the extensive literature describing circulating antisperm antibodies in subfertile or infertile men with no apparent primary disease suggests that intentional immunosuppression of fertility merits further study.

The major problem inherent in the interpretation of the presence of circulating antisperm antibodies is antigen identification. Years ago, attempts to identify sperm antigens involved measuring and counting precipitin bands from immunodiffusion assays. More recently, 1-D and 2-D gel electrophoresis under denaturing and nondenaturing conditions and Western blotting with monoclonal antibodies have provided more sensitive technologies to, at least, demonstrate cross-reaction of some antibodies with molecular constituents of spermatozoa and testes. Nevertheless, it is clear that the presence of circulating sperm-agglutinating and cytotoxic antibodies does not correlate in any consistent way with male infertility.

Obviously, autoimmune disease with complete disruption of spermatogenesis, as described elsewhere in this volume, represents an immune response of a magnitude that would not be acceptable for contraceptive practice. Whether more moderate intervention with antibodies that compromise sperm function can be achieved represents the central problem in this area. This problem may be approached at least operationally, with a well-defined antigen that will provoke antibodies of absolute specificity. One such antigen is the sperm-specific form of lactate dehydrogenase (LDH-X, LDH-C$_4$), which is present in testes and spermatozoa of most mammalian species, including human beings.

LDH-C$_4$ was first described several years ago in extracts of human testes and human spermatozoa as an additional zone of enzyme activity on electro-

Research from this laboratory was supported in part by Grant HD-05863 from the National Institutes of Health and by the Agency for International Development through the Program for Applied Research on Fertility Regulation, PARFR.

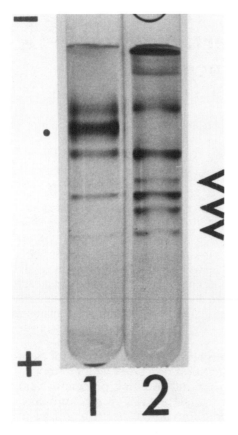

FIG. 42-1. Gel electropherogram resolving LDH isozyme activity in an extract of human sperm. Gel 1, untreated extract; gel 2, after incubation of extract with rabbit anti-mouse LDH-C_4; < designates serum isozymes; ● designates LDH-C_4. Also, note the specificity of antibody binding.

pherograms (Fig. 42-1).[4,10] LDH is a tetrameric enzyme of two somatic subunit types, A and B, that form homotetrameric or heterotetrameric molecules. It is now well established that each of these peptides is a separate gene product and that the differential expression of these genes is responsible for the distinctive LDH isozyme pattern of different tissues. The C subunit of LDH is also a unique gene product; of special interest is the fact that the *Ldh-c* gene is expressed only in the germinal epithelium of postpuberal testes. More precisely, this gene is "turned on" in the primary spermatocyte during mid-pachytene of the first meiotic division. The gene is not expressed in any somatic cell type, including the nongerminal cells of the testes nor in any cell of the female. As a consequence, immunization of both males and females with LDH-C_4 will provoke highly specific antibodies to this protein. These antibodies have been used to localize LDH-C_4 in sperm and testes (Fig. 42-2) by immunofluorescence. It is readily apparent from such studies that LDH-C_4 is predominantly cytosolic, that it increases in concentration in the developing germ cells and that it can be detected on the surfaces of spermatozoa. Figure 42-3 shows the distribution of LDH-C_4 in human sperm with the enzyme concentrated in the principal piece of the tail.

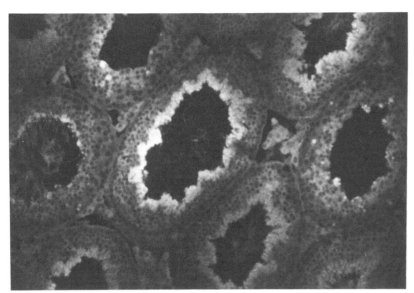

FIG. 42-2. Distribution of LDH-C$_4$ in a cross-section of mouse testis. Specific immunofluorescence can be seen in the spermatocytes and spermatids of the germinal epithelium. LDH-C$_4$ increases in concentration from the primary spermatocyte to the spermatid.

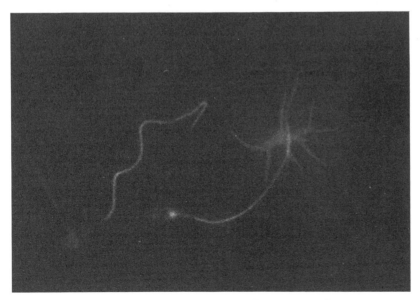

FIG. 42-3. Immunofluorescent localization of LDH-C$_4$ on human spermatozoa incubated with specific antiserum.

It is especially relevant from the standpoint of immunocontraception that LDH-C_4 is on the surface of the spermatozoon. For reasons that are presently obscure, but that may be related to the high degree of hydrophobicity of this protein, and to peculiar properties of the sperm plasma membrane, LDH-C_4 may diffuse from the cytosolic compartment and coat the sperm surface. In the mouse, LDH-C_4 was detected but not recognized as such on the luminal surface of epithelial cells of the body segment of the epididymis only when sperm were present.[1] Experiments by Zinkham and colleagues clearly showed that washing caused a release of LDH-C_4 from human sperm and suggested this as the basis for the depression of both aerobic and anaerobic glycolysis in washed bovine sperm.[47]

The primary catalytic function of LDH-C_4 is the same as that of somatic lactate dehydrogenases, the reversible interconversion of lactate and pyruvate in the presence of coenzyme to store or release reducing equivalents. Subtle differences in kinetic parameters, as well as substrate and coenzyme specificities, however, imply that LDH-C_4 is particularly suited to the metabolic requirements of spermatozoa.

LDH-C_4 is more sensitive to pyruvate inhibition and less sensitive to lactate than the other isozymes of LDH, although differences among species exist.[3,11,19] Spermatozoa may encounter high lactate concentrations in both the male and female reproductive tract fluids, making this adaptation physiologically relevant. In addition, round spermatids in the germinal epithelium prefer lactate as an energy source by a factor of three to four over glucose, fructose, and pyruvate to generate ATP.[26] Lactate also may serve as an energy source to support protein synthesis in spermatids. Some investigators have proposed an intramitochondrial localization for LDH-C_4 to explain certain metabolic data; however, the evidence is indirect and the question remains open to definitive analysis.[42] In any case, only a small fraction (less than 10%) of the total LDH-C_4 is reported to be associated with mitochondria.[38]

Although LDH-C_4 possesses unique catalytic properties, its three-dimensional structure is markedly similar to that of LDH-A_4 and LDH-B_4.[29] This finding is consistent with the observation that A, B, and C subunits can associate in vitro and in some species, in vivo.[12,14] Amino acid sequence analysis of the mouse LDH-C_4 suggested to Pan and co-workers that LDH-A and LDH-B genes are related more to each other than either is to the LDH-C gene.[31] Li and others proposed that the duplication giving rise to the gene encoding the testis-specific LDH of mammals preceded that producing the LDH-A and LDH-B genes.[23] This question is discussed eloquently by Whitt, who proposes a more recent origin of *Ldh-c* but a more rapid rate of evolution than for the somatic isozymes.[45] For this discussion, the immunochemical relatedness is the most relevant question.

As noted above, antisera developed to mouse LDH-C_4 do not cross-react with LDH-A_4 or LDH-B_4 (see Fig. 42-1).[13] Similarly, LDH-A_4 and LDH-B_4 are immunochemically distinct, even though there is as much as 38% conservation of amino acid sequences in the external regions among the LDH molecules.[6,23] The absolute specificity of antibodies to LDH-C_4 and their lack of cross-reactivity with somatic cells is absolutely crucial to use of this antigen for contraception. Recently, Wright and Swofford presented results that seemed to challenge this specificity.[46] They reported that mouse antisera to mouse or

TABLE 42-1. Effect of Antisera to LDH-C$_4$ on Mouse In Vitro Fertilization

ADDITION*	TRIALS	FERTILIZED OVA/ TOTAL OVA	PERCENT
None	5	61/76	80.2
Nonimmune serum	4	13/22	59.1
Antiserum	5	0/56	0
Antiserum plus LDH-C$_4$	1	11/14	78.6

From Beyler SA, Goldberg E: Unpublished data, 1982

* Individual incubations received 50 μl serum and 1×10^4 capacitated mouse epididymal spermatozoa.

rat LDH-C are cross reactive with LDH-A or LDH-B from the mouse, but that rabbit antisera to mouse LDH-C are specific to this isozyme. Aside from the internal inconsistency of this result, the cross-reactivity with mouse antisera very likely represents nonspecific protein–protein interaction at high serum concentrations and/or cross-reactions with denatured protein. Nevertheless, it was important to repeat these studies using comparable methodology as well as an additional procedure to establish specificity or cross-reactivity of antisera. A solid-matrix radioimmunoassay (RIA) was used. This assay is virtually identical to the ELISA procedure employed by Wright and Swofford except that the second antibody is labeled with ^{125}I rather than with phosphatase.[46] No cross-reaction between mouse anti-mouse LDH-C$_4$ sera and the purified A$_4$ and B$_4$ isozymes was detected at a dilution as low as 1:100 in contrast to the results of Wright and Swofford.[46] Furthermore, the purified A$_4$ and B$_4$ isozymes did not compete for binding with mouse or rabbit antisera to radiolabeled LDH-C$_4$ in a liquid-phase RIA even at a 15,000-fold higher concentration.[24] This latter result is especially persuasive that antibodies to LDH-C$_4$ are immunospecific and that this rationale for contraceptive vaccine development is not compromised.

Active immunization of female mice, rabbits, and baboons with LDH-C$_4$ reduces fertility.[16] The mechanism of immunosuppression of fertility probably involves inhibition of fertilization by anti-LDH-C$_4$ antibodies binding directly to the sperm membrane. The surface of the spermatozoon displays numerous binding sites for anti-LDH-C$_4$.[15] In vitro tests demonstrate that rabbit antimouse LDH-C$_4$ agglutinates mouse spermatozoa, and antibody-mediated, complement-dependent lysis is readily observed.[16] These specific immunoglobulins inhibit in vitro fertilization of mouse ova by mouse sperm (Table 42-1).

Systemic immunization with LDH-C$_4$ also provokes a cell-mediated cytotoxic response that may contribute to fertility suppression.[35] Female SJL/J strain mice given a single subcutaneous injection of 100 μg LDH-C$_4$ in Freund's complete adjuvant will respond by producing cytotoxic cells in the spleen that are specific for LDH-C$_4$ coated tumor cells. These cytotoxic cells would be capable of lysing spermatozoa as well.

Antibodies to LDH-C$_4$ have been detected in oviductal fluid.[21] Furthermore, the transport of sperm is virtually eliminated in the oviducts of rabbits immunized with LDH-C$_4$.[22] Therefore, fertilization can be prevented by a

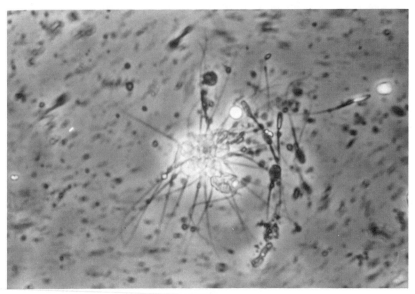

FIG. 42-4. Agglutinated rabbit sperm recovered from the oviducts of rabbits immunized with LDH-C$_4$. No agglutination was detected in appropriate controls.[22]

high concentration of anti-LDH-C$_4$ in the female reproductive tract. Presumably, antibodies to LDH-C$_4$ that agglutinate spermatozoa (Fig. 42-4) access reproductive tract fluids as a transudate of serum.[21] This also can be accomplished by local immunization to stimulate the secretory immune system, an approach that may be applicable to the male.

The local immune response involves the secretion of IgA specific to the immunogen by cells residing in the mucosal lining. This response can be elicited by direct immunization of the local area. Alternatively, because the mucosal immune system seems to be linked throughout the body,[27] it may be possible to elicit a response at the reproductive tract mucosa by indirect immunization of the gut or bronchial mucosa. Stimulation of a local secretory response to LDH-C$_4$ would ensure the high antibody levels in the reproductive tract necessary for complete abrogation of fertility. We have obtained results with female mice and monkeys that suggest manipulation of the secretory immune system could enhance the immunocontraceptive effects of LDH-C$_4$.

These studies of immunocontraception in the female serve as a useful model for development of a male vaccine. It is likely that a higher level of antibody is necessary in the male to neutralize all of the LDH-C$_4$ available for binding. In this regard, males respond to immunization with LDH-C$_4$ by producing significantly less antibody than do females.[25] Our model requires interaction of humoral or locally produced antibodies to LDH-C$_4$ with spermatozoa in the male reproductive tract or in semen. As long as the blood–testes barrier is intact, it prevents antigen from exiting into the general circulation, and to

TABLE 42-2. Levels of Anti-LDH-C₄ in Samples from the WHO Human Serum Bank*

	N	x̄	SD	ELEVATED VALUES†
Males with unexplained infertility	78	5.4	7.8	17, 17, 18, 19, 20, 36, 37
Vasectomized males	15	9.7	8.4	18, 20, 27

* Results are expressed as ng ^{125}I-labelled LDH-C₄ bound/ml of serum. Background binding was the mean binding for fertile male and fertile female sera, which was subtracted from all values.

† Values greater than 2 SD (15.6) from the fertile population mean.

some extent it also prevents antibodies and cells from entering the tract. It is well known, however, that when this barrier is breached by, for example, infection or tubular obstruction (*e.g.*, vasectomy), antibodies to sperm are made and do enter the reproductive tract.[2,33,39] In fact, even in the absence of any observable perturbations of the barrier, antibodies to sperm antigens have been found in male reproductive fluids and in serum from both fertile and infertile patients.[8,28] Antisperm antibodies of the IgM class have been found in serum of some subjects but not in seminal fluids.[7,34] IgG antibodies, on the other hand, have been found both in sera and in ejaculates. This class of antibody may enter the male reproductive tract from the circulation by means of transudation into the prostate gland secretions.[34] IgA and secretory IgA (sIgA) also have been found in both sera and ejaculates; however, the source is more controversial. It may be diffusing in from the circulation.[20] Alternatively, IgA may be secreted locally at the mucosal lining of the tract.[40] The latter is favored by cases in which sperm-agglutinating antibodies are of higher titer in the semen than in the serum, and also when the antibody class in semen is IgA, and differs from that in serum, in which it is IgG or IgM.[40] Friberg found that IgA antisperm antibodies were the majority class in ejaculates, with some IgG class antibodies also present.[7]

Antibodies that react with LDH-C₄ have not been implicated directly as the cause of naturally occurring infertility. Recently, however, samples of human sera from the World Health Organization (WHO) reference bank were examined for antibodies to LDH-C₄.[36] These sera were tested with a liquid-phase RIA employing purified radiolabeled mouse LDH-C₄. Two of the categories tested, males with unexplained infertility and vasectomized males, are of interest here. Table 42-2 shows the mean levels of anti-LDH-C₄ present in the two populations and individual values that were elevated. In the liquid-phase RIA, the counts per minute (cpm) bound by a pool of nonimmune sera is typically subtracted from the cpm bound by the sample being assayed to determine the specific antibody binding to radiolabeled LDH-C₄. In this study, however, a nonimmune pool was unavailable. Therefore, the mean cpm bound by sera from a group of fertile males and fertile females was considered the background binding of normal sera and was subtracted from values recorded for the other samples. Values were considered elevated if they were two standard deviations or higher above the fertile population mean. Among males with unexplained infertility, 7 of 78 subjects, or 10%, of the sera showed elevated levels by our criteria. Vasectomized males had higher values as a group than other categories tested. The mean value was 9.7, and 20% of the individual values were elevated. Although a much larger group must be tested before any clinical relevance can be placed on these values, it is of interest that $LDH-C_4$–specific antibodies can be detected in these subjects.

Based on this information, a model for male contraception would include two major routes of attack: systemic immunization to provoke IgG production, possibly with cell-mediated immunity, and local immunization to elicit sIgA antibodies. The advantages of using a defined, purified, sperm-specific antigen such as $LDH-C_4$ rather than whole sperm become apparent when these studies are outlined. The problem of interfering reactions with somatic cells is precluded because $LDH-C_4$ is absolutely sperm specific. $LDH-C_4$ immunization allows the resulting immune response to be evaluated accurately by reproducible assays and also permits the dosage regimens to be rigidly controlled. In addition, the restricted localization of $LDH-C_4$ to germinal elements suggests that an immune response specific for this antigen would be unlikely to result in severe pathologic damage to the male reproductive system. Furthermore, the contraceptive effects are likely to be reversible.

Systemic immunization with $LDH-C_4$ can be monitored by quantitative radioimmunoassay of $LDH-C_4$–specific humoral IgG antibodies and especially antibodies in prostate secretions and seminal plasma. This is particularly important because circulating antibody levels are not highly correlated with antibody levels in these secretions. Spleen and draining lymph nodes also may be examined for the presence of cytotoxic cells reactive against $LDH-C_4$ on sperm cells. We have established a methodology for detecting the presence of cytotoxic cells by their ability to lyse specifically ^{51}Cr-labeled tumor cells that have been coated with $LDH-C_4$.[35]

Local immunization to elicit production of a secretory IgA response in the reproductive tract may in fact be the most promising approach. In addition to the likelihood of producing the higher levels of antibody necessary in the male, the secretory component of this antibody class may render it less susceptible to the proteolytic enzymes that are abundantly present in seminal plasma.

Local immunization with $LDH-C_4$ is possible by two routes. Successful production of IgA against other antigens suggests direct immunization to the reproductive tract or in the vicinity of its draining lymph nodes. The latter could be accomplished by an intraperitoneal immunization. An alternate, and perhaps even more effective route, would be to immunize by way of the gut by administering the antigen in an enteric-coated capsule. There is a high concentration of IgA precursors in the Peyer's patches of the gut. Following gut stimulation, these cells would migrate to the mucosal lining of the reproductive tract, where they would encounter antigen on sperm, proliferate, and secrete anti-$LDH-C_4$ IgA.

The local immunization protocol may be designed to include some recent procedures that would enhance the response. Cox and Taubman reported that soluble antigens are better at eliciting local immunity than are particulate ones.[5] This procedure is readily tested with regard to the reproductive tract, using $LDH-C_4$. Also, Pierce and Gowans demonstrated that cholera toxoid is highly stimulatory of gut-associated lymphatic tissues.[32] This suggests that linking the antigen with cholera toxoid or administering it simultaneously with cholera toxoid may increase sIgA production. Stimulation of a secretory immune response to sperm antigens by remote-site immunization of the linked mucosal immune system affords a number of obvious advantages. The question arises, however, that if the response capabilities of the system are linked, then is the apparent "natural" tolerance of the reproductive tract mucosa to sperm antigens it is in constant contact with also linked? In other words, although the humoral immune system does not recognize sperm antigens as "self," does the mucosal system? Does the occurrence of antisperm IgA antibodies represent some sort of breakage of this tolerance? These are the kinds of questions that can be addressed more readily using a purified, sperm-specific, antigenic model than by using whole sperm or sperm extracts.

A third possible route for male contraception is by passive immunization with a specific antibody to LDH-C₄ that is attached to a spermicide or a liposome containing spermicide. This method is designed to target the drug to sperm in the reproductive tract. Specificity could be further ensured by using a monoclonal antibody to LDH-C₄. Monoclonal antibodies linked to cytotoxic agents and targeted to specific antigens have been used with some success in treating solid tumors.[9,30] The monoclonal antibody technology in combination with a defined sperm antigen also would allow directing an antibody to a functionally relevant, specific determinant site on the antigen. In the case of LDH-C₄, an antibody directed against the catalytic site would inhibit enzymatic activity and virtually immobilize sperm. We have generated a monoclonal antibody that binds the amino acid sequence 97-110 in LDH-C₄.[18] This sequence comprises the coenzyme binding loop of the enzyme.[29] When this monoclonal antibody is reacted with LDH-C₄ in the presence of substrate and coenzyme, enzymatic activity is inhibited.[37]

Synthesis of a peptide fragment that encompasses the 97-110 sequence would allow active immunization to accomplish sperm inactivation. This approach has the advantage of allowing one to construct a synthetic vaccine, especially because the amount of LDH-C₄ that can be isolated from natural sources is incompatible with a widely used contraceptive. Small, synthetic peptides representing antigenic domains of LDH-C₄ have now been identified. These peptides could be substituted for the natural product. They consist of surface residues that are directly linked to one another by peptide bonds and include eight regions of the LDH-C₄ subunit,[42,43] which are identified in Table 42-3. Thus far, we have established that synthetic peptides representing regions 1 (5–15) and 3 (211–220) are immunogenic in that they provoke antibodies that cross-react with native LDH-C₄.[44] Furthermore, fertility is significantly reduced in female baboons immunized with the synthetic peptide MC5-15 conjugated to diphtheria toxoid, and the effect appears to be reversible.[17] These findings confirm the utility of our strategy for replacing the natural product antigen in a contraceptive vaccine. The best peptide or combination of peptides remains to be defined. Nevertheless, with this approach, it should be possible to perform rigorous and quantitative analyses that will confirm or reject the potential for development of immunocontraceptive technology applicable to the male.

This report on the potential for development of a male contraceptive vaccine based on LDH-C₄ reflects a long series of experiments from the first observation of a unique LDH isozyme in human sperm and testes. The immune response to LDH-C₄ has been described, and immunosuppression of fertility in the female has been demonstrated. A practical strategy for the

TABLE 42-3. Antigenic Regions of the LDH-C Subunit

REGION	STRUCTURE AND LOCATION
1	5 10 14a 14b Glu-Gln-Leu-Ile-Gln-Asn-Leu-Val-Pro-Glu-Asp-Lys
2	41 50 55 Gly-Leu-Ala-Asp-Glu-Leu-Ala-Leu-Val-Asp-Ala-Asp-Asp-Thr-Asp-Lys
3	211 220 Ser-Leu-Asn-Pro-Ala-Ile-Gly-Thr-Asp-Lys
4	221 230 Asn-Lys-Gln-His-Trp-Lys-Asn-Val-His-Lys
5	231 240 243 Gln-Val-Val-Glu-Gly-Gly-Tyr-Glu-Val-Leu-Asp-Met-Lys
6	283 290 300 303 Glu-Glu-Val-Phe-Leu-Ser-Ile-Pro-Cys-Val-Leu-Gly-Glu-Ser-Gly-Ile-Thr-Asp-Phe-Val-Lys
7	304 310 316 Val-Asn-Met-Thr-Ala-Glu-Glu-Glu-Gly-Leu-Leu-Lys-Lys
8	317 320 330 Ser-Val-Asp-Thr-Leu-Trp-Asn-Met-Gln-Lys-Asn-Leu-Glu-Leu

replacement of the natural product enzyme with a synthetic antigen has evolved from the determination of the antigenic structure. Construction of a model for a male contraceptive around this well-defined sperm-specific antigen allows modification of proven immunization protocols that have successfully suppressed fertility in the female. Such modifications would not only adapt the protocols to the male physiology but would enhance exposure of the various arms of the immune system to the antigen, ensuring both high production of sperm-specific antibodies and access to the male reproductive system.

REFERENCES

1. ALLEN JM: Multiple forms of lactic dehydrogenase in tissues of the mouse: Their specificity, cellular localization, and response to altered physiological conditions. Ann NY Acad Sci 94:937, 1961
2. ANSBACHER R, HODGE P, WILLIAMS A, MUMFORD DM: Vas ligation: Humoral sperm antibodies. Int J Fertil 21:250, 1976
3. BATTELIINO LJ, JAMES FR, BLANCO A: Kinetic properties of rabbit testicular lactate dehydrogenase enzyme. J Biol Chem 243:5158, 1968
4. BLANCO A, ZINKHAM WH: Lactate dehydrogenase in human testes. Science 139:601, 1963
5. COX D, TAUBMAN MA: Salivary antibody response and priming stimulated by soluble or particulate antigens injected at a remote secretory site. Mol Immunol 19:171, 1982
6. EVENTOFF W, ROSSMANN MG, TAYLOR SS, TORFF HJ, MEYER H, KEIL W, KILTZ HH: Structural adaptations of lactate dehydrogenase isozymes. Proc Natl Acad Sci USA 74:2677, 1977
7. FRIBERG J: Relation between sperm-agglutinating antibodies in serum and seminal fluid. Acta Obstet Gynecol Scand 36 (Suppl):73, 1974
8. FRIBERG J: Seminal immunoglobulins, autoagglutination in ejaculates, and infertility in men, p 423. In GLEICHER N (ed): Progress in Clinical and Biological Research, Vol 70. Reproductive Immunology. New York, Alan R. Liss, 1981
9. GHOSE T, BLAIR AH: Antibody linked cytotoxic agents in the treatment of cancer: Current status and future prospects. JNCI 61:657, 1980

10. GOLDBERG E: Lactic and malic dehydrogenases in human spermatozoa. Science 139:602, 1963
11. GOLDBERG E: Lactate dehydrogenases and malate dehydrogenases in sperm: Studied by polyacrylamide gel electrophoresis. Ann NY Acad Sci 127:560, 1964
12. GOLDBERG E: Lactate dehydrogenases in spermatozoa: Subunit interactions *in vitro.* Arch Biochem Biophys 109:134, 1965
13. GOLDBERG E: Immunochemical specificity of lactate dehydrogenase-X. Proc Natl Acad Sci USA 68:349, 1971
14. GOLDBERG E: Molecular basis for multiple forms of LDH-X. J Exp Zool 186:273, 1973
15. GOLDBERG E: Isozymes in testes and spermatozoa. In RATTAZZI MS, SCANDALIOS JG, WHITT GS (eds): Isozymes: Current Topics in Biological and Medical Research, Vol 1, p 79. New York, Alan R. Liss, 1977
16. GOLDBERG E: Current status of research on sperm antigens: potential applications as contraceptive vaccines. In ZATUCHNI GI (ed): Research Frontiers in Fertility Regulation, Vol 2, No 6. Chicago, Program for Applied Research in Fertility Regulation, 1983
17. GOLDBERG E: Unpublished data, 1985
18. GOLDMAN-LEIKIN R, GOLDBERG E: Characterization of monoclonal antibodies to sperm-specific lactate dehydrogenase isozyme. Proc Natl Acad Sci USA 80:3774, 1983
19. HAWTREY CO, GOLDBERG E: Some kinetic aspects of sperm specific lactate dehydrogenase in mice. J Exp Zool 174:451, 1970
20. HEKMAN A, RUMKE P: Seminal antigens and autoimmunity. In HAFEZ ESE (ed): Human Semen and Fertility Regulation in Men, p 245. St. Louis, CV Mosby, 1976
21. KILLE JW, GOLDBERG E: Female reproductive tract immunoglobulin responses to a purified sperm-specific antigen (LDH-C₄). Biol Reprod 20:863, 1979
22. KILLE JW, GOLDBERG E: Inhibition of oviductal sperm transport in rabbits immunized against sperm-specific lactate dehydrogenase (LDH-C₄). J Reprod Immunol 2:15, 1980
23. LI SS-L, FELDMAN RJ, OKABE M, PAN Y-CE: Molecular features and immunological properties of lactate dehydrogenase C₄ isozymes from mouse and rat testes. J Biol Chem 258:7017, 1983
24. LIANG ZG, SHELTON JA, GOLDBERG E: Unpublished data
25. MARSH JA, O'HERN P, GOLDBERG E: The role of the X-linked gene in the regulation of secondary humoral response kinetics to sperm-specific LDH-C₄ antigen. J Immunol 126:100, 1981
26. MITA M, HALL PF: Metabolism of round spermatids from rats: Lactate as the preferred substrate. Biol Reprod 26:445, 1982
27. MONTGOMERY PC, LEMAITRE-COELHO IM, VAER J-P: A common mucosal immune system. Antibody expression in secretions following gastrointestinal stimulation. Immunol Communications 9:705, 1980
28. MUMFORD DM: Immunology and male infertility. Urol Clin North Am 5(3):463, 1978
29. MUSICK WDL, ROSSMANN MG: The structure of mouse testicular lactate dehydrogenase isoenzyme C₄ at 2.9 Å resolution. J Biol Chem 254:7611, 1979
30. OLSNES S: Directing toxins to cancer cells. Nature 290:84, 1981
31. PAN Y-CE, HUANG S, MARCINSZYN JP JR., LEE C-Y, LI SS-L: The preliminary amino acid sequence of mouse testicular lactate dehydrogenase. Hoppe-Seyler's Z Physiol Chem 361:795, 1980
32. PIERCE NF, GOWANS JL: Cellular kinetics of the intestinal immune response to cholera toxoid in rats. J Exp Med 142:1550, 1976
33. QUESADA EM, DUKES CD, DEEN GH, *et al:* Genital infections and sperm agglutinating antibodies in infertile men. J Urol 99:106, 1968
34. RUMKE P: The origin of immunoglobulins in semen. Clin Exp Immunol 17:287, 1974
35. SHELTON JA, GOLDBERG E: Induction of cell-mediated cytotoxic immunity to sperm-specific lactate dehydrogenase-C₄ in SJL/J female mice. Biol Reprod 32:556, 1985
36. SHELTON JA, GOLDBERG E: Serum antibodies to LDH-C₄. J Reprod Immunol (in press)
37. SHELTON JA, GOLDBERG E: Unpublished data, 1985
38. STOREY BT, KAYNE FJ: Energy metabolism of spermatozoa. VI. Direct intramitochondrial lactate oxidation by rabbit sperm mitochondria. Biol Reprod 16:549, 1977
39. TUNG KSK: Human sperm antigens and antisperm antibodies. I. Studies on vasectomy patients. Clin Exp Immunol 20:93, 1975
40. VEHLING DT: Secretory IgA in seminal fluid. Fertil Steril 22:769, 1971

41. WHEAT TE, GOLDBERG E: Sperm-specific lactate dehydrogenase C_4: Antigenic structure and immunosuppression of fertility. In RATTAZZI MC, SCANDALIOS JG, WHITT GS (eds): Isozymes: Current Topics in Biological and Medical Research, Vol 7, p 113. New York, Alan R. Liss, 1983

42. WHEAT TE, GOLDBERG E: Antigenic domains of the sperm-specific lactate dehydrogenase. Molec Immunol 22:643, 1985

43. WHEAT TE, GOLDBERG E: Immunochemical dissection of the testes-specific isozyme, lactate dehydrogenase. Ann NY Acad Sci 438:156, 1985

44. WHEAT TE, SHELTON JA, GONZALES-PREVATT VB, GOLDBERG E: The antigenicity of synthetic peptide fragments of lactate dehydrogenase C_4. Molec Immunol 22:1195, 1985

45. WHITT GS: Isozymes as probes and participants in developmental and evolutionary genetics. In RATTAZZI MC, SCANDALIOS JG, WHITT GS (eds): Isozymes: Current topics in Biological and Medical Research, Vol 10, p 1. Genetics and Evolution. New York, Alan R. Liss, 1983

46. WRIGHT LL, SWOFFORD JH: Mouse lactate dehydrogenase LDH-C_4 (testis) is immunochemically cross-reactive with LDH-A_4 (muscle) and LDH-B_4 (heart). Scand J Immunol 19:247, 1984

47. ZINKHAM WH, BLANCO A, KUPCHYK L: Lactate dehydrogenase in pigeon testes: genetic control by three loci. Science 144:1353, 1964

43
Discussion: Immunologic Approaches

MODERATORS: NANCY J. ALEXANDER

KENNETH S. K. TUNG

HAVE ANY STEROIDS BEEN FOUND THAT ACT SELECTIVELY ON LH OR FSH?

Investigators recently have isolated a steroid from Sertoli cells that has taken quite a while to identify. It is produced by Sertoli cells but not by Leydig cells, and has also been found in ovaries and the human brain. It is a highly reactive, labile alelic steroid that is destroyed at body temperature, by blowing nitrogen on it, or when placed under fluorescent light. It has not been synthesized but it has been studied in several biologic systems. In vivo, in gonadectomized or intact male and female rats, it selectively suppresses FSH and in some cases stimulates LH. In animals of certain ages, threefold increases in LH have been seen. This appears to be the first time a steroid has selectively suppressed FSH.

IS CIRCULATING IMMUNE COMPLEX DAMAGE A PROBLEM IN MEN IMMUNIZED WITH SPERMATOZOA?

Circulating immune complex damage in men or in male animals immunized with sperm antigen has not been reported. What has been seen in some species is an immune complex formation, localized exclusively in the testis, which may be a consequence of immunologic injury resulting in leakage of sperm antigen and a reaction of loose antigen with the antibody along the basement membrane of the seminiferous tubules; this may then exacerbate the immunologic injury rather than cause the disease. The cause may be T cell mediated.

DID THE ANTIBODY TITER OBSERVED BY ALEXANDER RELATE TO THE TIME SINCE VASECTOMY WAS PERFORMED?

No. It seems that some people develop antibodies against sperm and some do not; and once a certain titer per subject is reached, it is retained, even after vasovasostomy. We could predict before vasovasostomy which subjects would

---

Panelists: Deborah J. Anderson, C. Wayne Bardin, Paul Franchimont, Erwin Goldberg, Eberhard Nieschlag; *Discussants:* Andrzej Bartke, Marcos Paulo P. deCastro, Douglas Huber, Kamran S. Moghissi, C. Alvin Paulsen, Malcolm Potts, Carlos A. Schaffenberg, Sherman J. Silber, John P. Wiebe, Lourens J. D. Zaneveld, Gerald I. Zatuchni

have the best chance of conception, because antibody titers after vasovasostomy remained about the same. The only difference seen after vasovasostomy was an increase in the percentage of men who had antibodies in their seminal plasma.

IS INFERTILITY CAUSED BY ANTIBODIES OR BY POOR REVERSAL TECHNIQUE?

The infertility might be caused by a poor reversal technique, so that the worse the obstruction after reversal, the more antibodies will be seen. This could be true but it probably is not; probably the infertility has to do with the antibody titers because similar titers are found in men who are thought to be immunologically infertile but have not had a vasectomy. Antibodies may not interfere absolutely with fertility, but they probably play a role and may cause a reduction in the fertility of some persons.

At this time, it is not possible to prove cause and effect. A physiologic factor may induce the antibodies and also the infertility, rather than that the antibodies cause the infertility. Vasovasostomy per se did not cause gross changes in the antibody titers. Certainly, the immune response varies from subject to subject. All vasectomized men do not get antibodies. We would expect that certain types of antisperm antibodies impede fertility much more than other types, but at this time we cannot define which type is being seen. In the study being discussed, all men were eliminated who had poor anastomoses based on sperm return and sperm motility so that the sperm count seemed morphologically normal; they also had other characteristics that would put them in a normal group. Dr. Alexander's prednisone studies would support the fact that if the antibodies are suppressed, there is an enhancement to fertility, again pointing to the fact that the antibodies appear to play a strong role.

IS THERE A CORRELATION BETWEEN PREGNANCY RATES AND HIGH ANTIBODY TITERS?

Unlike the studies discussed above, investigators at the Cleveland Clinic found no correlation between pregnancy rates and high antibody titers. There is a strong possibility that the antibodies are a serum marker for epididymal breakdown, because most of the vasectomies have been performed with the closed-ended cautery approach. It is likely that most patients who have antibodies in the serum have had epididymal damage caused by sperm leakage at the vasectomy site, due to the closed-ended cautery vasectomy technique, so if the antibodies are predictive of infertility, this is probably because of epididymal structural damage.

In any case of infertility, it is important to evaluate the female partner carefully, because many women have an unrecognized poor luteal phase, ovulatory dysfunction, microcystic ovaries, poor cervical mucus, and other problems. Too often, the man and woman are studied as individuals, not as a couple.

One investigator found that pregnancy correlated well with traditional semen parameters, motility being the most important. When motility was normal and traditional semen patterns were normal but infertility persisted, often the woman had either poor luteal phase, poor mucus, or ovulatory dysfunction.

Some investigators believe that the existence of antibodies is not a significant problem in reversal of sterilization, considering that, in several animal models in which unilateral vasectomy has been performed, the animals had no decrease in their fertility. This correlates also with the human experience of unilateral vasectomy in unilateral herniorrhaphy repair in infants or unilateral congenital absence of the vas deferens, in which there is no decrease in fertility. Possibly in the group presently under study, the high antibody group with the high pregnancy rate were men who did not have much epididymal damage. Antibodies may, however, be one of several causes of infertility, although not a major factor in most subjects.

CAN THE CONCENTRATION OF ANTIBODY IN FEMALE REPRODUCTIVE TRACT FLUIDS BE ENHANCED TO BLOCK FERTILITY?

It appears that when animals or humans are actively immunized, the level of antibody in the female reproductive tract is relatively low. The three animals in Goldberg's study that became pregnant may possibly have had a lower level of antibody in their reproductive tract fluids. The correlation between circulating titer and the level of oviduct fluid or oviduct washings is not as well defined as would be wished. A technology needs to be devised by which a local immune response can be stimulated. In fact, some investigators have accomplished this by an intrauterine immunization in mice; there are also some data on monkeys, in which, using a gastric path of immunization, a local immune response has been achieved. This area needs further study but seems promising.

WHAT ADDITIONAL INFORMATION IS NEEDED BEFORE VACCINATION OF WOMEN IS POSSIBLE USING THE LDH-C$_4$ CONTRACEPTIVE VACCINE?

We need to know how to accomplish the immunization itself. A major problem is finding a suitable vehicle for administration. A problem with an antigen that is not cross-reactive and is not going to produce immune disease is to determine which members of the population are responders and which are nonresponders, by means of a dipstick or similar test. Another major problem impeding progress in this area is definition of the antigen. Whether LDH-C$_4$ will be *the* ideal antigen no one knows, but at the moment it is available, we can exploit its properties, and it looks promising.

WHAT IS THE MAJOR CONSTRAINT IN THE DEVELOPMENT OF A NEW MALE CONTRACEPTIVE?

What is required in terms of Goldberg's LDH-C_4 vaccine and the other promising research is the necessary funding to continue research programs. PARFR has prepared a vaccine development program with Goldberg to bring the LDH-C_4 research to preclinical studies within the next 3 years. Unfortunately, funding may not be available for that particular work. Inadequate funding is the major constraint in the field of male fertility control.

A final observation is that it took Gregory Pincus and many other contributors approximately 20 years to develop a female contraceptive pill, at a cost that has been estimated at approximately $30 to $40 million, during the 1940s and 1950s. When we look at the meager amounts of funding for male contraception in terms of research support, it is no wonder that a male fertility control mechanism is not yet available.

CONTRIBUTING AUTHORS

Joel W. Ager, Ph.D.
Chapter 13
Professor, Department of Psychology/
  Obstetrics/Gynecology
Wayne State University
Detroit, Michigan

R. John Aitken, Ph.D.
Chapters 11, 15, 22
Senior Scientist, Reproductive Biology Unit
Medical Research Council
Edinburgh, Scotland

Nancy J. Alexander, Ph.D.
Chapters 8, 41, 43
Professor and Scientist, Reproductive Physiology
Oregon Regional Primate Research Center
Beaverton, Oregon

Deborah J. Anderson, Ph.D.
Chapter 40
Assistant Professor of Pathology, Division of
  Immunogenetics
Harvard Medical School and Dana–Farber
  Cancer Institute
Boston, Massachusetts

Harry Anderson
Chapter 38
Peptide Biology Laboratory
Salk Institute
La Jolla, California

Ricardo H. Asch, M.D.
Chapter 32
Professor, Department of Obstetrics and
  Gynecology
The University of Texas Health Science Center
  at San Antonio
San Antonio, Texas

C. Wayne Bardin, M.D.
Chapters 23, 38
Director, Center for Biomedical Research
The Population Council
New York, New York

Kevin J. Barr, B.Sc.
Chapter 24
Research Associate, Department of Zoology
University of Western Ontario
London, Ontario, Canada

Andrzej Bartke, Ph.D.
Chapters 17, 35
Professor and Chairman, Department of
  Physiology
Southern Illinois University
Carbondale, Illinois

Ludwig Bauer, Ph.D.
Chapter 20
Professor, Department of Medicinal Chemistry
  and Pharmacognosy
University of Illinois at Chicago
Chicago, Illinois

Lee R. Beck, Ph.D.
Chapter 31
Executive Vice President
Stolle Research and Development Corporation
Cincinnati, Ohio

Hermann Behre
Chapter 29
Max Planck Clinical Research Unit for
  Reproductive Medicine
Münster, Federal Republic of Germany

Lutz Belkien, Ph.D.
Chapter 29
Max Planck Clinical Research Unit for
  Reproductive Medicine
Münster, Federal Republic of Germany

Hinrich Bents
Chapter 29
Max Planck Clinical Research Unit for
  Reproductive Medicine
Münster, Federal Republic of Germany

Karen K. Bergström, B.S.
Chapter 25
Biologist II, Department of Physiology
Syntex Research
Palo Alto, California

Stan A. Beyler, Ph.D.
Chapter 19
Assistant Professor, Department of Obstetrics
  and Gynecology
William Beaumont Hospital
Royal Oaks, Michigan

Shalender Bhasin, M.D.
Chapter 30
Assistant Professor, Division of Endocrinology
Harbor-UCLA Medical Center
Torrance, California

William J. Bremner, M.D., Ph.D.
Chapters 9, 33
Associate Professor, Division of Endocrinology/
Metabolism
University of Washington
Seattle, Washington

Kevin D. Buckingham, B.Sc.
Chapter 24
Research Associate, Department of Zoology
University of Western Ontario
London, Ontario, Canada

James W. Burns, Ph.D.
Chapter 19
Research Associate, Department of Material
Science and Engineering
University of Florida
Gainesville, Florida

C. Yan Cheng, Ph.D.
Chapter 38
Staff Scientist
The Population Council
New York, New York

Valerio Cioli, M.D.
Chapter 23
Head, Pharmacology Department
F. Angelini Research Institute
Rome, Italy

Jane S. Clarkson
Chapter 15
Research Assistant, Reproductive Biology Unit
Medical Research Council
Edinburgh, Scotland

Cesare De Martino, M.D.
Chapter 23
Assistant Professor
Regina Elena Institute for Cancer Research
Rome, Italy

William A. Depel, B.S.
Chapter 19
Director of Research and Development
Bivona, Inc.
Gary, Indiana

Rune Eliasson, M.D., Ph.D.
Chapter 12
Department of Physiology, Reproductive
Physiology Unit
Karolinska Institute
Stockholm, Sweden

Larry L. Ewing, Ph.D.
Chapter 28
Professor, Department of Population Dynamics
The Johns Hopkins University
Baltimore, Maryland

Thomas J. Fielder, B.Sc.
Chapter 30
Research Technician, Division of Endocrinology
Harbor-UCLA Medical Center
Torrance, California

Robin G. Foldesy, Ph.D.
Chapter 17
Senior Scientist, Division of Biological Research
Ortho Pharmaceutical Corporation
Raritan, New Jersey

**William Christopher Liberty Ford,
Ph.D.**
Chapter 10
Department of Physiology and Biochemistry
The University of Reading
Reading, England

Paul Franchimont, M.D.
Chapter 39
Professor, Department of Pathology
Universite de Liège
Liège, Belgium

P. Douglas Geddes, B.Sc.
Chapter 24
Research Assistant, Department of Zoology
University of Western Ontario
London, Ontario, Canada

Paul T. Giblin, Ph.D.
Chapter 13
Assistant Professor, Department of Pediatrics
Wayne State University School of Medicine
Detroit, Michigan

Richard M. Gilley
Chapter 32
Research Chemist, Microencapsulation Division
Southern Research Institute
Birmingham, Alabama

Erwin Goldberg, Ph.D.
Chapter 42
Professor, Department of Biochemistry,
 Molecular Biology, and Cell Biology
Northwestern University
Evanston, Illinois

Alfredo Goldsmith, M.D., M.P.H.
Chapter 7
Associate Professor, Department of Obstetrics
 and Gynecology
Head, Research Project Development, Program
 for Applied Research on Fertility Regulation
Northwestern University Medical School
Chicago, Illinois

Jessie C. Goodpasture, Ph.D.
Chapter 25
Staff Researcher II, Department of Physiology
Syntex Research
Palo Alto, California

Martha B. Grigg, B.S.
Chapter 25
Biologist II, Department of Physiology
Syntex Research
Palo Alto, California

Kenneth M. Gross, M.D.
Chapter 33
Senior Research Fellow, Department of
 Endocrinology
Veterans Administration Medical Center
Seattle, Washington

Do Won Hahn, Ph.D.
Chapters 17, 21
Assistant Director, Reproductive/Endocrine
 Research
Ortho Pharmaceutical Corporation
Raritan, New Jersey

Teri O. Heitman, B.S.
Chapter 32
Research Associate, Department of Obstetrics
 and Gynecology
The University of Texas Health Science Center
 at San Antonio
San Antonio, Texas

Sawon Hong, Ph.D.
Chapter 2
Research Associate
Association for Voluntary Sterilization, Inc.
New York, New York

Douglas H. Huber, M.D., M.Sc.
Chapter 2
Medical Director
Association for Voluntary Sterilization, Inc.
New York, New York

Stewart Irvine, B.Sc., M.B., Ch.B.
Chapter 15
Medical Practitioner, Reproductive Biology Unit
Medical Research Council
Edinburgh, Scotland

Joanne Kaminski, Ph.D.
Chapter 20
Instructor, Department of Obstetrics and
 Gynecology
Rush-Presbyterian-St. Luke's Medical Center
Chicago, Illinois

Inchull Kim, Ph.D.
Chapter 18
Research Associate, College of Pharmacy
University of Illinois at Chicago
Chicago, Illinois

Ulrich A. Knuth, M.D.
Chapter 29
Max Planck Clinical Research Unit for
 Reproductive Medicine
Münster, Federal Republic of Germany

Patricia A. Kudo, B.Sc.
Chapter 24
Research Assistant, Department of Zoology
University of Western Ontario
London, Ontario, Canada

Danny H. Lewis, Ph.D.
Chapter 31
Vice President, New Product Development
Stolle Research and Development Corporation
Cincinnati, Ohio

Alvin M. Matsumoto, M.D.
Chapters 9, 33
Assistant Professor, Department of Medicine
University of Washington
Seattle, Washington

Richard McClintock
Chapter 38
Peptide Biology Laboratory
Salk Institute
La Jolla, California

John L. McGuire, Ph.D.
Chapters 17, 21
Vice President, Department of Basic Sciences
Ortho Pharmaceutical Corporation
Raritan, New Jersey

Eric Michel, M. D.
Chapter 34
Max Planck Clinical Research Unit for
Reproductive Medicine
Münster, Federal Republic of Germany

Kamran S. Moghissi, M.D.
Chapter 13
Professor and Associate Chairman of
Gynecology/Obstetrics
Director, Division of Reproductive
Endocrinology and Infertility
Wayne State University School of Medicine
Detroit, Michigan

John J. Nestor, Jr., Ph.D.
Chapter 33
Department of BioOrganic Chemistry
Syntex Research
Palo Alto, California

Eberhard Nieschlag, M.D.
Chapters 29, 34, 35, 37
Professor
Max Planck Clinical Research Unit for
Reproductive Medicine
Münster, Federal Republic of Germany

Xin-yi Niu, Ph.D.
Chapter 18
Associate Professor
Institute of Materia Medica
Chinese Academy of Sciences
Beijing, People's Republic of China

Erik Odeblad, M.D., Ph.D.
Chapter 14
Professor, Department of Medical Biophysics
University of Umea
Umea, Sweden

Jane M. Olson, B.A.
Chapter 13
Research Assistant, Department of Obstetrics
and Gynecology
Hutzel Hospital/Wayne State University
Detroit, Michigan

C. Alvin Paulsen, M.D.
Chapters 26, 27
Professor, Department of Medicine
University of Washington School of Medicine
Seattle, Washington

Diana B. Petitti, M.D.
Chapter 4
Assistant Professor, Family and Community
Medicine
University of California at San Francisco
San Francisco, California

Eric C. Petrie, M.S.
Chapter 33
University of Washington
Seattle, Washington

Marilyn L. Poland, Ph.D., R.N.
Chapter 13
Department of Obstetrics and Gynecology
Wayne State University School of Medicine
Detroit, Michigan

D. Malcolm Potts, M.B., B.Chir., Ph.D.
Chapter 1
President
Family Health International
Research Triangle Park, North Carolina

David William Richardson, M.S., M.Sc.
Chapter 15
Chief Research Officer, Reproductive Biology
Unit
Medical Research Council
Edinburgh, Scotland

Jean Rivier, Ph.D.
Chapter 38
Associate Professor, Peptide Biology Laboratory
Salk Institute
La Jolla, California

John A. Ross, Ph.D.
Chapter 2
Center for Population and Family Health
Columbia University
New York, New York

John J. Sciarra, M.D., Ph.D.
Chapter 3
Professor and Chairman, Department of
  Obstetrics and Gynecology
Program Director, Program for Applied
  Research on Fertility Regulation
Northwestern University Medical School
Chicago, Illinois

Patrizio Scorza Barcellona, Ph.D.
Chapter 23
Head, Toxicology Department
F. Angelini Research Institute
Rome, Italy

Rochelle N. Shain, Ph.D.
Chapter 5
Associate Professor, Department of Obstetrics
  and Gynecology
The University of Texas Health Science Center
  at San Antonio
San Antonio, Texas

Seymour W. Shapiro, M.D.
Chapter 19
President
Bivona, Inc.
Gary, Indiana

Joyce A. Shelton, Ph.D.
Chapter 42
Research Associate, Department of
  Biochemistry, Molecular Biology, and Cell
  Biology
Northwestern University
Evanston, Illinois

Sherman J. Silber, M.D.
Chapter 6
Urologist and Microsurgeon
St. Luke's Hospital-West
St. Louis, Missouri

Molly B. Southworth, M.D.
Chapter 33
Senior Research Fellow, Department of
  Endocrinology
Veterans Administration Medical Center
Seattle, Washington

Jeffrey M. Spieler, M.Sc.
Chapter 26
Biologist, Research Division
Office of Population
Agency for International Development
Washington, D.C.

Joachim Spiess, M.D., Ph.D.
Chapter 38
Peptide Biology Laboratory
Salk Institute
La Jolla, California

Irving M. Spitz, M.D.
Chapter 23
Coordinator, Clinical Research
Center for Biomedical Research
The Population Council
New York, New York

Emil Steinberger, M.D.
Chapter 16
President
Texas Institute for Reproductive Medicine and
  Endocrinology, P.A.
Houston, Texas

Ronald S. Swerdloff, M.D.
Chapter 30
Professor, Department of Medicine
Harbor-UCLA Medical Center
Torrance, California

Thomas R. Tice, Ph.D.
Chapters 31, 32
Head, Microencapsulation Division
Southern Research Institute
Birmingham, Alabama

Kenneth S. K. Tung, M.D.
Chapters 36, 43
Professor, Department of Pathology
University of New Mexico School of Medicine
Albuquerque, New Mexico

Wylie Vale, Ph.D.
Chapter 38
Peptide Biology Laboratory
Salk Institute
La Jolla, California

Joan Vaughan
Chapter 38
Peptide Biology Laboratory
Salk Institute
La Jolla, California

Brian H. Vickery, Ph.D.
Chapters 25, 33
Head, Department of Physiology
Syntex Research
Palo Alto, California

Josef Voglmayr, Ph.D.
Chapter 38
M.R.I. Division of Reproductive Biology
Florida Institute of Technology
Melbourne, Florida

Geoffrey M. H. Waites, Ph.D., D.Sc.
Chapter 10
Special Programme of Research in Human
  Reproduction
World Health Organization
Geneva, Switzerland

Keith A. M. Walker, Ph.D.
Chapter 25
Principal Scientist, Basic Research
Syntex Research
Palo Alto, California

Donald P. Waller, Ph.D.
Chapters 18, 20
Associate Professor, Department of
  Pharmacodynamics
University of Illinois at Chicago
Chicago, Illinois

Gerhard F. Weinbauer, Ph.D.
Chapter 34
Max Planck Clinical Research Unit for
  Reproductive Medicine
Münster, Federal Republic of Germany

David R. White, B.Sc.
Chapter 22
Reproductive Biology Unit
Medical Research Council
Edinburgh, Scotland

John P. Wiebe, Ph.D.
Chapter 24
Professor, Department of Zoology
The University of Western Ontario
London, Ontario, Canada

Gayle Yamamoto
Chapter 38
Peptide Biology Laboratory
Salk Institute
La Jolla, California

Lourens J. D. Zaneveld, D.V.M., Ph.D.
Chapters 19, 20
Professor, Department of Obstetrics-
  Gynecology and Biochemistry
Rush-Presbyterian-St. Luke's Medical Center
Chicago, Illinois

WORKSHOP PARTICIPANTS

R. John Aitken, Ph.D.
Senior Scientist, Medical Research Council
Center for Reproductive Biology
Edinburgh, Scotland

Nancy J. Alexander, Ph.D.
Professor and Scientist
Oregon Regional Primate Research Center
Beaverton, Oregon

Deborah J. Anderson, Ph.D.
Assistant Professor of Pathology, Division of
Immunogenetics
Harvard Medical School and Dana-Farber
Cancer Institute
Boston, Massachusetts

Ricardo H. Asch, M.D.
Professor, Department of Obstetrics and
Gynecology
The University of Texas Health Science Center
at San Antonio
San Antonio, Texas

Alain Audebert, M.D.
Institut Aquitain
Bordeaux, France

C. Wayne Bardin
Director, Center for Biomedical Research
The Population Council
New York, New York

Andrzej Bartke, Ph.D.
Professor and Chairman, Department of
Physiology
Southern Illinois University
Carbondale, Illinois

B. Norman Barwin, M.D.
Ottawa, Ontario, Canada

Giuseppe Benagiano, M.D.
Professor and Director
Institute of Obstetrics and Gynecology
University of Rome
Rome, Italy

Shalender Bhasin, M.D.
Assistant Professor, Division of Endocrinology
Harbor-UCLA Medical Center
Torrance, California

Philippe Bouchard, M.D.
Center Hospitalier de Bicêtre
Le Kremlin-Bicêtre, France

Blaise Bourrit, M.D.
Geneva, Switzerland

William J. Bremner, M.D., Ph.D.
Associate Professor, Division of Endocrinology/
Metabolism
University of Washington
Seattle, Washington

Eric N. Chantler, Ph.D.
Lecturer, Department of Obstetrics and
Gynecology
University Hospital of South Manchester
West Didsbury, Manchester, United Kingdom

Jean Cohen, M.D.
Editor-in-Chief
Contraception Fertilité-Sexualité
Paris, France

Marcos Paulo P. de Castro, M.D.,
M.Sc.
Director
PRO-PATER Institute
Sao Paulo, Brasil

Rune Eliasson, M.D., Ph.D.
Department of Physiology, Reproductive
Physiology Unit
Karolinska Institute
Stockholm, Sweden

Larry L. Ewing, Ph.D.
Professor, Department of Population Dynamics
The Johns Hopkins University
Baltimore, Maryland

Timothy Farley, Ph.D.
Statistician, Special Programme of Research in
Human Reproduction
World Health Organization
Geneva, Switzerland

William Christopher Liberty Ford, Ph.D.
Department of Physiology and Biochemistry
The University of Reading
Reading, England

Paul Franchimont, M.D.
Professor, Department of Pathology
Université de Liège
Liège, Belgium

Erwin Goldberg, Ph.D.
Professor, Department of Biochemistry,
 Molecular Biology, and Cell Biology
Northwestern University
Evanston, Illinois

Alfredo Goldsmith, M.D., M.P.H.
Associate Professor, Department of Obstetrics
 and Gynecology
Northwestern University Medical School
Head, Research Project Development, Program
 for Applied Research on Fertility Regulation
Chicago, Illinois

Nicolai Goncharov, M.D.
Scientist, Special Programme of Research in
 Human Reproduction
World Health Organization
Geneva, Switzerland

David Griffin, M.A.
Scientist, Special Programme of Research in
 Human Reproduction
World Health Organization
Geneva, Switzerland

Do Won Hahn, Ph.D.
Assistant Director, Reproductive/Endocrine
 Research
Ortho Pharmaceutical Corporation
Raritan, New Jersey

Mr. Peter E. Hall
Scientist, Special Programme of Research in
 Human Reproduction
World Health Organization
Geneva, Switzerland

Harrith M. Hasson, M.D.
Associate Professor, Department of Obstetrics
 and Gynecology
Rush Medical College
Chicago, Illinois

Walter L. Herrmann, M.D.
Professor and Chairman, Department of
 Obstetrics and Gynecology
Hôpital Cantonal, Universitaire de Genève
Geneva, Switzerland

Erkki Hirvonen, M.D.
Senior Lecturer, Departments I and II,
 Obstetrics and Gynecology
University Central Hospital
Helsinki, Finland

Douglas H. Huber, M.D., M.Sc.
Medical Director
Association for Voluntary Sterilization, Inc.
New York, New York

Ulrich A. Knuth, M.D.
Max Planck Clinical Research Unit for
 Reproductive Medicine
Münster, Federal Republic of Germany

Dr. B. Leibundgut
Liestal, Switzerland

Danny H. Lewis, Ph.D.
Vice President, New Product Development
Stolle Research and Development Corporation
Cincinnati, Ohio

Kamran S. Moghissi, M.D.
Professor and Associate Chairman of
 Gynecology/Obstetrics
Director, Division of Reproductive
 Endocrinology and Infertility
Wayne State University School of Medicine
Detroit, Michigan

Eberhard Nieschlag, M.D.
Professor
Max Planck Clinical Research Unit for
 Reproductive Medicine
Münster, Federal Republic of Germany

Erik Odeblad, M.D., Ph.D.
Professor, Department of Medical Biophysics
University of Umea
Umea, Sweden

C. Alvin Paulsen, M.D.
Professor, Department of Medicine
University of Washington School of Medicine
Seattle, Washington

Diana B. Petitti, M.D.
Assistant Professor, Family and Community
  Medicine
University of California at San Francisco
San Francisco, California

D. Malcolm Potts, M.B., B.Chir., Ph.D.
President
Family Health International
Research Triangle Park, North Carolina

Patrick J. Rowe, M.B.B.S., M.R.C.O.G.
Medical Officer, Special Programme of
  Research in Human Reproduction
World Health Organization
Geneva, Switzerland

Ichel Samberg, M.D.
Chief of Clinic, Department of Obstetrics and
  Gynecology
Hôpital Cantonal
Geneva, Switzerland

Carlos A. Schaffenburg, M.D.
Medical Officer, Bureau of Drugs
Division of Metabolic and Endocrinology Drug
  Products
Food and Drug Administration
Rockville, Maryland

Paul C. Schwallie, M.D.
Clinical Research Physician, Fertility Research
The Upjohn Company
Kalamazoo, Michigan

John J. Sciarra, M.D., Ph.D.
Professor and Chairman, Department of
  Obstetrics and Gynecology
Director, Program for Applied Research on
  Fertility Regulation
Northwestern University Medical School
Chicago, Illinois

Patrizio Scorza Barcellona, Ph.D.
Head, Toxicology Department
F. Angelini Research Institute
Rome, Italy

Rochelle N. Shain, Ph.D.
Associate Professor, Department of Obstetrics
  and Gynecology
The University of Texas Health Science Center
  at San Antonio
San Antonio, Texas

Sherman J. Silber, M.D.
Urologist and Microsurgeon
St. Luke's Hospital-West
St. Louis, Missouri

Jeffrey M. Spieler, M.Sc.
Biologist, Research Division
Office of Population
Agency for International Development
Washington, D.C.

Irving M. Spitz, M.D.
Coordinator, Clinical Research
Center for Biomedical Research
The Population Council
New York, New York

Anna Steinberger, Ph.D.
Professor, Department of Obstetrics,
  Gynecology and Reproductive Sciences
The University of Texas Health Science Center
  at Houston
Houston, Texas

Emil Steinberger, M.D.
President
Texas Institute for Reproductive Medicine and
  Endocrinology, P.A.
University of Texas Medical School
Houston, Texas

Michel Thiery, M.D., Ph.D.
Department Head and Professor, Division of
  Obstetrics
University of Ghent
Ghent, Belgium

Kenneth S. K. Tung, M.D.
Professor, Department of Pathology
University of New Mexico School of Medicine
Albuquerque, New Mexico

P. A. Van Keep, M.D.
Medical Director
Organon International
Oss, The Netherlands

Willem A. A. van Os, M.D.
Gynecological and Obstetrical Department
Elizabeth's Gasthuis
Haarlem, Holland

Brian H. Vickery, Ph.D.
Head, Department of Physiology
Syntex Research
Palo Alto, California

Donald P. Waller, Ph.D.
Associate Professor, Department of
Pharmacodynamics
University of Illinois at Chicago
Chicago, Illinois

John P. Wiebe, Ph.D.
Professor, Department of Zoology
The University of Western Ontario
London, Ontario, Canada

Lillian Yin, Ph.D.
Director, Division of OB-GYN, ENT, and
Dental Devices
Food and Drug Administration
Silver Springs, Maryland

Lourens J. D. Zaneveld, D.V.M., Ph.D.
Professor, Department of Obstetrics-
Gynecology and Biochemistry
Rush-Presbyterian-St. Luke's Medical Center
Chicago, Illinois

Gerald I. Zatuchni, M.D., M.Sc.
Professor, Department of Obstetrics and
Gynecology
Director of Technical Assistance, Program for
Applied Research on Fertility Regulation
Northwestern University Medical School
Chicago, Illinois

Index

An *f* following a page number represents a figure; a *t* indicates tabular material.